CARE OF THE CRITICALLY ILL

THIRD EDITION

3 September 1991

CARE OF THE CRITICALLY ILL

THIRD EDITION

STEPHEN M. AYRES, M.D.
Dean, School of Medicine
Professor, Internal Medicine
Professor of Medicine
Virginia Commonwealth University
Medical College of Virginia
Richmond, Virginia

ROBERT SCHLICHTIG, M.D.
Assistant Professor, Anesthesiology and Critical Care Medicine
Director, Surgical ICU
Medical Director, Respiratory Therapy
Oakland Veterans Administration Medical Center
Pittsburgh, Pennsylvania

MICHAEL J. STERLING, M.D.
Director, Medical-Surgical ICU
Medical Director, Respiratory Therapy
North County Hospital
Newport, Vermont

Illustrated by
and with the assistance of
META E. BUEHLER, R.N., B.S.

YEAR BOOK MEDICAL PUBLISHERS, INC.

Chicago • London • Boca Raton

1 2 3 4 5 6 7 8 9 0 MP 92 91 90 89 88

Library of Congress Cataloging-in-Publication Data

Care of the critically ill.

Rev. ed. of: Care of the critically ill/Stephen M. Ayres, Stanley Giannelli, Jr., Hiltrud S. Mueller. 2nd ed. 1974.
Bibliography: p.
Includes index.
1. Critical care medicine. I. Ayres, Stephen M. II. Ayres, Stephen M. Care of the critically ill.
RC86.7.C374 1988 616'.028 87-21625
ISBN 0-8151-0349-2

Sponsoring Editor: David K. Marshall
Assistant Director, Manuscript Services: Frances M. Perveiler
Production Manager, Text and Reference/Periodicals: Etta Worthington

To My Family

Dolores Kobrick Ayres
Stephen
Elizabeth Ann
Margaret Louise

PREFACE TO THE FIRST EDITION

This book evolved from our experience in caring for cardiac surgical patients. The lessons learned from these patients were applied to other critically ill individuals who shared the common problem of cardiorespiratory collapse. It soon became apparent that although certain well-established concepts provided the basis for treatment of such patients, they could not be applied unless continuous quantitative observations were made. We have emphasized circulatory and respiratory derangements because they are usually present in the critically ill. Hence, we have presented basic physiologic concepts together with methods of measurement and have discussed plans of therapy which seem reasonable in light of present knowledge. Our goal has been to present a workable framework enabling the physician to reevaluate continually his treatment by constant observation of his own efforts and critical assessment of the growing literature in this area.

The modern care of the critically ill patient is a team effort. Many dedicated individuals were responsible for the development and execution of the concepts presented in this book. The authors gratefully acknowledge the assistance of:

Sister Anthony Marie, Administrator of Saint Vincent's Hospital and Medical Center, Dr. William J. Grace, Director of Medicine, and Dr. Louis M. Rousselot, Director of Surgery, who have provided a hospital environment fostering the aggressive care of the sick patient. We thank Dr. Grace, a pioneer in the field of cardiac monitoring, for contributing his chapter on the electrical management of heart disease.

Antoinette Criscitiello who developed a technical staff capable of performing sophisticated laboratory procedures, and who personally spent many long hours at bedside and laboratory bench testing the concepts presented in these pages. Her devoted service is appreciated.

The Sisters of Charity and the Nursing Staff of Saint Vincent's Hospital and Medical Center, and particularly Sister Richard Maureen, Mary Dowd, Rita Roland, and Kathleen Brown. They have supervised a group of dedicated women and taught them to blend technical excellence with human understanding.

Sally West for skillful supervision of the cardiac surgical patient. Most of the concepts presented are based on experience with these patients, and her constant creative suggestions have molded our thinking. In addition, she has introduced pulmonary physiotherapy techniques to our hospital.

Drs. Foster Conklin, John Gregory, Peter Fleming, and John Penny who have been stimulating professional colleagues.

Jeffrey Schneider, Ethel Beggs, and

Carolyn Jurasits for their preparation of the manuscript and Rudolph Henning for photographic aid.

Ruth Greus Armstrong and Meta E. Buehler who have served as loyal associates in developing a staff of nurses and technicians capable of studying and treating critically ill patients. We particularly acknowledge our indebtedness to Donald Armstrong, Jane Griesbach, Sarah Solan, Elizabeth Stuart, and Judith Sweetzer.

The editorial and art staffs of the Medical Department of Appleton-Century-Crofts for their direction and guidance.

STEPHEN M. AYRES, M.D.
STANLEY GIANNELLI, JR., M.D.

PREFACE TO THE THIRD EDITION

The number of hospital beds specifically reserved for the care of critically ill patients has multiplied many times over since we began preparing material for the first edition of this book in 1965. Prior to 1960, almost all hospitalized patients received the same type of medical care regardless of the complexity of their illness. The stratification of patients by intensity of nursing and medical care requirements is a relatively recent practice. Governmental decisions to control cost rather than quality has led to a dramatic shift in the types of patients admitted to hospitals. Only the sickest patients are eligible for admission, and their care is compressed into the shortest possible time because of the need to reduce length of stay and make the predetermined flat-rate reimbursement profitable to the hospital. Incredibly, the diagnosis-related grouping system was embraced by the Federal Government without considering the severity of illness within each grouping. Careful evaluation of physiologic status of patients within specific diagnostic groupings have demonstrated wide variation in the severity and expected mortality of individual patients. The need for early detection and prevention of potentially lethal situations is more urgent at this moment than ever before.

Recent studies have shown that the quality of critical care varies widely from hospital to hospital. Unfortunately, practice too often lags behind theory, and inappropriate use of high technology too often becomes a substitute for careful diagnostic and treatment planning. More than fifteen years ago, Senator Abraham Ribicoff, in an important essay entitled "The American Medical Machine," told of patients dying in intensive care units because of clogged tracheostomy tubes or accidentally disconnected respirators. The key to better performance in the treatment of such patients lies in the development of an organized system for the delivery of intensive care. Important as well-engineered hardware is, the success of a system for the care of the critically ill depends upon the availability of an experienced team of physicians, nurses, and other health professionals, interacting and growing together, and continuously evaluating their performance as they attempt to translate basic physiologic information into better patient care. Here more than anywhere else in the hospital, patient survival depends upon nurses who have been educated to observe, question, diagnose, and initiate independent action; and upon physicians who have been educated to function as team members—not as infallible despots.

This book has been written for all concerned with the care of extremely sick people, for practicing physicians, house officers, medical students, intensive care nurses, general staff nurses, and allied health personnel. These individuals share a common-knowledge base, and the authors believe that the concepts presented here are as useful to a nurse preparing for certification in critical care nursing as to a physician preparing for subspecialty certification in medicine, surgery, or anesthesiology.

One of the authors (S.M.A.) has been actively involved in the practice of critical care medicine since 1961, and most of the material presented in this third edition has resulted from personal observation and almost continuous communication with colleagues throughout the world. An incomplete list of those whose own ideas have contributed to this book include: Diane C. Adler, Roger C. Bone, Frank Cerra, Jacqueline Coalson, Foster Conklin, John B. Downs, Alpha Fowler, Frank Gafford, Stanley Giannelli, Thomas Hyers, Robert Kirby, William Knaus, Joanne Lagerson, Ian Ledingham, Sally Millar, Hiltrud Mueller, Joseph Parrillo, Norma Shoemaker, William Shoemaker, Peter Safar, William Sibbald, Harvey Sugerman, Joan Stoklosa, Max Weil, Robert Wilson, Harold Young, and Jack Zimmerman.

The third edition could not have been written without the editorial expertise of Meta Buehler, who illustrated and edited most of the text, and Ann Ramey, who typed and supervised the final preparation of the manuscript.

Stephen M. Ayres, M.D.
Robert Schlichtig, M.D.
Michael J. Sterling, M.D.

INTRODUCTION

THE EMERGENCE OF THE CRITICAL CARE CONCEPT

The life of an individual experiencing critical injury or illness hangs in a delicate balance between the forces promoting life and those leading to death. Not so long ago the physician stood helpless as the balance shifted away from life, and death became inevitable. Step by labored step an understanding of the life-promoting forces evolved, and, at some moment in the very recent past, an extremely ill individual could be said to profit more by medical action than by medical inaction.

The newest health care specialties, critical care medicine and critical care nursing, practiced informally for many years, have rapidly acquired theoretical foundation, state-of-the-art expectations, and organizational structure. Like almost all new socioscientific enterprises, they have also become focal points of significant controversy. Arriving on the American scene at a time when there was public concern over the high cost of medical technology, ethical questions over the initiation and termination of life-support measures, and increasing pressure for improved accountability of health professionals, these specialties now provide the health care system with important opportunities and vexing problems.

A historical paradigm summarizes how critical care medicine began and how it could mature or even disappear. For many years, poliomyelitis was frequently fatal because the failure to breathe was considered synonomous with the failure to survive. The introduction of the negative-pressure whole body ventilator or "iron lung" in the years following World War II saved many lives as communities acquired hardware and professional expertise. The very first acute care units arose in Scandinavia in the early 1950s[1] to centralize the use of these respirators, and similar respirator clusters arose in the United States. The number of respirators necessary was illustrated in a recent edition of the *Journal of the American Medical Association*. It republished as a Landmark Article the 1929 description by Drinker and McKhann of the first tank respiratory or iron lung.[2] Accompanying the actual article was a startling photograph showing more than 50 iron lungs in a Los Angeles County Hospital during a poliomyelitis epidemic in the 1950s. The economic problems of long-term care for ventilator-dependent patients were frequently solved by sideshow techniques. Vans carrying a "man in the iron lung" traveled from town to town and charged admission to wide-eyed youngsters and adults. Parallel progress in immunology and microbiology ended the need for iron lungs as widespread immunization prevented poliomyelitis.

Much of the present practice of critical care is rooted in experiences gained from the two World Wars, the Korean War, and Vietnam War. Wiggers et al.,[3] in a series of papers published between 1942 and 1945, showed that experimental bleeding of 4% of an animal's body weight produced irreversible shock if restoration of blood volume was delayed. Reinfusion during the first one to two hours of hemorrhagic hypotension could lead to complete restoration of health, but reinfusion after that time led to a syndrome of vascular collapse and death. The balance point between reversibility and irreversibility was named the "critical stage" and focused attention on the importance of prompt restoration of volume and flow to prevent death (Fig I–1).

At about the same time, Cournand et al.[4] studied human traumatic shock at Bellevue Hospital. They used right atrial catheterization to obtain mixed venous blood, and they calculated cardiac output from the arterial-venous oxygen content difference and calculated oxygen consumption using the Fick equation. They concluded that traumatic shock in humans was a "rapid or precipitate failure of the circulation, usually associated with inadequate return flow of blood to the heart. The chief findings were decreased cardiac output, low pressure in the right auricle, low arterial pressure, and decreased blood volume." They found that oxygen delivery was markedly reduced and that oxygen consumption was maintained at a lower-than-normal level by increased oxygen extraction at the expense of a reduction in mixed venous oxyhemoglobin saturation.

In the beginning, anesthesiologists played a leading role in the application of advanced technology to seriously ill patients. They were in the hospital for much of each day, were skilled at intubation, and were accustomed to dealing with seriously ill patients after surgery. Peter

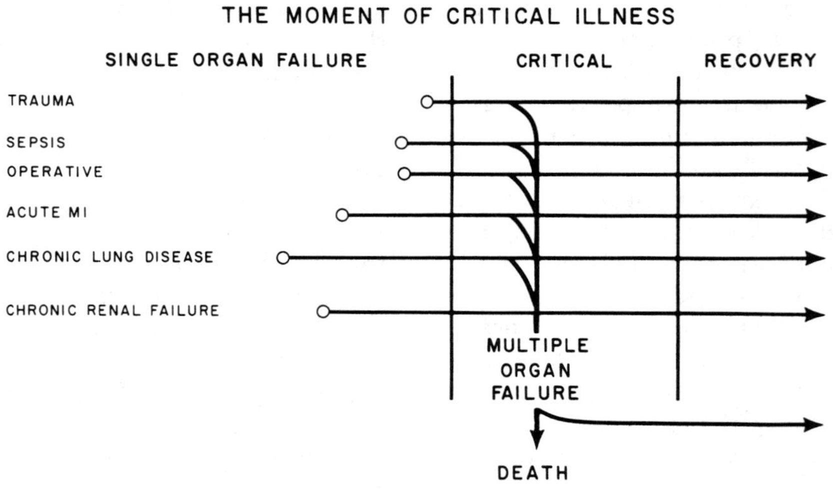

FIG I–1.
The forces leading to life or death hang in critical balance during the moments of critical illness. A variety of morbific (etiologic) processes can lead to single organ failure. Many patients rapidly recover from single organ failure, but others develop multiple organ failure and require highly organized specialized care in critical care units. A large number of these patients die, but early identification and treatment allow some to recover.

Safar, an anesthesiologist, organized the first special care unit in the United States at the Baltimore City Hospital in 1958 and called it an "intensive care" unit.[5] Internists soon became involved when it was discovered that apparent death from myocardial infarction could be successfully treated by electrical defibrillation. The observation that resuscitation was possible only if a trained team of health professionals armed with endotracheal tube and defibrillator arrived on the scene within several minutes led to the emergence of the coronary care unit and institutionalized the involvement of internists in critical care units.

The coronary care units introduced in the 1960s revolutionized the care of hospitalized patients.[6] Special observational techniques, the availability of skilled nursing care, and the regular assignments of physicians knowledgeable about the care of the extremely ill patient were necessary to reduce complications and improve survival. Technology forced the stratification of patients by severity and type of illness because expensive equipment could not be widely dispersed throughout the hospital. Such equipment was frequently too costly for general use and required special training. The direct current defibrillator was an important addition to patient care but was of little use unless immediately available. When the diagnostic value of ventricular premature contractions in patients with acute myocardial infarction was identified, the coronary care unit, with continuous electrocardiographic monitoring, resuscitation equipment including defibrillators, and specially trained personnel, became necessary. Amazing as the new technology seemed to be, the changes in utilization of health personnel were even more earth shattering. Registered nurses were suddenly propelled into the forefront of coronary care, since physicians were frequently not available on a 24-hour basis in many hospitals. They made electrocardiographic observations, diagnosed the specific types of cardiac arrhythmias, and prescribed electrical therapy, frequently in the total absence of physician support. A new era arrived as physicians delegated major diagnostic and decision-making responsibility to well-trained nurses.

Coronary care units have markedly improved the care of patients with acute myocardial infarction and reduced the mortality from cardiac arrhythmias. They became a prototype of intensive care limited to a specific problem. While patients rarely died from electrical problems associated with equipment, many continued to die from ventricular failure, forcing the cardiologist to acquire new skills as limited cardiac care became more generalized and included care of other failing physiologic systems. Patients with acute pulmonary edema were intubated, and hemodynamic measurements with bedside catheterization techniques were made in patients suffering from shock.[7] Perhaps the most significant change was the routine use and interpretation of arterial blood respiratory gas analysis to determine the level of pulmonary venoarterial shunting and the adequacy of alveolar ventilation. The acute respiratory care unit was born, and chest physicians joined cardiologists in the application of new techniques to old clinical problems.

In 1967, Ayres, Giannelli, and Mueller[8] published the first edition of *Care of the Critically Ill* based on their experiences caring for cardiac surgical patients at Saint Vincent's Hospital in New York City. "The lessons learned from these patients were applied to other critically ill patients who shared the common problem of cardio-respiratory collapse," they wrote in the preface. "It soon became apparent that although certain well-established concepts provided the basis for treatment of such patients, they could not be applied unless continuous quantitative observations were made.. . .The modern care of the critically ill patient is a team effort." The publication of that text and an article published the same year by Max Harry Weil[9] entitled "A New Look at the Critically Ill" provided a new name for the organized care of such individuals. Safar[10] had called the science of emergency life-support "resuscitation" or "reanimation" and used "intensive care" to mean long-term resuscitation in special units. The term "critical care" is now used to describe the entire continuum from emergency treatment at the scene of illness or accident to the special care provided in the hospital.

The first coronary care and medical-surgical intensive care units were located in large nonuniversity hospitals and arose because of obvious patient need. A new literature was created, and organizations to educate and motivate health professionals working in critical care units became necessary. The American Association of Cardiovascular Nurses, first incorporated in 1969, changed their name to the American Association of Critical Care Nurses (both organization abbreviated AACN) in 1971. They had 2,800 members at the time of the name change and grew to 58,000 in 1987. In 1971, 26 individual physicians representing medicine, anesthesiology, pediatrics, and surgery founded the Society of Critical Care Medicine. The society journal, *Critical Care Medicine*, skillfully edited by William Shoemaker, has become an important focus for scientific communication in the field. Another journal, *Heart and Lung*, reaches thousands of nurses and other health professionals, including physicians, and is a major educational source for high standards in critical care.

Critical care medicine was at one time focused on the heart and the lungs. The once secure belief, however, that the problems experienced by the patient of an organ specialist would remain conveniently limited to that organ was shaken by the growing realization that multiple organ failure frequently followed critical illness. A multi-institutional study organized by the Division of Lung Diseases of the National Institutes of Health[11] to study extracorporeal membrane oxygenation for acute respiratory failure found that two-thirds of the 490 patients studied had failure of other organ systems besides the lung. Mortality rates were 40% when only the lung was involved; however, rates rose to 85% in the 162 patients with renal failure, to 79% in the 143 patients with central nervous system involvement, and to 77% in the 116 patients with sepsis. The *number* of additional organs involved, not the *nature* of the organ system itself, appeared to determine mortality, so that involvement of one additional organ led to 55% mortality, three additional to 85%, and four additional to 100%. Had traditional deployment of medical specialists been followed, many patients would have required at least five subspecialists in addition to their primary physician.

A group of subsequent studies, most of them in the surgical literature, emphasized the need for comprehensively trained generalists ("intensivists") able to deal with the simultaneous or sequential malfunction of multiple organ systems. It was soon recognized that a rising creatinine, bilirubin, or fibrin split products in apparently stable patients might herald disaster even though they were frequently ignored. While precise knowledge of etiology permitted early application of corrective action, an expanding experience suggested that analysis of physiologic abnormalities provided a parallel and sometimes more predictive indicator of ultimate outcome. Cumulative scoring of physiologic abnormalities in the first few hours of care generated a predictive index that could be used to determine optimal treatment and allocation of scarce resources.[12]

The long-held clinical belief that a relatively stable "golden" period is often interposed between the inciting event and subsequent deterioration probably began with the important work of Wiggers et al.[3] The importance of early intervention has been buttressed by the gradual understanding that a group of primary etiologic factors seem to produce diffuse vascular injury with sluggish regional blood flow and leakage of plasma contents into interstitial spaces.[13] Animal models of all sorts suggest that early treatment may prevent multiple organ failure and may help expand the concept of critical care medicine to include on-site stabilization, safe transport to a hospital, and immediate care in emergency room and intensive care units.

Early recognition of life-threatening illness has become a major challenge for the medical community. At the moment, the advance of technology appears to have outdistanced the available human resources; better ways must be found for the recruitment, training, and organization of the people necessary to master this new technology. Medical care is traditionally delivered by office-based, primary care physicians or organ-focused specialists who spend a relatively small portion of their time in the hospital. While organ-oriented medical or surgical specialists perform superbly in situations involving their own areas of expertise, bedside care frequently becomes suboptimal when an unmanageable group of consultants attempt to forge a cohesive plan of action. Training and continued experience in the *comprehensive* care of critically ill patients, with emphasis on total function rather than a more parochial concern for organ protectionism, are essential.

The American Board of Medical Specialties recently attempted to define the boundaries of critical care medicine by examination and prescribed training. In 1980, the American Boards of Internal Medicine, Anesthesiology, Surgery, and Pediatrics joined together to offer a certificate of special competence in critical care medicine. Of novel design, an identical examination was proposed for all applicants—internists, surgeons, anesthesiologists, and pediatricians. The vision of the 26 founders of the Society of Critical Care Medicine seemed imminent. However, after several years of discussion, the Joint committee for Critical Care Medicine (JCCCM) fell apart. The proximate cause of dissolution was disagreement over training standards, but more important concerns actually undergirded the ultimate decision. The concept of critical care had simply become too important and too vital to allow transfer to a new, transdisciplinary, certifying authority. Within months after conversations ended, the American Boards of Anesthesiology and Internal Medicine announced their own plans for independent examination and certification. The anesthesiologists and surgeons gave their first examination in 1986, and the internists gave theirs in the fall of 1987. Critical care had entered the mainstream of American medicine.

A systematic assessment of the role of critical care medicine was undertaken by the Office of Medical Applications of Research (OMAR) of the National Institutes of Health. A Consensus Development Conference was held in Washington, D.C. in March 1983; the official Consensus Development Report was written by a panel that included biomedical investigators, critical care physicians, other medical specialists, nurses, a biostatistician, and a jurist. The panel report was published widely, and the entire proceedings were later presented in book form.[14] The panel concluded that modern therapeutic interventions benefit many patients admitted to critical care units but that the evidence of benefit was equivocal in another larger group of patients. The weight of clinical opinion supported the belief that intensive care was useful for this larger population, but the risk of iatrogenic illnesses and complications could outweigh any potential benefit. Many patients, the report emphasized, were admitted to intensive care units because they were at risk of becoming critically ill. In these patients, mortality might well be decreased if the likelihood of critical illness was strong and the benefits of treatment substantial. The panel emphasized that limited resources should not be devoted to patients "without reasonable prospects of significant recovery when patients who need those services, and who have significant prospect of recovery from acutely life-threatening disease or injury, are being turned away due to lack of capacity."

The Consensus Development Conference identified a number of perplexing systems problems that demand early solutions. Highly trained experts in critical care are of little use to the critically ill patient unless these people are available almost immediately. The staffing of emergency rooms and critical care units in the thousands of small hospitals that provide first-contact care in the United States is of great concern. At the very least, a physician with broad training, that is, who is able to intubate and initiate vascular monitoring, should be on the premises in any hospital receiving ambulance patients.

The sociopolitical uncertainties that have hindered the optimal organization of human resources for the care of the critically ill have also had an impact on other aspects of the health care system. Philosophers, politicians, ethicists, and other designers of public policy have had great difficulty deciding whether health care is a right or a luxury. Many shrink from orderly consideration of the allocation of scarce and expensive resources, but certain vexing questions must be faced.

The quality of critical care becomes an important issue. Recently published studies have emphasized the complications and errors of medical practice. Knaus, Draper, and Wagner[15] have recently published an important study evaluating outcome following admission to critical care units in 14 American hospitals. The severity of illness has determined by their APACHE scoring system, and expected mortality was derived from the overall experience of the involved hospital centers. Several of the hospitals had mortality rates significantly lower than predicted, while others had mortality rates significantly greater than the other hospitals. The hospital with the best mortality rate was characterized by the use of standard protocols, the presence of a medical director with considerable authority, a high level of educational achievement for staff nurses, and a collegial relationship among physicians and nurses. Interestingly, in the hospital with the best mortality rate, nursing personnel rather than physicians made the decisions to cancel elective surgery when the unit became crowded.

Consider the following the questions: Should all individuals have access to high-quality critical care medicine? How can seriously ill and sometimes unconscious patients reach appropriately staffed units within minutes of the onset of illness? How can those patients who appear too sick to benefit from treatment in a full-service intensive care unit receive sensitive and appropriate care in alternate settings? How can family members of a critically ill individual learn more about serious illness, prognosis, cost, and subsequent rehabilitative care. The Foundation for Critical Care was recently founded to explore these complex social issues. Members of the foundation board include representatives from the Society of Critical

Care Medicine and the American Association for Critical Care Nurses, as well as public-minded citizens without health care backgrounds.

This text deals with the science and art of critical care. Reliance on high-technology life-support systems should soon be replaced by techniques that can prevent or lessen the impact of serious illness at an early stage. The promise of cell and molecular biological research, demonstrated perhaps best in the eradication of poliomyelitis, may soon prevent the vascular damage that is a common pathogenic pathway for most serious illness. The fruits of molecular biology have rapidly influenced almost every area of medical science. Prestitious journals regularly publish important studies on the nature of critical illness, studies that were impossible even to contemplate when experimental design was limited to physiologic study. The endothelial cell and the capillary-interstitial interface have moved to center stage. Endothelial cells secrete proteins such as (1) the von Willebrand factor, which promotes platelet adhesion and aggregation, (2) prostacyclin, and (3) protein S and thrombomodulin, which amplify the anticoagulant activity of protein C. These cells also secrete both plasminogen activators and activator inhibitors. Ribes, Francis, and Wagner[16] recently demonstrated that the fibrin produced by vascular injury modulated endothelial cell behavior and promoted the release of the von Willebrand factor. This amplification of the coagulation cascade-platelet-endothelial cell interaction takes on special importance since thrombin increase lung vascular permeability. Another newly explored group of molecules—the reactive oxygen species, or free radicals—appears to mediate granulocyte-dependent, thrombin-induced lung injury. Johnson et al.[17] have shown that the protective enzyme, superoxide dysmutase, reduces the permeability response to thrombin. The endothelium is normally thrombo-resistant, but in certain pathologic states, such as gram-negative sepsis, the balance may shift to thrombosis. Moore et al.,[18] for example, have demonstrated that sepsis stimulates a tissue factor that profoundly decreases the thrombomodulin activity on endothelial cell surfaces, promoting coagulation.

The evolution of new methods permitting the scientist to examine the inner workings of the cell itself has led to the discovery of a specific macrophage product that appears to have a powerful tumor necrosis effect. This substance, which is called tumor necrosis factor or cachectin, has been analyzed and found to be a peptide that normally exists as an innocuous prohormone until it is activated. The activation process appears closely controlled so that inadvertent release is minimized. Beutler and Cerami[19] recently reviewed the properties of this cell destroyer and concluded that

> Thus it would seem possible that neutralizing monoclonal antibodies directed against human cachectin may prove useful in the treatment of sepsis, particularly in its early stages. It remains to be seen whether such antibodies (or other cachectin antagonists) will also prove useful in the treatment of other pathologic states in which inflammation has a role. However, it is anticipated that specific neutralization of cachectin and of related cytokines may offer new therapeutic directives with which to treat a broad spectrum of diseases.

None of these studies could have been performed until quite recently. While it is likely that continued study of the cell and its organelles will provide the intensivist with agents that will dramatically interrupt the pathogenetic cascade leading to multiple organ failure, problems of access and skilled care will remain. The immunization against poliomyelitis led to the virtual disappearance of that disease from the United States, but reduction in mortality from critical illness will require the skillful application of precise pharmacological remedies by skilled health care professionals.

The acquired immune deficiency syndrome (AIDS) has replaced poliomyelitis as a paradigm for critical care medicine. Admissions for AIDS and its associated infections have increased geometrically, and it is likely that there will be 150,000 patients per year admitted with Pneumocystis carinii pneumonia by 1990.[20] The use of scarce and expensive resources for patients with fatal illnesses will come under increased national scrutiny. Already, for example, physicians in areas of high prevalence have decided not to admit seriously ill patients with Pneumocystic pneumonia to intensive care units. The number of admissions to the ICU at San Francisco General Hospital[21] actually decreased from 17 during the second quarter of 1984 to 5 per quarter in 1985, even though hospital admissions for that condition were increasing. The need for better understanding of cell function, the development of vaccines, attempts to augment natural immunity, an understanding of a group of infectious agents once considered rare, the allocation of scare resources, and the possibility of recommending the termination of life support systems in relatively young individuals are important issues that place AIDS in the center of any discussion of critical illness. As iron lungs and then vaccines conquered poliomyelitis, so must highly organized critical care and modern cell biology learn to control the consequences of infection with the human immunodeficiency virus (HIV) and any of the newer infectious agents certain to follow.

It is probably fortunate that HIV did not emerge from its murky cradle any sooner. Biomedical science and health care professionals are almost ready for the challenge. Organized hospital care is an important part of the solution to this and other human maladies that will almost certainly follow the containment of AIDS. Comprehensive critical care is an idea that was born in the high technology that emerged following World War II. Its maturation reflects the important shifts from medical art to medical science that have marked the latter part of this century. It represents the concentration of sustaining resources gathered together where they can be most useful, and it is a concept rather than a specialty. Many can understand the value of early and rapid correction of disordered physiology; only those with training, continuing experience, and availability should attempt to practice those concepts at the bedside.

REFERENCES

1. Ibsen B: The anesthetist's viewpoint on treatment of respiratory complications in poliomyelitis during the epidemic in Copenhagen, 1954. *Proc R Soc Med* 1954; 47:72–74.

2. Drinker P, McKhann CF: The use of a new apparatus for the prolonged administration of artificial respiration. I. A fatal case of poliomyelitis. *JAMA* 1929; 92:1658. Reprinted *JAMA* 1986; 255:1473.

3. Wiggers CA: *Physiology of Shock*. New York, The Commonwealth Fund, 1950.

4. Cournand A, Riley RL, Bradley SE, et al: Studies of the circulation in clinical shock. *Surgery* 1943; 13:964–995.

5. Safar P, De Kornfeld T, Pearson J, et al: Intensive care unit. *Anaesthesia* 1961; 16:275–284.

6. Day HW: An intensive coronary care area. *Dis Chest* 1963; 44:423.

7. Mueller H, Ayres SM, Gregory JJ, et al: Hemodynamics, coronary blood flow, and myocardial metabolism in coronary shock. *J Clin Invest* 1970; 49:1885.

8. Ayres SM, Giannelli S Jr, Mueller HS. *Care of the Critically Ill*, ed 1. New York, Appleton-Century-Crofts, 1967.

9. Weil MH: A new look at the critically ill. *Hosp Pract* 1967; 2:27–37.

10. Safar P: Reanimatology—the science of resuscitation. *Crit Care Med* 1982; 10:134–136.

11. Extracorporeal Support for Respiratory Insufficiency. A Collaborative Study in Response to RFP-NHLI-7320. National Heart, Lung and Blood Institute, 1979.

12. Knaus WA, Zimmerman JE, Wagner DP, et al: APACHE: acute physiology and chronic health evaluation: a physiologically based classification system. *Crit Care Med* 1981; 9:591.

13. Shasby DM, Shasby SS, Peach MJ: Granulocytes and phorbol myristate acetate increase permeability to albumin of cultured endothelial monolayers and isolated perfused lungs. *Am Rev Resp Dis* 1984; 127:72.

14. Parrillo JE, Ayres SM (eds): *Major issues in Critical Care Medicine Consensus Conference.* Baltimore, Williams & Wilkins Co, 1984.

15. Knaus WA, Draper EA, Wagner DP: An evaluation of outcome from intensive care in major medical centers. *Ann Intern Med* 1986; 104:410.

16. Ribes JA, Francis CW, Wagner DD: Fibrin induces release of von Willebrand factor from endothelial cells. *J Clin Invest* 1987; 79:117–123.

17. Johnson A, Perlman MB, Blumenstock FA, et al: Superoxide dismutase prevents the thrombin-induced increase in lung vascular permeability: role of superoxide in mediating the alterations in lung fluid balance. *Circ Res* 1986; 59:404.

18. Moore KL, Andreoli SP, Esmon NL, et al: Endotoxin enhances tissue factor and suppresses thrombomodulin expression of human vascular endothelium in vitro. *J Clin Invest* 1987; 79:124–130.

19. Beutler B, Cerami A: Cachectin: More than a tumor necrosis factor. *N Engl J Med* 1987; 316:379.

20. Centers for Disease Control Update: Acquired Immunodeficiency Syndrome—United States. *MMWR* 1986; 35:757.

21. Wachter RM, Luce JM, Turner J, et al: Intensive care of patients with the acquired immunodeficiency syndrome, outcome and changing patterns of utilization. *Am Rev Resp Dis* 1986; 134:891–896.

CONTENTS

Preface to the First Edition vii

Preface to the Third Edition ix

Introduction xi

1 **Oxygen Delivery and the Cellular Response to Injury** 1

- Cellular Respiration and the Generation of ATP 2
- Cell Regulation, Defense, and Injury 15

2 **Multiple Organ Failure, Sepsis and Septic Shock** 26

- Injury, Sepsis, and Multiple Organ Failure 28
- Outcome 37
- Treatment 37
- Septic Shock 40

3 **Circulatory Monitoring** 43

- The Relationship Between Oxygen Supply and Oxygen Demand 46
- Assessment of Circulatory Compensation 49
- Evaluation of Systemic Oxygen Delivery 59
- Improving Oxygen Delivery and Consumption in the Critically Ill 63

4 **The Normal Cardiovascular System and Its Regulation** 67

- Introduction to Biophysics 67
- The Heart 69
- Circulatory Response to Exercise 81
- Regional Circulation 85
- Physiology and Pharmacology of the Autonomic Nervous System 99

5 **Cardiovascular Dysfunction, Failure, and Shock** 115

- The Shock Syndrome 116
- Shock Associated with Acute Myocardial Infarction 125
- Non-Coronary Cardiogenic Shock 144
- Hypertensive Emergencies 148
- Cardiac Arrhythmias in the Critically Ill 149
- Physiologic Consequences of Arrhythmias 155

6 **The Normal Respiratory System** 175

- General Behavior of Gases 175
- Structure of the Normal Lung 179

7 Respiratory Dysfunction and Failure 206

Pathophysiologic Considerations 207
Determinants of Arterial Carbon Dioxide Tension 209
Physiologic Effects of Hypoxia 211
Physiologic Effects of Changes in Carbon Dioxide Tension 214
Specific Forms of Acute Respiratory Failure 216
The Adult Respiratory Distress Syndrome (ARDS) 217
Respiratory Failure Associated with Chronic Airway Obstruction 240
Chronic Airway Obstruction 241

8 The Kidney and Body Fluids 268

Body Fluids 269
Renal Regulation of Body Composition 273
Acute Renal Failure 276
Disturbances of Salt, Water, and Electrolyte Balance 283
Regulation of Hydrogen Ion Concentration 292
Acidosis and Alkalosis 301
Disturbances of Calcium and Magnesium Homeostasis 306

9 The Central Nervous System in the Critically Ill 311

Structural Arrangements within the Brain 311
Neurotransmitter Control of Synaptic Transmission 312
Cerebral Metabolism and Blood Flow 314
Cerebral Edema and the Blood-Drain Barrier 316
Cerebral Ischemic Syndromes 317
Alterations in Consciousness 319
Care of the Brain-Damaged Patient 320
Brain Death 322
Permanently Lost Consciousness 325
Ethical and Legal Considerations in the Care of Brain-Damaged Patients 326

10 Nutritional Support of Critically Ill Patients 335

Protein Catabolism in Health and Critical Illness 332
Clinical Studies 335
Nutritional Support in Critical Illness 337
Modes of Delivery 344
Complications Caused by Nutritional Support 347

11 Specific Etiologic Factors in Critical Illness 352

Sepsis 352
Care of the Burned Patient 358
Trauma 364
The Acquired Immunodeficiency Syndrome (AIDS) and Pneumocystic Pneumonia 367

12 Dysfunction of Other Organs 380

The Liver 380
The Splanchnic Circulation 382
The Pancreas 383
Hemostasis and Disseminated Intravascular Coagulation 383
Endocrine Dysfunction 387

13 The Care of the Critically Ill 389

Appendix 405

Index 406

1 OXYGEN DELIVERY AND THE CELLULAR RESPONSE TO INJURY

Acute blood loss, severe diarrhea with dehydration, severe pulmonary disease, acute myocardial infarction, sepsis, and trauma may all lead to collapse of cellular respiration. Changes in cerebral function, agitation, mental confusion or coma, deep rapid breathing, blue nail beds, cold pale skin, decrease in urine output, and low blood pressure with poorly palpable peripheral pulses bear external evidence of the body's progressively more agonal attempts to distribute oxygen to the more vital organs as cellular metabolism of vital organs fails. This syndrome—the expression of severe oxidative failure—is traditionally subdivided into respiratory failure or shock depending upon whether the respiratory or circulatory system is primarily at fault. It is characterized biochemically by failure of mitochondrial oxidation, depletion of high-energy phosphates, and accumulation of unmetabolized substrate and unoxidized enzymes. Cell death progresses inexorably unless causal factors are corrected and tissue oxygen delivery restored.

One of the central themes of critical care medicine is the direct relationship between tissue integrity and the amount of oxygen consumed by the mitochondria. In turn, mitochondrial oxygen consumption is determined by the amount of oxygen required by and the amount of oxygen delivered to those subcellular organelles. While oxygen has long held center stage as a key determinant of mitochondrial ATP synthesis, the general equation for oxidative phosphorylation shown below emphasizes that substrate as well as oxygen is necessary for energy production. Both oxygen and substrate delivery determine cell integrity, but the former is much more easily monitored.

The cellular utilization of oxygen and substrate for energy production and the associated production of carbon dioxide are properly called *respiration*. The oxygen requirements of the single-celled organism were met in the earliest stages of biologic evolution by simple diffusion from the environment across the cellular membrane. The simplest multicellular forms were later able to accomplish oxygen transport by a concentric arrangement of cells around a central fluid-conducting chamber. Increasing complexity of development created a requirement for a system to transport oxygen to cells not in direct contact with the external environment. This led to the evolution of the cardiovascular and respiratory systems. Oxygen is transferred by the lungs from the atmosphere to the circulatory system, which then distributes the gas to individual cells. Carbon dioxide, the gaseous product of cellular respiration, is then carried by the circulation to the lungs and is eliminated into the atmosphere.

CELLULAR RESPIRATION AND THE GENERATION OF ATP

Life is made possible by the continuing production of energy by living cells. Energy cannot be piped from a site of production to a site of utilization but must be generated by each cell for its own use. Not only is energy necessary for gross muscular actions such as walking, lifting, or running, but it is also required for breathing, contraction, and maintaining the organization of body tissues.[1]

A general use of energy is the maintenance of concentration gradients that oppose the physical tendency toward equilibrium.[2] The low intracellular sodium concentration of all human cells and the high intracellular hydrogen ion concentration of the specialized gastric mucosal cells, for example, are made possible by an energy-produced concentration gradient. Following depolarization of muscle cells, intracellular potassium falls as potassium flows out of and sodium flows into the cell. An energy-dependent sodium pump pushes sodium out following contraction and restores the concentration gradient.[3] Energy is thus necessary for intracellular function and the maintenance of membrane integrity. Since loss of membrane function signals imminent cell death, it is likely that cell metabolism can be down-regulated so that ATP may be reserved for membrane stabilization during periods of energy restriction. Creatine phosphate serves as a storage compound for high-energy phosphate bonds that are transferred between creatine phosphate and ATP. These high-energy bonds may be considered the "coin of the realm" since they are required for all cellular transactions. Energy is derived from the oxidative breakdown of carbon compounds that enter the body as carbohydrate, fat, and protein. The combustion of carbohydrate in a bomb calorimeter rapidly converts all stored energy into heat:

$$CHO + O_2 = H_2O + \text{heat}$$

Direct generation of heat and water is obviously useless for providing energy to biologic systems. Instead, energy is released in a stepwise manner in biologic oxidation, as hydrogen and electrons are sequentially stripped from metabolic substrate and transferred to the coenzyme nicotinamide adenine dinucleotide or NAD. Reduced NAD (NADH) then transfers its electrons to a series of respiratory enzymes (flavoproteins, coenzyme Q, and the cytochromes), each of which are reduced in sequence as they oxidize the reduced product transferred to them. This modulated electron loss from substrate (oxidation) transfers and stores energy in the high-energy phosphate linkages of ATP. The general equation for oxidative phosphorylation basically demonstrates that two electrons join the six orbital electrons in the oxygen atom to complete the outer ring, while hydrogen ions combine with the oxygen atom to form water. The two substrate electrons pass through three coupling sites so that three moles of ATP are produced for each pair of electrons

$$NADH + \tfrac{1}{2}O_2 + H^+ + 3ADP + 3P_i = 3ATP + NAD^+ + H_2O$$

and stores energy as high-energy phosphate linkages in ATP. High-energy phosphate bonds are produced in both the cytoplasmic glycolytic cycle and the mitochondrial citric acid cycle. The former generates a small amount of ATP and is able to function for short periods of time without oxygen (anaerobic metabolism). The end metabolic product of this glycolytic cycle is transferred to the citric acid cycle, which generates a larger quantity of high-energy phosphates. Many of these chemical steps have been understood for some time, but the availability of electron microscopy and newer analytic techniques, including magnetic resonance spectroscopy, has provided new insight into the reduction of oxygen and the production of high-energy phosphates.

The internal anatomy of the mitochondria could only be studied when electron microscopy became generally available. The outer mitochondrial membrane is basically an invagination of the cell membrane and appears as a smooth closed bag. The inner mitochondrial membrane is invaginated to form dimples or cristae that contain respiratory transport enzymes. Spherical particles on stalks arising from the inner membrane contain the enzymes of oxidative metabolism. These enzymes are in close contact with the surrounding aqueous "stew," which contains ADP and inorganic phosphate. The general equation shown previously for oxidative phosphorylation demonstrates the important relationship between ADP and ATP. When ATP concentrations are low, the reaction moves to the right, following the laws of mass action, and increases the production of more ATP. When ATP concentration is high, the reaction moves back to the left, decreasing the production of ATP. This negative feedback mechanism permits the cell to match high-energy phosphate generation to metabolic need. The ADP/ATP ratio becomes a good index of cellular metabolic integrity.

Chance and Williams in 1955[4] showed that this feedback regulation could be demonstrated in isolated mitochondria; an increase in ADP increased the production of ATP and the consumption of oxygen. Chance and Hollunger[5] demonstrated that this "phosphate potential" was a useful indicator of mitochondrial energy conservation.

$$\text{phosphate potential} = \text{ATP}/(\text{ADP} \times \text{P}_i)$$

This equation becomes of practical importance to the intensivist because of the recent demonstration that magnetic resonance spectroscopy permits the measurement of various phosphate compounds in the intact subject. When organs or tissue samples are placed in a pulsed magnetic field, their phosphate nuclei absorb energy. Energy is released following cessation of the pulse and analyzed as a radio-frequency spectrogram, which exhibits peaks for tissue phosphate compounds such as ATP, ADP, creatine phosphate, and inorganic phosphate. Since the phosphate potential is a description of the relationship between phosphocreatine and inorganic phosphate, an estimate of respiratory chain function may be obtained.[6]

Chance[7] had used optical methods to study the state of respiratory enzyme oxidation for many years and immediately realized that magnetic resonance spectroscopy could provide a noninvasive measure of oxidative metabolism. He demonstrated that the ratio of inorganic phosphate to phosphocreatine was closely related to his earlier derivation of the phosphate potential. He pointed out that the P_i/CrP ratio actually measured the "capability of the respiratory chain" to produce ATP since the enzymes translocase and ATP synthetase were not rate-limiting. Figure 1–1, based on this work, demonstrates that a decrease in mitochondrial oxygen tension to progressively lower levels leads to rapidly increasing P_i/PCr ratios. The form of the relationship is a rectangular hyperbola, a function often observed in physiologic systems.

Significant decreases in mitochondrial Po_2 have little effect on the P_i/PCr ratio until a critical point is reached. At that point, a further small reduction in oxygen tension produces a very large increase in the ratio indicating almost complete anoxia. Obviously, the converse direction suggests that only a little therapeutic oxygen given in such a critical situation could dramatically improve cell function. Chance et al.[7] also pointed out that oxidative phosphorylation requires NADH (substrate) and phosphate as well as oxygen.

The Generation of NADH

Adequate reserves of creatine phosphate and ATP require substrate in the form of NADH and phosphate. Glucose is converted to pyruvic acid* in the glycolytic cycle with the production of two molecules of ATP for each molecule of glucose (Fig 1–2). The reaction does not require oxygen directly but is made possible by a coenzyme, nicotinamide adenine dinucleotide (NAD, or DPN in the older terminology), which accepts hydrogen atoms and is itself reduced to NADH (DPNH). The continuing function of the glycolytic cycle depends on an adequate supply of NAD, which is produced by the oxidation of NADH. NADH is reoxidized by reduction of pyruvate to lactate in the cytoplasm. NADH is also oxidized in the mitochondrium, but there the glycolytic pathway is in part dependent upon a supply of oxygen.

Pyruvate and two-carbon fragments from amino and fatty acids enter the mitochondrial citric acid cycle, where hydrogen atoms are peeled off (dehydrogenation) and transferred to NAD or another group of coenzymes, the flavoproteins (FLAV). Carbon dioxide is produced in the citric acid cycle by decarboxylation of intermediates; energy, however, is not produced by this reaction. The entire available energy is stored in the hydrogen bonds of NADH and FLAVH. This stored energy is gradually made available in the form of high-energy phosphates by the production of a series of compounds with successively lower- energy contents intermediate between the high-energy content of NADH and FLAVH and the low-energy content of the simple hydrogen-oxygen linkage in water.

The cytoplasmic glycolytic cycle provides an emergency pathway for the temporary production of ATP in the absence of oxygen. When oxygen is plentiful, pyruvate enters the citric acid cycle and NADH is oxidized by molecular oxygen to NAD. Fortunately, NADH can facilitate the reduction of pyruvate to lactate and, in doing so, is itself oxidized to NAD. During periods of hypoxia or relative hypoxia due to increased energy demands, pyruvate is converted to lactate and NADH oxidized to NAD, which in turn facilitates continued glycolysis (Fig 1–3). The adequacy of the anaerobic emergency pathway varies among organs. In the heart, for example, anaerobic metabolism is capable of sustaining effective contraction for only several beats following total deprivation of oxygen.

The accumulation of lactic acid in tissue indicates the onset of anaerobic

*Lactic acid and pyruvic acid are in equilibrium with their respective anions, lactate and pyruvate. The lactic acid/lactate and pyruvic acid/pyruvate ratios are fixed for a given pH as described in Chapter 8. When either lactic or pyruvic acid is formed, the following reaction is driven toward the right, shown here for lactic acid:

$$\text{H lactate} + \text{cation}^+ + \text{buffer}^- \rightleftharpoons \text{H buffer} + \text{cation}^+ + \text{lactate}^-$$

In the literature the terms lactate and lactic acid, and pyruvate and pyruvic acid, are usually employed interchangeably. Strictly speaking, this is incorrect. However, if there is increased production of either acid, the respective salts also increase according to the above equation. Laboratory determinations measure both the acid and salt forms, giving "total" lactate or pyruvate.

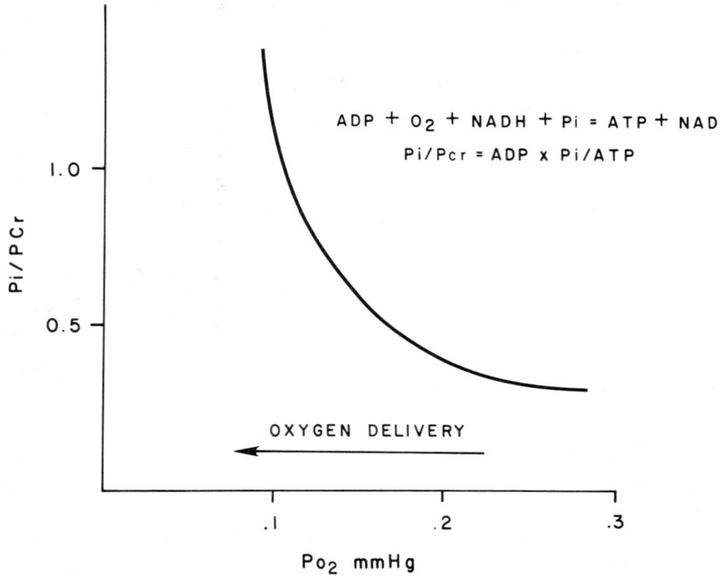

FIG 1–1.
Magnetic resonance spectroscopy demonstrates that the production of high-energy phosphates is a function of mitochondrial oxygen tension. As oxygen delivery falls, the ratio of inorganic phosphate (P_i) to phosphocreatine (PCr) rises. The relationship is that of a rectangular hyperbola where each arm approaches the straight line asymptotically. When oxygen delivery falls to critical levels, cell energetics become destabilized and concentrations of inorganic phosphate rise. (Adapted from Chance B, et al: Control of oxidative metabolism and oxygen delivery in human skeletal muscle. A steady-state analysis of the work/energy cost transfer function. *Proc Natl Acad Sci USA* 1985; 82:8384.)

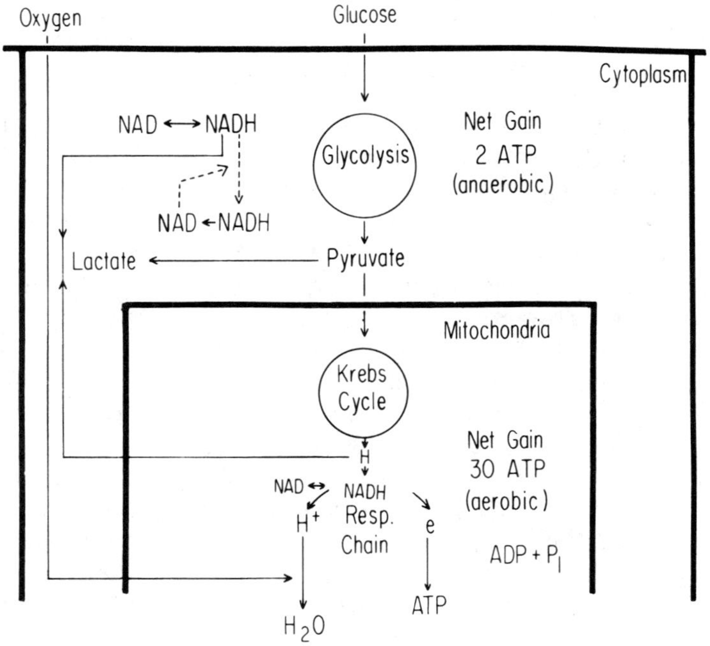

FIG 1–2.
Glucose, fatty acids, and amino acids cross the cellular membrane and enter the cytoplasm. Glucose is enzymatically oxidized to pyruvate, which enters the mitochondria along with other substrate. Hydrogen atoms and carbon dioxide molecules are peeled off in the mitochondrial citric acid cycle. The energy-rich hydrogen atoms are transferred to the respiratory enzymes, which successively decrease in energy content as they transfer energy to ADP to produce ATP. (From Ayres S, Gregory: *Cardiology: A Clinicophysiologic Approach*, Appleton-Century-Crofts, 1971.Used by permission.)

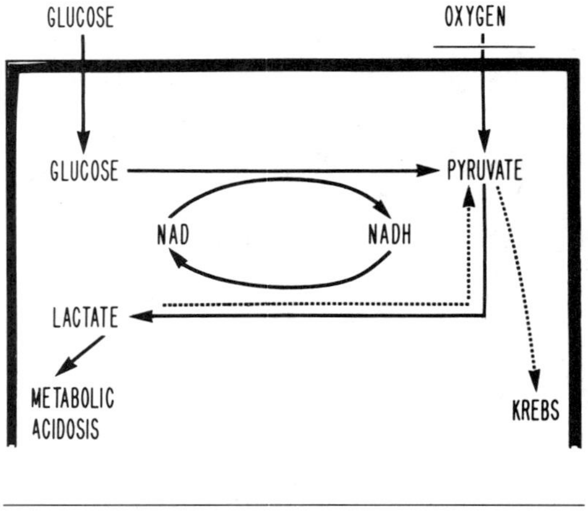

FIG 1–3.
Magnification of the cytoplasmic events of Figure 1–2 shows that glucose is oxidized to pyruvate by NAD, which itself is reduced to NADH. A modest amount of high-energy phosphate, ATP, is produced by this anaerobic step. Under conditions of normal oxygen availability, pyruvate then enters the Krebs citric acid cycle where it is further degraded; NADH is then oxidized to NAD by the respiratory chain of enzymes, which transfer the hydrogen ion to oxygen to form water. If oxygen supply is insufficient, pyruvate is reduced to lactate by NADH. This reduction process oxidizes NADH to NAD, making the enzyme available for further anaerobic conversion of glucose to pyruvate. Energy is thus produced in the absence of oxygen, but acid metabolites rapidly accumulate, producing intracellular metabolic acidosis.

metabolism. The ratio of blood lactate to pyruvate may be used as a rough estimate of the ratio of NADH to NAD and thus the adequacy of tissue oxygenation.[8] Although quantitation of the oxidation-reduction status of the cell has been attempted by measurement of blood lactate/pyruvate ratios, precise correlation is impossible because intracellular and extracellular lactate content are not in equilibrium, and small amounts of lactate may be produced under aerobic as well as anaerobic conditions. The anaerobic production of ATP in the glycolytic cycle is the only method available to the body for energy production during periods of deficient oxygen supply to the tissues. It is called upon in many normal everyday situations requiring sudden increases in energy production. Heavy exercise usually results in some anaerobic ATP production and lactic acid formation. The hyperventilation following heavy exercise is partly related to the continued higher-than-normal resting oxygen consumption to repay the so-called oxygen debt incurred during exercise.

Following circulatory collapse or cardiac arrest, lactate accumulates rapidly and overwhelms the buffering capacity of tissue and blood. Successful therapy, therefore, must include infusion of alkalinizing solution to restore the hydrogen ion concentration to normal.

The actual concentration of lactate in plasma (and the L/P ratio) is dependent upon both the rate of lactate production from the periphery and the rate of lactate uptake and metabolism by the liver. Anaerobic metabolism may occur before plasma levels increase and may remain elevated after improvement of tissue oxygenation or with hepatocellular liver damage.

Transport of Oxygen and Carbon Dioxide in the Blood

In a resting man the processes of cellular respiration that have been described require an average of 200 ml of oxygen per minute. If the respiratory quotient—which is a ratio showing the relation between the volume of carbon dioxide expired and the volume of oxygen inspired per unit of time during respiration—is 0.8, 160 ml of carbon dioxide is produced in a resting man and must be removed from the body.[9]

The blood transports these gases used and produced in the processes of cellular respiration. Oxygen molecules pass from alveoli into interstitial fluid and then cross the pulmonary capillary wall to enter the blood. In the peripheral tissue beds the molecules cross the capillary wall, pass through interstitial fluid, and enter the cells. Carbon dioxide molecules trace this path in the opposite direction. The partial pressure of the gas is about the same on either side of the capillary—in the interstitial fluid and in the plasma. However, with respect to oxygen, if the sole reliance for oxygen transport were placed on the physical solution of oxygen in plasma water ($\alpha = 0.0232$), only 3 ml of oxygen could be carried in each liter of circulating fluid, and the heart would have to pump at least 200/3 or 67 liters of fluid per minute. Moreover, the oxygen tension of the fluid leaving the cells would be close to zero and many cells would be perpetually hypoxic. Therefore, the development of a carrier which binds large amounts of oxygen and releases it at relatively high oxygen tensions has been a critical evolutionary feature of larger organisms.

In man, oxygen is carried by hemoglobin, a complex molecule containing four iron-heme units combined with a large protein molecule. These four units reversibly combine with oxygen in an unusual reaction unlike most ordinary chemical interactions. The mechanism of oxygen exchange in resting man is seen in Figure 1– 4. The right ventricle pumps an average of 5 liters of blood per minute through the pulmonary capillaries, which combines with about 200 ml of oxygen each minute. Since each gram of fully saturated hemoglobin binds 1.34 ml of oxygen, a normal adult with 15 g of hemoglobin per 100 ml of blood could carry 20 ml of oxygen in each 100 ml of blood. Actual measurements, however, indicate that arterial blood in normal man contains but 19 ml of oxygen due to reasons described later in this chapter. The hemoglobin is said to be 19/20 or 95% saturated. The oxygen capacity is said to be 20 ml/100 ml; the oxygen content is 19 ml/100 ml or 19 volumes percent (vol %). Each liter of blood thus contains 190 ml of oxygen as it reaches the tissues, of which 40 ml/liter (or 4 ml/100 ml)

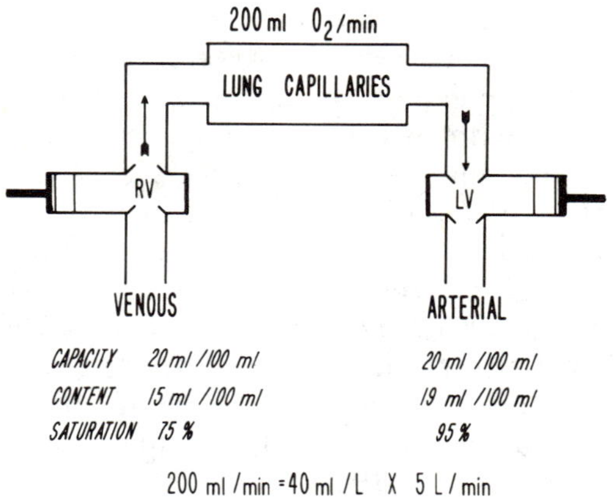

FIG 1–4
Overall cardiopulmonary oxygen exchange is shown by a double pump model. Each minute, 200 ml of oxygen is transferred to the pulmonary capillaries and distributed to the peripheral tissues by the action of both ventricles, which pump 5 liters of blood each minute through the pulmonary and systemic capillaries. Arterial blood entering the peipheral capillaries contains 19m /100ml of blood and is 95 percent saturated. Four milliliters of oxygen is extracted from each 100 ml of blood by the peripheral tissues; the venous blood is but 75 percent saturated. In order to balance the Fick equation dimensionally, the arteriovenous oxygen difference is expressed as 40 ml/liter of blood rather than 4 ml/100 ml.

are released to the tissues. As shown in the equation of Figure 1–4, the total amount of oxygen delivered to the tissues must be equal to the amount given up by each liter of blood multiplied by the total liters of blood flowing each minute. Knowing any two of these three variables, the third can be easily calculated. In practice, cardiac output is usually calculated by dividing oxygen consumption by arteriovenous oxygen difference*(Fick principle).

$$\text{cardiac output} = \frac{\text{oxygen consumption}}{\text{arterial } O_2 \text{ content} - \text{venous } O_2 \text{ content}}$$

$$5 \text{ liters/minute} = \frac{200\text{ml/minute}}{40\text{ml/minute}}$$

*The arteriovenous oxygen difference is generally abbreviated $Ca_{O_2} - C\bar{v}_{O_2}$.

Note that the arteriovenous oxygen difference is expressed as milliliters per liter.

The amount of oxygen chemically combined with hemoglobin is determined by the partial pressure of oxygen in the red blood cell. Either oxygen content or oxygen saturation may be plotted as a function of arterial tension (Fig 1–5); oxygen saturation may be easily obtained by dividing content by capacity. Alveolar and capillary oxygen tensions average about 100 mm Hg in normal man and permit approximately 19 ml of oxygen to be combined with each 100 ml of whole blood containing 15 g of hemoglobin. (Hemoglobin at pH 7.4 is 100% saturated at an oxygen tension of 300 mm Hg.) Blood oxygen tension decreases to about 90 mm Hg as arterial blood leaves the left ventricle because of the admixture of a small amount of venous blood (venoarterial shunting).

Figure 1–5 demonstrates the change in oxygen tension as blood traverses systemic capillaries. Hemoglobin entering the capillary contains 19 ml of oxygen per 100 ml of blood and is at an oxygen tension of 80 mm Hg (point **A**); 4 ml of oxygen (hatched area) are released to the tissues so that hemoglobin leaving the capillary contains 15 ml of oxygen per 100 ml at an oxygen tension of 41 mm Hg (point **B**).

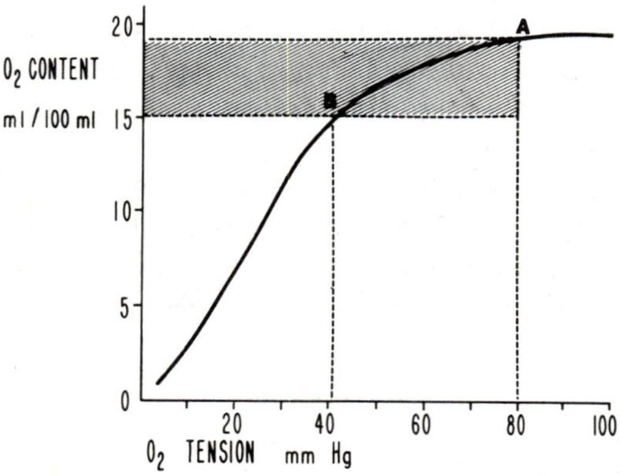

FIG 1–5.
The relationship between oxygen content and oxygen tension is termed the oxyhemoglobin dissociation curve. The shaded area shows the oxygen released by 100 ml of blood as it traverses the systemic capillary.

The shape of the oxyhemoglobin dissociation curve determines the efficiency of pulmonary and tissue oxygen exchange. The relatively flat upper region ensures that a 10 percent drop in alveolar oxygen tension is accompanied by less than a 2 percent drop in oxygen content. Should alveolar oxygen tension decrease from 100 to 60 mm Hg, for example, arterial oxygen content would decrease only from 19 to 18 ml/100 ml. The steep lower region, in contrast to the flat upper region, permits rapid decreases in content with lesser decreases in oxygen tension facilitating oxygen unloading to the tissues.

Two measurements have been used to describe these two strikingly different areas of the oxyhemoglobin dissociation curve. Figure 1–6 shows the same curve presented in Figure 1–5, but oxygen concentration is now expressed as saturation rather than content. The loading tension is the oxygen tension which saturates 95% of the hemoglobin with oxygen. The unloading tension (P-50) is the tension which saturates 50% of the hemoglobin with oxygen and expresses the ease of oxygen unloading to the peripheral tissues. Note that factors which shift the oxyhemoglobin dissociation curve to the left lower the tension required for 50% oxygen unloading, while factors shifting the curve to the right increase the tension for unloading.

Acidosis, increased carbon dioxide tension, and increased body temperature shift the curve to the right and raise the P-50, while alkalosis, decreased carbon dioxide tension, and lowered temperatures shift the curve to the left, lowering the P-50. Rightward shifts may be considered helpful adaptations which assist the

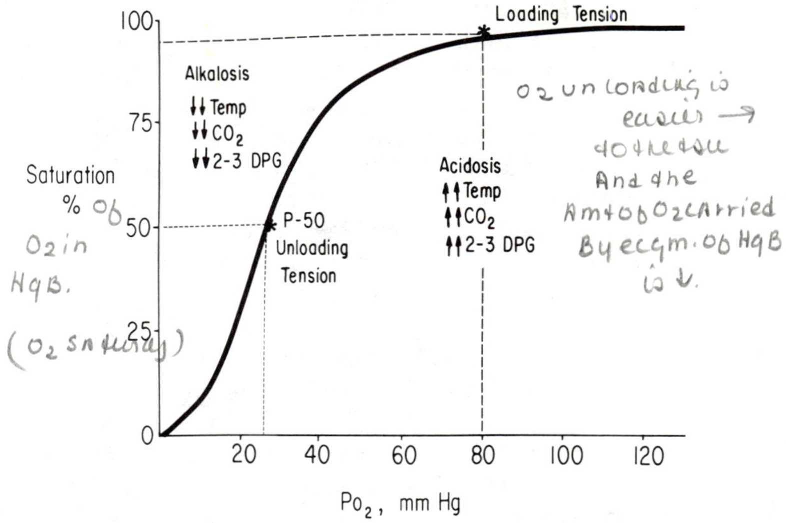

FIG 1–6.
Oxyhemoglobin dissociation curve. P-50 is oxygen tension corresponding to 50 percent oxyhemoglobin saturation. Factors shown on the right shift the curve to the right; factors shown on the left shift the curve to the left. (From Ayres S: *Resp Care* 1972; 17:291. Used by permission.)

organism in coping with decreased oxygen availability, as they make oxygen unloading easier. In contrast, leftward shifts are potentially damaging since a lower oxygen tension is necessary for the same degree of oxygen unloading.

A property of a product of carbohydrate metabolism has given considerable insight into the importance of shifts in P-50 and of the shape of the oxyhemoglobin dissociation curve. Glucose is normally metabolized to carbon dioxide and water with the production of the high-energy compound ATP. When oxygen tensions fall, certain intermediary products such as lactic acid accumulate in the cell. One of these products—2,3-diphosphoglyceric acid—has a direct effect on the shape of the dissociation curve.[10] Decreasing oxygen supply increases the concentration of 2,3-diphosphoglyceric acid, which in turn shifts the curve to the right, making it easier to unload oxygen.[11] In contrast, decreased concentrations of 2,3-diphosphoglycerate shift the curve to the left, making it more difficult to release oxygen to the tissues.

The variability of the position of the oxyhemoglobin dissociation curve has important implications in the treatment of the critically ill patient. A rightward shift of the curve raises the P-50 or unloading tension, but raises the loading tension. While the increase in loading tension is not biologically important in normal man, it may be of great significance in the patient with a reduced arterial oxygen tension. A rightward shift associated with reduction of pH from 7.4 to 7.2, for example, has little effect on oxyhemoglobin saturation at high oxygen tensions but significantly reduces the amount of oxygen carried by the arterial blood at lower oxygen tensions. The oxyhemoglobin saturation resulting from an oxygen tension of 60 mm Hg would be 89.7% at pH 7.4: the saturation would fall to 83.3 at pH 7.2. A saturation of 84.3 percent at an oxygen tension of 50 mm Hg would fall to 76.2 if the pH dropped to 7.2. Thus rightward shifts, while improving oxygen release to the tissues, decrease the amount of oxygen carried by each gram of hemoglobin. Knowledge of the hemoglobin concentration and position of the oxyhemoglobin dissociation curve are necessary in order to decide the optimal arterial oxygen tension in any individual patient.

These shifts in the position of the oxyhemoglobin dissociation curve require 6–12 hours and are easily obscured by associated changes in hemoglobin concentration or blood flow. While some authorities have tended to minimize their significance in many critically ill patients[12] it seems likely that decreased tissue oxygen unloading can further decrease cellular oxygenation in certain subsets of critically ill patients.

The carbon dioxide tension of the plasma is equal to that of the surrounding media—that is, the alveoli in the lung and interstitial fluid in the periphery. As with oxygen, carbon dioxide can be carried in blood at a much lower gas tension than would be the case if it were only in physical solution. A carbon dioxide dissociation curve can be constructed which relates the carbon dioxide content of the blood to the tension of carbon dioxide in the plasma (Fig 1–7).

Carbon dioxide (CO_2) is carried in the blood by several methods. The gas diffuses into the plasma from the tissues, and a fraction hydrates at once to form carbonic acid.

$$H_2O + CO_2 \rightarrow H_2CO_3$$

Carbonic acid reacts in the plasma with protein and phosphates to form bicarbonate (chapter 8).

$$H_2CO_3 + Na^+ + Pr^- \rightarrow HPr + Na^+ + HCO_3^-$$

$$H_2CO_3 + 3Na^+ + PO_4^{\equiv} \rightarrow 3Na^+ + HCO_3^- + HPO_4^=$$

$$H_2CO_3 + 2Na^+ + HPO_4^= \rightarrow 2Na^+ + HCO_3^- + H_2PO_4$$

Most of the CO_2 from the tissues, however, passes through the plasma into the red blood cells, where it reacts in either of two ways with hemoglobin.

CO_2 reacts with amide groups to form carbamino compounds.

$$CO_2 + HbNH \rightarrow HbNHCO_2$$

The reduced hemoglobin of venous blood can accept more CO_2 in the carbamino form at the same CO_2 tension than oxygenated hemoglobin.

The remaining CO_2 reacts with basic hemoglobin radicals. (K^+ is the predominant cation and is included to obtain electrical neutrality in the equation.)

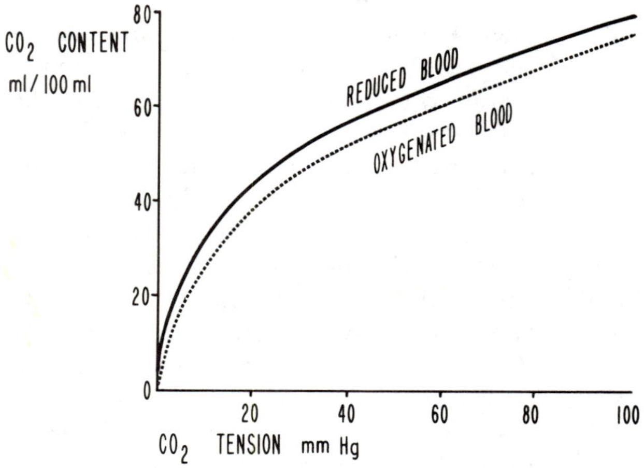

FIG 1–7.
The carbon dioxide–hemoglobin dissociation curve is essentially linear in the physiologic range. Reduced hemoglobin can carry significantly more carbon dioxide than can oxygenated hemoglobin at the same carbon dioxide tension (Haldane effect).

$$H_2CO_3 \rightleftharpoons H^+ + HCO_3^-$$

$$H^+ + HCO_3^- + K^+ + Hb^- \rightleftharpoons HCO_3^- + K^+ + HHb$$

Reduced hemoglobin more readily reacts with H_2CO_3 in this manner than oxygenated hemoglobin because reduced hemoglobin is a stronger base (weaker acid) than the oxygenated form.

Haldane first described the increased CO_2 carrying capacity of reduced hemoglobin versus the oxygenated form at the same P_{CO_2}, and the effect bears his name.

Oxygen Delivery to the Tissues

The amount of oxygen actually delivered to the tissues and available for metabolic and other purposes depends upon the oxygen content of arterial blood, the rate of blood flow to each organ system, and the distribution of blood flow within that organ system. Oxygen delivery may be calculated as the product of oxygen content and cardiac output. The oxygen extraction ratio is the percentage of delivered oxygen actually extracted by the peripheral tissues and is a useful indicator of cellular oxygen transport; a high extraction ratio generally indicates inadequate oxygen transport under resting conditions and is a mechanism to maintain oxygen consumption in the face of decreased blood flow. Hemoglobin concentration, hydrogen ion concentration (pH), temperature, the shape of the oxyhemoglobin dissociation curve, and arterial oxygen tension all determine the arterial oxygen content (see Table 1–1).

Blood flow to the individual tissues is determined by the output of the left ventricle and by the resistance of the peripheral vessels. Resistances may vary widely from organ to organ so that one region may be underperfused while another is normally perfused or actually overperfused. In the shock syndrome, for example, renal vascular resistance may be quite high and renal blood flow markedly reduced while brain resistance and blood flow remain relatively normal. Not only cardiac output, but also the flow rate of each organ system is important in determining cellular oxygen delivery. Another example of this may be seen in the effect of hyperventilation on brain metabolism in certain older individuals. Inadvertent hyperventilation during controlled ventilation may well decrease arterial carbon dioxide tension to low levels, increasing cerebral vascular tension and decreasing cerebral blood flow. Although arterial oxygen content and cardiac output are normal, localized cerebral ischemia may occur even to the point of depriving the brain of adequate oxygen delivery; the patient might suffer irreversible brain damage.

The first edition of this text, published in 1967, presented a diagrammatic view of oxygen delivery to the cell that attempted to remind bedside therapists of the integration of the lung, the heart, and the peripheral circulation (Fig 1–8). It was published at a time when cardiologists and pulmonologists were generally unaware of the importance of each others' areas of knowledge to their own critically ill patients; cardiologists tended to ignore the significance of pulmonary abnormalities to cardiac function, while pulmonologists often failed to recognize the fundamental importance of the circulation in delivering oxygen to the periphery. It has since become clear that, in the intensive

TABLE 1–1.
Determinants of Oxygen Delivery

Cardiac output
Arterial oxygen content
Arterial oxygen tension
Hemoglobin concentration
Position of the oxyhemoglobin dissociation curve (P–50)

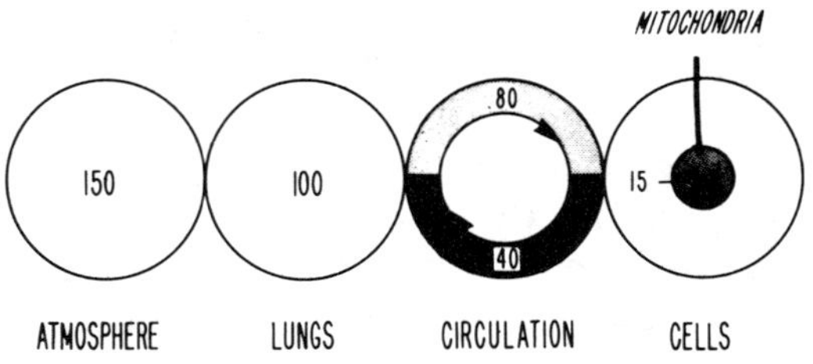

FIG 1–8.
An oxygen tension of 150 mm Hg in the atmosphere is necessary to produce an oxygen tension of 1 to 2 mm Hg in the mitochondria. Oxygen is delivered by the serial transportation system involving the lungs and circulation.

care unit at least, a sound understanding of both fields of expertise is necessary.

A recent study by Kawakami et al.[13] demonstrates this important interaction. Survivorship in chronic obstructive pulmonary disease was not predicted by forced expiratory volume measurements, hematocrit, or pulmonary arterial resistance. Arterial and mixed venous oxygen tensions were lower in the group of nonsurvivors. Oxygen delivery was lower and had less variability in the nonsurvivors, although the difference between groups did not reach statistical significance. The breathing of pure oxygen produced an increase in arterial and mixed venous carbon dioxide tension in both groups; cardiac index fell by 1.39 and 1.01 $L/min/M^2$ in survivors and nonsurvivors respectively, suggesting that cardiac function was maintained by the hypoxic state. Whether oxygen therapy affected mortality directly was not addressed. Bergofsky[14] summarized the important findings in an editorial: spirometric measurements "... no longer differentiate survivors from nonsurvivors. At the same time, the analysis of factors governing oxygen carriage from lung to tissues has gained prognostic importance in advanced disease."

Oxygen delivery is a relatively inefficient process since oxygen molecules at a partial pressure of 150 mm Hg in the atmosphere are transported to the mitochondria where a partial pressure of less than 0.5 mm Hg is adequate for the generation of ATP from ADP. *Oxygen delivery* ($\dot{D}O_2$) is the product of blood flow in ml/min times oxygen content in ml/100 ml of blood. In the equations dealing with oxygen transportation, the abbreviation, $\dot{Q}$ and C are used for flow and content, respectively. A small dot over $\dot{Q}$ means that it is a time derivative (see standard abbreviations in appendix).

$$\dot{D}O_2 = \dot{Q}O_2 \text{ x } CO_2$$

Oxygen content is the amount of oxygen contained in a sample of blood and includes oxygen bound to hemoglobin and a small amount dissolved in the plasma. With the virtual disappearance of the Van Slyke manometric method for measuring oxygen content and the general availability of accurate spectrophotometric methods for measuring oxyhemoglobin saturation, oxygen content is usually approximated from oxygen saturation in the following manner. Since the saturation is predicted from a "standard" oxyhemoglobin saturation curve, significant error is commonly introduced.

$$SO_2 = \frac{CO_2 - 0.031\text{ml}/100\text{ml}}{\text{oxygen capacity} - 0.6\text{ml}/100\text{ml}}$$

where 0.031 is the amount of dissolved oxygen in arterial blood and 0.6 is the amount dissolved when arterial blood is equilibrated with sufficient oxygen to completely saturate hemoglobin. Rearrangement of this equation permits the calculation of oxygen content if one assumes that the oxygen capacity is equal to the hemoglobin concentration times

1.34 ml of oxygen for each gram of hemoglobin.

$$So_2 = \text{Hgb Concentration} \times 1.34\text{ml/gram} \times \text{oxyhemoglobin saturation}$$

The 965 ml of oxygen leaving the left ventricle per minute is distributed to the various regional vascular beds. The total body oxygen consumption is about 200 ml/minute so that roughly only 20 to 25 percent of the delivered oxygen is extracted by the peripheral tissues. Venous saturation and oxygen tension are therefore about 75 percent and 40 mm Hg, respectively. Arterial hypoxemia lowers the oxygen delivery as shown above. Lowering arterial oxygen tension to 40 mm Hg reduces oxygen delivery from 965 to 750 ml (Fig 1–9). Removal of 200 ml/minute reduces the venous saturation to 53 pecent and the venous oxygen tension to 27 mm Hg. Oxygen consumption is maintained, but venous oxygen tension (an index of tissue oxygen tension) drops to potentially dangerous levels. Arterial hypoxemia (lowered arterial oxygen ten sion) thus leads to tissue hypoxia. The distinction between hypoxia and hypoxemia is more than academic since either one can exist without the other (see below).

Figure 1–9 emphasizes the importance of the circulating hemoglobin concentration on oxygen delivery. A decrease in hemoglobin concentration to either 10 or 5 g/100 ml decreases oxygen delivery and tissue oxygen tension in exactly the same way as does hypoxemia. Since arterial oxygen tension is normal in the presence of anemia unless pulmonary problems coexist, hypoxia exists without hypoxemia.

Tissue Hypoxia and Reduced Oxygen Delivery

The ultimate reason for individual or multiple organ failure in the critically ill patient is usually major reduction in regional blood flow. While direct parenchymal damage may at times destroy the ability of an organ to function at an adequate level, potentially reversible decreases in organ oxygen delivery appear to be the rule so that inter-

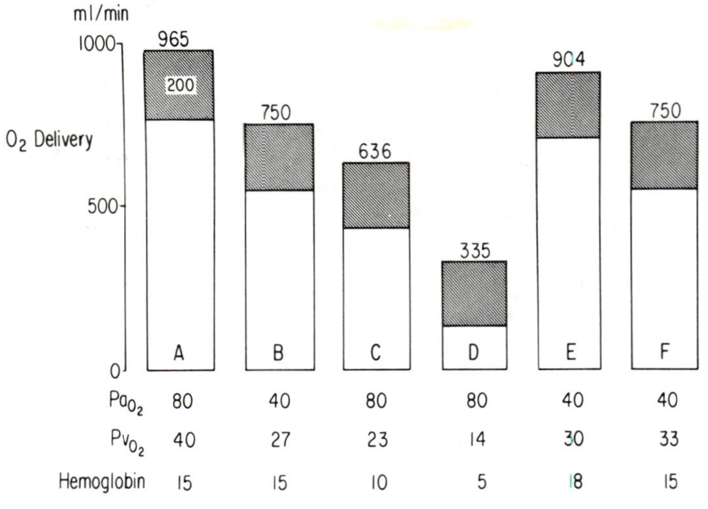

FIG 1–9.
Oxygen delivery in a number of clinical situations. Total height of bar and value above bar indicate total amount of oxygen delivered to the tissues. Hatched area represents 200 ml of oxygen extracted by the tissues. Arterial oxygen tension, venous oxygen tension, and hemoglobin are shown below. **A,** normal situation **B,** arterial hypoxemia. **C,** hemoglobin of 10 g/100 ml. **D,** hemoglobin of 5 g/100 ml. **E,** Polycythemia with hemoglobin of 18 g/100 ml. **F,** shift of oxyhemoglobin dissociation curve to right.

ventions that increase organ blood flow might restore organ function in many clinical situations. Shoemaker, Appel, and Kram,[15] for example, pioneered the view that the increased metabolic needs of critical illness require increased, rather than merely normal, systemic oxygen delivery. Their randomized studies have shown remarkable decreases in mortality from over 30% to less than 5% when oxygen delivery to the whole body was increased to at least 50% greater than normal. Whether these patients do better because of increased oxygen requirements or inefficient use of oxygen is unclear. These observations and a group of important experimental studies suggest that in many clinical situations oxygen consumption by the cell is limited by the amount of oxygen available.

Normal tissue oxygen tension is much higher than the minimum requirements of the mitochondria[16] so that much more oxygen than needed is normally available to the mitochondria. Viewed from another perspective, oxygen delivery does not limit oxygen consumption under normal circumstances so long as oxygen delivery is above a critical level; above this critical level, oxygen consumption is normally maintained, when necessary, by increasing oxygen extraction.[17] Guitierrez and Pohil,[18] however, and a number of other investigators have identified a puzzling phenomenon in critically ill patients that appears inconsistent with this classical teaching. They described 30 critically ill patients who had 8 or more determinations of oxygen delivery and consumption in whom a plateau level of oxygen consumption was never reached. Oxygen consumption was linearly related to oxygen delivery at all levels of oxygen delivery. These patients were further subdivided into a group of 20 patients where the relationship between $\dot{V}O_2$ and $\dot{D}O_2$ was quite steep. Oxygen consumption was high in this group, and oxygen extraction failed to increase with a decrease in oxygen delivery. Most of these patients had either the adult respiratory distress syndrome, sepsis, or gastrointestinal bleeding and their mortality rate was 70%. In the remaining patients, the relationship between $\dot{V}O_2$ and $\dot{D}O_2$ less steep, oxygen consumption was lower, oxygen extraction was increased at lower levels of oxygen delivery, and the mortality rate was only 30%. The investigators concluded that the relationship between $\dot{V}O_2$ and $\dot{D}O_2$ was linear for all of their patients and that oxygen consumption was always dependent upon oxygen delivery in critically ill patients.

An alternative explanation seems equally plausible. The high oxygen consumption observed in the first group of patients suggests that they were seriously ill and presumably catabolic. Oxygen delivery may never have been raised high enough to demonstrate a plateau. It is possible that failure to reach the level at which oxygen consumption became independent of oxygen delivery may explain the high mortality in that group. In contrast, patients in the second group may actually be near a plateau at which oxygen consumption is independent of oxygen delivery. Several possible relationships between these variables are shown in Figure 1–10.

These pathophysiologic issues are more than academic. If a critical level for oxygen does exist, as suggested by Shoemaker, Appel, and Kram,[15] that level of oxygen delivery must be achieved if oxygen deprivation and death are to be avoided. A linear relationship at all levels of oxygen delivery would require reexamination of basic assumptions and might suggest that part of the delivered oxygen is used for extramitochondrial purposes, such as the production of superoxide anion and free oxygen radicals.

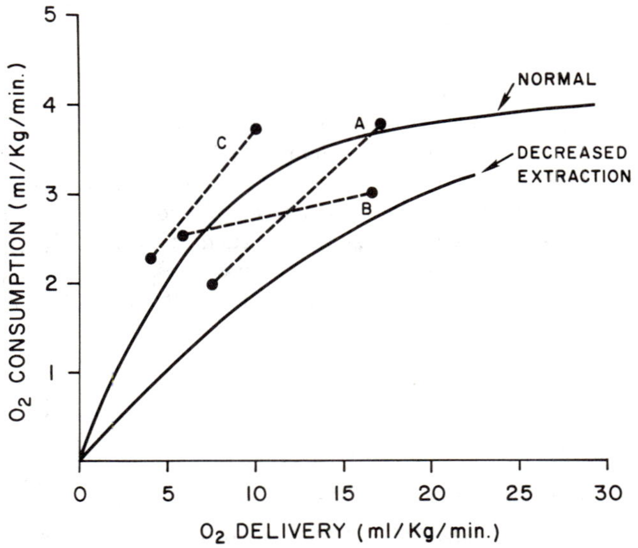

FIG 1–10.
Oxygen consumption becomes supply-dependent when oxygen delivery falls below a critical level. The dashed lines show clinical data from Gutierrez et al (**A** and **B**) and experimental data from Cain et al (**C**). While supply-dependency is shown in **A** and **C**, **B** shows that oxygen consumption does not increase with increased oxygen delivery because of decreased extraction in certain clinical situations. The solid line (normal) attempts to summarize existing information and suggests that there is a supply-independent region during circumstances of high oxygen delivery and a supply-dependent relationships below a critical level of oxygen delivery. During pathologic states, extraction is decreased and oxygen consumption is dependent upon oxygen delivery at higher oxygen delivery rates than in the normal situation. The normal relationship is shown here as a rectangular hyperbola since available information suggests that relationship.

CELL REGULATION, DEFENSE AND INJURY

Why do cells die? Two obvious causes are direct physical injury and loss of oxygen supply. Neurons are particularly sensitive to oxygen deprivation; a minute or two of circulatory arrest, and brain function appears to be irreversibly damaged. Presumably, loss of ATP leads to loss of membrane function, and the ionic gradients necessary for neural function are rapidly lost. Accumulation of hydrogen ions from unoxidized metabolites produces a massive intracellular acidosis further damaging cellular function. While cell death appears to be an obvious consequence of oxygen deprivation, the failure of tissues to respond completely to early reperfusion suggests the operation of other mechanisms.

It seems increasingly likely that critical illness initiates a series of defensive responses with mobilization of soluble humoral substances, protein cascades, and a variety of cellular elements that may lead to cell injury. Studies beginning in the early years of this century demonstrated the importance of the sympathetic nervous system as the mediator of the "fight or flight" responses described by Walter Cannon. [19] An understanding of cell-to-cell communication followed Ahlquist's[20] postulation of alpha and beta adrenergic receptors in 1948 and led to the important introduction of "sympathomimetic" drugs into the care of the critically ill patient (see chapter 4). The past decade has seen the growing understanding of a group of control molecules that dramatically affect cell function. While these substances have evolved because of their importance in cell defense, their inappropriate secretion may actually initiate cell damage (see also adult respiratory distress syndrome, chapter 7). Lewis Thomas, the elegant contemporary philosopher-scientist, summarized the risk-benefit values of a highly organized defense network:[21]

> (It's) our response to their presence (bacteria) that makes the disease. Our arsenals for fighting off bacteria are so powerful, and

> involve so many different defense mechanisms, that we are in more danger from them than from the invaders. We live in the midst of explosive devices; we are mined.
>
> When we sense lipopolysaccharide, we are likely to turn on every defense at our disposal; we will bomb, defoliate, blockade, seal off, and destroy all tissues in the area. Leukocytes become more actively phagocytic, release lysomal enzymes, turn sticky, and aggregate together in dense masses, occluding capillaries and shutting off the blood supply.
>
> Lewis Thomas, The Lives of a Cell New York, The Viking Press, 1974.

Sometimes, of course, direct toxic or traumatic damage may produce immediate cell death. The possibility that many instances of organ failure in the days following critical illness may be due to uncontrolled mediator release suggests an important leverage point for therapeutic intervention.

Cell Regulation

The cell membrane, or plasmalemma, controls all communication between the cell and its environment. Its lipid composition provides a diffusion barrier for the entrance of water-soluble substances, but lipid-soluble materials and gases such as oxygen, carbon dioxide, and nitrogen penetrate it with ease. Protein molecules lying across the entire membrane allow water-soluble substances to enter the cell either through ion channels, carriers for specific metabolites, or "pumps" that maintain a concentration gradient. Control molecules such as catecholamines, other neurotransmitters, or peptide hormones (e.g., angiotensin and insulin) combine with specialized receptors within the membrane. These circulating molecules have long been known as chemical messengers and are important regulators of cell function.

The space within the plasmalemma is highly compartmentalized. The endoplasmic reticulum is a network of channels that permits rapid intracellular communication. The small pathways connect expanded reservoirs or cisternae. Calcium is alternately stored and released by the endoplasmic reticulum and provides an important intracellular control opportunity.

The recognition by Sutherland and Rall[22] that cyclic AMP (cAMP) functioned as an intracellular messenger led to the expression "second" chemical messenger. These investigators demonstrated that adrenergic stimulation activated the enzyme adenyl cyclase, which catalyzed the loss of two phosphates from adenosine triphosphate and converted it into cAMP. The receptor-adenyl cyclase system is imbedded in the cell membrane; the receptor component faces outward and responds to the environment, while the adenyl cyclase component faces inward toward the cytoplasm. The amount of cAMP product is modulated by guanine-nucleotide binding proteins, which affect adenylate cyclase activity, and by cytoplasmic phosphodiesterases, which inactivate cAMP soon after it is formed.[23]

The discovery that enzymes known as protein kinases (after the Greek "to move") change cell function by phosphorylating specific proteins is an important unifying theme for cell regulation. Rapid phosphorylation by a protein kinase and dephosphorylation by phosphoprotein phosphatases allow for rapid changes in cell function. Cyclic AMP controls cell function by phosphorylating a specific protein kinase. Calcium-activated calmodulin-dependent protein kinases such as myosin light chain kinase, phosphorylase b kinase, and calmodulin-dependent kinase regulate smooth muscle tone and a variety of other cell functions. A recently discovered calcium-activated phospholipid-dependent protein kinase—protein kinase C—is responsible for the activation of a variety of receptors including those for thrombin, platelet activating factor, metabolites of arachadonic acid (prostaglandins and leukotrienes), insulin, interleukin-2, and others. The ubiquitous nature of calcium control makes it another important second intracellular or second chemical messenger. The two branches of the calcium messenger system, C kinase and calmodulin-dependent kinase, work together with cyclic AMP to regulate cell function. Since the complexity of these pathways provides opportunities for therapeutic intervention, several examples are presented.

Epstein[24] presents two examples of such interaction. Thrombin binds to platelets and leads to the hydrolysis of a group of phosphatidyl compounds releasing diacylglycerol and arachadonic acid metabolites. Intracellular calcium rises, both because of intracellular release and influx. A group of kinases is activated and phosphorylate specific proteins that are believed to initiate the platelet-release reaction. The system is amplified by the generation of thromboxane A_2 from the released arachadonic acid, which binds to the platelet surface and stimulates the production of additional phospholipase C. As in most biologic systems, a parallel generation of PGI_2 tends to restrain the response and prevent a generalized platelet release response. In general, the calmodulin branch mediates initial responses and the C-kinase branch permits more sustained reactions. In addition, Epstein points out that "in many systems calcium and cAMP serve as synarchic messengers, acting together to rule the intercellular domain." The interactions are complex and variable. An increase in cAMP amplifies the effects of glucose-induced insulin secretion or angiotensin II–mediated aldosterone secretion, but it decreases the smooth muscle contractile response to angiotensin II.

Mediators of the Systemic Defense Response

Work over the past century by Walter Cannon[19] with the autonomic nervous system mediated "fight or flight" response, Claude Bernard[25] with the defense of the "milieu interior," and Hans Selye[26] with his concept of stress and disease has generated the concept of the systemic defense response. The organism responds to loss of blood volume, hypotension, and hypoxemia (physiologic stress) in one way and to infectious or particulate stress in another. Trauma is an obvious example of physiologic and particulate stress occurring either at once or in tandem. A large number of mediators (including catecholamines, angiotensin, vasopressin, thromboxanes, prostaglandins, leukotrienes, the complement and coagulation cascades, macrophage products, and concentrations of calcium, magnesium and other ions, and a group of yet uncharacterized myocardial and vascular depressant factors) have all been identified and suggested as possible causes of critical illness. It is likely that different primary mediators are responsible for the syndromes associated with different inciting events, although the interactive nature of the systemic-defense response results in the involvement of other branches of the network as the syndromes evolve and become more life-threatening. It is as if a single sentry analogous to the baroreceptor system or the macrophage signals an alarm that ultimately involves the mobilization of an entire nation.

Products of Arachidonic Acid Metabolism

The study of prostaglandins has so dominated the field of cell regulation that some cynics have even asked "are they important?" Almost 25 years have passed since the discovery of the chemical structure of the prostaglandins and the subsequent elucidation of certain of their biologic functions. Arachidonic acid is one of the naturally occurring unsaturated acids like oleic acid (18 carbons and one double bond) or linolenic acid (18 carbons and 3 double bonds). It contains 20 carbons and 4 double bonds and is formally described as eicosatetraenoic (Greek for 20) acid. Figure 1–11 shows that the hydrolysis by phospholipase A_2 produces a variety of biologically active molecules that include the prostaglandins, thromboxanes, and leukotrienes. These products may be called either arachidonic acid metabolites or eicosanoids. The enzyme cyclooxygenase converts arachidonic acid into a parent compound, PGH_2, which is then further metabolized to PGI_2 or prostacyclin—a group of three prostaglandins—or to thromboxane A_2. Fifty percent of the stored body fatty acids are unsaturated, and much of this lipid pool is used for energy purposes as two carbon fragments are produced by beta oxidation. Membrane lipids perform important structural and control functions. Cyclooxygenase, the enzyme blocked by aspirin, does not produce beta oxidation but catalyzes lipid *peroxidation* producing the unstable endoperoxide intermediate, PGH_2. Since arachidonic acid is believed to be present in almost all plasma membranes, the availability of specific metabolites depends only on the existence of specific intracellular enzymes. More primitive cells, such as macrophages and monocytes, appear to contain a relatively full complement of enzymes so that many eicosanoids may be produced. Other cells, such as neutrophils, are "de-differentiated" and can only produce certain eicosanoids.[27]

Prostacyclin or PGI_2 is identified by measurement of its metabolite 6-keto-

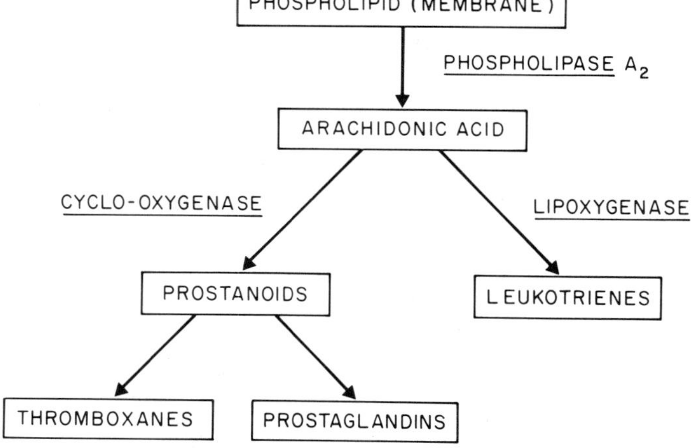

FIG 1–11.
The hydrolysis of membrane phospholipid by phospholipase A_2 generates arachidonic acid, which serves as a precursor for a variety of important regulatory substances. Cyclooxygenase, an enzyme inhibited by aspirin and nonsteroidal anti-inflammatory agent, converts arachidonic acid into a cyclized endoperoxide intermediate, PGH_2. This prostanoid intermediate is then enzymatically converted to two groups of prostaglandins, PGI_2 (prostacyclin) and the classic prostaglandins, PGE_2, PGD_2, and $PGF_{2\alpha}$. A specific thromboxane synthetase found mainly in platelets converts the PGH_2 precursor to thromboxane A_2. 5-Lipoxygenase catalyzes the formation of leukotriene A_4 from arachidonic acid. LTA_4 then generates LTB_4, LTC_4, and LTD_4.

$PGF_{1\alpha}$. Produced by endothelial and other cells including platelets, it is a powerful vasodilator and inhibits platelet aggregation. It appears to act by stimulating adenyl cyclase and the production of cAMP. Thromboxane A_2 decreases the production of cAMP and has effects directly opposite to those of PGI_2; it is a powerful vasoconstrictor and enhances platelet aggregation. PGE_2 is a moderate vasoconstrictor in some vascular beds but a vasodilator in others, such as the coronary circulation. $PGF_{2\alpha}$ is a vasoconstrictor for all vascular beds.[28]

The more recently discovered lipoxygenase pathway produces a group of molecules known as leukotrienes (LTs) because they were first thought to be formed mainly from granular leukocytes. The individual molecules bear the designations A, B, C, and D; the subscript 4 refers to a shared structural configuration. LTA is the precursor of LTB, and the other three leukotrienes are similar to the mysterious "slow-reacting substance of anaphylaxis," which has been known to exist for many years. LTB_4 causes cells to become sticky and adhere to blood vessels. LTC_4 and LTD_4 produce vasoconstriction and bronchoconstriction, while LTB_4, LTC_4, and LTD_4 all cause increased vascular permeability.[29]

Lefer[30] has reviewed the role of eicosanoids in ischemia and shock. Increases in most of them have been observed in the shock syndrome; and Lefer has suggested that the leukotrienes B_4, C_4, D_4, PGH_2, thromboxane A_2 and $PGF_{2\alpha}$ may be "putative" mediators of critical illness. A variety of specific enzyme inhibitors and receptor antagonists may be useful in the early treatment of shock.

Opioids and Other Neuropeptides

A large list of regulatory peptides, some of them containing but several amino acids, were originally named for their obvious function. They are found in the central nervous system as well as peripherally and include substances such as thyroid releasing hormone (TRH), somatostatin, adrenocorticotrophin (ACTH), prolactin, cholecystokinin, gastrin, glucagon, vasopressin, the opioid peptides, and others. They exist in much smaller quantities than the classical hormones and act both locally (autocrines) and systemically (endocrines).

The observation by Holaday and Faden[31] that the opioid antagonist naloxone raised blood pressure in experimental endotoxin shock suggested that opioids might be significant mediators of the shock syndrome. At least eight endogenous opioids and five opioid receptors have been identified in the central nervous system. Two contain just five amino acids each. Methionine-enkephalin (Met-enk) and leucine-enkephalin (Leu-enk) differ only by one amino acid. Beta endorphin contains 31 amino acids and is found in distinct regions of the central nervous system. Some of the opioid receptors have been particularly well characterized. The mu receptor recognizes the drug morphine, is blocked by naloxone, and produces euphoria, analgesia, and respiratory depression. The delta receptor has great affinity for Leu-enk and may be the mechanism for hypotension in experimental endotoxin shock. TRH is a three–amino acid peptide that appears to have important neurotransmitter actions in addition to its effect on the pituitary release of thyrotropin. It is a physiologic opiate antagonist that is additive to naloxone in reversing the hypotension of experimental endotoxin shock, but it does not reverse the narcotic effects of morphine. It is believed to have its own independent receptor and, unlike naloxone, reverses leukotriene D_4 hypotension.[32]

The Particulate (Immune) Response Network

A burst of incredibly productive research over the past quarter century has unravelled many of the complex components of the human immune system and has identified the important participation of two key branches: the thymus-dependent system, through specific T-lymphocytes, is responsible for the delayed tissue responses to infectious agents; and the closely integrated B cell branch produces specific antibodies that combine with foreign antigens and trigger the complement cascade. It now seems likely that the concept proposed by Metchnikoff in the early years of this century[33] is correct and that the macrophage is the key cell in initiating the host defense system. While Metchnikoff emphasized the phagocytic and digestive function of the macrophage, more recent studies have shown that the macrophage is also an incredibly versatile secretory cell.

The reticulo-endothelial system described by Aschoff in 1924[34] included a diffuse network of vascular conduits and both fixed and circulating mononuclear cells called histiocytes. The liver and spleen are the primary organs responsible for particulate clearance. Diminished hepatic blood flow or other kinds of hepatic injury reduce the activity of the hepatic reticuloendothelial system, and the bone marrow and kidney may respond by increasing uptake of particulate material. Macrophages possess the biochemical capacity to generate reactive oxygen when they meet a variety of particulate materials, phorbol esters, or microorganisms coated with IgG.[35] Oxygen is enzymatically converted to superoxide ion with the rapid formation of hydrogen peroxide, hydroxyl radicals, and other reactive substances. This respiratory burst enhances the microcidal capacity of activated macrophages and makes them extremely dangerous elements.

The macrophage also possesses a rich enzymatic endowment that allows it to produce a variety of soluble substances (monokines) for general systemic exportation.[36] Many of these substances were first thought to be generated by granulocytes but are now known to arise from either macrophages, monocytes, or lymphocytes. Four general categories have been identified thus far: (1) thermoregulatory monokines, (2) immunoregulatory monokines, (3) metabolic regulatory monokines, and (4) endocrine regulatory monokines. In addition, macrophages oxidize arachidonic acid to produce PGE_2, PGI_2, thromboxane A_2, leukotrienes B_4 and C_4, and irritant hydroxy fatty acids.[37]

Interleukin-1 is a monokine that is probably similar, if not identical, to previously studied leukocytic pyrogen (LP) and LEM (leukocytic endogenous mediator). The low molecular substance-weight (10,000 to 15,000 MW) produces fever, leukocytosis, protein degradation, and increased hepatic synthesis of acute-phase proteins (see chapter 2, multiple organ failure). It also influences lymphocyte maturation and stimulates other elements of the immune system. Interleukin-2 is a lymphokine that initiates lymphocyte proliferation[38] and has been shown to produce the adult respiratory distress syndrome when used therapeutically in patients with advanced malignancies (see chapter 7).[39]

Cell Injury and Death

The recognition that multiple organ failure frequently follows critical episodes involving one organ has given new importance to the question of why cells die. Ischemic damage may occur due to uneven distribution of regional blood flow, even when overall cardiac output is close to normal. Cheung et al.[40] have recently pointed out that many factors including ATP depletion, plasmalemma phospholipid depletion, release of autolytic enzymes, cellular acidosis, mitochondrial dysfunction, cellular calcium accumulation, and generation of toxic oxygen species may damage cells during ischemic injury.

The complement cascade has long been assumed to produce cell damage by some mechanism and Craddock et al.[41] demonstrated in 1977 the complement-activated leukocytes could produce hypoxemia during hemodialysis. The eleven classical and four alternate complement components are proteins that circulate as inactive precursors and are sequentially activated, usually by limited proteolytic cleavage, by sequential members of the cascade. This cascade could be likened to a series of Chinese boxes, one within another, or to a gradually arousing infantry squad with each member in turn becoming increasingly concerned. Some members of the squad call for additional assistance (chemotaxis mediated by C5a and immune adherence by C3b). While help is on the way, other members of the squad unlimber their machine guns and begin firing at the presumed enemy (the membrane attack complex, C5b to C9). The attack complex has been visualized as a group of five seperate complement fragments attaching to a cell membrane and damaging its integrity. Depletion of either complement or granulocytes prevents lung vascular injury produced by cobra venom factor,[42] but it is not clear whether granulocyte elastase, the complement attack complex, or the generation of oxygen-derived free radicals is most responsible for the observed cellular damage. Bacterial toxins themselves maydirectly injure cells; Meyrick[43] has shown, for example, that endotoxin directly damages endothelial cells but that complement and neutrophil activation increases the injury. In a somewhat different system, Smedly et al.[44] have shown that neutrophil-derived elastase is the major agent of endothelial injury induced by the lipopolysaccharide fraction of endotoxin.

Fibronectin

Fibronectin is a glycoprotein that has been called "tissue glue" since it is necessary for the maintenance of intact cell-to-cell relationships. Loss of tissue fibronectin may well play an important pathogenetic role in cell injury and the development of multiple organ system failure. Saba and Jaffe[45] demonstrated that plasma fibronectin functions as an opsonic protein necessary for normal phagocytosis. Plasma fibronectin has a half-life of less than 20 hours, and reduced plasma concentrations have been observed in malnourished individuals prior to decreases in albumin and transferrin. It is synthesized in the liver; tissue fibronectin, the material used for cell-to-cell adhesion, may also be made in the liver but the precise location for its synthesis is not known. Linden et al.[46] have confirmed that inadequate nutrition decreases plasma fibronectin concentration in human volunteers. They also observed reduced concentrations in stressed and septic patients. A substantial increase in plasma fibronectin was found after administration of total parenteral nutrition to malnourished patients for seven days. The effects of a mixture containing branched-chain amino acids (15.6% BCAA) were not different from mixtures without branched-chain amino acids. Plasma cryoprecipitate contains fibronectin and has been shown to increase plasma levels and improve cardiopulmonary function. The use of nutritional support and other measures to reduce cell death are discussed in Chapters 2 and 10.

Superoxide anion

A rapidly growing body of information suggests that an amplified and uncontrolled reduction of molecular oxygen to superoxide anion may be responsible for

THE LONELY OXYGEN ATOM

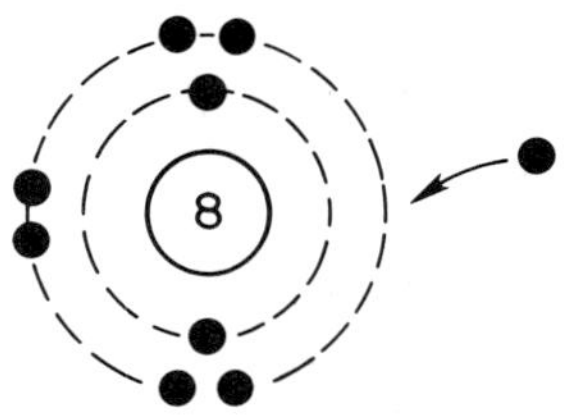

$$O_2 + NADPH \rightarrow O_2^- + NADP^+ + H^+$$
$$2\,O_2^- + 2H^+ \rightarrow H_2O_2 + O_2$$

FIG 1–12.
The oxygen atom has two vacant electron positions on its outer ring. Two electrons are shared covalently in the oxygen molecule. An electron carried by NADPH can partially reduce molecular oxygen to form the superoxide anion, O_2^-. This anion is rapidly converted to hydrogen peroxide and other irritant-free radicals.

much of the cell damage observed in critical illness.[47] In itself it is harmless, but it reacts with itself to produce hydrogen peroxide, which is an essential building block for the synthesis of oxidized halogens and oxidizing radicals. Superoxide anion is normally generated in the respiratory burst of granulocytes and is necessary for microbicidal activity; unleashed it may also turn on nonmicrobial proteins. The outer ring of the oxygen atom contains six electrons instead of the eight necessary for chemical stability (see Fig 1–12). Under most circumstances, oxygen atoms share electrons with another oxygen atom producing a stable compound. When exposed to bacteria or other materials, oxygen is reduced (an electron is added) to superoxide anion.

The electron carrier, NADPH, in the presence of an enzyme, NADPH-oxidase, generates superoxide anion.

$$O_2 + NADPH \ = O_2^- + NADP^+ + H^+$$

The equation above should be compared with the general equation for oxidative phosphorylation.

$$NADH + \tfrac{1}{2}O_2 + 3ADP + 3P_i = 3ATP + NAD^+ + H_2O$$

Both require oxygen and either NADH or NADPH. One leads to the synthesis of ATP, the other to the production of superoxide anion. Neutrophils, eosinophils, and macrophages increase their oxygen consumption more than 50-fold when generating the superoxide anion, and it is not difficult to believe that under certain circumstances a substantial fraction of delivered oxygen is diverted to the generation of superoxide anion rather than for oxidative phosphorylation. A number of substances, including bacteria, particulate material, arachidonic acid, and chemical substances known as phorbol esters, may activate the respiratory burst. NADPH is derived from the hexose monophosphate shunt, which is stimulated to pro vide increased substrate. The phorbol esters are potent stimulators of oxygen consumption and activate the protein kinase C cascade. Recent evidence suggests that this cascade may directly activate NADPH oxidase.[48] Prostaglandin hydroperoxidase also catalyzes the generation of superoxide anion indicating a linkage between toxic oxygen species, prostanoids, and leukotrienes. The key synthetic enzyme, NADPH oxidase, is central to the production of superoxide anion and provides an important locus for pharmacologic inhibition of toxic oxygen radical production. Another important aspect of oxygen products is their role in inactivating antiproteases and producing proteolysis by other mechanisms.

An understanding of the synthesis and consequences of free radical generation provides an important opportunity for pharmacologic intervention. Superoxide dysmutase converts superoxide anion to hydrogen peroxide, and catalase converts hydrogen peroxide to molecular oxygen and water. Both have been shown to reduce pulmonary injury from complement-activated neutrophils. Treatment with free radical scavengers such as N-acetyl cysteine (Mucomyst),[49] dimethyl sulfoxide and iron chelators also protects against complement and neutrophil cell injury.[50] The presence of iron enhances the generation of *hydroxyl radical* from hydrogen peroxide. Ibuprofen inhibits the production of superoxide anion from granulocytes in *in vitro* studies. Fixed tissue cells also may produce oxygen metabolites when stimulated; Adler et al.[51] showed that the complement membrane attack complex stimulated glomerular mesangial cells to produce toxic oxygen metabolites, providing a partial explanation for the pathogenesis of immune renal disease.

The development of multiple organ failure in the patient with sepsis is stark evidence that the mediated response to infection may, like a runaway engine, drive the organism to destruction, even if the offending bacterial infection has been controlled. At some unknown moment the mediated process becomes autonomous; the equivalent of the "dead man's switch" used in railroad locomotives to prevent a driverless train is inoperative. A number of these cytolytic steps have been presented in this chapter. Protein catabolism of skeletal muscle with marked wasting, atrophy, and a massive negative nitrogen balance may be directly due to the action of certain monokines. Human leukocyte pyrogen in the presence of PGE produces significant proteolysis in the rat soleus muscle,[52] and Clowes et al.[53] have identified a peptide monokine in patients with sepsis that may be a fragment of IL-1. Besedovsky et al.[54] have used recombinant techniques to synthesize a human tumor necrosis factor known as cachectin. Injection of cachectin into rabbits produces a febrile response with the release of PGE_2 and IL-1.

Restoration of perfusion deficits and elimination of infected foci may stop the process of progressive cell death if instituted at a sufficiently early time. The development of pharmacologic agents to inhibit the process at later stages seems close at hand.

REFERENCES

1. Jobis FF: Basic processes in cellular respiration. In *Handbook of Physiology*. Section 3, Respiration. Washington, DC, American Physiological Society, 1964, Vol 1, chap 2.

2. Hodgkin AL, Keynes RD: Active transport of cations in giant axons from sepia and loliga. *J Physiol* (Lond) 1955; 128:28.

3. Dahl JL, Hokin LE: The sodium-potassium adenosine-triphosphatase. *Annu Rev Biochem* 1974; 43:327.

4. Chance B, Williams G: Respiratory enzymes in oxidative phosphorylation. *J Biol Chem* 1955; 217:383–393.

5. Chance B, Hollunger G: Inhibition of electron and energy transfer in mitochondria: IV Inhibition of energy-linked diphosphopyridine nucleotide reduction by uncoupling agents. *J Biol Chem* 1963; 238:445.

6. Veech RL, Lawson JWR, Cornell NW, Krebs HA: Cytosolic phosphorylation potential. *J Biol Chem* 1979; 254:6538–6547.

7. Chance B, Leigh JS Jr, Clark BJ, et al: Control of oxidative metabolism and oxygen delivery in human skeletal muscle. A steady-state analysis of the work/energy cost transfer function. *Proc Natl Acad Sci USA 1985; 82:8384.*

8. Huckabee WE: Relationships of pyruvate and lactate during anaerobic metabolism. I Effects of infusion of pyruvate or glucose and of hyperventilation. *J Clin Invest* 1958; 37:244.

9. Roughton FJW: Transport of oxygen and carbon dioxide, in *Handbook of Physiology*, Section 3, Respiration, Washington, DC, American Physiological Society 1964; Section 3, Respiration, Vol 1, Chap 31.

10. Benesch RE, Benesch R, Ing Yu C: The oxygenation of hemoglobin in the presence

of 2,3-diphosphoglycerate: effect of temperature, pH, ionic strength, and hemoglobin concentration. *Biochemistry* 1969; 8:2567.

11. Lenfant C, Torrance J, English E, et al: Effect of altitude on oxygen binding by hemoglobin and on organic phosphate levels. *J Clin Invest* 1968; 47:2652.

12. Klocke RA: Oxygen transfer from the red cell to the mitochondrion, in Bryan-Brown CW, Ayres SM (eds): *Oxygen Transport and Utilization*. Fullerton, CA, Soc Crit Care Med, 1987.

13. Kawakami Y, Kishi F, Yamamoto H, et al: Relation of oxygen delivery, mixed venous oxygenation, and pulmonary hemodynamics to prognosis in chronic obstructive pulmonary disease. *N Engl J Med* 1983; 308:1045.

14. Bergofsky EH: Tissue oxygen delivery and cor pulmonale in chronic obstructive pulmonary disease (editorial). *N Engl J Med* 1983; 308:1092.

15. Shoemaker WC, Appel PL, Kram HB: Comparison of two monitoring methods (central venous pressure versus pulmonary artery catheter) and two protocols as therapeutic goals (normal values versus values of survivors) in a prospective randomized clinical trial of critically ill surgical patients. *Crit Care Med* 1985; 13:304(abst).

16. Nylander E, Lund N, Wranne B: Effect of increased blood oxygen affinity on skeletal muscle surface oxygen pressure fields. *J Appl Physiol* 1983; 54:99.

17. Cain SM: Peripheral oxygen uptake and delivery in health and disease. *Clin Chest Med* 1983; 4:139.

18. Gutierrez G, Pohil RJ: Oxygen consumption is linearly related to O_2 supply in critically ill patients. *J Crit Care* 1986; 1:45.

19. Cannon WB: *Bodily Changes in Pain, Hunger, Fear and Rage*. New York, Appleton, 1929.

20. Ahlquist RP: A study of the adrenotropic receptors. *Am J Physiol* 1948; 153:586.

21. Thomas L: *The Lives of a Cell*. New York, The Viking Press, 1974.

22. Sutherland EW, Rall TW: The relation of adenosine-3′,5′ phosphate and phosphorylase to the action of catecholamines and other hormones. *Pharmacol Rev* 1960; 12:265.

23. Cuatrecasas P: Hormone receptors, membrane phospholipids, and protein kinases. *Harvey Lect* 1986; 80:89.

24. Epstein FH: Mechanisms of disease. The calcium messenger system (two parts). *N Engl J Med* 1986; 314:1094,1164.

25. Bernard C: *An Introduction to the Study of Experimental Medicine*. Paris, Flammarion, 1865. Reprinted by permission of Abelard-Schuman Ltd, 1949.

26. Selye H: The evolution of the stress concept. *Am J Cardiol* 1970; 26:289–299.

27. Mason RJ, Stossel TP, Vaughan M: Lipids of alveolar macrophages, polymorphonuclear leukocytes, and their phagocytic vesicles. *J Clin Invest* 1972; 51:2399–2407.

28. McGiff JC: New developments in prostaglandin and thromboxane research. *Fed Proc* 1979: 79:64.

29. Ford-Hutchinson AW: Leukotrienes: their formation and role as inflammatory mediators. *Fed Proc* 1985; 44:25.

30. Lefer AM: Eicosanoids as mediators of ischemia and shock. *Fed Proc* 1985; 44:275–280.

31. Holaday JW, Faden AI: Nalozone reversal of endotoxic hypotension suggests role of endorphins in shock. *Nature (London)* 1978; 275:450–451.

32. Lux WE, Feuerstein G, Faden AI: Alteration of leukotriene D_4 hypotension by thyrotropin releasing hormone. *Nature* 1983; 302:822–824.

33. Metchnikoff E: *Immunity in Infective Diseases*. London, Cambridge University Press, 1907:1–591.

34. Aschoff L: Das reticulo-endotheliale System. *Ergeb Inn Med Kinderheilkd* 1924; 26:1–24.

35. Bianco C, Griffin FM, Jr, Silverstein SD. Studies of the macrophage complement receptor: alteration of receptor function upon macrophage activities. *J Exp Med* 1975; 141:1278–1290.

36. Filkins JP: Monokines and the metabolic pathophysiology of septic shock. *Fed Proc* 1985; 44:25.

37. Bonney RJ, Opas EE, Humes JL: Lipoxygenase pathways of macrophages. *Fed Proc* 1985; 44:25.

38. Ognibene FP, Rosenberg SA, Skibber J, et al: Interleukin-2 hemodynamics mimic septic shock. *Clin Res* 1986; 34:413A.

39. Filkins JP, Yelich MR: Mechanism of hyperinsulinemia after reticuloendothelial system phagocytosis. *Am J Physiol* 1982; 242 (Endocrinol Metab 5):E–115.

40. Cheung JY, Bonventre JV, Malis CD, et al: Calcium and ischemic injury. *N Engl J Med* 1986; 314:1670.

41. Craddock PR, Fehr J, Brigham KL, Kronenberg RS, Jacob HS: Complement and leukocyte-mediated pulmonary dysfunction in hemodialysis. *N Engl J Med* 1977; 296:769–774.

42. Till GO, Ward PA: Systemic complement activation and acute lung injury. *Fed Proc* 1986; 45:13.

43. Meyrick BO: Endotoxin-mediated pulmonary endothelial cell injury. *Fed Proc* 1986; 45:19.

44. Smedly LA, Tonneson MG, Sandhaus RA, et al: Neutrophil- mediated injury to endothelial cells. Enhancement by endotoxin and essential role of neutrophil elastase. *J Clin Invest* 1986; 77:1233.

45. Saba TM, Jaffe E: Plasma fibronectin (opsonic glycoprotein): Its synthesis by vascular endothelial cells and role in cardiopulmonary integrity after trauma as related to reticuloendothelial function. *Am J Med* 1980; 68:577–594.

46. Linden CJVD, Buurman WA, Spronken EEM, et al: Fibronectin levels in stressed and septic patients fed with total parenteral nutrition. *JPEN* 1986; 10:360.

47. Babior BM: The respiratory burst of phagocytes. *J Clin Invest* 1984; 73:599.

48. Cox JA, Jeng AY, Sharkey NA, et al: Activation of human neutrophil nicotinamide adenine dinucleotide phosphate (NADPH)-oxidase by protein kinase C. *J Clin Invest* 1985; 76:1932.

49. Bernard GR, Lucht WD, Niedermeyer ME, et al: Effect of N-acetylcysteine on the pulmonary response to endotoxin in the awake sheep and upon in vitro granulocyte function. *J Clin Invest* 1984; 73:1772.

50. Ward PA, Till GO, Kunkel R, Beauchamp C: Evidence for role of hydroxyl radical in complement and neutrophil-dependent tissue injury. *J Clin Invest* 1983; 72:789–801.

51. Adler S, Baker PJ, Johnson RJ, et al: Complement membrane attack complex stimulates production of reactive oxygen metabolites by cultured rat mesangial cells. *J Clin Invest* 1986; 77:762.

52. Baracos VE, Rodemann HP, Dinarello CA, Goldberg AL: Stimulation of muscle protein degradation and prostaglandin E_2 release by leukocytic pyrogen: a mechanism for the increased degradation of muscle proteins during fever. *N Engl J Med* 1983; 308:553–558.

53. Clowes GHA Jr, George BC, Villee CA Jr, et al: Muscle proteolysis induced by a circulating peptide in patients with sepsis or trauma. *N Engl J Med* 1983; 308:545.

54. Besedovsky H, del Rey A, Sorkin E, et al: Immunoregulatory feed-back between interleukin-1 and glucocorticoid hormones. *Science* 1986; 233:652–654.

2 MULTIPLE ORGAN FAILURE, SEPSIS, AND SEPTIC SHOCK

Progressive dysfunction of lungs, liver, kidneys, and other organs has become an increasingly prevalent problem in the modern intensive care unit. Clinical observations recorded over the past 15 years have shown that impaired oxygen delivery to the tissues and sepsis are the key factors responsible for this ultimately fatal clinical course. One of the central themes of critical care medicine is the direct relationship between tissue integrity and the amount of oxygen and fuel consumed by the mitochondria. In turn, mitochondrial oxygen consumption is determined by the amount of oxygen and fuel required by and delivered to those subcellular organelles. Multiple organ systems failure (MOSF) is a paradigm of critical care medicine because it expresses the importance of early identification of oxygen deficits, the need for aggressive monitoring and treatment, the importance of broadly trained specialists in critical care medicine, and the ethical problems associated with long hospital stays and inevitable death. The first chapter dealt with the determinants of cell oxygenation and the causes of cell death. This chapter, dealing with the damage of cells in a variety of organs, appropriately precedes chapters dealing with individual organ system abnormalities.

Tilney, Bailey, and Morgan,[1] in 1973, described the hospital course of 18 patients with ruptured abdominal aneurysms who were treated by hemodialysis and survived for at least five postoperative days. Seventeen patients died between the fifth and forty-eighth postoperative days. The authors noted that "a similar progression of organ system failure was observed in all. The sequence unfolded more slowly in patients who survived longer, and developed quickly in those surviving for shorter periods, but most patients developed all components of the pattern in approximately the same order before death occurred." They coined the term "sequential system failure" and noted that, after the onset of renal failure, sequential failure of additional organs appeared in an almost stereotypic manner. Pancreatic and respiratory failure appeared an average of two days after rupture, hepatic failure in five days, central nervous system in six days, heart failure in nine days and gastrointestinal hemorrhage in 13 days. Sepsis was believed to be an important cause of death in 10 patients. Almost all had preexisting systemic disease; 50% had chronic pulmonary disease, 78% had heart disease, and 56% had hypertension. Eighty percent of the group were hypotensive during the emergency surgical procedure. This series of symptoms provides the basis for an understanding of the syndrome. A major deficit in oxygen delivery, even though corrected surgically, leads to sequential organ failure. Sepsis and preexisting organ dysfunction appear to be major pathogenetic factors.

Suprisingly, the implications of Tilney's observations were not generally understood. Baue in 1975,[2] Eiseman, Beart, and Norton in 1977,[3] and Fry et al.[4] in 1980 published articles in the surgical literature that further defined the syndrome of multiple or sequential organ failure. Fry et al.[4] emphasized the importance of uncontrolled infection and demonstrated that the number of organ systems involved was a better determinant of outcome than the specific organ systems involved. Mortality was 30% when single organ dysfunction was present, 60% with two organ systems involved, 85% with three, and 100% with four organ system failures. Mortality rates similar to those published by Fry et al.[4] were found in the collaborative extracorporeal support for respiratory insufficiency (ECMO) study supported by the National Institutes of Health.[5] The mortality for respiratory failure alone was 40%. It rose to 56% with one additional organ system involved, 73% with two additional organ system failures, 82% with three, and 100% with four organ system failures.

One of the reasons for the failure to understand the importance of sepsis was the belief that positive blood cultures were necessary for its diagnosis. Polk and Shields[6] had suggested that "remote organ failure" was an important sign of intra-abdominal infection, and Fry found clinical evidence of sepsis in 34 of 87 patients with multiple organ failure; 50% of these had primary pulmonary and 44% primary intra-abdominal foci of infection.[4] Many of these patients with silent sepsis exhibited hypoxemia, hyperbilirubinemia, gastric bleeding, renal failure, thrombocytopenia, abnormal mentation, and transient hypotension. Meakins et al.[7] used these clinical signs as evidence of "nonbacteremic clinical sepsis," and found that only 22 of 42 patients with clinical evidence of sepsis had positive blood cultures!

Multiple organ systems failure first received attention in a journal regularly read by internists 10 years after the publication of Tilney's original observations. Bell et al.[8] had studied a group of patients with the adult respiratory distress syndrome and found that 40% of nonsurvivors with the syndrome had an unsuspected major focus of infection at autopsy. Again, the lung and peritoneum were the most common sites for infection. Coalson[9] carefully studied the 77 autopsies performed on patients reported by Bell et al.[8], and found that the histopathologic findings were much more extensive than those found in either experimental models of septic shock or in patients with sepsis or septic shock who died early in their hospital course. Infected organ sites revealed a classic suppurative inflammatory response; other organs revealed degenerative and necrotic changes. Severe liver lesions were common, and included severe hepatic necrosis and fatty infiltration. "Widened sinusoids lined by prominent Kupfer cells were occasionally filled with numerous PMNs, and sites of bile stasis were frequently prominent. Severe cellular degeneration was observed in the pancreas (16% had clinically unsuspected acute pancreatitis), gastrointestinal tract, adrenal glands, heart, lung, and kidneys. Thirteen patients with single organ failure showed little evidence of remote organ degeneration, and only one had an intra-abdominal infection. Remote organ degenerative or necrotic changes were common in the 64 patients with multiple organ failure; 72% had pulmonary and 50% had abdominal sites of sepsis. Coalson concluded that "pathologic analysis supports the concept of a blood-borne cytotoxic agent(s) indiscriminately delivered to the various organ systems in proportion to their perfusion."[9]

The syndrome of multiple organ systems failure is all too common in most intensive care units. While silent septic foci with nonbacteremic sepsis appear to be a major causal factor in producing remote organ degeneration, the initial inciting factor is usually a decrease in organ oxygen delivery. All of Tilney's patients experienced profound hypovolemia, and subsequent studies have emphasized the central importance of hypoperfusion to the development of multiple organ failure. After sepsis, Fry et al.[4] listed hypovolemic shock and massive fluid or blood therapy as major risk factors for the development of the syndrome. These, of course, are the same risk factors associated with the acute respiratory distress syndrome. Patients with cardiogenic shock or severe blood loss may initially respond to vigorous treatment but soon develop sequential organ dysfunction. An altered immune status, manifested as cutaneous anergy, has been found in patients with burns, multiple trauma, malignancies, and other critical illness, and clearly predisposes to sepsis. Whether the inciting factor is impaired oxygen transport due to low cardiac output or to sepsis-induced regional hypoperfusion and impaired fuel utilization, the ultimate limiting factor appears to be impaired oxidative phosphorylation and synthesis of ATP. Thus, many patients suffer a seemingly reversible injury, but subsequently develop progressive organ dysfunction due to a septic focus. In such patients, it is often difficult to separate these etiologic factors. In other patients, sepsis followed by septic shock directly initiates the syndrome. Whether the inciting factor is hypoperfusion due to a number of causes or sepsis with increased oxygen requirements and decreased tissue perfusion, the ultimate limiting factor is cellular oxygen delivery.

An important animal model demonstrating the importance of early replacement of perfusion deficits was developed by Wiggers[10] during World War II. Rapid removal of blood, amounting to 2–4% of body weight, produced profound but reversible hypotension in dogs. A syndrome of irreversible shock with generalized vasodilatation, however, developed if reperfusion was delayed for more than 60 to 90 minutes. These seminal studies had great relevance to wartime battle injuries and set the stage for understanding the importance of the first few hours after injury in producing irreversible illness. Correction of deficits during this "golden hour" has become the cornerstone of critical care medicine.

INJURY, SEPSIS, AND MULTIPLE ORGAN FAILURE

A classic description of sepsis was given by Sir William Osler in his 1892 treatise, *The Principles and Practice of Medicine.* The identification of the factor responsible for initiating the host response to infection, a low molecular weight molecule now called interleukin-1 but previously termed endogenous pyrogen or leukocyte endogenous mediator, followed Osler's description by almost one hundred years.

> In cases of wound infection, prior to the onset of the characteristic symptoms, there may be signs of local trouble, and, if a discharging wound, the pus may change in character. The onset of the disease is marked by a severe rigor, during which the temperature rises to 103°–104° and is followed by a profuse sweat. These chills are repeated at intervals, either daily or every other day. In the intervals there may be

slight pyrexia. The constitutional evidence is marked and there are loss of appetite, nausea, vomiting, and, as the disease progresses, rapid loss of flesh.[11]

Host Factors in Sepsis

Sepsis may be defined as the systemic response to dividing and invading microorganisms of all types—gram-negative and gram-positive bacteria, fungi, and viruses. Sepsis in a previously healthy person should be readily correctible. The classic presentation may be attenuated, diagnosis more difficult, and complications more common in individuals with altered host responses following surgery, trauma, and acute illness, or in patients with preexisting chronic illness. Host-related phenomena, rather than the type of invasive microorganism, appear to determine the septic response.

Both surgery and injury have been shown to alter host responses. Meakins et al.[12] showed that age and the severity of injury increase the prevalence of cutaneous anergy and of changes in neutrophil chemotaxis and adherence. These changes occur immediately after injury, are related to the severity of physiologic abnormalities, and are not necessarily a result of diminished nutritional status, since these deficiencies resolve spontaneously even in the absence of nutritional supplementation after weeks of convalescence. Similar changes in immune status are observed after major surgery. Immune function can be shown to relate temporally to infective foci in the post-operative patient. Skin anergy associated with abscess formation recovered within several days after drainage of abscesses, infected common bile ducts, or other inflammatory processes. Neutrophil function measured by chemotaxis and adherence also returned to normal. These patients did not receive nutritional support, so that rapid improvement in immune function was clearly due to control of infection.

The Hemodynamic Responses to Sepsis

The American physiologist Eugene DuBois[13] demonstrated in the 1940s that the metabolic rate averaged an increase of 13% for each degree centigrade of fever in a variety of infectious diseases. Considerable variation was noted, however; metabolic rates in patients with typhoid fever were much greater relative to the level of fever than those in patients with tuberculosis. Kinney and Roe[14] demonstrated in 1962 that the relationship between body temperature and sepsis was much more complicated than previously suspected; in some patients, for example, an elevated temperature might be due to decreased heat loss rather than to increased heat production. These enhanced rates of metabolism are not dissimilar to those associated with exercise, and suggest the adaptive recruitment of body reserves for increased transport and synthesis of antimicrobial defenses, rapid cell replication, and accelerated cardiorespiratory function. Increased metabolic needs are served by generalized vasodilatation with resultant increases in vascular capacity, which may rise to twice the normal circulating blood volume by increased oxygen consumption, by increased heart rate, and by increased cardiac output.

Sepsis imposes a stress on the organism. In the early stages of sepsis, relatively small decreases in vascular resistance and increases in cardiac output and oxygen consumption are observed; the arteriovenous oxygen difference is unchanged or increases slightly. As the septic state progresses, there is evidence of a complex disturbance in vasomotor tone (peripheral vasculopathy) characterized by nonspecific systemic vasodilatation, pulmonary vasoconstriction, and increased capillary permeability. Pinsky and Matuschak[15] showed that endotoxemia in a canine model produced a marked increase in peripheral vascular capacitance without a change in peripheral vascular compliance that was unrelated to level of endogenous autonomic tone. This peripheral vascular "paralysis" leads to an inability to regulate the distribution of blood flow to the peripheral circulation. In addition, blood pressure falls because the peripheral resistance is inappropriately low for the cardiac output. The decreased systolic arterial pressure allows the ventricles to empty more rapidly. This high cardiac output systemic arterial resistance state is the cardiovascular hallmark of sepsis. Since the capacitance of the peripheral vasculature increases during sepsis, what was once an adequate circulating blood volume is now inadequate to fill all the newly perfused or overperfused vascular channels. This, coupled with an increased microvascular permeability, results in a relative and progressive hypovolemia that requires a rapid and massive fluid resuscitation effort. The hyperdynamic response to sepsis does not always occur. Carroll and Snyder demonstrated that if intravascular volume is not adequately replaced, a hypodynamic shock state ensues.[16] Similarly, if preexisting myocardial dysfunction or myocardial failure due to sepsis is present, the heart may be unable to increase its output despite the decrease in afterload. In physiologic terms, either decreased ventricular preload or reduced myocardial contractility may prevent the hyperdynamic cardiovascular response from occurring during sepsis. Such limitations are particularly common in patients following trauma, surgery, or prolonged serious illness.

At some point, adaptive responses are unable to cope with continuing cellular damage and death. Tissues are no longer able to extract oxygen, and the vascular bed becomes close to being maximally dilated. Interpretation of a rising mixed venous oxyhemoglobin saturation and a falling arteriovenous oxygen content difference is complicated by two abnormalities which change in the same direction. Vasodilatation in excess of tissue oxygen needs in the septic patient produces a rise in venous oxyhemoglobin saturation, and the inability of septic tissue to utilize oxygen produces an even greater increase in the oxyhemoglobin saturation of venous blood. Both clinical observations and studies with animal models have suggested this shift from "compensated" sepsis to "decompensated" sepsis, or, "septic shock," is characterized by a fall in oxygen consumption relative to need; there is a diminished ability to extract oxygen in spite of increased oxygen delivery. The actually measured consumption may be within normal limits for a nonstressed individual but is inadequate for meeting the rising metabolic requirements of advanced sepsis. Oxygen consumption becomes dependent upon blood flow and the ability of tissues to extract oxygen. Anaerobic conditions lead to the conversion of pyruvate to lactate in an attempt to increase the availability of oxidized NAD. Rising lactate and lactate/pyruvate ratios herald the development of metabolic acidosis. The transition from compensated sepsis to septic shock was described by MacLean et al.,[17] who identified two basic hemodynamic patterns. The increased cardiac output and decreased arteriovenous oxygen difference were in striking contrast to the low output and wide arteriovenous oxygen difference of hypovolemic and cardiogenic shock. The authors also described patients with septic shock and low cardiac output and considered this an advanced stage with extremely poor prognosis.

Metabolic and Hormonal Responses to Critical Illness

Hypoperfusion and sepsis lead to a group of immunologic, hematologic, and metabolic symptoms. These responses include fever, depressed levels of serum zinc and iron, increased gluconeogenesis and glycogenolysis, protein catabolism causing a negative nitrogen balance, and a marked increase in the hepatic synthesis of acute-phase proteins (see Fig 2–1).

Under normal circumstances, the utilization and synthesis of glucose and glycogen are carefully balanced to maintain blood glucose concentrations. The reversible glycogenetic/glycogenolytic and glucogenetic/glycolytic pathways store glycogen for emergency situations and maintain blood glucose in the face of varying carbohydrate uptake and metabolic need. Insulin promotes the synthesis of glycogen, triglycerides, and protein. It also facilitates glucose uptake in insulin-sensitive tissues such as muscle. The counterregulatory hormones, in contrast, may be visualized as preparing the body for a vigorous response to external threat by the rapid release of stored carbohydrate and lipid. Glucagon, secreted by pancreatic alpha cells, stimulates the hepatic gluconeogenic reactions which convert pyruvate to phosphoenolpyruvate and also activates hepatic lipase leading to an elevation of free fatty acids. Catecholamine release has a dual effect on insulin secretion; beta-adrenergic agonist activity stimulates the pancreatic secretion of insulin while alpha-adrenergic agonist activity inhibits insulin secretion and stimulates glucagon secretion by the pancreas.

THE NEUROHUMORAL STRESS RESPONSE

↓

EPINEPHRINE, GLUCAGON, CORTISOL

↓

INCREASED OXYGEN CONSUMPTION
GLYCOGENOLYSIS
VASOREGULATION
SHIFT IN GLUCOSE FLUX
GLUCONEOGENESIS

FIG. 2–1
Hypothalamic activation by hypotension, sepsis and other morbific processes initiates the neuro-humoral stress response. The counter-regulatory hormones; (cortisol, epinephrine, and glucagon); increase oxygen consumption, shift blood flow to vital organ structures by regional vasoconstriction, decrease insulin activity favoring its delivery to noninsulin-dependent tissues, and provide ready energy sources by glycogenolysis and gluconeogenesis.

Measurement of counter-regulatory hormones in plasma demonstrate the intensity of these adaptive responses. How a presumably adaptive response becomes counterproductive is not entirely clear. The importance of catecholamine release has been known since the early part of this century. Plasma epinephrine and norepinephrine increase in patients with injury, hemorrhage, hypothermia, and acute myocardial infarction. Experimental hemorrhagic shock provides an experimental model for these responses.[18] The adrenal medulla appears to be the major source of catecholamines; a 50-fold increase in epinephrine and a 10-fold increase in norepinephrine are observed, and removal of the adrenal medulla eliminates the epinephrine response and blunts the norepinephrine response. Epinephrine concentrations rise rapidly to a plateau while norepinephrine concentrations steadily increase. A variety of catecholamine responses have been observed in clinical studies. Up to 10-fold increases in plasma epinephrine and norepinephrine concentrations have been observed in injured patients, and the increases are closely related to the severity of trauma.[19] Catecholamine concentrations increase in acute myocardial infarction and become much higher as cardiac output falls and shock develops. The endocrine nature of the heart is demonstrated by high concentrations of coronary sinus catecholamines observed in myocardial infarction. Cold pressor stress and a vaso-vagal response during coronary arteriography dramatically increased catecholamines in both arterial and coronary sinus blood.[20] In contrast, catecholamine concentrations rise much more slowly in sepsis, and there is evidence of down-regulation of adrenergic receptors. The differing temporal responses of the sympathetic nervous system to hypoperfusion and sepsis suggest different initial activating systems.

Rises in other counter-regulatory hormones have also been measured. Hume, Nelson, and Miller,[21] in a classic study published in 1956, demonstrated increases in urinary excretion of corticosteroids in patients with severe burns. Recently Vaughan, Becker, and Allen[22] observed 5-fold to 15-fold increases in plasma cortisol concentrations in patients with severe burns. The increases were related to the extent of burn and remained elevated in patients who did not survive. Elevation of ACTH and cortisol confirms experimental conclusions that the catecholamine response to injury is initiated by the hypothalamus.

Problems in assay development have limited the measurement of regulatory or anabolic hormones until quite recently. Plasma insulin is modestly decreased in acute myocardial infarction, but is increased in sepsis, presumably because of macrophage secretion of insulinlike molecules. Epinephrine blocks the peripheral utilization of glucose and redirects it to noninsulin-dependent tissues, such as the central nervous system. Large exogenous infusions of insulin fail to increase skeletal muscle glucose uptake, but markedly reduce the rate of muscle protein breakdown.[23] Human growth hormone is an anabolic factor that may reduce amino acid loss during critical illness. Dahn et al.[24] observed reduced mortality in seriously ill individuals who exhibited increased growth hormone secretion in response to glucose infusion compared to another group who did not demonstrate hypersecretion. Plasma concentrations of epinephrine, glucagon, and cortisol were elevated but similar in both groups. Stimulated norepinephrine levels were significantly higher in the group with reduced growth hormone responsiveness, suggesting that, in these patients, the balance had shifted from regulatory or anabolic control to counter-regulatory or catabolic state.

The humoral stress response was simulated by Eigler, Sacca, and Sherwin,[25] who infused physiologic concentrations of glucagon, epinephrine, and cortisol into the conscious dog and noted that the combined effect of all three hormones demonstrated hormone-hormone synergism. Glucagon alone produced a transient elevation in plasma glucose due to an increase in glucose production by the liver, while epinephrine alone produced a much greater increase in plasma glucose because decreased peripheral utilization was coupled with increased hepatic glucose production. When glucose and epinephrine were infused simultaneously, synergism was demonstrated, since the increase in blood glucose was 50% greater than with individual infusions. Cortisol alone had little hyperglycemic effect but, when infused with epinephrine and glucagon, produced a sustained hyperglycemic effect.

The counter-regulatory hormones also have been shown to increase metabolism in normal volunteers. Bessey et al.[26] infused a mixture of cortisol, glucagon, and epinephrine, and observed increased oxygen consumption, hyperglycemia, hyperinsulinemia, diminished insulin-mediated glucose disposal, skeletal muscle insulin resistance, accelerated protein catabolism, and a modest negative nitrogen balance. Although hyperinsulinemia is a feature of sepsis, epinephrine blunts its effect on peripheral utilization and leads to a redirection of the glucose flux to noninsulin-dependent tissues, such as the central nervous system. Whether flux redirection is more profound under ischemic conditions where alpha-adrenergic stimulation decreases pancreatic insulin release is not known.

The effect which counter-regulatory hormones exert on protein catabolism has received the greatest attention. Studies beginning in the 1930s[27] identified disturbances in protein metabolism. More recent studies have demonstrated protein depletion, increased urea production, and release of amino acids into the circulation. Oxidation of amino acids may account for up to 30% of total energy cost; a proportion of these are consumed directly by oxidative deamination while others are converted to glucose. Glucose oxidation is slightly higher than normal; the glucose consumed is ultimately derived from amino acids, glycerol and lactate.[28]

Studies by Siegel and Cerra[29] and Cerra et al.[30] have emphasized increased skeletal muscle oxidation of the branched-chain amino acids: valine, leucine, and isoleucine. The branched-chain amino acids transfer amino groups to alpha-keto glutaric acid, which is then transferred to glutamate or used for alanine synthesis. Greater amounts of alanine and glutamine, and lesser amounts of branched-chain amino acids are released into the circulation from septic skeletal muscle than are present in intact skeletal muscle. This pattern is not significantly different from that seen during starvation, but occurs at a much faster rate. The phenomenon appears to be restricted to muscle tissue. Glutamine derived from proteolysis is transported to the liver and gastrointestinal tract and plays an important role in the synthesis of ammonia; alanine serves primarily as a gluconeogenic precursor but is also a substrate for the synthesis of acute-phase proteins. There is increasing evidence that gastrointestinal tract metabolism may be critically dependent on glutamine availability.

Uncontrollable gluconeogenesis from protein is an important feature of septic metabolism, and presumably results from both increased peripheral release of amino acids and from the nonsuppressibility of gluconeogenesis by conventional quantities of glucose. Recall that glycolysis converts one mole of glucose into two moles of lactate and yields two moles of ATP, while gluconeogenesis reverses the process by producing glucose from lactate and other noncarbohydrate sources. The concentration of oxaloacetic acid regulates the rate of gluconeogenesis; the catabolism of proteins and deamination of the free amino acids increases its concentration. Free fatty acids enter the Krebs cycle directly via acetyl CoA, and both alanine and lactate may be converted to pyruvate and stimulate the Krebs cycle. Hepatic gluconeogenesis requires energy and is favored when ATP concentrations are high and AMP and ADP concentrations low. When oxygen availability is reduced, low hepatic ATP concentrations favor glycolysis and gluconeogenesis is turned off.

Cerra et al.[30] have presented data based on plasma levels of amino acids that suggest that leucine, isoleucine, and valine may be preferentially utilized by muscle in decreasing order. Pittiruti et al.,[31] from Siegel's laboratory, subsequently demonstrated increased oxidation of branched-chain amino acids but diminished clearance of other amino acids in posttraumatic septic patients who developed fatal multiple organ system failure. This pattern was not observed in survivors. They proposed that an increased leucine-to-tyrosine clearance ratio in nonsurvivors indicated impairment of hepatic amino acid uptake and oxidation, with an increased skeletal muscle uptake of branched-chain amino acids, especially leucine. Valine enters the Krebs cycle through succinyl CoA only, while leucine and isoleucine enter at several sites. Utilization of other fuel substrates may be limited due to impairment of pyruvate dehydrogenase and/or malate shuttle activity. It must be emphasized that the shift to branched-chain amino acid utilization occurs mainly in skeletal muscle. The entrance through acetyl CoA for leucine and isoleucine remains intact until the end, so that a rising concentration of these two amino acids indicates imminent death. Cerra's group coined the term "autocannibalism" because protein catabolism "proceeds unabated by exogenous metabolic support until death ensues."[30] Their studies suggested the possible use of branched-chain amino acid solutions, acetoacetate, and fatty acids for nutritional support in patients with septic metabolic failure (see chapter 10).

Recent studies of forearm glucose and amino acid fluxes in normal and injured individuals suggest that exogenous insulin might decrease protein catabolism in skeletal muscle.[23] It is known that insulin has an important sparing effect in critically ill patients, even though it does not reverse the characteristic decrease in glucose uptake by skeletal muscle. Insulin administered to four moderately injured patients without evidence of infection dramatically reversed the sevenfold increase in nitrogen flux from forearm muscle. Significant declines in arterial levels of valine, isoleucine, leucine, and glutamine were observed; the flux of aspartic acid, alanine, lysine, and all three branched-chain amino acids shifted from release to uptake. The authors suggested that a combination of branched-chain amino acid and insulin administration might reverse the catabolism of injury.

The driving force behind protein catabolism is still not understood with certainty. Infusion of three counterregulatory hormones as discussed above produces a negative nitrogen balance, but other humoral factors also may be important. Two important reports published in 1983 suggest that a recently discovered monokine may be responsible. Human leukocyte pyrogen (LP) had been associated with the development of fever and the induction of prostaglandin synthesis in the brain; Baracos et al.[32] studied its effect on protein metabolism. They were able to show that human leukocytic pyrogen acted on rat muscle to stimulate intralysosomal proteolysis by increasing the production of prostaglandin E_2 within muscle. Indomethacin, a cyclooxygenase inhibitor, prevented LP-induced catabolism. Clowes et al.,[33] studying patients with critical illness, identified a plasma factor that induced proteolysis when incubated with normal rat skeletal muscle. The concentration of the factor was significantly increased in patients with trauma, whether or not infection was present, and was highest in those with sepsis and hepatic failure.

Work from Loda et al.[34] in Clowes' group has led to a general understanding of the pathogenesis of the catabolic state. The proteolysis-inducing factor (PIF) appears to be a 4,000 molecular weight fragment of interleukin-1 (MW, 16,000 daltons) and may be a cleavage fragment of interleukin-1. Interleukin-1 is produced by activated macrophages, and produces muscle proteolysis and increased hepatic uptake of amino acids. Thus, the release of amino acids into the circulation may be viewed as an adaptive mechanism sup-

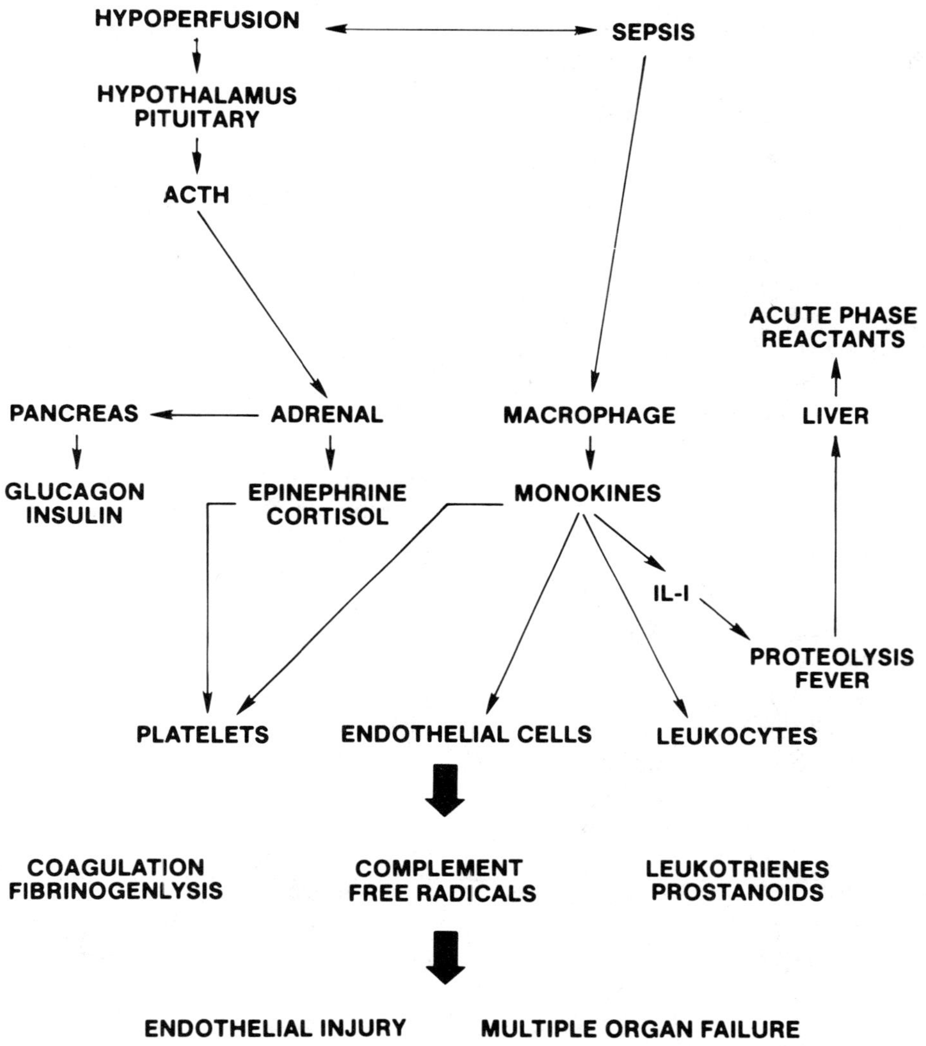

FIG. 2–2

Hypoperfusion and tissue hypoxia initiate the neurohumoral stress response by releasing ACTH and other centrally derived humoral factors. The carotid-sinus reflex and other baroreceptor responses release catecholamines when arterial blood pressure falls. The sepsis syndrome is initiated by macrophage activation associated with particulate phagocytosis. Cortisol, epinephrine, norepinephrine, and glucagon are released in response to hypoperfusion and hypotension; activated macrophages release a group of monokines. The counter-regulatory hormones and macrophage-derived IL-I stimulate platelets, leukocytes, and endothelial cells. These cells then synthesize and release or activate a group of adaptive humoral agents that may produce endothelial injury, cell death, and multiple organ failure. IL-I liberates amino acids into the circulation by a direct proteolytic effect on muscle protein. These amino acids are transported to the liver for synthesis of acute phase reactants.

plying building materials for the accelerated hepatic synthesis of protein that is necessary to support the humoral, phagocytic, and cellular aspects of the immunologic system. Increased synthesis of acute-phase proteins such as alpha-2 macroglobulin, C-reactive protein, serum amyloid A, and fibrinogen all appear to be part of the adaptive response to serious injury. Measurement of hepatic protein synthesis in liver biopsies from seriously ill patients suggests that survival was closely linked to the ability to increase protein production.

The Pathogenesis of Multiple Organ Systems Failure

The humoral and metabolic responses to severe injury serve important adaptive purposes. Figure 2–2 presents the pathogenetic network leading to the final common pathway of organ system destruction. While initially triggered by different activating systems, the neurosympathetic axis following hypoperfusion and the reticulo-endothelial-macrophage system following sepsis, the subsequent responses are strikingly similar. Hypoperfusion, secondary to reduced cardiac output, hypovolemia, or hypoxemia triggers the release of ACTH, cortisol, epinephrine and norepinephrine, and glucagon. These stress hormones attempt to preserve vital organ function. Constriction of the renal vascular bed and the vascular beds in other less vital organs allows the available blood volume and flow to perfuse the heart and brain. Glycogenolysis raises blood glucose and hormonally produced insulin resistance decreases glucose uptake in muscle and fat, redirecting the glucose flux to the brain. Microbial agents initiate the mediated septic response by activating fixed and circulating macrophages, which release a variety of soluble monokines. One of these, interleukin-1, activates immune defense systems, produces fever, and begins protein catabolism. Another monokine presumably activates the hypophyseal-pituitary-adrenal axis and initiates a somewhat delayed and blunted catecholamine response. The action of these counterregulatory hormones soon exhausts glycogen stores and initiates glucose production from protein (gluconeogenesis). Amino acids are released by muscle breakdown and transferred to the liver for the production of fuel and new protein synthesis. When tissue oxygen requirements are not met by oxygen delivery capability in the patient with sepsis, the catecholamine response is additionally enhanced. If the inciting factor is controlled, and if vascular volume, flow, and biochemical milieu are speedily corrected, the counterregulatory response is turned off and anabolism replaces catabolism. It is not clear whether oxygen delivery or lack of substrate limits cell survival; but, in any event, failure of ATP synthesis prevents restoration of normal function. Continued production of counterregulatory hormones, including interleukin-1, leads to continued catabolism. Protein catabolism progressively weakens skeletal, diaphragmatic, and cardiac muscle. Amino acids released from these organs are not metabolized appropriately, as the liver loses it synthetic ability to produce the badly needed phase-phase reactants. The striking autocannibalism, therefore, becomes a progressively less effective response to protein synthetic needs. Metabolic blockade may impair fuel utilization—the other vital requirement for oxidative phosphorylation. Eventually, cytolytic and catabolic influences lead to vital organ dysfunction; the number of organ systems under assault is roughly proportional to the intensity of the mediated response. The roles of complement activation, granulocyte degranulation and free-radical generation are presented in chapter one.

OUTCOME

The studies reviewed earlier presented a dismal outcome, which recently has been confirmed by Knaus et al.[35] These investigators have developed an important functional scoring system for evaluating the severity of critical illness. As part of that multihospital study, they presented criteria for identifying cardiovascular, respiratory, renal, hematologic, and neurologic failure; and they evaluated prognosis in 5,677 consecutive admissions to 19 intensive care units in 13 hospitals. Mortality was closely related to the number of failed organ systems and the duration of individual system failure, and ranged from 22% for individuals with single organ failure lasting one day to 100% in individuals with three or more failed systems for five or more days. Mortality rates were greater than 50% whenever two organs were involved for any period of time. Patients over the age of 65 had higher mortality rates for any combination of failed organ systems and days of failure.

Shoemaker, Appel, and Kram[36] have recently tested the hypothesis that oxygen deficit may be a critically important determinant of death from multiple organ failure. They had previously shown that oxygen consumption and cardiac output were higher than normal in patients surviving a wide variety of critical illnesses, and postulated that increased oxygen delivery in response to increased oxygen demands was related to recovery. They identified 88 high risk preoperative patients and randomized them to three groups. One group was monitored with central venous pressure catheters only, another group received pulmonary artery catheters, and a third group was monitored with pulmonary artery catheters and treated by a protocol that attepted to raise cardiac output and oxygen consumption to 50% and 30% greater than usually predicted normal values. There were 10 deaths in the 28 patients randomized to the group where the goal of therapy was restoration to published normal values. In contrast, there was only one death in the 27 patients in the group where cardiac output and oxygen consumption were raised to greater than normal levels ($\leq$ 0.02).

TREATMENT

The studies of Shoemaker, Appel, and Kram indicate that prevention may be the best treatment for multiple system organ failure[36]. The prevention and treatment of critically ill patients, those with single organ failure as well as those with multiple organ failure, are based on the early removal of *inciting* or *activating* causes. Restoration of blood volume, cardiac output, and vascular integrity so that oxygen delivery can be maintained to all organ beds are simply the *sina qua non* of modern treatment. In most cases, careful clinical observation should be combined with measurement of cardiac filling pressures (right and left arterial pressures) and cardiac output. Hemodynamic monitoring is not always necessary in all patients with single organ failure, but is almost always necessary in patients with multiple organ failure; treatment directed to one system may have adverse hemodynamic consequences for another.

Vigorous volume loading should be employed initially, and cardiac output determinations obtained at increments in pulmonary artery capillary wedge pressure (PCWP) to obtain the optimal filling pressures. In general, the PCWP should not be allowed to exceed 15 mm Hg in the patients who are not intubated. Many critically ill patients have stiff (noncompliant) ventricles so that a higher PCWP is necessary to attain adequate ventricular filling volumes. Crystalloid containing solutions may be used for initial therapy in many situations, but it must be remembered that infused crystalloid fills the entire extracellular space, which is three times the vascular space. Plasma volume can be successfully restored after acute volume loss if sufficient crystalloid is present, but edema results when more than 50% of the plasma volume is given as crystalloid.[37] Colloid solutions—such as blood, albumin, or hetastarch—should be considered when filling pressures cannot be raised by crystalloid, but their precise role remains controversial (see chapter 8). Shoemaker's results presented above were achieved with colloid solutions, however, and have not been equalled by similar studies with crystalloid.

Although volume loading generally improves cardiac output, administration of an inotrope-vasodilator such as dobutamine is generally necessary. Vasoconstrictor inotropes such as norepinephrine or "high dose" dopamine should be held in reserve for patients who are extremely vasodilated or who do not respond to fluid administration. A mean blood pressure of at least 60 mm Hg generally is required to maintain perfusion of most organs, so that vasoconstrictors are occasionally life-saving. The peripheral effects of vasoconstrictors may be monitored by observing urine flow rate and the development of skin mottling. Prolonged vasoconstrictor therapy is rarely useful and should be avoided. Vasoconstrictor support is especially important for hypotensive patients with coronary or cerebral arterial disease. Organ flow in these patients is dependent upon perfusion pressure, and an arterial pressure that prevents mentational or electrocardiographic abnormalities must be achieved. Low concentrations of norepinephrine are usually preferable to dopamine for this purpose, since they have less proclivity for increasing heart rate. Vasopressor therapy is still a trade-off since raising arterial blood pressure maintains coronary or cerebral artery flow but decreases the flow and oxygen delivery to many organ systems. Vasodilators may occasionally be required in some patients with severe vasoconstriction, although the vasodilating capability of dobutamine is usually sufficient.

A vigorous search for infectious agents should be maintained throughout the hospital course. Pulmonary foci are more common in patients on medical services, abdominal foci in patients on surgical services. Clinical sepsis should be diagnosed when the symptoms suggest sepsis regardless of negative blood cultures. Early and aggressive surgical drainage of septic foci corrects abnormal immune status and is an important way to prevent and treat multiple organ failure. Protocols for the management of monitoring and hyperalimentation lines must be assiduously followed, and lines replaced whenever unexplained infection occurs. Pulmonary infections are common and their prevention depends upon rigorous adherence to appropriate airway care, clearance of secretions, maintaining airway patency, handwashing by attendants before and after each patient encounter, and maintenance of an adequate functional residual capacity. Upright positions in bed and early ambulation, even when on a ventilator, reduce pulmonary atelectasis and infection.

Antibiotics are widely used in patients with suspected sepsis; their indiscriminate use may actually lead to the development of resistant infections, since they quickly break down the resistance to colonization provided by a normal bacterial flora. Other side effects, such as malabsorption syndromes, particularly with broad-spectrum antibiotics, hypersensitivity reactions, and a variety of direct toxic effects make it important to limit their use to situations where beneficial effects clearly outweigh possible untoward actions. Sheagren[38] suggests that they be used when a microbial agent is capable of either causing local tissue damage or entering the circulation causing metastatic abscesses or leading to generalized sepsis. They should never be administered until adequate biologic material for culture is obtained, and their empiric use may be guided by a group of algorithms.

Perhaps one of the most exciting therapeutic possibilities for the early treatment of multiple organ failure is the use of agents which block the mediated stress response that follows serious injury or illness. The first antimediator agents were corticosteroids. Hinshaw, Beller-Todd, and Archer[39] used slow infusions of *E. coli* in a baboon model and demonstrated 100% survival when antibiotics and corticosteroids were used together. Timing was important in their study: a two-hour delay before institution of combined therapy produced a 15% mortality, while a four-hour delay associated with one to three hours of hypotension produced a 35% mortality. A group of clinical studies has produced conflicting results. Kreger, Craven, and McCabe[40] found that large doses of corticosteroids increased mortality from septic shock, while Shumer[41] reported a prospective study with the early administration of either desamethasone (3 mg/kg) or methylprednisolone (30 mg/kg) repeated in four hours. Mortality was 38.4%; in the saline-treated controls and 10.4% in the steroid groups ($p \leq 0.01$). Schein, Long, and Sprung[42] concluded that "steroids used as adjunctive therapy should be given early in shock for them to be helpful." Hinshaw, Beller-Todd, and Archer[39] concluded that "we believe as others do that steroids are efficacious if used early in shock."

Unfortunately, the broad action of corticosteroids may produce unwanted immunologic and circulatory effects, and they should be used clinically with extreme caution. Better clinical results with fewer side effects might be expected with more specific mediator inhibitors, and it is likely that the use of steroids in critically ill patients will shortly become a historical curiosity. Cyclooxygenase inhibitors, thromboxane synthetase inhibitors, opiate antagonists, inhibitors of leukotriene synthesis, and antioxidants all have been shown to be useful in experimental models (see chapter 1). Perhaps the "last word" is found in a recent multi-institutional randomized and prospective study which revealed increased mortality in certain subsets of patients (see page 224).

Frequently, therapy for multiple organ failure is ineffective, perhaps either because oxygen deficits were restored too late or because etiologic factors such as hidden septic foci or continued hypoperfusion have not been corrected. Treatment of individual organ failure is then essential. Almost all therapeutic interventions used to support individual organ function may produce undesirable effects on other organ systems. Positive end-expiratory pressure is necessary to maintain lung expansion and improve arterial oxygenation, but it may decrease vital organ perfusion and increase cerebral venous pressure. Norepinephrine or other alpha agonist agents are indicated to raise coronary perfusion pressure in patients with acute myocardial infarction, but increase ventricular afterload and decrease organ perfusion. Vasodilators unload both ventricles but may produce hypotension, and fluid administration improves the peripheral circulation but can lead to pulmonary edema in certain clinical situations. Aminoglycosides may effectively treat septic foci but can directly injure the kidney. The key to this complicated network of desired and undesired effects is a continuing risk-benefit ratio considered each time the patient's status changes. Frequently, failure of a single organ system becomes the limiting factor for survival, and therapeutic agents must be initiated that may well injure other noncritical organ systems. The concept of the *rate-limiting (survival limiting) organ system is an important guide to the treatment of end-organ failure in patients with multiple organ systems failure.*

SEPTIC SHOCK

The syndrome of septic shock is a specific subset of the spectrum that begins with sepsis and ends in multiple organ failure. A majority of instances of septic shock are in patients with gram-negative infections, and it has been estimated that shock develops in about 25% of the 330,000 gram-negative bacteremias that occur each year in the United States.[40] Shock, of course, can occur in patients with gram-positive bacteremia and also with viruses, fungi, rickettsiae, and protozoa. Bacteremic shock was understood long before the problem of multiple organ failure was reported. Udhoji and Weil[43] presented hemodynamic observations on 16 patients in 1965, and subsequent studies have led to the description of an easily recognized but frequently underdiagnosed syndrome.[17,44] Fever, hyperventilation, and respiratory alkalosis follow therapeutic instrumentation such as urethral catheterization. Peripheral resistance falls, cardiac output rises, and a characteristic increase of mixed venous oxyhemoglobin saturation is observed. Vigorous fluid replacement is indicated, and many clinicians would institute high dose corticosteroid treatment to blunt mediator responses if the diagnosis is made early (see above). The infection must be quickly treated with appropriate antibiotics or surgical drainage. Pure septic shock appears to be less common than sepsis and multiple organ failure in the critical care unit. Sepsis following prolonged intubation, accidental trauma, or serious illness is usually overshadowed by the organ failure that accompanied the initial critical event. Hypovolemia or cardiac dysfunction may prevent the appearance of the classical hyperdynamic phase; serious illness or age may produce hypothermia instead of hyperthermia. Septic shock is a major clinical problem and should be recognized as early as possible. Excessive reliance on classical indicators, however, will lead to the underdiagnosis of the more common "silent sepsis" that appears to lead inexorably to multiple organ failure.

REFERENCES

1. Tilney NL, Bailey GL, Morgan AP: Sequential system failure after rupture of abdominal aortic aneurysms: An unsolved problem in postoperative care. *Ann Surg* 1973; 178:117–112.

2. Baue AE: Multiple, progressive, or sequential systems failure—a syndrome of the 1970s. *Arch Surg* 1975; 110:779–781.

3. Eiseman B, Beart R, Norton L: Multiple organ failure. *Surg Gynecol Obstet* 1977; 144:323–326.

4. Fry DE, Pearlstein L, Fulton RL, et al: Multiple system organ failure: The role of uncontrolled infection. *Arch Surg* 1980; 115:136–140.

5. *Extracorporeal Support for Respiratory Insufficiency: A Collaborative Study in Response to RFP-NHLI-7320.* National Heart, Lung and Blood Institute, 1979.

6. Polk HC Jr, Shields CL: Remote organ failure: A valid sign of occult intraabdominal infection. *Surgery* 1977; 81:310–313.

7. Meakins JL, Wicklund B, Forse RA, et al: The surgical intensive care unit: Current con-

cepts in infection. *Surg Clin North Am* 1980; 60:117–132.

8. Bell RC, Coalson JJ, Smith JD, et al: Multiple organ system failure and infection in adult respiratory distress syndrome. *Ann Intern Med* 1983; 99:293–298.

9. Coalson JJ: Pathology of sepsis, septic shock, and multiple organ failure, in Sibbald SJ, Sprung CL (eds): *New Horizons. Perspectives in Sepsis and Septic Shock*, vol 1. Fullerton, CA, Society of Critical Care Medicine, 1985.

10. Wiggers CA: *Physiology of Shock*. New York, The Commonwealth Fund, 1950.

11. Osler W: *The Principles and Practice of Medicine*. New York, D Appleton and Co, 1892.

12. Meakins JL, Christou NV, Shizgal HM, et al: Therapeutic approaches to anergy in surgical patients. Surgery and levamisole. *Ann Surg* 1979; 190:285–296.

13. DuBois EF: *Fever and The Regulation of Body Temperature*. Springfield, IL, Charles C Thomas, 1984.

14. Kinney JM, Roe CF: Calorie equivalent of fever. 1. Patterns of postoperative response. *Ann Surg* 1962; 156:610.

15. Pinsky MR, Matuschak GM: Is endotoxemia a peripheral vascular disease? Studies in an intact canine model. *Am Rev Respir Dis* 1984; 131:A148.

16. Carroll G, Snyder J: Hyperdynamic severe intravascular sepsis depends on fluid administration in cynomolgus monkeys. *Am J Physiol* 1982; 243:R131–R141.

17. MacLean LD, Mulligan WG, McLean APH, et al: Patterns of septic shock in man—A detailed study of 56 patients. *Ann Surg* 1967; 166:543–562.

18. Chernow B, Rainey TG, Lake CR: Endogenous and exogenous catecholamines in critical care medicine. *Crit Care Med* 1982; 10:409.

19. Davies CL, Newman RJ, Molyneux SG, et al: The relationship between plasma catecholamines and severity of injury in man. *J Trauma* 1984; 24:99.

20. Mueller HS, Ayres SM: Propranolol decreases sympathetic nervous activity reflected by plasma catecholamines during evolution of myocardial infarction in man. *J Clin Invest* 1980; 65:338–346.

21. Hume DM, Nelson DH, Miller DW: Blood and urinary 17- hydroxycorticosteroids in patients with severe burns. *Ann Surg* 1956; 143:316–329.

22. Vaughan GM, Becker RA, Allen JP: Cortisol and corticotrophin in burned patients. *J Trauma* 1982; 22:263.

23. Brooks DC, Bessey PQ, Black PR: Insulin stimulates branched-chain amino acid uptake and diminshes nitrogen flux from skeletal muscle of injured patients. *J Surg Res* 1986; 40:395–405.

24. Dahn MS, Jacobs LA, Lange MP, et al: Endocrine mediators of metabolism associated with injury and sepsis. *JPEN* 1986; 10:253.

25. Eigler N, Sacca L, Sherwin RS: Synergistic interactions of physiologic increments of glucagon, epinephrine, and cortisol in the dog. *J Clin Invest* 1979; 63:114–123.

26. Bessey PQ, Watters JM, Aoki TT, et al: Combined hormone infusion simulates the metabolic response to injury. *Ann Surg* 1984; 200:264–281.

27. Cuthbertson DP: The disturbance of metabolism produced by bony and non-bony injury, with notes on certain abnormal conditions of the bone. *Biochem J* 1930; 24:1244–1263.

28. Duke HJ Jr, Jorgensen SB, Broell JR, et al: Contribution of protein to caloric expenditure following injury. *Surgery* 1970; 68:168–174.

29. Siegel JH, Cerra FB: Physiological and metabolic correlations in human sepsis. *Surgery* 1979; 86:163.

30. Cerra FB, Siegel JH, Coleman B, et al: Septic autocannibalism: A failure of exogenous nutritional support. *Ann Surg* 1980; 192:570–580.

31. Pittiruti M, Siegel JH, Sganga G, et al: Increased dependence of leucine in posttraumatic sepsis: Leucine/tyrosine clearance ratio as an indicator of heparin impairment in sep-

tic multiple organ failure syndrome. *Surgery* 1983; 98:378.

32. Baracos V, Rodemann HP, Dinarello CA, et al: Stimulation of muscle protein degradation and prostaglandin E2 release by leukocytic pyrogen (interleukin-1). *N Engl J Med* 1983; 308:533–558.

33. Clowes GHA, George BC, Ville CA, et al: Muscle proteolysis induced by a circulating peptide in patients with sepsis or trauma. *N Engl J Med* 1983; 308:545–552.

34. Loda M, Clowes GHA Jr, Dinarello CA, et al: Induction of hepatic protein synthesis by a peptide in blood plasma of patients with sepsis and trauma. *Surgery* 1984; 96:204.

35. Knaus WA, Draper, EA, Wagner DP, et al: Prognosis in acute organ-system failure. *Ann Surg* 1985; 202:685.

36. Shoemaker WC, Appel PL, Kram, HB: Comparison of two monitoring methods (central venous pressure versus pulmonary artery catheter) and two protocols as therapeutic goals (normal values versus values of survivors) in a prospective randomized clinical trial of critically ill surgical patients. *Crit Care Med* 1985; 13:304(abst).

37. Demling RH: Colloid or crystalloid resuscitation in sepsis, in Sibbald WJ, Sprung CL (eds): *New Horizons. Perspective in Sepsis and Septic Shock*, vol 1. Fullerton, CA, Society of Critical Care Medicine, 1985.

38. Sheagren JN: Controversies in the management of sepsis and septic shock: Empiric antimicrobial therapy, in Sibbald WJ, Srpung CL (eds): *New Horizons. Perspectives in Sepsis and Septic Shock*, vol 1. Fullerton, CA, Society of Critical Care Medicine, 1985.

39. Hinshaw LB, Beller-Todd BK, Archer LT: Current management of the septic shock patient—experimental basis for treatment. *Shock* 1982; 9:543–553.

40. Kreger BE, Craven DE, McCabe WR: Gram-negative bacteremia. IV. Re-evaluation of clinical features and treatment in 612 patients. *Am J Med* 1980; 58:344–355.

41. Schumer W: Steroids in the therapy of clinical septic shock. *Ann Surg* 1976; 184:333–341.

42. Schein RMH, Long WM, Sprung CL: Controversies in the management of sepsis and septic shock: Corticosteroids, naloxone and non-steroidal antinflammatory agents, in Sibbald WJ, Sprung CL (eds): *New Horizons. Perspectives in Sepsis and Septic Shock*, vol 1. Fullerton, CA, Society of Critical Care Medicine, 1985.

43. Udhoji VN, Weil MH: Hemodynamic and metabolic studies on shock associated with bacteremia; observations on sixteen patients. *Ann Intern Med* 1965; 62:966.

44. Winslow EJ, Loeb HS, Rahimtoola SH, et al: Hemodynamic studies and results of therapy in 50 patients with bacteremic shock. *Am J Med* 1973; 54:421.

3 CIRCULATORY MONITORING

Recognition of impending cardiopulmonary disaster is not as easy as one might imagine. The coronary care unit was born when it was realized that instability of cardiac rhythm could foretell the sudden appearance of ventricular fibrillation. Increasing experience with extremely ill patients has shown that seemingly inconsequential findings may presage disaster. The gravity of the situation may not be readily apparent, even though there is serious malfunction of one or more organ systems. An elevated creatinine, a reduction in hematocrit, or moderately severe volume contraction may occur without obvious signs or symptoms. Subtle changes in physical status may be the only indication of imminent collapse. Unfortunately, early warning signs are frequently overlooked or dismissed unless both physician and nurse are ever vigilant. There is a recurring tendency, even in experienced physicians, to dismiss an abnormal finding by attributing it to an unimportant cause. It is not enough to recognize that a physical sign *could* indicate serious difficulty. The weakest link in patient care is the misplaced optimism that everything will be all right or the equally inappropriate view that nothing will help!

Richards and Cournand,[1] and their many associates at Columbia University and Bellevue Hospital, were clinical cardiopulmonary physiologists who dealt with the heart and lungs as a single transport system. "Studies of the Circulation in Clinical Shock" appeared in a surgical journal in 1943.[2] The carefully documented experimental study listed eight authors and six technical assistants and still serves as a model for the scientific investigation of the critically ill patient. The authors rescued Forssmann's[3] technique of right atrial catheterization from academic oblivion, and used it to obtain right atrial blood samples, which they demonstrated to represent "mixed venous blood." Oxygen consumption was calculated from expired oxygen and carbon dioxide concentrations; cardiac output was determined by the direct Fick method (see Chap ter 1). Arterial and venous oxygen and carbon dioxide contents, blood volume, hemoglobin, blood lactic acid concentration, pulmonary ventilation and respiratory gas exchange, and the clearance of substances by the kidney were measured in 36 patients. The investigators were charting unexplored territory, and their "methods" section required more than half of the article's 31 pages.

The studies demonstrated that traumatic shock in man was "a rapid or precipitate failure of the circulation, usually associated with inadequate return flow of blood to the heart. The chief findings were decreased cardiac output, low pressure in the right auricle, low arterial pressure, and decreased blood volume." In addition, the investigators noted "marked reduction in effective renal blood flow, out of proportion to the decrease in the systemic blood flow, with a filtration fraction either normal or low," as well as severe metabolic acidosis due to accumulation of lactic acid. Measurements of this sort were not to be repeated in critically ill patients for several decades, and oxygen content is rarely measured at the present time. For reasons perhaps related to the desire for rapid publication of research findings, the elegant Van Slyke-Neill manometric technique was discarded, and investigators estimated arterial oxygen content from oxygen tension and a "standard" oxyhemoglobin dissociation curve (if there ever was one). Cournand et al[2] found that oxygen delivery was 568 ml/min/M^2 in normal individuals, 243 patients with shock associated with skeletal trauma, 388 in those with shock and blunt abdominal injury, and 326 in burned patients in shock. They weighed and measured their patients so that they could present their findings in relationship to body surface area. Several of their extremely ill patients demonstrated what has now been identified as the adult respiratory distress syndrome and flow-limited oxygen consumption. One injured patient had an arterial oxyhemoglobin saturation of 83%, while a burned individual had an oxygen delivery of 129 ml/min/M^2 and an oxygen consumption of 109 ml/min/M^2. That unfortunate person extracted 84% of his available oxygen supply, but still could not maintain an adequate oxygen consumption!

Almost inexplicably, the concepts of systemic oxygen delivery and consumption lay fallow during the twenty-five years that followed the publication of Cournand and Richards' important studies. Part of the problem was methodologic. The nineteen sixties were dominated by continuous electrocardiographic monitoring (by the cardiologists) and repeated measurement of arterial oxygen and carbon dioxide tensions (by the chest physicians). Surgeons and anesthesiologists, however, needed better techniques for intra-operative monitoring, and a group of clinical scientists, most notably William Shoemaker,[4] began to make measurements of oxygen delivery in seriously ill surgical patients. Shoemaker and his associates soon demonstrated that a low oxygen delivery during the intra-operative and post-operative periods was a predictor of death. A few years later, Clement Finch, a hematologist, and Claude Lenfant, a surgeon turned pulmonary physiologist (now director of the National Heart Lung and Blood Institute) gave oxygen transport national attention in their *Medical Progress* contribution published in the New England Journal of Medicine in February 1972.[5] "Oxygen transport is a corporate process involving several organs," they emphasized, "each with its own regulatory system." They listed the essential components of oxygen delivery as pulmonary gas exchange, blood flow, hemoglobin concentration, and hemoglobin affinity for oxygen. Echoing Cournand and Richards, they concluded that "Evaluation of available oxygen in shock thus requires the measurement of arterial oxygen content, the in-vivo oxygen dissociation (including allowance for body temperature) and information concerning cardiac output. The adequacy of supply may be monitored by the mixed venous oxygen tension."

Justification of the high cost and potential risk of invasive ICU monitoring is based on the belief that it facilitates earlier recognition and better treatment of physiologic abnormalities than would be possible by clinical evaluation alone.

Evidence that morbidity or mortality can be influenced is sparse because of the difficulty in performing prospective randomized trials. One convincing randomized trial is that of Shoemaker, Appel, and Kram,[6] who used specific treatment protocols to raise cardiac output and oxygen consumption to levels 50% and 30% greater than predicted normal values, respectively. There were 10 deaths in the 28 patients randomized to the group where the goal of therapy was restoration to published normal values. In contrast, there was only one death in the 27 patients in the group where cardiac output and oxygen consumption were raised to greater than normal levels ($p<0.02$).

While many investigators believe that the physiologic principles pioneered by Cournand and others are so compelling that clinical trials might be unethical, not everyone has accepted the value of hemodynamic monitoring for the evaluation of oxygen delivery. Eugene Robin,[7] for example, has recently suggested that the use of hemodynamic monitoring to guide treatment in critically ill patients has become a cult. He took the trouble to quote Webster: "Cult: A system for the cure of disease based on dogma set forth by its promulgators . . . great and faddish devotion." Wiggers, Cournand, and Richards—the founders of a cult—interesting suggestion! Robin was certainly correct in suggesting the need for solid clinical trials, and such a plea was made by the National Institutes of Health Consensus Conference on Critical Care[8] more than one year before the publication of his polemic. But Robin misses the point in not properly understanding the great value of measuring blood flow and oxygen delivery in individuals who are at risk of death. Admittedly, catheters have been inserted by inexperienced physicians and the derived data not properly utilized for decision making, but such maturational problems require constructive support rather than blanket condemnation. Parrillo[9] recently reviewed his experience in an intensive care unit at the National Institutes of Health where pulmonary artery catheters are changed every 3 to 4 days because many of their patients are immunosuppressed. They place and remove 700 to 800 catheters each year and have an autopsy rate of 90%. An autopsy proven infectious endocarditis was not encountered in 2000 catheter placements and none of their patients developed clinically significant arrhythmias due to catheter insertion. In discussing a recent case report in the literature, he emphasizes the importance of training and supervision: "In our ICU, physicians in training are given substantial experience before they are allowed to perform this important procedure (pulmonary artery catheter insertion) without supervision. With appropriate supervision, the spinal canal placement would never have occurred."

Almost all monitoring techniques except the experimental magnetic resonance spectroscopy discussed in Chapter 1 indirectly estimate the rate of energy generation by measuring the determinants of oxygen delivery to the tissues. The generation of adequate amounts of high-energy phosphates, however, is dependent upon metabolic *need* as well as oxygen and nutrient delivery. Too often, oxygen requirements are assumed to be normal even though it is well known that restlessness, respiratory distress with increased work of breathing, sepsis, and fever all increase metabolic demands. *There is no single level of oxygen or nutrient delivery that is adequate for all patients or all clinical circumstances.*

Monitoring techniques must never be used as a substitute for good clinical judgment. There will probably never be enough mechanical sensors to measure oxygen delivery to all organ systems, and continuous clinical observations by physicians and nurses remain the most useful global monitoring technique. Brain metabolism, for example, is estimated better by a careful evaluation of mental status, although other techniques may be necessary in states of disordered consciousness. In general, careful evaluation of clinical information frequently provides better information of early abnormalities, since they tend to integrate the balance between oxygen demand and availability.

The principles of oxygen delivery have been presented in Chapter 1. The general focus has been on oxygen rather than fuel delivery to the tissues, since the determinants of oxygen delivery are easier to measure and control. In addition, most clinicians are unfamiliar with disease states (other than hypoglycemic coma) where the primary deficit is that of fuel substrate. Preliminary data is beginning to suggest that inability to mobilize or utilize available species of fuels may characterize certain disease states such as sepsis,[10] and even acute myocardial infarction.[4] Chapter 1 also emphasized that processes other than insufficient generation of high-energy intermediates may lead to cellular damage. Oxygen delivery and oxidative phosphorylation remain the most useful principles underlying physiologic monitoring, however, and remain the basis for physiologic monitoring.

THE RELATIONSHIP BETWEEN OXYGEN SUPPLY AND OXYGEN DEMAND

Although the need for high-energy intermediates varies widely from minute-to-minute and hour-to-hour, and can rise rapidly with physical exercise, oxygen delivery is closely matched to these needs so that energy stores remain within normal limits. There may be brief periods of disequilibrium in the concentration of individual high-energy phosphates as creatine phosphate is temporarily depleted, but increased oxygen supplies quickly restore a new balance point. Total body oxygen consumption ($\dot{V}O_2$), at any moment, is defined by the product of cardiac output and the arterial-venous oxygen content difference. Oxygen content, as discussed above, is the amount of oxygen carried in blood; most of it is in the form of oxyhemoglobin while a small amount is dissolved in plasma. Oxygen content can be directly measured by the Van Slyke manometric or other techniques, but is usually calculated from oxyhemoglobin saturation for most purposes. The following equation requires saturations calculated from oxygen tension measurements by a standard oxyhemoglobin dissociation curve:

$$\dot{V}O_2 = 13.4(Hb)(\dot{Q}s)(Sa_{O_2} - Sv_{O_2}) + 0.0031(\dot{Q}s)(Pa_{O_2} - Pv_{O_2})$$

where Hb is hemoglobin, $\dot{Q}s$ is systemic blood flow (cardiac output), Sa_{O_2} and Sv_{O_2} are arterial and venous mixed saturations respectively, and Pa_{O_2} and Pv_{O_2} are arterial and mixed venous oxygen tensions, respectively. The first part of the equation accounts for oxygen carried by hemoglobin, and the latter for that carried by plasma. A decline in oxygen consumption for any reason below the minimum required for metabolic function results in a slowing of metabolism; extra-mitochondrial anaerobic metabolism inefficiently attempts to maintain ATP generation, and lactic acid is produced. When deficient oxygen consumption is prolonged, end-organ damage results. Until recently, it was assumed that all oxygen consumed was used for the generation of ATP. Studies into free radical generation described in Chapter

1 suggest that significant amounts of oxygen may be reduced to superoxide anion and converted to irritant oxygen species. The sudden restoration of blood flow to ischemic tissue appears to increase free radical production (reperfusion injury); damage may be prevented by pretreatment with free radical scavengers.

Oxygen consumption can be rapidly calculated from cardiac output and arterial and venous saturations. The use of standard curves to determine oxyhemoglobin saturation neglects the possible shifts of the dissociation curve in various clinical situations. Giannelli, Lambright, and Martin[11] found that the P-50 differed by as much as 8.5 mm Hg on different days in normal laboratory personnel. The change was not due to changes in the concentration of 2,3 DPG and might be expected to be substantially greater in unstable patients with critical illness. Spectrophotometric measurement of saturation may be somewhat more accurate than calculation from oxygen tensions, but some spectrophotometers are not linear and are particularly inaccurate with low mixed venous saturations.

An important determinant of the rate of oxygen consumption, the rate of oxygen delivery ($\dot{D}O_2$) to the tissues, is the basis for most hemodynamic monitoring. It is simply the product of cardiac output and arterial oxygen content, and is described by the following equation:

$$\dot{D}O_2 = 13.4(Hb)(\dot{Q}s)(Sa_{O_2}) + 0.0031(\dot{Q}s)(Pa_{O_2}).$$

Hemoglobin concentration, cardiac output, and arterial oxygen saturation are each equally important; a decrease in hemoglobin by half, for example, assuming that the remaining factors remain constant, is equally as deleterious as a decline in cardiac output by one half. Note, in addition, that the major difference between the above two equations is the absence from the latter of values for mixed venous oxygenation. The oxygen which is left over in the blood after it has filtered through the systemic circulation is not considered. The amount of oxygen leaving the left ventricle (oxygen delivery) is actually compared with that taken up by the periphery (oxygen consumption). Oxygen consumption can be maintained in the face of a decline in oxygen delivery only by increasing the fraction of oxygen extracted by the tissues. An increased extraction obviously leads to a reduction in venous oxyhemoglobin saturation which may place the peripheral tissues in additional jeopardy. A useful indicator of oxygen extraction, the actual volume of oxygen extracted, is the oxygen extraction ratio which is defined as:

$$O_2\,\text{extraction} = \dot{V}O_2/\dot{D}O_2$$

Cardiac output appears in the calculation of each of these measurements so that the oxygen extraction ratio may be calculated from the arterial-venous oxygen content difference divided by the arterial oxygen content.

Measurement of Systemic Oxygen Extraction

The ability of peripheral tissues to increase oxygen extraction from the circulating blood is an important mechanism for survival in the face of diminished oxygen delivery. Oxygen extraction was the best predictor of survival in a large series of post-operative surgical patients.[12] Although some tissues (brain, heart) normally extract the maximal degree of oxygen from their arterial blood, others (kidney, skeletal muscle, skin, gastrointestinal tract) receive a good deal of "non-nutritive" blood flow and extract relatively little oxygen.[5] The consequence is that blood flowing from the coronary sinus or jugular vein has very low venous oxygen saturation (37%) while the venous effluent from the kidneys, skin and gastrointestinal tract is highly saturated with oxygen. (Table 3–1.)

The mixture of these various venous effluents results in a normal resting mixed venous oxygen saturation of 70–75%. As oxygen delivery to the tissue declines, however, the pattern of blood flow is rerouted to vital tissues, producing the clinical signs of a cold ashen skin and diminished urine flow. Diminished flow in turn is due to sympathetic nervous system–mediated vasoconstriction and to angiotensin release.[13] Oxygen consumption and therefore viability of these organs may, however, be maintained in spite of diminished flow by increased oxygen extraction in these organs. The value of this rationing of blood flow to various organs is that all organs may then receive the minimal quantity of oxygen necessary for survival. The mechanism whereby increased extraction is achieved at the level of the various organs probably varies somewhat, but appears generally to involve an increase in capillary density; since the distance which oxygen must travel from the capillary to the cell is then shorter, oxygen is more readily extracted.[14] Increased capillary density, in turn, may be secondary to dilatation of precapillary sphincters, which may respond to local vasodilators or to hypoxemia.[15]

The increased oxygen extraction, which occurs as oxygen delivery declines, is due to diminished blood flow in a number of organs that normally receive considerable non-nutritive flow; these organs may compensate for diminished flow by increasing their extraction of oxygen; identification of increased extraction is valuable evidence for decreased blood flow.

Pulmonary arterial blood represents "mixed" venous blood and describes total body oxygen extraction at any given moment. Other sampling sites are less useful because of inadequate mixing of various venous streams. Peripheral venous blood reflects limb metabolism inferior vena caval blood being lower than superior vena caval blood. Inferior vena caval blood obtained below the entrance of hepatic veins is high, however, because of the contribution of renal venous effluent and the exclusion of hepatic venous blood.

TABLE 3–1.
Regional Venous Oxygen Saturation and Tension

ORGAN	SATURATION	TENSION
Heart	24%	23 mm Hg.
Muscle	44	34
Brain	58	33
Liver	72	43
Kidney	91	56
Skin	93	60
Mixed	75	40

It would be useful to identify "critical" values of Sv_{O_2} that signal a decrease in oxygen consumption as consumption becomes dependent upon oxygen supply. Cain[14] demonstrated that the critical Sv_{O_2} in hypoxic animals is close to 20% but near 70% in anemic animals. The critical venous saturation is near 50% with acute depression of cardiac output. It is difficult to identify critical levels of venous saturations in patients, although a falling venous saturation indicates increasing difficulty with oxygen delivery.

Even though the critical level for mixed venous saturation differed widely in the studies of Cain,[14] oxygen extraction was about the same (80%). The different critical levels of mixed venous saturation are due in part to the differing arterial saturation. The oxyhemoglobin dissociation curve becomes quite steep with arterial saturations below 80%;

extraction of normal quantities of oxygen results in low mixed venous saturations which become dramatically lower if cardiac output is reduced. The level of oxygen extraction may vary further with different disease states; patients with chronic low oxygen delivery states enhance their ability to extract oxygen at the tissue level by increased levels of 2,3 DPG within their erythrocytes[5] and other mechanisms. Individuals with chronic low cardiac output, for example, may survive for prolonged periods with considerably lower Sv_{O_2} due to extraordinarily high rates of oxygen extraction.[16]

Defective Oxygen Extraction

Factors that impair the redistribution of arterial blood during declining total body oxygen delivery will impair total body oxygen extraction. The most obvious example is implantation of an artificial arterial-venous shunt; introduction of arterial blood directly into the venous circulation makes it unavailable for peripheral utilization. Arteriovenous shunting is identified by an increased Sv_{O_2} and decreased oxygen extraction. Under normal circumstances, such shunting of arterial blood is tolerated to the extent that cardiac output can increase sufficiently to perfuse both the shunt and the remaining circulation; cardiac output must rise to a level high enough to raise the pressure within the shunt (recall that pressure equals flow times resistance) to the minimum level required for autoregulation of flow in the remaining vascular beds. If systemic oxygen delivery is reduced, however, preservation of flow through the shunt may compromise the delivery of oxygen to the periphery.

A number of conditions mimic arteriovenous shunts. Alpha-adrenergic blockade, for example, impairs the vasoconstrictor response to severe hypoxia and diminishes the maximal degree of oxygen extraction.[17] Early phases of sepsis are characterized by pathologic vasodilatation in one or more vascular beds.[10] Patients with hepatic failure exhibit hemodynamics similar to those with sepsis,[18] certain anaesthetic agents[19] interfere with oxygen extraction either by causing direct vasodilatation or by impairing sympathetic nervous system activity. Acute dilatation of the atria produces increased (presumably non-nutritive) renal blood flow by neural and hormonal pathways.[20] The adult respiratory distress syndrome is frequently associated with defective oxygen extracting ability in the face of declining oxygen delivery, due possibly to plugging of capillaries with agglutinated granulocytes. A large number of additional syndromes characterized by vasodilatation and diminished systemic vascular resistance are similarly characterized by impaired ability to extract oxygen from the bulk of oxygen delivered to the systemic circulation. When systemic pressure falls below that required for flow through vascular beds with normal vascular resistance, blood flow is shunted through pathologically dilated vessels.

ASSESSMENT OF CIRCULATORY COMPENSATION

The methods available for monitoring physiologic functions of critically ill patients have expanded tremendously over the past decade, adding a considerable degree of sophistication and complexity to ICU technology. As discussed above, the effect of monitoring on patient outcome has not been proven in most cases; cost/benefit and risk/benefit ratios must be considered in each clinical situation. Excessive use of monitoring that does not alter patient treatment decisions leads to unnecessary complications, patient discomfort, and increased costs. Failure to initiate adequate monitoring techniques, on the other hand, will lead to increased morbidity and likelihood of death in seriously ill patients with reversible disease. The patient may survive a delay in initiating appropriate therapy but might spend considerably more time in the hospital than would have been otherwise necessary. In the absence of cost/benefit and risk/benefit information for most patient groups, monitoring decisions must be based on basic pathophysiology considerations and the likelihood that an individual patient either exhibits or will develop an oxygen deficiency syndrome.

The Indirect Assessment of Oxygen Delivery

A "gold standard" does not yet exist for monitoring the ability of a critically ill patient's circulation to deliver the necessary quantities of nutrients. Calculation of oxygen delivery and consumption is extremely useful, but does not by itself provide a complete description of the state of cellular oxygenation. Moreover, such sophisticated and expensive measurements are not always required, because clinical methods such as physical examination, blood pressure monitoring, and measurement of urine flow are often sufficient for many clinical situations.

The Physical Examination

A decrease in oxygen delivery can frequently be identified by a careful physical examination, even though a number of studies have shown that physicians at all levels of training have considerable difficulty in estimating left ventricular filling pressure.[21,22] Careful clinical evaluation should suggest the need for obtaining precise information because the redistribution of flow to vital organ systems in low flow states provides important objective evidence of decreased cardiac output. Reduced skeletal muscle and skin blood flow produce profound weakness and decreased skin temperature. Slowing of bowel sounds reflects diminished mesenteric flow. The radial pulse and pedal pulses become weak and thready. Respiratory effort becomes labored in those individuals with pulmonary congestion. Underperfusion of the central nervous system produces first lethargy, then confusion, and finally unconsciousness. Increased oxygen extraction produces cyanosis of the lips and nailbeds (peripheral cyanosis). Air hunger is often evident in conscious individuals as tachypnea and utilization of accessory muscles of respiration. Altered mentation becomes evident as arterial saturation declines; unconsciousness usually occurs when the arterial P_{O_2} falls below 30 mm Hg.[5] Even moderately severe anemia may not produce generalized pallor if the cardiac function is normal because the increased cardiac output necessary to maintain oxygen delivery leads to relatively normal perfusion of the skin. Close examination of the mucous membranes, however, permits inspection of small blood vessels and reveals pallor. The circulation is hyperdynamic and "high output failure" may occur. Patients with diseases characterized by ineffective oxygen extraction often behave differently. Septic individuals frequently exhibit warm, well-perfused skin because of generalized vasodilatation. Cerebral hypoperfusion may be present as confusion and a general "toxic" appearance. Marked hyperventilation, even in the absence of metabolic acidosis or hypoxia, is almost invariably present. Similarly, patients with inferior myocardial infarction may manifest "warm shock" due to relative cutaneous and renal hyperperfusion due to increased vagal activity.

Although few of the findings of the physical exam are specific for any disease state, it is often important to take quick action based on clinical judgment. At these critical moments, the time lost in inserting a Swan-Ganz catheter or in waiting for an arterial blood gas could lead to increasing deterioration; action based on clinical evidence may prevent the patient's death.

Monitoring of Arterial Blood Pressure

Autoregulation of cerebral, coronary, renal, and other vital vascular beds maintains blood flow and oxygen delivery within broad limits of mean arterial pressure, generally between 60 to 180 mm Hg. Flow is reduced, however, below a mean arterial pressure of 60 mm Hg. The range of autoregulation depends upon the ability of regional vascular beds to dilate under stress. In some patients, especially in the young, normal mental status and urine flow are maintained at even lower arterial pressures. In the elderly and in patients with atherosclerosis, organ dysfunction may occur at substantially higher mean arterial pressures.

Although hypotension suggests underperfusion, an arterial pressure within normal limits does not necessarily imply optimal perfusion of all vascular beds, since the pressure may be maintained by arteriolar vasoconstriction. Pressure is maintained at the expense of flow. Blood pressure in individuals with chronic congestive heart failure, for example, is commonly in the normal range, despite very low cardiac outputs, because of increased peripheral vasoconstriction. Renal blood flow and glomerular filtration in such individuals has been found to be as low as 50% of normal.[23] The sensitivity of blood pressure measurements for identifying hypovolemia may be improved by evaluating orthostatic changes.

Profound diminution in regional blood flow may occur with normal blood pressures when the areas of vascular beds are pathologically reduced by atherosclerosis or other conditions. Rapid drops in arterial blood pressure produced by either disease or therapy may lead to myocardial, renal, or cerebral ischemia. Vascular resistance is inversely proportional to the fourth power of its radius, and increased resistance to flow may be overcome most readily by raising perfusion pressures. Failure to understand this obvious physiologic principle frequently leads to iatrogenic cerebral infarctions in the treatment of hypertension. Blood pressure should not be lowered rapidly unless the patient is known to be at a well-defined risk for an acute complication of hypertension. Even patients without focal cerebral vascular disease (especially those with severe longstanding hypertension) may experience vascular accidents when blood pressure is rapidly lowered.[24] Conversely, raising blood pressure rapidly when such individuals develop neurologic deficits may reverse an ischemic deficit and thereby preserve brain tissue. Abnormal blood pressure may have other adverse effects in addition to its effects on oxygen delivery. Elevated blood pressure may disrupt vascular anastomoses and lead to increased bleeding in patients with vascular dissections. Reduced systemic blood pressure in patients with Eisenmenger's syndrome may increase right to left shunting. Malignant hypertension represents the opposite end of the spectrum of autoregulation, as the capacity of the arterioles to protect capillary beds from a high perfusion pressure is exhausted.

Sphygmomanometry Cuff pressures are generally taken at the level of the brachial or popliteal arteries. The first sound audible as the cuff is deflated represents turbulent blood flow past the external constriction during systole; damping of the sound occurs as the cuff is deflated and blood flows freely through the unimpeded artery. Errors are introduced by the use of improper cuff size, failure to calibrate the mercury column, or by taking measurements downstream from a stenotic lesion. Automated devices are available at most institutions, and may substitute for invasive monitoring for patients who are relatively stable. These devices are rather uncomfortable, however, and may produce ischemia of a limb with severe atheroschlerotic disease.

Invasive Monitoring Cannulation of radial, brachial, dorsalis pedis, or femoral artery permits continuous monitoring of arterial pressure. Sites of cannulation vary according to local preference. In general, however, it may be safest to avoid cannulation of vessels without anastomotic flow, since thrombosis may lead to necrosis of an extremity. For the most severely compromised individuals, pressure recorded from the femoral artery may be higher than that recorded distally due to vasoconstriction or stenosis of smaller distal arteries.[25] Pressure waves transmitted within the connecting tubing are converted to an electrical signal by a transducer; this information is then converted to a visual signal. Visualization of the waveform is important in order to judge its quality; damping may be due to air in the transducer or connecting tubing, to a defective transducer, to a "kink" in the catheter, to impingement of the catheter tip on a vessel wall, or to adherent thrombus. Pressure measured through a catheter may often exceed that measured by a cuff, since the peak of an unusually rapid and narrow upstroke may be sensed by the electrical device but not heard by the human examiner. Mean arterial pressure is measured as area under the curve, and should therefore be accurate. Pressure measured by a sphygmomanometer should never exceed that measured by the electrical device; this observation should prompt recalibration, a check to insure that the transducer is at the level of the left atrium, and examination of the pressure tracing for damping.

Complications of arterial catheterization include catheter sepsis, thrombosis, and embolization. Sepsis is most commonly the result of migration of bacteria down the dermal tunnel and may be reduced by aseptic insertion and meticulously sterile care of the insertion site; radial lines cared for in this manner should be rotated every four days (see chapter 1). Larger catheters appear no more likely to become infected. The percutaneous technique is always preferred; the incidence of catheter sepsis is ninefold greater for catheters placed by cutdown.[26] The incidence of occlusion of an artery increases with increasing catheter radius, cannulation longer than three days,[27] and use of pharmacologic vasoconstrictor.[28] Clinically significant complications from radial artery cannulation occur less than 1% of the time.[29,30].

Urine Flow

Timed measurement of urine output may be of value in monitoring circulatory adequacy of a hemodynamically unstable patient if changes in systematic circulation are reflected by those in renal perfusion. Few other observations assess the degree of circulatory compensation under such a wide variety of conditions. Renal blood flow and glomerular filtration rate vary together due to autoregulatory processes (see chapter 8). As renal perfusion pressure falls, urine flow diminishes, due at first to increased tubular reabsorption (reflected in low urine sodium, high urine creatinine), and then to decreased GFR as renal perfusion falls further. With the possible exceptions of nonoliguric renal insufficiency and diabetes insipidus, a urine flow of 0.5 cc/kg/hr in adults and 1.0 cc/kg/hr for children is generally accepted as evidence that the kidneys are adequately perfused; this is minimal quantity of urine required for the removal of solute at the rate at which it is delivered (assuming normal concentrating abiblity). On the other hand, low urine flow, increased concentration, and low urine sodium is often observed in stressed ICU patients with normal or high cardiac output, mixed venous oxygen saturation, and other measures of circulatory adequacy. This may be related to increased ("appropriate") secretion of antidiuretic hormone in response to stress, although other factors also appear to be involved.[31] Thus, while normal urine flow may generally be taken as a sign that the circulation is adequate, low urine volume is generally nonspecific. For a patient with diminished urine flow and other signs of circulatory insufficiency, additional monitoring devices may be required.

Measurement of Individual Determinants of Oxygen Transport

Each of the primary determinants of oxygen delivery—hemoglobin concentration, cardiac output, and arterial oxygen saturation—has an equal weight in determining oxygen transport, but frequently only a single determinant of oxygen transport, such as arterial saturation, is deficient and should be monitored.

Measurement of Oxygen Carrying and Releasing Capacity

Hemoglobin is, of course, the primary carrier of oxygen; the rate of its flow (cardiac output) and the degree of its saturation with oxygen (Sa_{O_2}) are clearly irrelevant unless the serum hemoglobin concentration is known. Consider, for example, that a circulatory system perfused by pure water could have a normal flow rate and oxygen *tension* but be useless for transporting oxygen.

Hemoglobin Concentration A plasma hemoglobin concentration as low as 3.8 gm/dl may be tolerated by an individual with normal cardiac reserve.[32] For a patient with impaired myocardial function, however, diminishing hemoglobin concentration is equally detrimental to systemic oxygen delivery as diminishing cardiac output. For individuals with normal or high intravascular volume but low serum hemoglobin, it is the concentration, not quantity, of blood in the intravascular space which is important to follow.

Serial hemoglobins are also commonly monitored for patients with acute blood loss. It must be recognized, however, that although normal hemoglobin concentration is important for tissue oxygenation for these individuals with hypovolemic low cardiac output, volume deficiency is generally their primary defect. In consequence, acute bleeding is often *not* associated with low hemoglobin concentration unless bloodless fluids have been administered. In the absence of volume infusion, serum hemoglobin concentration eventually falls following severe bleeding due to movement of water from the intracellular to the extracellular space; however, this process takes several hours. Assessment of intravascular volume by measuring the orthostatic blood pressure in addition to frequent serum hemoglobin concentration measurement is necessary when acute hemorrhage is suspected.

Affinity of Hemoglobin for Oxygen A number of critically ill individuals are so close to the critical level of systemic oxygen delivery that small increments in tissue oxygenation may constitute the difference between success and failure. Factors which shift the oxyhemoglobin dissociation curve to the right and increase the P-50 may enhance unloading of oxygen at the tissue level. This decreased affinity of hemoglobin for oxygen makes oxygen loading in the lung less effective, but the effect can be overcome by administering supplemental oxygen to raise the arterial Po_2 and maintain an adequate arterial So_2. The position of the oxyhemoglobin dissociation curve may be measured by tonometry or calculated by the Hill equation from mixed venous oxygen tension and saturation. A pocket calculator facilitates the logarithmic transformation necessary to describe the curvilinear relationship. The normal P-50 is 28, and an abnormal value might suggest the need for procedures aimed at returning it to normal.

$$P_{50} = \frac{\frac{Sv_{O_2}}{1-Sv_{O_2}} - 2.65(\text{Ln}Pv_{O_2})}{2.65}$$

In performing these calculations, Sv_{O_2} must be measured rather than estimated from nomograms.

Measurement of Arterial Oxygenation

The same arguments applied to serum hemoglobin above are also true for arterial saturation of oxygen; a normal serum hemoglobin and cardiac output are of little value unless the hemoglobin is not adequately saturated with oxygen. Attention to arterial saturation is especially important in low flow states, since raising saturation to normal may be one of the only ways to improve oxygen delivery. In consequence, it makes sense to routinely administer supplemental oxygen to patients with stenotic vascular lesions.

Arterial "Blood Gases" It may be difficult for recent graduates to understand that the routine measurement of respiratory gas tensions in blood and pH has only recently been possible. An analysis of arterial respiratory gases should be obtained in all unstable patients. Each of the reported measurements reflects the adequacy of systemic oxygen delivery. Metabolic acidosis may suggest anaerobic metabolism in one or more vascular beds. Progressive hypercarbia indicates deteriorating ventilation and impending respiratory arrest. A number of hospital laboratories do not directly measure oxygen saturation, but estimate using pH, Pco_2 and/or serum hemoglobin and standard nomograms; such values may be misleading for patients who have received large blood transfusions or who suffer from chronic low oxygen delivery states.[11] Oxygen tension only indirectly assesses hemoglobin saturation and therefore the quantity of oxygen carried by the blood.

Continuous Monitoring Devices Intermittent sampling of arterial blood is painful and may produce arterial damage. Values may change suddenly and without warning, so that the value available at the bedside may actually reflect *past* rather than *present* events. For example, the first evidence of hypoxemia due to worsening pulmonary edema in a patient with a large myocardial infarction may be a sudden cardiac dysrhythmia. Continuous monitoring is clearly indicated in patients with rapidly changing cardiopulmonary function. Two basic approaches have been developed. The first continuous sensors were arterial catheters equipped for fiberoptic reflectometry or for chemical measurement of oxygen tension. More recently, noninvasive oximetry has become available. Light of two or three wavelengths is passed through the skin of a digit or earlobe; the wavelength of light which is reflected from erythrocytes beneath the skin correlates well with the oxygen saturation. Since skin normally extracts only a small proportion of its blood flow, oxygen saturation of this vascular bed generally correlates well with that obtained from within an artery. At least one arterial sample should be obtained simultaneously in order to assess the accuracy of the noninvasive technique.

Measurement of Cardiac Hemodynamics

A common indication for measurement of cardiac output is unexplained hypotension; since pressure is equal to the product of flow times resistance, it is often unclear whether a catastrophic decline in blood pressure is due to diminished cardiac output or to pathologic vasodilatation. Treatment with a primary vasoconstrictor would generally be inappropriate for an individual with volume depletion and low cardiac output, for example, while a primary inotropic agent may not be the optimal form of therapy for the patient with high cardiac output and low vascular resistance. Information obtained from a pulmonary artery balloon flotation catheter indicates whether preload, afterload, or contractility are abnormal and whether they should be manipulated.

Another indication for measurement of cardiac output is the peri-operative monitoring of patients with impaired myocardial reserve. These patients frequently experience fluid shifts as vascular resistances change with anesthesia and surgery. They are often dependent upon preload to maintain stroke output, and may easily experience serious oxygen deficits if the abnormalities are not recognized and corrected. In addition, major operative stress may impair myocardial contractility and compliance. The frequent measurement of cardiac output allows detection of major trends in physiologic status so that appropriate treatment may be instituted before clinical deterioration occurs.

Monitoring of cardiac output is indicated in a number of clinical situations. The optimal treatment of patients with acute renal failure, for example, requires adequate cardiac output and atrial filling pressures to assure that renal perfusion is optimal. In such a patient, a fall in urine output might lead to rapid administration of fluid ("fluid challenge") if the patient is believed to be hypovolemic. If the estimate of volume status is incorrect, pulmonary edema requiring mechanical ventilation and emergency dialysis might well occur. Thus pulmonary artery balloon flotation catheters are frequently used, on the basis of sound theoretical reasoning, without solid evidence that they improve outcome.

Cardiac output measurements may be misleading unless metabolic need and vascular function are also considered. Although specific levels of cardiac index have been shown to separate survivors from nonsurvivors in certain situations (2.2 $L/min/M^2$,[33] for example), reported levels of cardiac output may be grossly inadequate for individuals with defective peripheral extraction or elevated oxygen requirements. Cardiac output determinations for such individuals are relatively meaningless unless considered together with additional data.

Noninvasive Measurement of Cardiac Function

Noninvasive methodology now available includes Doppler echocardiography and electrical impedance cardiography. The Doppler method measures the surface area of the aortic root and the velocity of blood flowing through this area; cardiac output is then velocity times surface area. Changes in the electrical impedance as an electrical current is passed through the skin from systole to diastole form the basis for the latter method.[34,35] Whether noninvasive measurement will find a role in acute management of critically ill patients remains to be determined; conceivably one might utilize these methods to judge the efficacy of therapeutic maneuvers such as volume expansion of the intravascular space or infusion of inotropic agents. However, an isolated cardiac output determination generally does not, in the absence of additional data, give information regarding the cause or consequence of reduced cardiac output. If reliable methodology for noninvasive determination of end diastolic volume and pulmonary capillary wedge pressure were also developed, invasive hemodynamic monitoring might become less necessary.

Direct Measurement of Cardiac Hemodynamics

Cardiac output is most commonly measured using a pulmonary artery balloon flotation catheter with a proximal port for infusion of saline and a temperature-sensing device at the tip. As saline is injected into the superior vena cava or right atrium, a time-temperature curve is generated. The mathematical equation which translates this information into cardiac output is complex, but is, in essence, a variation of the equation used for indicator-dilution methods where the cardiac output is calculated from the ratio of the injected volume to the average concentration of the indicator multiplied by time. The area under the indicator dilution curve (time-temperature curve for thermal dilution methods) is a reflection of the average concentration of the indicator. Since the volume of indicator is in the numerator, injection of less than the calculated amount through leakage would produce an erroneously high measured output because the curve would be smaller than predicted. Errors in estimating the area under the curve are greatest in patients with extremely low outputs, severe mitral or aortic regurgitation, or intracardiac shunts. Errors in the intensive care unit are encountered when an incorrect computer calibration factor is used or when the saline is injected at a variable rate; computers have recently been introduced which display the time-temperature curve graphically so that the operator may evaluate the quality of the curve. It is important to recognize that pressure changes within the thoracic cavity markedly affect cardiac output; injection of the saline bolus at various times in the respiratory cycle may introduce substantial variability in the measurements. For patients with large respiratory variation, it is wise to average three to five determinations.

Pulmonary Capillary Wedge Pressure

The importance of left and right ventricular filling volumes to evaluate the determinants of myocardial performance is discussed in Chapter 4. Since ventricular volume measurements were almost impossible to obtain in the intact human until recently, end-diastolic pressures have been used to estimate end-diastolic volumes. Measurement of left ventricular filling pressures via the pulmonary vascular bed takes advantage of the low resistance in most segments of that bed. The earliest hemodynamic technique was the wedging of cardiac catheters in pulmonary arteries to sample events in the left atrium. This pressure was termed either the pulmonary wedge pressure or the pulmonary capillary pressure. The balloon catheter permits isolation of a direct low-resistance pathway to the left atrium, which has a surprisingly close approximation of pressures in the left atrium. A number of names have been given to these indirect measurements: wedge pressure, capillary pressure, or pulmonary artery occlusion pressure. While the measurement is not really one of pulmonary "capillary" pressure, the terms pulmonary capillary wedge pressure (PCWP) and ventricular filling pressure will be used in this text. It cannot be overemphasized, however, that the PCWP, or even the directly measured left ventricular end-diastolic pressure, is not necessarily equivalent to left ventricular preload.[36] The Frank-Starling law described in Chapter 4 relates stroke output to ventricular fiber length or volume. The PCWP is, at best, an indirect reflection of length; the degree to which pressure and length are related depends on the degree to which compliance (dV/dP) remains constant. The left ventricle in patients with severe ischemic cardiomyopathy, for example, is very stiff (noncompliant). A change in wedge pressure of 5 mm Hg in these patients is associated with a much smaller increment in left ventricular muscular fiber length than would be observed in patients with a normally compliant ventricle at normal physiologic ranges of PCWP. It is becoming increasingly apparent that critically ill patients with a wide variety of disease processes other than primary cardiac disease such as sepsis or hemorrhage are characterized by considerable, though reversible, changes in myocardial compliance; in addition, many pharmacologic manipulations similarly affect ventricular compliances.[37] Since ventricular compliance may vary widely from patient to patient and from moment to moment in the same patient, interpretations of single pressure measurements must be made with great care. There is no single wedge pressure that identifies an optimal preload which is applicable to all patients or even to the same patient under differing conditions.

Effect of Respiratory Variation on PCWP Measurements: It is often difficult to determine the PCWP in critically ill patients because of the wide respiratory pressure swings observed in the tracing. The digital readout of most bedside monitors is reliable, but both positive and negative intrathoracic pressures may be transmitted to the tip of the pulmonary artery catheter in a different way than they are transmitted to the ventricular surfaces. These respiratory variations may profoundly affect left ventricular filling, but the pressure recorded during respiratory swings does not necessarily reflect preload. For example, during spontaneous inspiration, the measured PCWP will fall, sometimes to negative levels, even though left ventricular end-diastolic filling is actually increasing. Alternatively, during positive pressure mechanical ventilation, PCWP rises while ventricular filling is decreasing. The most reliable part of the PCWP tracing is the end-expiratory segment, where the tracing is stable and is close to the end-diastolic pressure.[38] Electronic devices that average pressures over several seconds do not discriminate respiratory variation from baseline. It is necessary to examine directly the oscilloscopic pressure tracing or, better yet, to measure hard copy obtained from a strip recorder. The value obtained at end-expiration can then be compared to the value obtained from the digital readout. Unfortunately, some patients exhibit such a large degree of respiratory variation that accurate measurement of the PCWP tracing is not possible without using neueromuscular blocking agents (although this is rarely wise). Strict reliance on digital readout will frequently reflect changes in respiratory variation to a greater degree than changes in left ventricular filling pressure; in other words, the values are most reflective of pressure changes in the wrong cavity!

Effect of PEEP on PCWP Measurement: Positive intrathoracic pressure, arising from either a mechanically delivered inspiration or positive end-expiratory pressure (PEEP), directly affects the PCWP, further complicating interpretation of the tracing. The cardiovascular effects of positive pressure ventilation are described in Chapter 7; this section deals with the estimation of left ventricular filling pressures in the presence of positive intrathoracic pressure. Decreases in compliance limit the transmission of airway pressures to the pleural space and blunt its effects on cardiac function; the lower the compliance, the less the transmission of airway pressure.[39] For example, 10 cm. PEEP may depress left ventricular filling in patients with normally compliant or those with the increased compliant lungs of chronic obstructive lung disease, while 20 cm. PEEP may not be transmitted to the catheter tip or pleural space in patients with severe homogenous ARDS and poorly compliant lungs. It is often difficult, however, to determine whether PEEP is transmitted to the pulmonary artery catheter tip of an individual patient. The catheter tip must be in zone III of West, where pulmonary artery and pulmonary vein are in open communication (chapter 6). A catheter tip in zone I would not be in communication with either the alveolar spaces or pulmonary veins, while one in zone II would directly reflect alveolar pressure. Lateral chest radiographs have been advocated for assurance that the catheter tip is in zone III,[40] but identification of the catheter tip is sometimes difficult. Other methods have been suggested for this purpose, but none seem completely satisfactory.[36]

Right Atrial Pressure

Isolated right ventricular dysfunction, or biventricular dysfunction, may be found in patients with cardiomyopathy, massive pulmonary embolus, right ventricular myocardial infarction, or those having had cardiac transplantation. Right atrial as well as PCWP must be carefully monitored in these patients. The right ventricle may dilate significantly as it responds to an increased pulmonary vascular resistance; at higher right ventricular end-diastolic pressures, the interventricular septum is pushed into the left ventricle, causing increased resistance to left ventricular filling (ventricular interdependence).[41] The elevated PCWP in this situation may reflect decreased left ventricular compliance rather than ventricular dilatation.

Stroke Work

The ready availability of hand-held computers at the bedside has led to the frequent calculation of stroke work. Oxygen requirements are directly related to work, so the calculation has some theoretic attractiveness. The work of moving an object along a plane is equal to force times distance; pressure and output are substituted for work. Left ventricular stroke work is calculated by the following equation:

$$\text{LVSW} = (\text{stroke volume})(\text{mean arterial pressure} - \text{PCWP})(0.0136)$$

where 0.0136 is a constant and work is expressed as gram meters (gm.M). The normal stroke work for the left ventricle using this calculation is 60–80 gm.M. Similar calculations may be made for the right ventricle using right atrial and mean pulmonary arterial pressure.

Volume work is much less oxygen costly than pressure work, and the calculation does not include heart rate. While a manipulation of primary data, it has been useful in studying overall cardiac performance.

Vascular Resistance

Pulmonary and systemic vascular resistances may also be calculated from the same pressure and flow data used for calculating work. In the work calculation they are multiplied together, in the resistance calculation the pressure drop across a vascular bed is divided by flow.

Vascular resistance calculations may be used to estimate afterload and classify patients into those with vasoconstriction or vasodilatation. These measurements do not really indicate afterload, since the internal geometric afterloading of the ventricle cannot be readily measured and is not included in the vascular resistance measurement.[41] Sequential measurements following pharmacologic intervention are generally quite useful.

Echocardiography

Availability of portable echocardiography for use at the bedside is occasionally lifesaving. Similar atrial and ventricular end-diastolic pressures suggest acute cardiac tamponade but intracardiac pressures are frequently difficult to interpret in the tachypneic or mechanically ventilated patient who has suddenly begun to deteriorate. An unexpectedly low cardiac output with elevated filling pressures in the absence of electrocardiographic evidence of acute myocardial ischemia or after insertion of venous catheters is a good indication for echocardiography. Cardiac perforations are more common in elderly patients.

EVALUATION OF SYSTEMIC OXYGEN DELIVERY

Many critically ill patients exhibit deficiencies of more than one determinant of oxygen delivery. An individual with a large mass of infarcted myocardium may, for example, exhibit hypoxic respiratory failure and dilutional anemia, as well as a low cardiac output. Raising cardiac output alone may not adequately increase oxygen delivery to the periphery. In addition, even raising oxygen delivery to levels considered normal for healthy individuals may not improve survival.[6]

At least three reasons account for the failure to improve survival when cardiac output, hemoglobin concentration, and oxygenation are raised to normal levels. While oxygen consumption is near normal in many critically ill patients, others must consume considerably more oxygen than normal in order to survive. An individual with a fixed cardiac index of 2.2 L/min/M^2 would not be capable of sustained strenuous activity, so it is not surprising that some critically ill patients with very high oxygen requirements are actually deficient in oxygen delivery even though values for all three determinants of O_2 delivery are "normal." Respiratory distress, anxiety and restlessness, convulsions, or inability to synchronize breathing with mechanical breathing aids may raise systemic oxygen consumption by 25%[42] because of increased respiratory muscle work. Severely burned patients frequently consume more than twice the amount of oxygen predicted for a healthy resting individual.[43]

Another reason for increasing oxygen delivery beyond normal levels is the failure of peripheral oxygen extraction. This is perhaps best demonstrated by the patient with sepsis, where a high output and low resistance state require high levels of systemic oxygen delivery for survival.[1] Marked increases in ventricular stroke work in these patients appear necessary to maintain arterial pressure, and may approach levels observed during maximal exercise. Finally, insufficient nutrient delivery, as well as oxygen delivery, may limit survival.

Recent clinical studies have shown striking relationships between systemic oxygen delivery, plasma lactic acid concentrations, and mortality.[6] Rashkin, Basken, and Baughman[44] have shown that lactic acid concentration remains normal until oxygen delivery falls to 8–10 ml/kg/min. At this point, lactic acid concentrations begin to rise and become more than fourfold elevated when oxygen delivery falls to 4 ml/kg/min. This rectangular hyperbola is similar to that shown for the production of high-energy phosphates and cellular oxygenation. Mortality was substantially greater at oxygen deliveries below the critical level of 8–10 ml/kg/min. A strategy for management of postoperative surgical patients, which has as its goal achievement of oxygen delivery and other hemodynamic variables, and which attempts to raise oxygen delivery and cardiac output to levels previously associated with survival has been proposed.[6]

There are problems with the application of oxygen delivery data in the clinical setting. Its calculation requires three independent measurements and is time consuming; oxygen delivery data may not be collected quickly enough to predict sudden deterioration in patient status. Peripheral oxygen sensors coupled to computer technology may, however, soon permit rapid monitoring of oxygen delivery. Even if rapid monitoring techniques were available, however, oxygen delivery data alone without consideration of oxygen consumption may be misleading.

Systemic Oxygen Consumption

Oxygen consumption can be calculated from the same data used for calculating oxygen delivery if mixed venous oxyhemoglobin saturation is available. The need for several independent measurements increases error, however, and oxygen consumption values can be expected to be accurate only to within approximately 20%. Apparatus for measuring oxygen consumption for ventilator-dependent patients is available and becoming increasingly accurate. Since energy requirements vary widely among critically ill patients, oxygen consumption measurements share the same limitations as those for oxygen delivery.

Plasma Lactic Acid Concentrations

The process of anaerobic glycolysis with the release of lactic acid has been discussed in Chapter 1. There is no question that metabolic acidosis associated with increased lactate production is associated with increased mortality.[44] A number of factors interfere with a more direct relationship between lactic acid concentrations and the mitochondrial energy state. Devices capable of measuring lactic acid levels rapidly at the bedside are now available[45] and may prove useful in determining the efficacy of various therapeutic interventions.

A rise is plasma lactic acid may be due to either an increase in its rate of generation or to a decrease in its rate of uptake by the liver. Since lactate is normally oxidized to pyruvate when oxygen is plentiful, the lactate to pyruvate (L/P) ratio has been used to estimate the oxidation-reduction status of the cell. This couplet is most active in the cytoplasm, however, and may not directly reflect mitochondrial events. Another couplet, beta-hydroxybutyric acid (BOHB) and acetoacetate (AcAc), is localized to the mitochondria and might be a more useful indicator of cellular oxygenation. Davies and Samuelson[46] studied the equilibrium of the two couplets during muscular exercise. Lactic acid rose fourfold, pyruvic acid twofold, and the L/P ratio doubled. In contrast, the BOHB/AcAc ratio was not significantly altered, suggesting that mitochondrial and cytoplasmic events might not be in equilibrium. The investigators then calculated the equilibrium ratio for each couplet and demonstrated that the relationship between the L/P and the BOHB/AcAc ratios was a useful indicator of oxygen delivery. Whether serum lactate levels or other plasma indicators will be shown to be sufficiently sensitive to detect clinically significant anaerobiasis and whether early detection improves outcome remains to be seen.

Mixed Venous Oxygen Saturation

Mixed venous Sv_{O_2} has been shown to predict mortality and systemic hemodynamics after open heart surgery or acute myocardial infarction. The recent introduction of fiberoptic reflectometry makes continuous monitoring of Sv_{O_2} readily available and requires evaluation of its overall usefulness.

Oxygen consumption ($\dot{V}_{O_2}$ cardiac output ($\dot{Q}s$), and oxygen extraction ($a - v_{O_2}$ difference) are all related by the Fick relationship ($\dot{Q}s = \dot{V}O_2/a{-}v_{O_2}$ difference) and Sv_{O_2} reflects oxygen extraction. An increase in Sv_{O_2} could be due to either an increase in oxygen consumption or a decrease in cardiac output. Since Sv_{O_2} is a good measure of oxygen extraction and also reflects tissue oxygenation, it might serve as an integrative approach to assessing oxygen delivery. Extraction rises and mixed venous saturation falls when oxygen need exceeds oxygen delivery, so Sv_{O_2} could be viewed as expressing the oxygen balance.

A cardiac output of 2.2, for example, is rarely adequate for a patient who has suffered massive multiple trauma, a large surface area burn, or severe respiratory distress. Such a cardiac output would certainly be associated with a significant decline in Sv_{O_2} (approximately 10%), which signals that increased systemic oxygen extraction has become necessary because oxygen delivery is inadequate. In general, Sv_{O_2} below 50% is a sign that oxygen delivery is becoming inadequate, and that compensatory mechanisms are becoming exhausted[16] although considerable variability is observed. Evaluation of the value of continuous Sv_{O_2} monitoring on morbidity and mortality is currently underway. Several groups of investigators have failed to find a correlation between Sv_{O_2} and individual determinants of oxygen delivery in patients.[47,48] Another group of investigators failed to find a correlation between Sv_{O_2} and lactic acidosis.[44] Availability of continuous information regarding oxygen extraction should allow the clinician to set therapeutic goals and judge the efficacy of individual therapeutic interventions.

Transcutaneous Oxygen Sensors

The transcutaneous oxygen sensing technique measures oxygen which diffuses through the skin. This value correlates best with arterial oxygen saturation, but becomes inaccurate during low cardiac output states[49] because of decreased dermal blood flow and increased dermal oxygen extraction. Transcutaneous oxygen sensors thus correlate well with systemic oxygen delivery in the patients studied thus far.

Monitoring Oxygen Transport in Regional Vascular Beds

Optimal care of the critically ill requires the maintenance of adequate oxygen supplies to all organ systems. Most of the methods available at present measure *total* rather than *regional* oxygen delivery.

Cerebral Circulation For awake individuals, cerebral perfusion can, of course, be assessed by frequent neurological exam. For anesthesized or comatose patients, however, current techniques, such as observation of pupil size or other cranial nerve function, lack specificity and sensitivity. Continuous monitoring technology would clearly be extremely useful since neural tissue is particularly sensitive to hypoxia; even quarter hourly neurological assessment of cranial nerve function may not be adequate. Monitoring is important in patients with head trauma and cerebral edema, where alterations in blood flow may suddenly and unexpectedly occur. A precise and reliable monitoring technique would be highly desirable in these clinical situations see chapter 9).

Continuous EEG monitoring is utilized in a number of centers during carotid endarterectomy, since the diseased vessel must be cross clamped during the procedure, and since the Circle of Willis is not always patent. The frequency of cerebral electrical activity is measured prior to and following cross clamping. Should activity slow significantly, a temporary shunt can be placed across the occluded vessel.

Conjunctival oxygen monitoring recently has been utilized to assess brain oxygenation. The conjunctivae are perfused by the ophthalmic artery; since this vessel is a branch of the internal carotid, a change in the oxygenation of the conjunctivae may reflect changes in the remainder of the ipsilateral brain. This technique appears valuable in the operating room and during CPR. It may prove useful in the intensive care unit.[50]

Intracranial pressure monitoring is an indirect measure of cerebral perfusion. Although blood flow through the brain is normally autoregulated within narrow limits over a broad range of blood pressure, swelling of the brain makes flow become pressure-dependent as blood vessels become compressed by the expanding brain. A higher perfusion pressure is required to maintain the same flow through vascular beds exhibiting increased resistance. Cerebral perfusion pressure is the difference between systemic pressure and intracranial pressure. When intracranial pressure rises to extremely high levels, blood flow may stop completely. While the measurement of intracranial pressure gives only partial information about cerebral perfusion, a rising pressure alerts the clinician to the likelihood that the brain is becoming hypoperfused. Measures to diminish intracranial pressure, to raise systemic pressure, or both may then be undertaken (chapter 9).

A more direct technique involves measurement of regional cerebral blood flow (rCBF). In this method, xenon 133 is injected into the internal carotid artery, and its arrival and clearance in the brain is monitored by eight scintillation detectors placed at the side of the patient's head. This technique has been found to give consistent results in patients with head injury, and to reflect therapeutic manipulations following head injury.[51]

Renal Circulation Although acute renal failure may be the consequence of many insults, hypoperfusion is a common etiology.[52] This may be the result of intense renal vasoconstriction during states of critically impaired system oxygen transport, leading to progressive diminution in renal oxygen supply and consumption. Oxygenation of the brain and myocardium is maintained at the expense of less important vascular beds. Following successful resuscitation, it is imperative that renal perfusion be maintained; two insults are rarely tolerated. Since these individuals are generally characterized by either low urine output or by a form of nephrogenic diabetes insipidus ("nonoliguric ATN"), invasive monitoring with a pulmonary artery balloon flotation catheter is occasionally employed for the reasons discussed.

Information regarding renal blood flow can be inferred from central hemodynamic monitoring. Prolonged depression of cardiac output has been associated with renal failure, while improvement of cardiac output is associated with improved renal function for postoperative cardiac bypass patients.

Skeletal Muscle Circulation within a Compartment Muscular injury following trauma, sustained compression, *circumferential* skin burns, or other insults may result in swelling with a fascial compartment. The pathophysiology of this syndrome is very similar to that described above for increased intracranial pressure. Elevated pressure within a compartment may lead to nerve compression, vascular insufficiency, and ultimately to rhabdomyolysis and death of the muscle. In the event of severe compression, only fasciotomy can preserve function. This procedure is, of course, unpleasant and incurs the risk of infection and prolonged convalescence. Physical findings suggesting the need for fasciotomy include pain, a feeling of tenseness on palpation, neurologic deficit, and myoglobinuria. Recent introduction of "wick" catheters represents an attempt to reduce the subjectivity required of the examining surgeon; hydrostatic pressure within the compartment may be assessed by measuring the height of a column of water within a thin glass tube inserted into the compartment.

Myocardial Circulation Perfusion of the myocardium is usually best assessed by the patient himself, who generally perceives pain during coronary insufficiency. Patients who are diabetic, sedated, intubated, or otherwise unable to communicate may, however, develop myocardial ischemia unexpectedly. Continuous EKG monitoring in most institutions is generally unreliable with regard to the sensitivity and specificity of ST segment changes. The increased secretion of catecholamines and other humoral mediators of the stress syndrome may produce secondary myocardial damage, and twelve-lead electrocardiographic recordings should be obtained at frequent intervals in patients suspected or known to have coronary artery disease. Individuals with peripheral vascular disease should be watched carefully, since they have a 10% chance of having triple vessel coronary disease even in the absence of a suspicious history or an abnormal electrocardiogram.

IMPROVING OXYGEN DELIVERY AND CONSUMPTION IN THE CRITICALLY ILL

Collection of data is of little value unless it affects therapeutic decisions. Methods for improving the determinants of oxygen delivery are detailed in this text; a summary of some of them follow.

Improving Oxygen Carrying and Releasing Capacity of the Blood

A reduction in hemoglobin is common in many clinical situations, and raising its concentration is an important option whenever acute or chronic blood loss appears to reduce oxygen delivery. Raising hemoglobin from 10 to 12 gm/dl, for example, increases oxygen delivery as much as increasing cardiac index from 1.8 to 2.2 L/min/M^2. Since fluorocarbons carry less than 25% of that carried by hemoglobin, human blood transfusion becomes the only useful approach. Unfortunately, blood is relatively scarce, expensive, and contaminated by potentially lethal infectious agents. Patients with normal myocardial and vascular reserves tolerate hematocrits as low as 20%. There is little agreement when blood should be administered in traumatic shock, and the decision in critically ill patients must balance the effect of oxygen delivery with the disadvantage of increasing blood viscosity. Increasing hematocrit to 30–35% seems sensible in patients with severe hypoperfusion due to hypovolemia or decreased myocardial contractility. On the other hand, reduction of hematocrits to levels below 30% salvages infarcted brain tissue[53] so that lower hematocrits are probably indicated in the presence of ischemic injury. The use of packed cells, fluids, and fresh frozen plasma to replace coagulation factor deficiencies is the most precise way of treating massive blood loss, but practical considerations usually dictate the use of some whole blood (see chapter 12).

Raising Arterial Oxyhemoglobin Saturation

Reversible atelectasis or alveolar edema are common causes of hypoxemia in critically ill patients. Reversing these fundamental abnormalities is the most direct way of raising arterial oxygen tension; attention to deep breathing, positioning, chair sitting where possible, and coughing dramatically increases arterial oxygenation. Supplemental oxygen or mechanical ventilation with positive-end expiratory pressure are necessary in many clinical situations (see chapter 7).

Increasing Regional Perfusion

Identifying and correcting hypovolemia rapidly improves oxygen delivery. Inotropes such as dobutamine and dopamine are indicated when a low cardiac output in a hypovolemic individual is identified. Maintainance of appropriate heart rates and normal sinus rhythm to take advantage of atrial contraction and afterload reduction are other important techniques for improving cardiac output. Intra-aortic balloon counterpulsation may be indicated in certain clinical situations (see chapter 5).

REFERENCES

1. Richards DW Jr, Cournand A, Darling RC, et al: Pressure of blood in the right auricle, in animals and in man: Under normal conditions and in right heart failure. *Am J Physiol* 1942; 136:115.

2. Cournand A, Riley RL, Bradley SE, et al: Studies of the circulation in clinical shock. *Surgery* 1943; 13:964–995.

3. Forssmann W: The catheterization of the right heart. *Klin Wochenschr* 1929; November:2085–2087.

4. Shoemaker WC, Montgomery ES, Kaplan E, et al: Physiologic patterns in surviving and nonsurviving shock patients. *Arch Surg* 1973; 106:630.

5. Finch CA, Lenfant C: Oxygen transport in man. *N Engl J Med* 1972; 286:407–415.

6. Shoemaker WC, Appel PL, Kram, HB: Comparison of two monitoring methods (central venous pressure versus pulmonary artery catheter and two protocols as therapeutic goals (normal values versus values of survivors) in a prospective randomized clinical trial of critically ill surgical patients. *Crit Care Med* 1985; 13:304(abst).

7. Robin ED: The cult of the Swan-Ganz catheter. *Ann Intern Med* 1985; 103:445–449.

8. Parrillo JE, Ayres SM: *Major Issues in Critical Care Medicine*. Baltimore, Williams & Wilkins, 1984.

9. Parrillo JE: Complications of central venous and flow-directed pulmonary artery catheters. *Crit Care Med* 1986; 1:1.

10. Siegel JH: Relations between circulatory and metabolic changes in sepsis. *Annu Rev Med* 1981; 32:175–194.

11. Giannelli S, Lambright BR, Marin MA: Spontaneous variability of the hemaglobin affinity for oxygen. *Crit Care Med* 1977; 5:150.

12. Shoemaker WC, Bland RD, Appel PL: Therapy of critically ill postoperative patients based on outcome prediction and prospective clinical trials. *Surg Clin North Am* 1985; 65:811–833.

13. Abboud FM, Helstad DD, Mark AL, et al: Reflex control of the peripheral circulation. *Prog Cardiovasc Dis* 1976; 18:371–403.

14. Cain SM: Peripheral oxygen uptake in health and disease. *Clin Chest Med* 1983; 4:139–148.

15. Guyton AC: Local control of blood flow by the tissues themselves, in *Textbook of Medical Physiology*. Philadelphia, WB Saunders, 1981.

16. Schlichtig R, Cowden WL, Chaitman BR: Tolerance of unusually low mixed venous oxygen saturation: adaptations in the chronic low cardiac output syndrome. *Am J Med* 1986; 80:813–818.

17. Wanman K, Shoemaker WC: Physiologic responses to massive intraoperative hemorrhage. *Arch Surg* 1982; 117:470–475.

18. Abelman WH, Kowalske H, McNeely W: The hemodynamic response to exercise in patients with Laennec's cirrhosis. *J Clin Invest* 1955; 34:690–695.

19. Shibutani K, Komatsu T, Kubal K, et al: Critical level of oxygen delivery in anaesthetized man. *Crit Care Med* 1983; 11:640–643.

20. Gorfinkel JH, Szidon JP, Hirsch LJ, et al: Renal performance in experimental cardiogenic shock. *Am J Physiol* 1972; 222:1260–1267.

21. Eisenberg PR, Jaffe AS, Schuster DP: Clinical evaluation compared to pulmonary artery catheterization in the hemodynamic assessment of critically ill patients. *Crit Care Med* 1984; 12:549–553.

22. Connors AF Jr, McCaffree DR, Gray BA: Evaluation of right-heart catheterization in the critically ill patient without acute myocardial infarction. *N Engl J Med* 1983; 308:263.

23. Maher JF: Pathophysiology of renal hemodynamics. *Nephron* 1981; 27:215–221.

24. Haas DC, Streeten DHP, Kim RC, et al: Death from cerebral hypoperfusion during nitropursside treatment of acute angiotensin-dependent hypertension M. *J Med* 1983; 95:1071–1076.

25. Cohn JN: Blood pressure measurement in shock. *JAMA* 1967; 199:118.

26. Maki DG: Infections associated with intravascular lines, in Remington J, Swartz M (eds): *Current Clinical Topics in Infectious Disease*. New York, McGraw-Hill, 1982.

27. Bedford RF: Long-term radial artery cannulation: effects on subsequent vessel function. *Crit Care Med* 1978; 6:64.

28. Gardner RM, Schwartz R, Wong HC, et al: Percutaneous indwelling radial artery catheters for monitoring cardiovascular function. *N Engl J Med* 1974; 290:1227.

29. Kim JM, Arakowa K, Bliss J: Arterial cannulation factors in the development of occlusion. *Anesth Analg* 1975; 54:836.

30. Bedford RF, Wallman H: Complications of percutaneous radial artery cannulation: An objective prospective study in man. *Anesthesiology* 1973; 38:228.

31. Morgan RJ, Martyn JAJ, Philbin DM, et al: Water metabolism and antidiuretic hormone response following thermal injury. *J Trauma* 1980; 20:468–472.

32. Duke M, Abelmann WH: The hemodynamic response to chronic anemia. *Circulation* 1969; 39:503–514.

33. Parr GV, Blackstone EH, Kirklin JW: Cardiac performance and mortality early after intracardiac surgery. *Circulation* 1975; 51:867–874.

34. Kubicek WG, Karnegis JN, Patterson RP, et al: Development and evaluation of an impedance cardiac output system. *Aerospace Med* 1976; 47:1046–1051.

35. Veigl VL, Judy WV: Reproducibility of haemodynamic measurements by impedence cardiography. *Cardiovasc Res* 1983; 17:728–734.

36. Raper R, Sibbald WJ: Mislead by the wedge? The Swan-Ganz catheter and left ventricular preload. *Chest* 1986; 89:427–434.

37. Sibbald WJ: Myocardial function in the critically ill: factors influencing left and right ventricular performance in patients with sepsis and trauma. *Surg Clin N A* 1985; 65:867–893.

38. Berryhill RE, Benumof JL, Rauscher LA: Pulmonary vascular pressure reading at end expiration. *Anesthesiology* 1978; 49:365–368.

39. Wallis TW, Robothom JL, Compean R, et al: Mechanical heart-lung interaction with positive end expiratory pressure. *J Appl Physiol* 1983; 54:1039–1047.

40. Shasby DM, Dauber IM, Pfister S, et al: Swan Ganz catheter location and left atrial

pressure determination. *Chest* 1981; 80:666–670.

41. Jardin FJ, Farcot JC, Boisante L, et al: Influence of positive end expiratory pressure on left ventricular performance. *N Engl J Med* 1981; 304:387–392.

42. Field S, Kelly SM, Macklem PT: The oxygen cost of breathing in patients with cardiorespiratory disease. *Am Rev Resp Dis* 1982; 126:9–13.

43. Saffle JR, Medina E, Raymond J, et al: Use of indirect calorimetry in the nutritional management of burned patients. *J Trauma* 1985; 25:32–39.

44. Rashkin MC, Basken C, Baughman RP: Oxygen delivery in critically ill patients: relationship to blood lactate and survival. *Chest* 1985; 87:580–584.

45. Clark LC, Noyes LK, Grooms TA, et al: Rapid micromeasurement of lactate in whole blood. *Crit Care Med* 1984; 12:461–464.

46. Davies AO, Samuelson WM: Assessing redox status in human plasma: Experience in critically ill patients. *Crit Care Med* 1986; 14:942–946.

47. Vaugn S, Puri V, Raheja R: Prediction of cardiac output changes from continuous mixed venous oxygen saturation measurements? *Crit Care Med* 1986; 14:339.

48. Astiz M, Rackow EC, Kaufman BS, et al: Relationship of mixed venous oxygen saturation to lactic acidosis in patients with circulatory shock. *Crit Care Med* 1986; 14:339.

49. Tremper KK, Shoemaker WC: Transcutaneous oxygen monitoring of critically ill adults, with and without low flow shock. *Crit Care Med* 1981; 9:706–709.

50. Abraham E, Smith M, Silver L: Conjunctival and transcutaneous oxygen monitoring during cardiac arrest and cardiopulmonary resuscitation. *Crit Care Med* 1984; 12:419–421.

51. OBrist WD, Langfitt TW, Jaggi JL, et al: Cerebral blood flow and metabolism in surgical patients with acute head injury. *J Neurosurg* 1984; 61:241–253.

52. Myers BD, Moran SM: Hemodynamically mediated acute renal failure. *N Engl J Med* 1986; 314:97–105.

53. Wood JH, Fleisher AS: Observations during hypervolemic hemodilution with acute focal cerebral ischemia. *JAMA* 1982; 248:2999–3004.

4 THE NORMAL CARDIOVASCULAR SYSTEM AND ITS REGULATION

Every aspect of the mammalian heart commands respect and demands admiration. The rhythmic shortening of each muscle, as myosin molecules embrace adjacent actin molecules in a tight but quickly reversible bond, is achieved by precise timing of disparate biochemical processes. A conducted electrical impulse opens the sodium and calcium channel gates and initiates the cardiac action potential, calcium influx releases stored calcium from the sarcoplasmic reticulum, a burst of energy is provided by calcium-mediated glycogenolysis, ionized calcium relieves the inhibitory action of tropomyosin (a specific enzyme located in the blunt end of each myosin molecule) and hydrolyzes adenosine triphosphate, and arms of myosin reach out and pull actin toward the parent myosin molecule, creating shortening and tension. And the entire process shifts from contraction to relaxation in a split second.

"There is a time when it moves, and a time when it is motionless," observed William Harvey more than 400 years ago.[1] He went on to note that the "motion of the heart consists in a certain universal tension" and that "the heart, at the moment of its action is at once constricted on all sides, rendered thicker in its parietes and smaller in its ventricles, and so made apt to project or expel its charge of blood." His iconoclastic and radical view that the "blood in the animal body is impelled in a circle, and is in a state of ceaseless motion; that this is the action or function which the heart performs by means of its pulse; and that is the sole and only end of the motion and contraction of the heart" set the stage for modern cardiovascular physiology. His observation that "when the heart begins to flag, to move more slowly, and as it were, to die," it "is soft, flaccid, exhausted, laying as it were, at rest," might be considered to have set the stage for modern critical care medicine.

The early physiologic studies of Frank in 1890[2] and Patterson, Piper, and Starling in 1914[3] were based on measurements of pressure, stroke output, and ventricular volumes. Studies beginning in the 1960s and culminating in the important volume published by Braunwald, Ross, and Sonnenblick in 1968,[4] borrowed concepts from the physical sciences and analyzed cardiac performance in terms of myocardial shortening and force development. These biophysical terms are now used daily by the practicing intensivist and have become the building blocks of cardiac physiology.

INTRODUCTION TO BIOPHYSICS

The fundamental quantities are mass, length, and time. All other quantities are derived from them. The following units are conventional in medical science: *mass*: grams (g); *length*: centimeters (cm); *time*: seconds. Certain derived qualities are important.

Velocity is the rate of change of distance with respect to time (t). It is actually dl/dt, or the first derivative (d) of length (l) (units: cm/second).

Acceleration is the rate of change of velocity (v), dv/dt, or the second derivative of length:

$$\frac{d^2l}{dt^2} \text{(units: cm/second}^2\text{)}$$

Force is an agent capable of accelerating a mass. The force required to give a mass of 1 g an acceleration of 1 cm/second^2 is 1 dyne. The gravitational attractive force of the earth upon a mass causes it to accelerate 980 cm/second^2. The force upon a 1 g mass is thus 1 g times 980 cm/second^2 or 980 dynes ($F = MA$; Newton's first law).

Pressure is force per unit area (units: dynes/cm^2). In medicine, pressure is generally expressed in the more common unit of the height of a column either of mercury or of water.

A column of mercury 10 cm high and of 1 cm^2 area contains 10 cm^3 of mercury that weighs 13.6 g/cm^3. The total column, weighing 136 g, constitutes a force acting on 1 cm^2 of area. Since force equals mass times gravitational acceleration, the total force in conventional units is 136 g times 980 cm/second^2. The pressure exerted is thus 133,280 dynes/cm^2. The force exerted by 1 mm Hg is the conversion factor for converting millimeters of mercury into dynes per square centimeter.

Work is an important physical and physiologic concept. Food material is metabolized to produce energy that is converted to mechanical work and heat. The efficiency of any engine is the ratio of useful mechanical work to total energy input. Many cardiac phenomena may be understood in terms of total work, external work, and efficiency. Work (*W*) is defined as force times distance (*L*). When a force is applied to a particle that is then moved, work is performed on that particle. If the force is constant over the period of application, the problem is relatively simple. A force of 1 dyne acting upon a body and moving it 1 cm performs 1 erg of work (1 erg = 1 dyne-cm). In physiology the force usually varies with distance, and work must then be calculated by integral calculus where:

$$W = \int FdL$$

The work done upon volumes of either blood or air is calculated by the equation:

$$W = \int PdV$$

where P equals pressure, V equals volume, and d equals first derivative.

Work is performed only if a body is moved some distance. While it is obvious that walking upstairs results in the performance of work, standing erect also requires work performance in maintaining muscle tension, imparting velocity to the blood, and for many other functions. Note that in general terms work always includes an intensity factor and a distance factor.

The history of the calculation of **cardiac work** emphasizes the difficulties in directly applying physical concepts to the human organism. **External cardiac work** is the work performed by the heart in pumping blood throughout the body. It is frequently calculated as:

$$W = (MAP - RAP)(SV)$$

where MAP equals mean arterial pressure, RAP equals right atrial pressure, and SV equals stroke volume. Suitable constants are included for dimensional accuracy. This is not strictly correct, since both pressure and cardiac volume change during systole. A more correct approximation of external work is given by the following expression derived from integral calculus:

$$W = \int PdV$$

where P is intraventricular pressure and V is cardiac volume.

A number of studies have shown that during the phase of isometric contraction, when no ejection occurs (no external work performed), oxygen is still required. The Hill concept described in this chapter suggests that even though the total length of a muscle fiber does not change, the contracting portion—the contractile element–does shorten as it generates tension.[5] Thus the most adequate description of work should include contractile element work performed when the total fiber remains isometric.

$$CEwork = \int FdL$$

where F is the force generated by the contractile element and L the length it shortens.

The heart muscle is essentially a biologic heat engine transforming energy from biologic oxidation (instead of burning fossil fuel). Cardiac function may also be analyzed in terms of the two general laws of thermodynamics:

Energy is the capacity to do work, and the first law describes the conservation of energy; energy can neither be created nor destroyed, but mechanical energy can be changed into heat energy where 4.18 joules is equivalent to one calorie.

The second law is based on the observation that heat cannot pass from a cold body to a hot body on its own accord. Systems tend to approach a state of equilibrium as the available energy in a system becomes unavailable. Entropy is the measure of the total quantity of unavailable energy. It, in theory, is always increasing as the amount of available energy in the universe is decreasing.

THE HEART

Cardiac muscle fibers originate and insert on the fibrous skeleton of the heart. Most of the ventricular fibers originate at the base of the heart (aortic and pulmonary annuli), spiral downward to the apex, and return as deeper fibers to be inserted at the site of origin. Each cardiac muscle fiber is actually a striated muscle cell ranging from 30 to 60 μ in length. Muscle cells connect to adjacent cells by a specialized derivative of the sarcolemma, termed the intercalated disc. Each cell is bounded by an anatomic sarcolemma, but since these cell boundaries offer little electrical resistance, the myocardium may be considered a functional syncytium.

Myocardial cells contain many strands called myofibrils that, under the light microscope, are seen to be crossbanded. Each myofibril is composed of a series of repeating elements, the sarcomeres, each delineated from its neighbor by dark lines, the Z lines. Another line, the M line, is observed in the center of each sarcomere, while a dark central zone is termed the A band. Lighter areas adjacent to the Z lines are termed I zones (see Fig 4–1).

Generously sprinkled between the myofibrils are cylindrically shaped structures, the mitochondria, which are the sites for oxidative phosphorylation. The tremendous oxygen requirements of the myocardium may be suspected from the observation that over one-fourth of the total myocardial mass is occupied by these mitochondria. The transverse tubular sys-

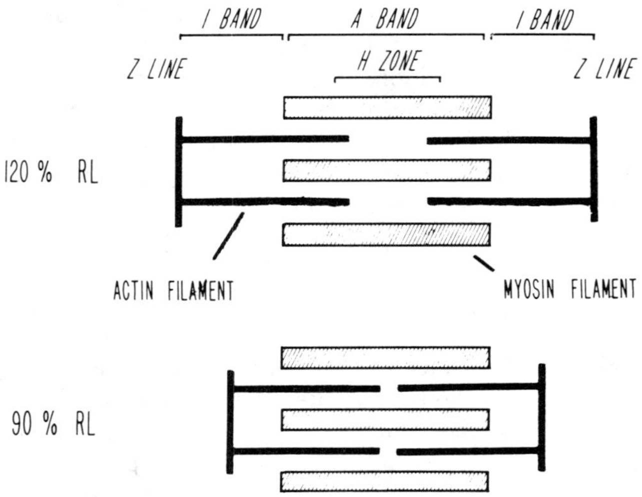

FIG 4–1.
Sliding model of contractile proteins. Contraction is initiated when the central myosin filament pulls adjacent actin filaments toward it, shortening the fiber. The *I* and *A* bands, the *Z* lines, and the *H* zone may be visualized by electron microscopy.

tem (*T* tubules) and the sarcoplasmic reticulum constitute an intracellular storage and transportation system. The *T* system is composed of sarcolemmal invaginations which arise near the *Z* lines and branch throughout the cell.[6] The sarcoplasmic reticulum, in contrast, is not continuous with the extracellular space, but expands into thin-walled cisternae as it approaches the *T* system. A relatively small proportion of the myocardial cell is allocated to the nucleus and the cytoplasm; important glycolytic enzymes are contained in the latter and constitute an important alternate source for energy generation, which may maintain membrane integrity during periods of stress.

The effector proteins, actin and myosin, and two regulatory proteins, troponin and tropomyosin, form the molecular basis of muscle contraction.[7] Each myosin molecule bears two heads that extend laterally and form crossbridges with the thinner filaments of actin during systole (Fig 4–1). These crossbridges propel the actin fibers toward the center of the sarcomere so that they shorten and develop tension in the same manner that many hands on a rope develop tension and ultimately take up on the rope in a tug of war. Depolarization of the sarcolemma releases calcium from the sarcoplasmic reticulum and initiates contraction by binding to troponin. Calcium binding to troponin produces conformational changes in tropomyosin, which make it shift out of the way so that actin-myosin bridges can form. Metaphorically, tropomyosin acts like a parent sitting between a teenage boy and girl. The parent exerts an inhibitory effect on romance. A phone call may be envisioned as calcium release, removing the parent from an inhibitory position and permitting a short-lived period of embrace.

The myosin heads have an additional function; they contain an enzyme ATPase, which is activated by contact with actin and hydrolyzes ATP, releasing energy for muscle contraction. Only ionized magnesium and ATP are needed to produce contraction in the absence of troponin and tropomyosin; when they are present, bridging does not occur unless ionized calcium is available. Recent studies have shown important relationships between myosin ATPase and velocity of muscle shortening, and it may function as an important regulator of myocardial contractility.[8] ATP seems to serve as a relaxing agent, or "plasticizer," as well as an energy source. When bound to the myosin heads, crossbridging is inhibited and the muscle is relaxed; when the bound ATP is hydrolyzed to ADP and inorganic phosphate, energy is released and muscle contraction occurs. The dead heart, for example, is in a state of rigor because ATP has been consumed and its inhibitory effect removed. Since unbridled ATPase activity would lead to a state of continued contraction, its dependence upon ionized calcium assumes great importance. Calcium not only relieves tropomyosin inhibition but also activates ATPase, so that ATP hydrolysis and actin-myosin bridging can occur simultaneously.

These events explain the effect of certain clinical states. A reduction in ionized calcium, which may not be evident from the more conventional measurement of total calcium, may decrease myocardial contractility. Acidosis produces the same effect, presumably by competing with calcium for binding sites on troponin. Catecholamines increase contractility by increasing calcium transport via a cyclic adenosine monophosphate (cAMP)-mediating mechanism;[9] they may do this in part by enhancing relaxation through increased activity of the sarcoplasmic reticulum. This would explain why catecholamines that increase cAMP (beta adrenergic agonists) relax vascular smooth muscle to cause vasodilatation.

The overall force of the contraction is a function of the number of binding sites between actin and myosin. Sonnenblick, Spiro, and Spotnitz[10] proposed that the Frank-Starling law of the heart is related do stretching of the sarcomere. The authors showed that the maximum muscular force is generated when the sarcomere is 2.2 μ in length, the length that theoretically provides the greatest area for actin and myosin interaction. If the sarcomere is shorter, there is less opportunity for actin and myosin interaction. If the fiber is stretched beyond the optimal length, the filaments are partially engaged, decreasing the force of contraction.

Mechanics of Isolated Muscle

The factors determining the stroke output and intraventricular pressure of a single contraction are best understood by considering the contraction of a single muscle fiber. The extent of shortening of that fiber is analogous to the stroke output; the force generated during shortening is the myocardial tension produced during cardiac contraction.

A number of aspects of muscular function are explained by the model for frog sartorius muscle proposed by Hill.[5] Figure 4–2 shows the three elements of

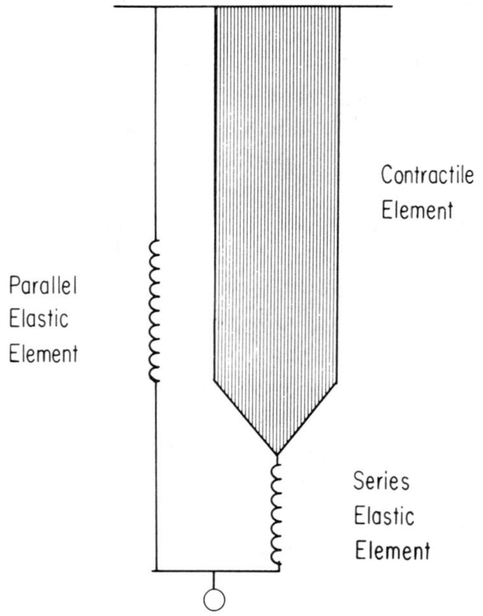

FIG 4–2.
Hill model of a muscle fiber shows a contractile element in series with an elastic element. Another elastic element is in parallel with the entire muscle fiber. (From Ayres and Gregory: *Cardiology: A Clinicophysiologic Approach*, East Norwalk, Conn., Appleton-Century-Crofts, 1981. Used by permission.)

this model. A contractile element (the myofibril) is in series with a passive elastic component, while another passive elastic component is in parallel with both the contractile element and the series elastic component. A general discussion of the model is beyond the framework of this book, but a single example may serve to explain the general utility of the concept. During isometric contraction the overall length of the fiber does not change, but according to model theory the contractile element does shorten and stretches the series elastic component. Since work is defined as force times distance, external work is not performed because the muscle does not shorten. A number of experiments demonstrated that isometric contraction with the production of muscle tension requires oxygen even though external work is not performed. The Hill model indicates that internal work—shortening of the contractile element—is performed and that this internal work requires oxygen consumption. Thus isometric contraction with the development of high degrees of muscle tension is costly in terms of oxygen consumption even though external work is not performed.

The properties of a single muscle fiber are generally studied by allowing it to contract under either isotonic or isometric conditions. Three basic attributes and three interrelationships are examined under these conditions:

Basic attributes: muscle length, force generated, velocity of shortening

Interrelationships: length-force relationship, force-velocity relationship, length-velocity relationship

Figure 4–3 illustrates the conduct of such a muscle experiment. The muscle fiber is fixed at the upper end, and a small weight or preload that determines its resting length is attached to the lower end. Another weight is attached to the lower end but is supported by a platform rather than the muscle. This weight is termed the afterload, since it is not sensed by the muscle until it begins to shorten. The rate of muscle shortening is maximum with minimal afterloads, and decreases as the afterload is increased. The experiment is continued by measuring the velocity of shortening with various afterloads, and a force-velocity curve is plotted. The force-velocity curve defines the function of the contractile element. Since force and veloc-

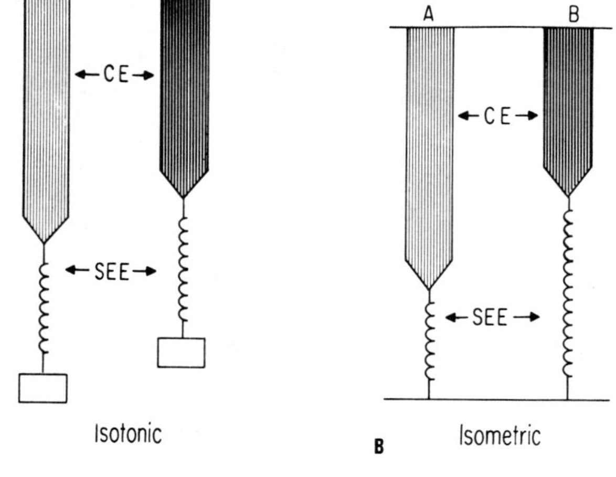

A

B

FIG 4–3.
Isotonic contraction (*A*) when the contractile element shortens and lifts a weight (afterload) attached to the lower end of the fiber. In an isometric contraction (*B*) the overall weight of the muscle is fixed but the contractile element shortens as it stretches the series elastic element. In both examples the contractile element performs work by shortening. (From Ayres and Gregory: *Cardiology: A Clinicophysiologic Approach*, East Norwalk, Conn., Appleton-Century-Crofts, 1971. Used by pemission.)

ity are related, neither may be used as an independent measure of the contractile state of the muscle fiber. Figure 4–4 shows such a force-velocity curve and demonstrates that the addition of an inotropic agent, such as norepinephrine, shifts the curve to the right and upward (increasing force for the same velocity), while the curve shifts to the left in situations associated with a decrease in myocardial contractility.

The contraction described above is termed isotonic because the load applied remains constant. When the load is so great that the muscle cannot shorten, maximum force is generated, and the contraction is termed isometric. Extrapolation of the force-velocity curve reveals that maximum velocity occurs as force approaches zero, while maximum force occurs as the velocity of shortening approaches zero.

The relationship between muscle length and force may be investigated by applying various preloads to the muscle and thereby varying initial length. The extremely important relationship demonstrated by this experiment is that increasing initial length increases both the force and extent of shortening of the subsequent contraction. The same preparation demonstrates that increasing initial length increases the velocity of shortening.

The effects of increasing muscle length (increasing preload), increasing the amount of developed tension (increasing afterload), and increasing the contractile state on the extent of muscle shortening have important implications for the function of the intact ventricle (Table 4–1).

Function of the Intact Ventricle

The principles outlined above for single muscle fibers apply equally well to the intact ventricle, but the disposition of muscle fibers around a central cham-

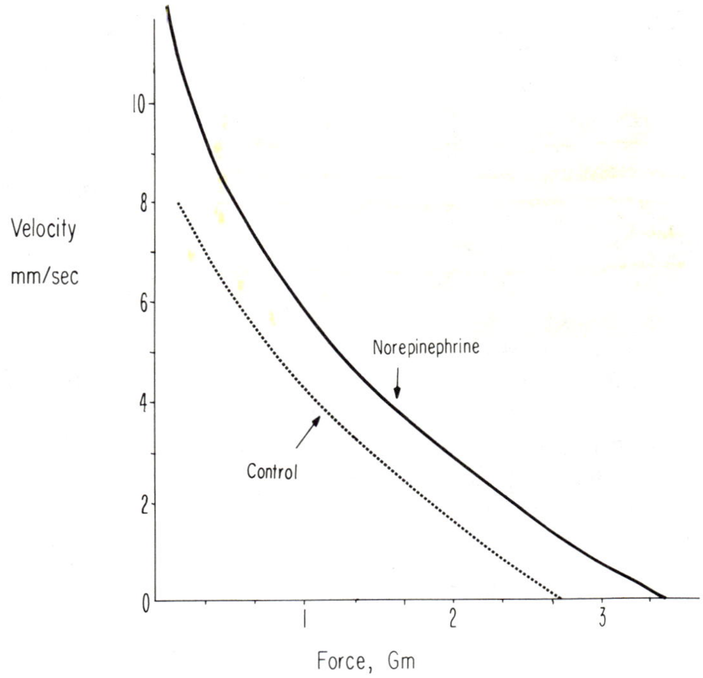

FIG 4–4.
Relationship between velocity of shortening and force or afterload during isotonic contraction. The velocity of contraction decreased with increasing afterload. The curve intersects the abscissa at the point of iscmetric contraction. Extrapolation of the curve to zero load allows calculation of the theoretic value *V max*, which represents the maximum velocity of shortening that would occur if no load was present. Addition of a positive isotropic agent, such as norepinephrine, shifts the curve to the right and upward. (From Ayres and Gregory: *Cardiology: A Clinicophysiologic Approach*, East Norwalk, Conn., Appleton-Century-Crofts, 1971. Used by permission.)

TABLE 4–1.
Effects of Manipulation on Ventricular Function

	INCREASED PRELOAD	INCREASED AFTERLOAD	INCREASED CONTRACTILITY
Extent of shortening (stroke volume)	Increases	Decreases	Increases
Velocity of shortening	Increases[a]	Decreases	Increases
Developed force	Increases	Increases	Increases

[a]V_{max} is not increased, but instantaneous velocities early in ventricular contraction are increased.

ber produces certain functional variations from that of simple fibers. Moreover, a number of assumptions must be made in order to study the intact ventricle in the same manner as a simple muscle fiber.

The initial phase of ventricular contraction, with both aortic and mitral valves closed, resembles isometric contraction in the isolated fiber. This is properly called isovolumic contraction because, although the length of individual fibers may change, ventricular volume is constant. The individual fibers develop tension, the contractile elements shorten and perform work, oxygen is consumed, but the overall dimensions are unchanged, and ejection does not occur.

The relationship between myocardial wall tension and intraventricular pressure is expressed by the LaPlace law, in which intraventricular pressure (P) is directly proportional to wall tension (T) and inversely proportional to the diameter (D) of the cavity ($P = 4T/D$). This relationship indicates that with increasing cardiac dilatation, greater tension is required to achieve a given intraventricular pressure. Thus, individual muscle fibers from a heart with myocardial failure may be required to generate several times as much tension as fibers from a nondilated heart.

The myocardium can increase its force of contraction either by increasing its initial fiber length or by an actual increase in myocardial contractility. In 1895 Frank first showed that the force-length relationship of skeletal muscle also applied to cardiac muscle.[11] Starling extended these observations and, in 1918, summarized the relationship between ventricular volume and stroke output.[12] Although initially Starling's law was accepted as the major cardiac control mechanism in the human, studies performed between 1920 and 1940 by other investigators minimized its importance in the intact heart and considered it to be primarily a property of the isolated heart preparation. Sarnoff and Berglund[13] rescued the Starling concept from oblivion by demonstrating that the end-diastolic pressure-stroke output relationship held if one considered that different relationships existed for different inotropic states.

A convenient method of describing the relationship between end-diastolic fiber length or end-diastolic volume and stroke work is shown in Figure 4–5. Stroke work (roughly equal to stroke volume multiplied by mean arterial pressure) is plotted on the ordinate against end-diastolic pressure. While end-diastolic fiber length or volume is the appropriate abscissal value, end-diastolic pressure is commonly substituted in human studies, since it is readily measured at cardiac catheterization. Note that stroke work increases considerably with little increase in end-diastolic pressure until

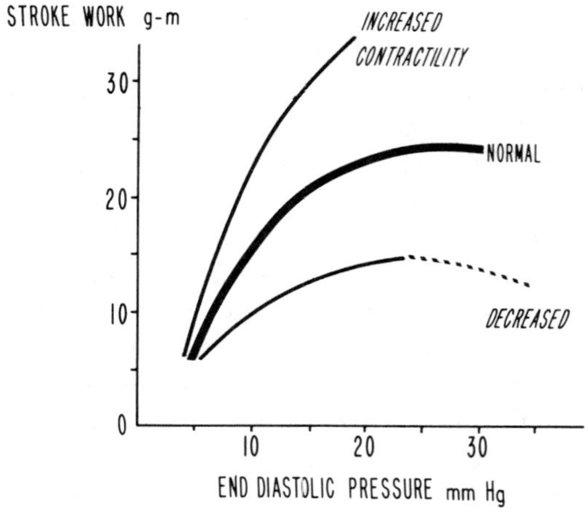

FIG 4–5.
An increase in stroke work for the same end-diastolic pressure indicates increased myocardial contractility and may be produced experimentally by the administration of catecholamines. A less than normal increase in stroke work with increasing end-diastolic pressure indicates decreased myocardial contractility. The dotted line is the so-called descending limb of the Frank-Starling curve. It is not clear whether such a descending limb occurs in human heart failure or shock.

the latter reaches 15 mm Hg. Above this point, further increase in end-diastolic pressure produces minimal increases in stroke work. Many diseased hearts appear to be on the upper portion of this curve in the region where increased end-diastolic volume might produce a decrease rather than an increase in stroke work.

The family of ventricular function curves was emphasized by Sarnoff and Berglund[13] in their restoration of the Starling concept (Fig 4–5). An inotropic influence, such as norepinephrine, causes a shift to the left, while decreased myocardial function produces a shift to the right.

Unfortunately, end-diastolic pressure is not a linear function of end-diastolic fiber length, although it is a useful clinical approximation. Considerable stretching of the fiber may occur before end-diastolic pressure rises appreciably (Fig 4–6). The relationship between end-diastolic pressure and fiber length is further complicated by alterations in ventricular distensibility (compliance). The curve on the left in Figure 4–6 is from a patient with concentric hypertrophy of the left ventricle and decreased ventricular distensibility. For the same end-diastolic fiber length, a much higher end-diasatolic pressure is observed. The patient might appear to be on the upper part of the Frank-Starling curve and to demonstrate ventricular failure if end-diastolic pressure were plotted against stroke work. Correct calculations, using end-diastolic fiber length, would indicate that the patient was still operating on a normal lower portion of the curve.

Ventricular end-diastolic volume has been demonstrated to be an important determinant of stroke output in many clinical situations. The relationships between end-diastolic volume, pulmonary capillary wedge pressure, and stroke output vary widely in critically ill patients, however, because of changes in ventricular compliance (see chapter 5).

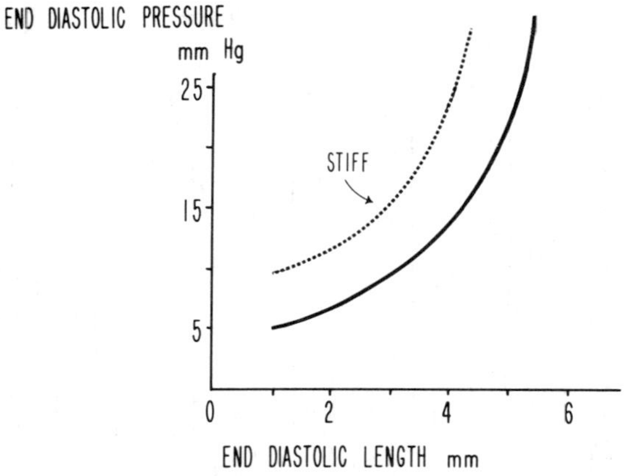

FIG 4–6.
Relationship of end-diastolic pressure to end-diastolic length. End-diastolic length cannot be readily predicted from measurements of end-diastolic pressure. End-diastolic pressure is significantly higher for the same fiber length in patients with stiff or noncompliant ventricles.

Ventricular Function in Man

Although obviously limited by constraints in experimental design, the properties shown to exist for both simple muscle fibers and the intact experimental ventricle have also been shown to exist for the human ventricle.

The ready accessibility of the cardiac chambers to the cardiac catheter permitted the design of a number of studies using end-diastolic pressure as an index of end-diastolic fiber length. Lewis et al.,[14] in a study whose results were subsequently confirmed by a number of laboratories, demonstrated a relationship between pulmonary wedge (left atrial) pressure and left ventricular stroke work in a series of patients with left ventricular malfunction. Both pulmonary wedge pressure and stroke work rose during exercise in patients with normal resting pressures, but stroke work generally did not increase in patients with elevated pressures at rest. These authors were able to construct curves relating stroke index to pulmonary wedge pressure and suggested that these curves were similar to the Starling curves obtained from the isolated heart preparation.

Other studies in which ventricular end-diastolic pressure was observed to vary spontaneously have also confirmed the presence of a relationship between end-diastolic fiber length and stroke output in man. Respiratory maneuvers, such as the Valsalva intervention, alter ventricular filling and change end-diastolic pressure. Left ventricular and aortic systolic pressure vary with end-diastolic pressure, as predicted from the Starling relationship. The changing diastolic filling time observed in atrial fibrillation changes end-diastolic volume, fiber length, and pressure. Figure 4–7 shows a series of left ventricular beats from a patient with atrial fibrillation, demonstrating that left ventricular systolic pressure varies with the end-diastolic pressure of the preceding diastolic interval.

Perhaps one of the most interesting demonstrations of the effect of end-

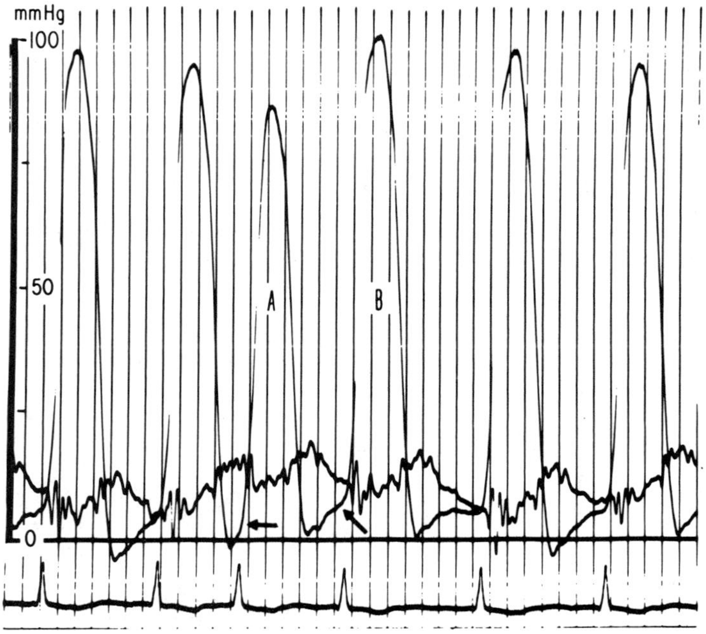

FIG 4–7.
Starling's law shown in a series of left ventricular beats from a patient with atrial fibrillation. The arrows indicate end-diastolic pressure following a short and a long diastolic filling period. The short filling period produces diminished ventricular volume, a low end-diastolic pressure, and a relatively low systolic pressure (A). A longer filling period increases diastolic volume, augmenting left ventricular end-diastolic and systolic pressure (B). (From Ayres and Gregory: *Cardiology: A Clinicophysiologic Approach*, East Norwalk, Conn., Appleton-Century-Crofts, 1971. Used by permission.)

diastolic pressure on ventricular pressure and stroke work is that observed with varying the position of atrial systole. Atrial systole normally augments cardiac output, and its relationship to ventricular systole determines, in part, the effect of an arrhythmia on cardiac output. Figure 4–8 shows the dependence of ventricular systolic pressure on the timing of the preceding atrial contraction wave in a patient with complete heart block. Complete atrioventricular dissocation was present, causing the relationship between atrial and ventricular contraction to vary from beat to beat. A properly timed atrial systole raises end-diastolic pressure and volume, increasing the force of the subsequent ventricular contraction. Systolic pressure is significantly lower with prolongation of the P-R interval or with delay of atrial contraction, so that it falls during ventricular systole.

Cardiac Volume

Left ventricular volume may be calculated from left ventricular angiocardiograms by considering the ventricle to be an ellipsoid. Dodge et al.[15] refined this technique, so that left ventricular volume may be accurately determined either from films exposed in a rapid film changer or from cineangiocardiograms. The cineangiocardiograms have the advantage of permitting more exposures per beat. Although somewhat laborious, instantaneous changes in cardiac diameters and volumes may be calculated throughout the cardiac cycle by the cineangiocardiographic technique.

A number of important measurements may be derived from the quantitative left ventricular angiocardiogram. End-diastolic volume (*EDV*) is the ventricular volume immediately prior to systole, while end-systolic volume (*ESV*) is the volume immediately following systolic ejection. The stroke volume may be calculated as the difference between *EDV* and *ESV*. The systolic ejection fraction, the ratio between stroke volume and *EDV*, may be readily calculated and appears to be a useful index of left ventricular function. Another index expressing the residual volume of the ventricle is the ratio between *ESV* and *EDV*. Regurgitant flow may be calculated using an independent technique for cardiac output, such as the Fick method or an indicator-dilution technique. Since these techniques measure forward flow while the angiographic technique measures total ventricular out-

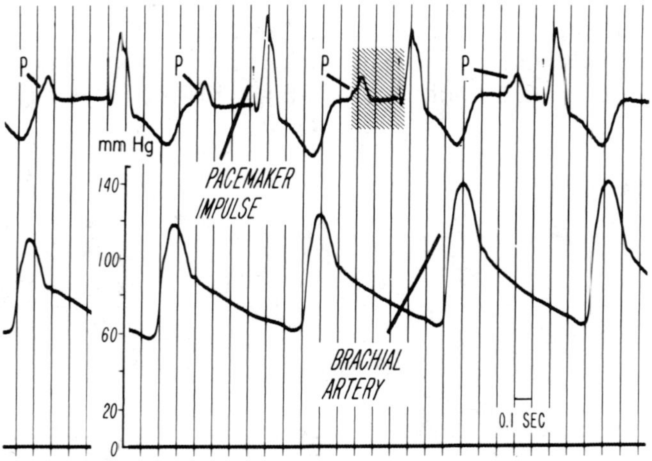

FIG 4–8.
Regular ventricular contractions were maintained in a patient with complete heart block by electrical pacemaking. A somewhat longer interval between the patient's spontaneously occurring atrial contraction waves permitted observation of the effect of P-R interval on the subsequent ventricular contraction. The highest arterial pulse pressure (reflecting stroke volume) is noted when atrial systole precedes ventricular systole by 0.1 to 0.3 second. The optimal P-R interval is shown by the hatched area.

put, the regurgitant flow is obtained by subtracting the angiocardiographic stroke volume from either the Fick or indicator-dilution stroke volume.

The following data were obtained by Kennedy et al[16] in 21 patients with normal left ventricles: *EDV* 124, *SV* 82, *ESV* 42, *SEF* 0.67, *SV* (Fick or dye) 87. All of the values are presented in milliliters per beat, except for the systolic ejection fraction, which is a ratio of stroke volume to end-diastolic volume. In practice, the volumes are expressed as milliliters per square meter of body surface.

The angiocardiographic techniques are not suitable for serially measuring changes in ventricular volume. In addition, the rapid injection of contrast media may significantly alter ventricular and peripheral vascular function. A number of investigators have evaluated the dilution of a single bolus of indicator injected into the left ventricle as a technique for measuring ventricular volume.

If a suitable sensing system and indicator are used, the concentration of indicator in the aorta falls in a stepwise manner following ventricular injection. Stated differently, indicator is washed out of the ventricle by each diastolic filling of blood not containing the indicator. The difference in aortic concentration of indicator on successive beats depends upon the end-diastolic volume and upon the stroke volume. In practice, the stroke volume is calculated from an independent measure of cardiac output, and end-diastolic volume is calculated from the following formula, where *A* and *B* are the concentration of indicator in the aorta corresponding to two succesive beats.

$$EDV = SV \div (1 - \frac{B}{A})$$

This technique is admirably suited to the measurement of serial ventricular volumes during experimental intervention. Unfortunately, because of poor dye mixing, estimates of end-diastolic volume by this technique are considerably larger than those obtained by the angiographic technique. Table 4–2[17] compares indicator-dilution and angiographic measurements in humans without myocardial disease.

A recently introduced right ventricular thermistor catheter has a much more rapid response time than the standard pulmonary artery flotation thermistor. This catheter demonstrates beat to beat changes in right ventricular temperature and can be used to calculate right ventricular end-diastolic volume. Simultaneous measurement of right ventricular stroke volume allows calculation of right ventricular ejection fraction and also the beat to beat display of the right ventricular end-diastolic volume and stroke output relationship. For the first time, the actual determinants of the Starling relationship may be plotted for a ventricle in the critically ill patient.

TABLE 4–2.
Indicator–Dilution and Angiographic Measurements in Patients Without Myocardial Disease

MEASUREMENT	EDV (ml/M^2)	ESV/EDV (%)
Angiography	80 ± 10	30 to 40
Indicator-dilution method	130 to 210	65 to 80

Data adapted from Sanmarco ME, Bartle SH: Left Ventricular volume determinations: comparison of angiocardiographic and thermal washout techniques. *Circulation.* 1964; 30(Suppl III): 151.)

Instantaneous Tension-Velocity-Length Relationships in the Intact Ventricle

Many of the techniques presented in the sections above are obviously unsuited to application in the conscious human subject. Gault, Ross, and Braunwald[18] measured instantaneous ventricular volume throughout the cardiac cycle by an angiocardiographic technique and intraventricular pressures by a pressure manometer positioned on the end of a cardiac catheter. A unique display system permitted left ventricular pressure, the first derivative of ventricular pressure, and brachial arterial pressure to be photographed on the same film strip as the angiocardiogram. Left ventricular wall tension was measured at frequent intervals during systole by a formula involving intraventricular pressure, and the instantaneous ventricular radius was obtained from the angiocardiogram. An index related to the velocity of shortening of isolated fibers—the circumferential fiber shortening velocity—was calculated for each interval using a geometric formula relating the shortening of the radius of a circle to the shortening of its circumference. Studies were performed on six normal subjects and on nine with left ventricular disease.

These studies demonstrated that, in the normal ventricle, left ventricular wall tension became maximal soon after ejection and then declined rapidly. The normal ventricle changed its dimensions rapidly during systole, so that the velocity of circumferential fiber shortening ranged from 1.66 to 2.71 circumferences per second. In the group with left ventricular disease, left ventricular wall tension did not fall rapidly during ejection and rose to considerably higher than normal levels with more severe grades of left ventricular disease because of the increased ventricular dimensions. The velocity of circumferential fiber shortening was consistently less in these patients and ranged from 0.22 to 1.11 circumferences per second.

The Regulation of Stroke Output

The amount of blood ejected by each systolic contraction is directly related to the extent of myocardial fiber shortening and reduction in circumferential size. Studies on isolated muscle fibers have shown that the extent of shortening is related to the initial stretch of the muscle (the preload), the load the muscle is asked to move as it shortens (the afterload), and the rate of generation of cross-linkages between actin and myosin (the state of contractility).[19]

Applying these determinants to the intact ventricle requires the measurement of volume. Pressure-volume curves were first described by Frank,[2] but were somewhat eclipsed by the studies of Patterson, Piper, and Starling,[3] who emphasized the relationships between end-diastolic pressure and stroke output. Much of this shift was methodologic because the latter group did not measure ventricular volumes. Carl Wiggers used ventricular volume measurements to describe the function of the heart in shock.[20] In a sense, the Starling emphasis was on the amount of blood ejected from the ventricle, while the Frank emphasis was on the amount remaining in the heart at the end of systole. Although many investigators made important contributions to the study of ventricular control, Braunwald, Ross and Sonnenblick developed an approach particularly useful for bedside evaluation. They demonstrated, both in isolated muscle and in intact animal and human hearts, that stroke output was determined by preload (ventricular end-diastolic fiber length), afterload (systemic vascular resistance and the internal resistance of the ventricle to contraction), and myocardial contractility (Fig 4–9). Sibbald, Calvin, and Driedge

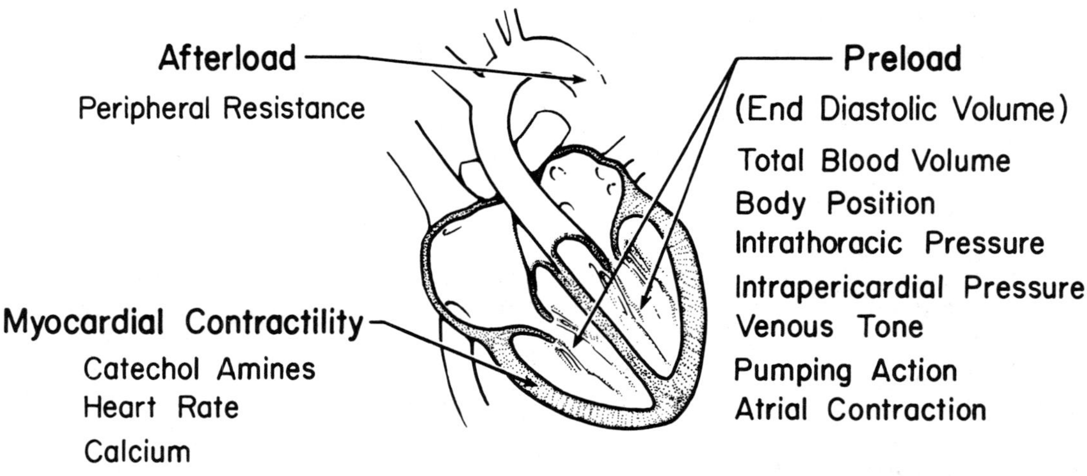

FIG 4–9.
Summary of the factors affecting the extent of muscle shortening and thus stroke output. Increasing either preload or myocardial contractility increases stroke volume, while increasing afterload decreases stroke volume. The stroke volume resulting from any given intervention depends on the effect of the intervention on preload, afterload, and myocardial contractility.

took the analysis one step further by pioneering the use of radionuclide ventriculography to measure ventricular preload and diastolic compliance in critically ill patients.[21] A detailed discussion of ventricular afterload may be found in Chapter 3.

The events of the cardiac cycle can be studied by means of pressure-volume curves (Fig 4–10). Left ventricular filling begins with mitral valve opening (*MVO*) as ventricular pressure falls below that of the atrium. The diastolic pressure-volume curve reflects the stiffness or compliance of the ventricle, and demonstrates the important point that pressure is not a linear function of volume. Pressure rises more steeply as the ventricle fills, and is proportionately lower in a dilated ventricle and higher in a rigid ventricle. For these reasons, left atrial pressure measurements must be interpreted with attention to diastolic volume and cardiac size.

The mitral valve closes (*MVC*) and pressure rises steeply during the phase of isovolumic contraction. The aortic valve opens (*AVO*) shortly thereafter and the stroke volume is ejected as pressure rises even higher. The aortic valve then closes (*AVC*) and ventricular pressure falls during the period of isovolumic relaxation. The blood remaining in the ventricle at the end of systole is the residual volume of the ventricle and averages 40–50 ml in the normal heart. The percentage of the end-diastolic volume ejected, the ejection fraction, averages 55–70% in the normal individual.

Changing diastolic compliance prevents pulmonary capillary wedge pressure from predicting volume in many critically ill patients. The alpha adrenergic blocking agent, phentolamine, and other vasodilators improve ventricular compliance so that PCWP falls without significant changes in left ventricular volume.[22] Thus, arterial vasodilators improve stroke output by increasing compliance as well as by decreasing afterload. Calvin, Driedger, and Sibbald[23] showed that several responses could be observed with fluid loading in critically ill patients. When ventricular volumes were low, a

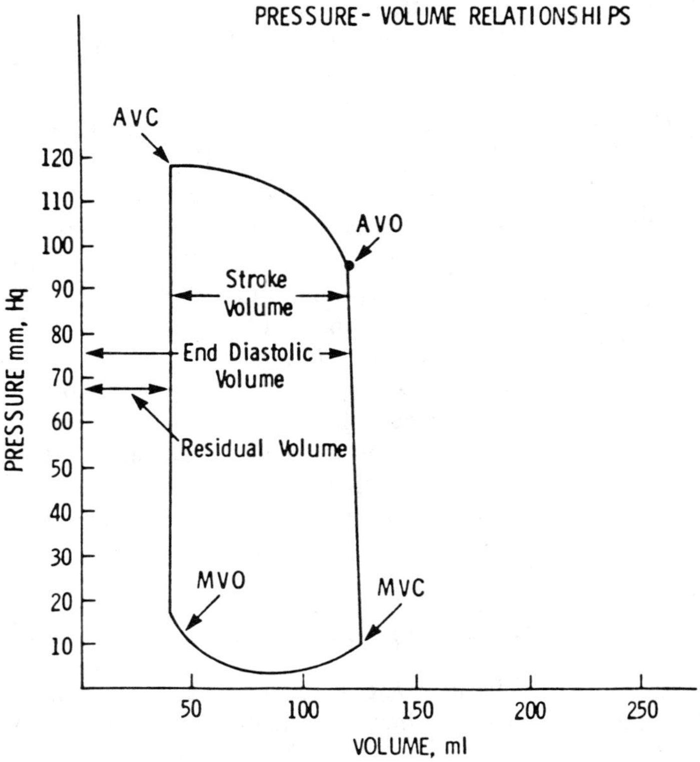

FIG 4–10.
The relationships among stroke volume, residual volume, and end-diastolic volume may be visualized in the pressure-volume diagram of the heart. See text for complete description.

20-minute infusion of 250 ml of albumin produced the expected increase in stroke output and end-diastolic volume. Wedge pressure, however, did not significantly change. In patients with abnormally large ventricular volumes and low pulmonary capillary wedge pressures, stroke volume increased in association with a statistically significant *decrease* in left ventricular end-diastolic volume. The increase in stroke output following fluid administration in patients with increased ventricular volumes suggests that fluid replacement may decrease afterload.

Ventricular interdependence can also produce changes in ventricular compliance. Increased right ventricular pressure and volumes due to pulmonary hypertension of positive end-expiratory pressure can cause the ventricular septum to bulge into the left ventricle. The septal shift alters left ventricle geometry and reduces its volume so that smaller volumes are accommodated at higher pressures and stroke output falls.[24] Left ventricular distension can produce a similar effect on right ventricular function.

CIRCULATORY RESPONSE TO EXERCISE

Successful adaptation to environmental stress characterizes mammalian evolution, and the ability to regulate oxygen consumption and cardiac output to metabolic need stands high in the list of evolutionary accomplishments. While a number of human and animal studies demonstrated that cardiac output is closely adjusted to oxygen demands, the precise description of the human response to exercise was delineated only recently. The cardiovascular response to exercise is complex and involves both the peripheral circulation and the heart.

Peripheral Circulatory Response to Exercise

Local arteriolar dilatation during exercise increases peripheral blood flow and oxygen availability. This local vasodilatation is believed to be due to either cellular hypoxia or the accumulation of unoxidized metabolites; it is termed autoregulation.[25] Adenosine diphosphate (ADP) is a potent vasodilator, for example, and accumulates in tissues during periods of hypoxia. The increase in cardiac output observed with exercise is commonly believed to be caused by generalized peripheral dilatation with decrease in ventricular afterload. One experiment in support of this thesis is the observation that cardiac output does not increase in an exercising experimental animal if peripheral vascular resistance is maintained at resting levels by inflating a balloon around the aorta.[26]

Two factors—an increase in peripheral venous tone and pumping action of the skeletal muscles—increase venous return and compensate for the venous pooling that occurs in the erect position. The increase in venous tone is due to the effect of muscle contraction externally compressing venous structures and to increased autonomic discharge that increases tone in both exercising and nonexercising veins.

Arteriolar tone depends upon the balance of peripheral metabolic autoregulation, tending to dilate arterioles, and autonomic discharge, tending to constrict them. Regional beds—such as those in the kidney, splanchnic system, and skin—constrict because autonomic constrictor forces are not balanced by autoregulatory dilator forces. In consequence, blood is shunted from these organ systems to skeletal muscle. The regulation of the peripheral circulation is considered in more detail in the section on the autonomic nervous system.

Cardiac Response to Exercise

The increase in cardiac output demanded by peripheral metabolic needs could be met by increasing either heart rate or stroke output.

The role of alterations in stroke volume in the response to exercise has caused a major controversy in the field of car-

TABLE 4–3.
Circulatory and Ventilatory Response to Standing and Exercise

PARAMETER	REST, SUPINE	REST, STANDING	Walking 3mph[a] 0	8%	16%
Minute ventilation (liters/minute/meter)	4.67	7.35	12.81	20.71	34.61
Oxygen consumption (ml/minute)	269	351	969	1,600	2,350
Cardiac output (liters/minute)	6.09	5.09	9.88	13.60	17.49
Stroke volume (ml/beat)	86	57	96	103	108
Heart rate (beats/minute)	72	91	102	131	161
Arteriovenous difference (ml/100ml)	4.5	7.0	9.8	11.8	13.5
Mean pulmonary arterial pressure (mm Hg)	15	15	21	27	29

[a]O = walking on flat surface; 8% and 16% = walking up 8% and 16% grades on treadmill.
Data adapted from Damato A.N., Galante J.G., Smith W.M.: Hemodynamic response to treadmill exercise in normal subjects. *Journal of Applied Physiology,* 1966; 21:959.

diac physiology. A rise in end-diastolic volume and an increase in stroke volume were predicted from considerations of the Frank-Starling relationship in the isolated heart-lung preparation. Rushmer,[27] however, demonstrated that end-diastolic volume actually decreased with exercise in the conscious dog, and that the increase in cardiac output associated with exercise was due primarily to an increase in heart rate.

Many of the discrepancies between various studies exist because of failure to consider two variables: (1) the degree of exercise, and (2) the position of the subject performing that exercise. As indicated above, resting supine and resting erect cardiac output and ventricular dimensions are quite different. A comparison of supine rest with supine exercise may thus be quite different from a comparison of erect rest with erect exercise.

Damato, Galante, and Smith[28] studied cardiac output in the supine and erect positions at rest and during various degrees of erect exercise in a group of 24 normal subjects. Their data emphasize the importance of body position and the effect of position and degree of exercise on the regulation of stroke volume.

The data in Table 4–3 should be studied in detail because they summarize the ventilatory and circulatory response to standing and exercise. Minute ventilation and oxygen consumption both increase with assumption of the erect position and progressively increase with increasing exercise. Heart rate also increases with both the erect position and with exercise. Studies performed by Robinson et al.[29] on the role of the autonomic nervous system in the control of the heart rate demonstrate that the tachycardia associated with mild exercise is due to withdrawal of parasympathetic tone (atropine-like effect), while the tachycardia found with more vigorous activity is due to increased sympathetic activity.

The observations on stroke volume are of great importance relative to the roles of increased heart rate and stroke volume during exercise. Stroke volume decreases strikingly as the subject stands erect, primarily because of venous pooling in the lower extremities and decreased venous return. Exercise leads to an increase in venous tone that, together with muscular pumping, augments venous return, leading to an increase in stroke volume with each increment of exercise. These data explain why stroke volume failed to increase during exercise in certain earlier studies. Stroke volume is maximal while supine, and increasing cardiac output during supine exercise is accomplished primarily by increasing heart rate. Comparison of supine and erect exercise at similar levels of oxygen consumption indicates that supine cardiac output is always somewhat higher than erect cardiac output.

The data in Table 4–3 also demonstrate that the arteriovenous oxygen difference increases while erect and progressively increases with exercise. Mean pulmonary arterial pressure rises with exercise to almost twice control levels with the highest grade of exercise.

Rushmer's observations that the canine ventricle decreased in size during exercise suggested that the Frank-Starling mechanism was not the cause of increased cardiac output.[27] Braunwald, Ross, and Sonnenblick[4] sutured tantalum clips to the left ventricle of patients undergoing cardiac surgery and studied them after recovery. Supine exercise in this group of patients led to a decrease in ventricular dimensions, confirming the results of the earlier animal studies.

If ventricular end-diastolic volume does not increase with exercise, what is the cause of the increase in stroke volume seen with erect exercise? Increased autonomic activity, with the release of norepinephrine from myocardial sympathetic fibers, leads to an increase in contractility, so that greater stroke work is generated from a shorter end-diastolic fiber length (a leftward shift of the Sarnoff ventricular function curve). The tantalum clip study reveals that the force-velocity curve is shifted upward and to the right, so that a greater velocity of shortening for a given developed force was present. Increased myocardial contractility results in an increase in the rate of aortic pressure development and a shortening of ventricular ejection time.

Not only does an augmented heart rate increase cardiac output by increasing the number of ejections each minute, it also directly enhances myocardial contractility. In 1869 Bowditch showed that successive stimuli at short intervals produce a progressive increase in the force of each resultant contraction.[30] This staircase or treppe suggests that each stimulus exerts a beneficial aftereffect on cardiac muscle. This force-frequency relationship is believed to obtain in the intact heart, so that increasing the heart rate increases myocardial contractility independent of the increased inotropism mediated through the sympathetic nervous system. Thus, increased adrenergic activity enhances myocardial contractility directly and also indirectly via an increase in ventricular rate.

Role of Venous System in Regulating Cardiac Output

Except during periods of re-equilibration, venous return to the right heart must be equal to the output of the left ventricle. Most investigations concerning the regulation of cardiac output have dealt with those factors influencing ventricular output. Guyton[31] pioneered the study of the importance of the venous system in regulating cardiac output and subsequent investigators have expanded his work. It is important for the intensivist to recognize that the heart is not solely responsible for maintaining its output; the peripheral circulation also regulates the flow of blood, independently of the heart, by regulating its return to the right ventricle. Blood may either be allowed to pool in the periphery or may be "squeezed" into the circulation by appropriate constrictor mechanisms. Pooling may lead to hypotension, abnormal venoconstriction may produce pulmonary edema. Certain of these concepts are additionally presented in the section dealing with the cardiovacular response to positive end-expiratory pressure (see chapter 7).

The resistances are low in the venous system unlike the arterial side of the systemic circulation. Small pressure gradients, however, are still required to produce flow from the periphery to the right heart. The other major difference between the venous and arterial systems is that the veins are quite distensible compared to the arteries.

Guyton performed animal experiments from which the characteristics of venous return could be described by a series of "venous return curves." The right side of the heart was bypassed via a circuit consisting of a reservoir of adjustable height and a pump to transfer blood from the right atrium to the pulmonary artery. This arrangement allows the factors affecting venous return to be studied independently of the influence of those factors on the pumping capability of the heart. Progressive increases in right atrial pressure influence the venous return (Fig 4–11). As "atrial pressure" (the pressure in the reservoir) is increased by raising the reservoir, the amount of blood returning to the reservoir progressively decreases until flow ceases at a pressure of 8 mm Hg. This occurs because the gradient of pressure between the small venules and the reservoir, the pressure gradient which drives blood from

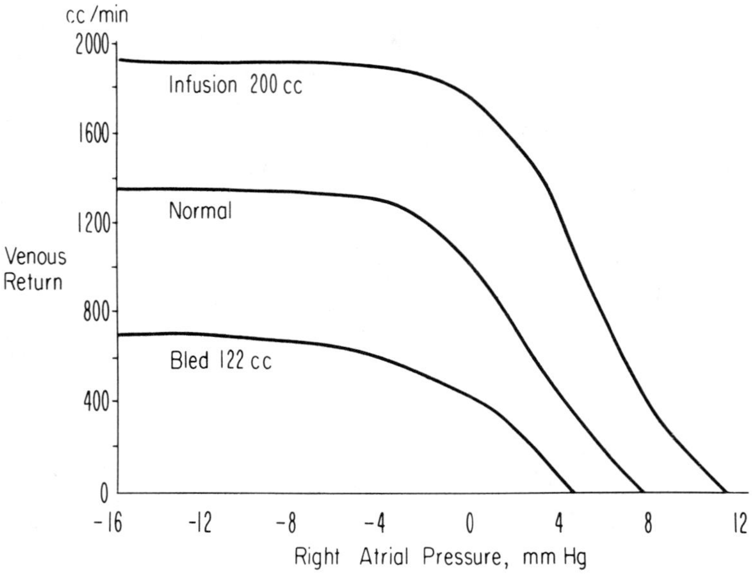

FIG 4-11.
The middle curve demonstrates the relationship of right atrial pressure to venous return in a normal dog. The other curves show the influence of changes in blood volume upon venous return. (Adapted from Guyton AC: Circulation. In: *Handbook of Physiology*, sec. 2. Washington, DC, *Am Physiol Soc* 1963; 2:32.)

the periphery to the heart, becomes zero. The level of pressure in the reservoir (relative to right atrial pressure) at which flow ceases is called the mean systemic pressure and is equal to the pressure in all regions of the systemic vascular bed—arteries, capillaries, and veins—if the heart had stopped beating. The anatomic location in the circulation where systemic pressure is equal to the actual pressure has been determined to be at the level of the small venules.

The normal venous return curve can be modified by several factors. Increased blood volume allows greater venous return to occur at any level of right atrial pressure because additional blood is available to provide a pressure gradient between capillaries and the right heart. Viewed from another perspective, increased blood volume increases the volume of the circulation and thereby raises mean systemic pressure. Constriction of the venous system by nervous or pharmacologic means also facilitates venous return by reducing venous distensibility. It squeezes blood from the small veins. Equally important is arteriolar constriction, particularly in the splanchnic bed, which decreases peripheral pooling.*

REGIONAL CIRCULATION

Oxygen requirements are different for different organs; even for a given organ it may vary widely, depending on its metabolic state. The actively working heart, for example, uses up to three times as much oxygen per unit of weight as the brain, and working skeletal muscle may require 40 times as much oxygen as resting skeletal muscle. These different oxygen requirements are met by the peripheral circulation, which is able to regulate the distribution of blood flow according to organ need. This is best typified by the stress reaction in which blood flow is preferentially shunted away from splanchnic and renal vascular beds in order to increase oxygen delivery to the heart, brain, and skeletal muscle.

Blood flow is governed by standard

*Venous return equals ventricular output under equilibrium conditions so that venous return curves become a convenient method for studying the simultaneous behavior of both ventricles and their venous return.

hydraulic principles, which state that flow is directly proportional to the driving pressure and inversely proportional to the resistance encountered. Fluid flow can be compared to electrical current flow, which is directly proportional to voltage and inversely proportional to resistance (Ohm's law).[32,33]

Resistance to flow in blood vessels depends upon blood vessel area, length, and the viscosity of the blood itself. These variables may be expressed in the Poiseuille equation (Fig 4–12), in which blood flow is directly proportional to the pressure drop across the tube (P_1-P_2) and the fourth power of the radius (R), but is inversely proportional to the length of the tubing (L) and the viscosity of the liquid (η). The role of viscosity may be best appreciated by considering that a much greater pressure head would be necessary to achieve the same flow rate with molasses as compared to water.

The Poiseuille relationship is useful for interpreting vascular dynamics, but cannot be quantitively applied to the circulatory system for several reasons. Blood vessels are not rigid pipes, but distensible tubes. No matter how much the pressure may increase in a lead pipe, the diameter is unchanged until the breaking point of the pipe is reached. Increasing the pressure in a blood vessel, however, distends the vessel, increases its diameter, and actually decreases its resistance. In consequence, flow increases linearly with pressure in a rigid tube but increases proportionately greater than pressure in a vascular tube (Fig 4–13).

The observation that increasing pressure within a vascular tube actually distends it and lowers its resistance to blood flow has given rise to the concept of transmural pressure.[33,34] The diameter of a blood vessel, and thus its resistance, is proportional to the pressure gradient across the vascular wall (intraluminal pressure minus extravascular pressure). Increasing intraluminal pressure decreases vascular resistance, while increasing extravascular pressure increases vascular resistance. This relationship is particularly important for the pulmonary vascular bed, and is described

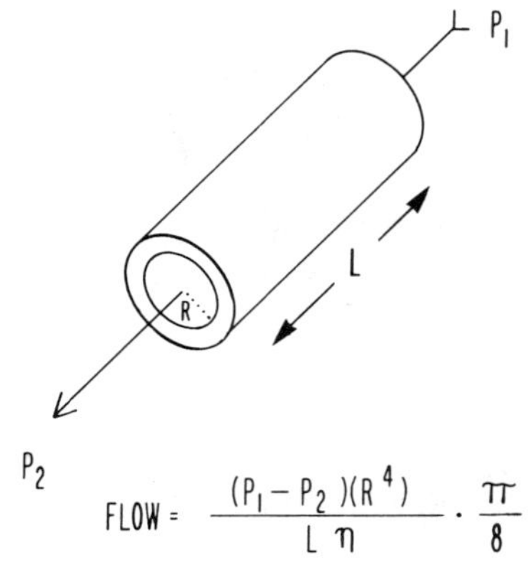

FIG 4–12.
nqc Poiseuille relationship. Flow rate of a liquid through a tube is directly proportional to the pressure drop ($P_1 -$ P_2) and the fourth power of the radius (R) but is inversely proportional to the length (L) and the viscosity of the fluid (η). The constant $\pi/8$ is a geometric factor.

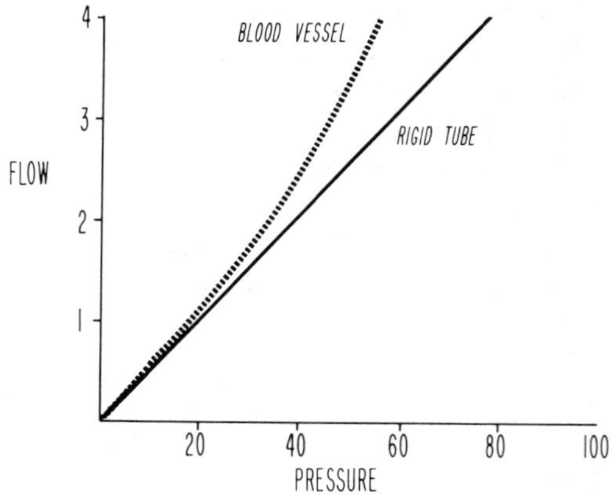

FIG 4–13.
Flow-pressure relationship depends on the distensibility of the conduit. In a rigid tube, flow increases proportionately with pressure. In a distensible tube, increasing pressure increases the diameter of the tube, and flow increases proportionately more than pressure. In consequence, vascular resistance decreases with increasing flow.

in detail below (under *Pulmonary Blood Flow*).

Furthermore, blood is not a true fluid, but a suspension of macromolecules and blood cells. In the larger blood vessels where flow is rapid, viscosity decreases with increasing flow rate. (In a true fluid, in contrast, viscosity does not change with changing flow rate.) In the smallest vessels of the microcirculation where blood flow is slowest, these suspended particles play a major role in determining the nature of blood flow. The prime example of this is the squeezing of erythrocytes through a capillary in rouleaux formation.

Mean arterial pressure is approximately the same in all organs. Since viscosity and vessel length are also relatively constant, regulation of blood flow may be achieved only by regulation of vessel diameter, which affects resistance according to the fourth power. The muscular arterioles regulate flow by constricting or dilating in response to organ requirements. The total vascular resistance of an organ is related to its total vascular cross-sectional area and length of the vascular components. The low resistance of the kidneys, for example, is due to the large number of blood vessels per unit of tissue.

The parallel arrangement of vascular beds may be compared to a parallel hydraulic system (Fig 4–14). The main conduit (aorta) delivers fluid to each lateral conduit at a mean pressure of about 100 mm Hg. The arterioles, shown in the figure as a valve, produce a variety of resistances. The flow of liquid leaving each lateral conduit is inversely related to the resistance and varies widely. Resistance units are given in the squares, and flow rate in milliliters per minute per 100 g of tissue in the circles. Note that the renal blood flow is approximately 150 times skeletal blood flow because of an extremely low resistance. Cerebral, splanchnic, and coronary blood flows are intermediate between these two extremes.

The Fick principle states that the ox-

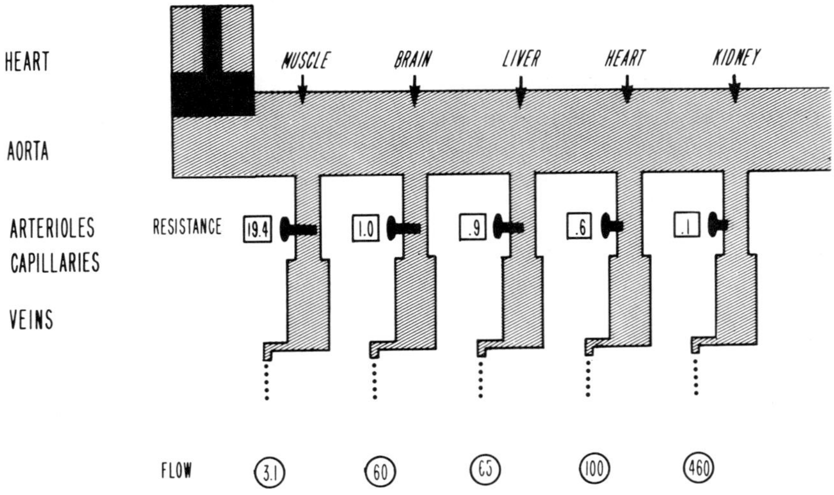

FIG 4–14.
The parallel arrangement of vascular beds may be compared to a parallel hydraulic system. Flow through each vascular bed (shown in circles and expressed as milliliters per 100 g of organ tissue) is determined by the vascular resistance of that organ (shown in squares and expressed as resistance per 100 g of tissue). The total vascular resistance of an organ is determined both by vascular tone and by the total cross-sectional area of the vascular supply per unit weight of tissue. The capacitance vessels or veins are situated distal to the capillaries and serve a reservoir function.

ygen uptake of an organ is equal to the blood flow multiplied by the arteriovenous oxygen difference. Table 4–4 shows the partition of total oxygen consumption by the various organ systems. Also shown is the flow rate in absolute units and the percentage of total cardiac output diverted to each organ. The differing patters of oxygen extraction may be seen by the variations in arteriovenous oxygen difference. The myocardium extracts 11.4 ml of oxygen while the kidney extracts but 1.3 ml of oxygen from each 100 ml of blood.

The increased oxygen requirement of exercise or stress may be met by either increasing organ flow or oxygen extraction. Most vascular beds rely on both of these mechanisms. The heart is unique, however, in that it extracts almost maximally at rest. Increased myocardial oxygen consumption is accomplished primarily by increasing coronary blood flow. This flow-limited system permits a high level of oxygen uptake with relatively low flow rates. It is extremely disadvantageous to the patient with coronary arterial disease, since he is unable to increase coronary flow in response to increased oxygen demands.

Figure 4–14 demonstrates another feature of the peripheral circulation. While the arterioles are considered the resistance vessels of the circulation and regulate the rate of organ blood flow, the veins are considered the reservoir or capacitance vessels and provide a storage area for the blood volume. Should volume be lost from the vascular space, the capacitance vessels contract and attempt to maintain venous pressure and diastolic cardiac filling.

Interposed between the resistance and capacitance vessels are the capillaries. The only purpose of the circulatory system is to facilitate transfer of material across the capillary walls in the lung and in the peripheral circulation. The capillaries are very permeable to water, and the amount of water which passes back and forth through the capillary walls is estimated to be many times greater than the flow through the vessels. There is also a relatively free passage of other molecules through the capillary walls, and in the splanchnic region there is evidence that the large serum albumin molecules rapidly equilibrate with an extravascular compartment.

The capillary bed or microcirculation (Fig 4–15)[35] received little attention until recently because of its relative inaccessibility to direct measurement. Of great importance is the concept that much of the capillary bed is unused at rest, most

TABLE 4–4.
Regional Distribution of Blood Flow*

SITE	BLOOD FLOW $\dot{Q}$ (ml/minute)	CARDIAC OUTPUT(%)	WEIGHT (kg)	OXYGEN CONSUMPTION, $\dot{V}O_2$ (ml/minute)	ARTERIOVENOUS OXYGEN DIFFERENCE, $CaO_2 - CvO_2$ (ml/100 ml)
Muscle	1,200	21	31.0	70	8.0
Brian	750	13	1.4	46	6.3
Splanchnic area	1,400	24	2.6	58	4.1
Heart	250	4	0.3	27	11.4
Kidney	1,100	19	0.3	16	1.3
Skin	500	9	5.6	5	1.0
Other organs	600	10	28.8	12	3.0

*Adapted from Wade OL, Bishop JM: Cardiac Output and Regional Blood Flow. Oxford, Blackwell Scientific Publication, 1962.

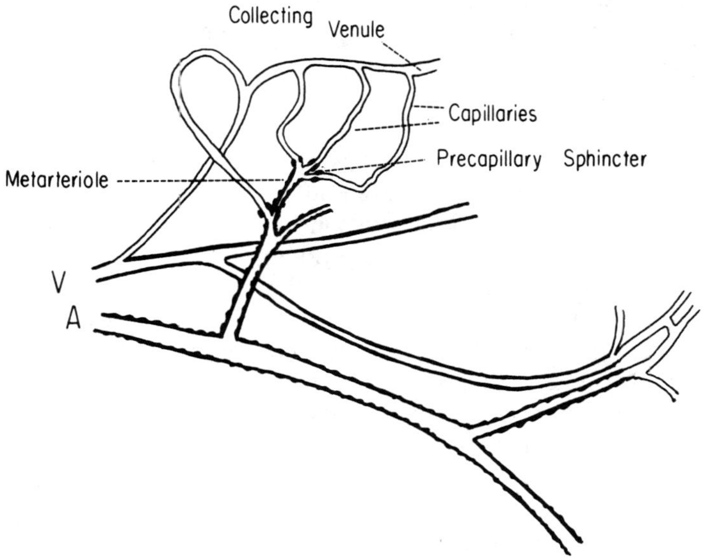

FIG 4–15.
The microcirculation. The muscular arteriole divides into several terminal arterioles. The terminal arteriole then divides into several metarterioles, the last vascular branch with a complete muscular wall. A group of capillaries arise from each metarteriole. Note the precapillary sphincters located at the origin of each capillary. Normally many of the precapillary sphincters are constricted, and blood from the arteriole follows a preferential pathway. In times of stress, the precapillary sphincters dilate, and all of the capillary bed is used. Shown also is an arteriovenous communication between a metarteriole and collecting venule. (Adapted from Zweifach BW: Basic mechanisms in peripheral vascular hemostasis, in *Third Conference on Factors Regulating Blood Pressure.* New York, Josiah Macy Jr Foundation, 1950.)

of the blood passing through preferential channels or metarterioles, which connect arterioles and venules. The metarterioles branch at almost right angles from arterioles and have an intermittent coating of smooth muscle cells. True capillaries—vessels without recognizable muscle tissue branch at right angles from the metarterioles. As each capillary branches from the parent metarteriole, it is embraced by one or two smooth muscle cells—the precapillary sphincter. Short muscular vessels also run directly from arteriole to venule and are considered to represent arteriovenous anastomoses. When dilated, blood is diverted *from* the capillary bed; when closed, *to* the capillary bed.

The presence of preferential channels, precapillary sphincters, and arteriovenous anastomoses provide considerable opportunity for control. Resting tissues may be provided with minimal blood supply, while actively working tissues may receive augmented volumes of capillary blood. Krogh[36] in 1929 estimated that the capillary bed of skeletal muscle could increase its cross-sectional area 100 times during vigorous exercise.

The net movement of water molecules in either direction depends upon the two sets of opposing forces described in Starling's law of the capillary. The net movement of water out of the capillary is caused by the hydrostatic pressure in the capillary and the osmotic pressure of the interstitial space. Movement of water into the capillary is caused by the hydrostatic pressure in the tissues and the osmotic pressure of the plasma.

Many disease states, physiologic adaptations, and therapeutic interventions affect the function of the microcirculation. Tissue hypoxia—either direct or through the production of certain metabolites such as adenosine diphosphate (ADP)—relaxes the precapillary sphincter and increases capillary blood flow. Alpha-adrenergic stimulation constricts precapillary sphincters and decreases capillary blood flow. If venoconstriction exceeds precapillary constriction, capillary pressure rises and fluid is lost into the surrounding tissues. Such a sequence is believed to occur during severe shock. Precapillary sphincters, after initial constriction, relax (perhaps in response to production of local humoral substances), while postcapillary venoconstriction persists, leading to transcapillary fluid shifts.

Man's ability to adapt to a wide variety of external requirements and internal metabolic states is based on the ability of the peripheral circulation to match neatly the delivery of oxygen and nutrient to the needs of the cells. Two basic mechanisms—local autoregulation and distant control by the autonomic nervous system—provide this adaptive ability.

Autoregulation is the ability of a tissue bed to increase its blood flow by a local vascular dilatation without the need for intercession by the autonomic nervous system. This is best typified by an experiment which produces reactive hyperemia. If the artery supplying the tissue bed is occluded for a short period of time and then released, vascular dilatation and increased blood flow distal to the occlusion is observed as soon as the occlusion is released. Presumably, local metabolites accumulate during the period of ischemia and act directly on the vascular walls. Myocardial autoregulation is thought to be mediated by adenosine nucleotides, which accumulate because of their inability to be oxidatively phosphorylated to adenosine triphosphate (ATP). A useful compensatory cycle thus develops. The failure of oxygen delivery to the mitochondria leads to a decrease in the production of high-energy phosphate (ATP) from adenosine. Adenosine nucleotides accumulate, lead to vascular dilatation, increase local blood flow, and increase the rate of oxygen delivery to the tissues.

A second level of adaptive response is provided by the autonomic nervous system. Alpha or constrictor receptors are found in most vascular beds, but are most active in the kidney, skin, and mesenteric arterial beds. Beta or dilator receptors, in contrast, are most active in skeletal muscle and myocardial beds. Central stimulation of the sympathetic nervous system produces the familiar stress reaction, with an increase in skeletal and myocardial blood flow, but a decrease in renal, cutaneous, and splanchnic blood flows. A similar type of response is observed in certain patients who develop the shock syndrome.

The capacitance vessels—the veins—are innervated by alpha-adrenergic receptors. If beta receptors are in fact also present, they are constrictor in nature. Stimulation of these receptors produces contraction of the venous reservoir and a rise in capillary pressure. Intense sympathetic constrictor activity may lead to such high capillary pressure that fluid is lost from the capillaries into the tissues.

Control of Circulation to Specific Organ Systems

The oxygen requirements of specific organ systems (Fig 4–14) vary widely not only in the basal state but in different stress situations. Physical exercise may result in a 20-fold increase in skeletal muscle blood flow, lesser increases in coronary blood flow, and little change in cerebral or splanchnic blood flow. Splanchnic, cutaneous, and cerebral blood flow, in contrast, are regulated by changing gastrointestinal, temperature regulation, and intellectual needs. Either extrinsic neurogenic and humoral influences or intrinsic autoregulatory influences regulate regional vascular resistance and play the major role in determining regional blood flow. The effectiveness of these adjustments is demonstrated by the relative independence of cerebral and renal blood flow from a wide range of shifts in arterial perfusion pressure.

Balancing the energy requirements of the several organ systems becomes extremely important in the care of the critically ill patient. Disease may interfere with the regulation of vascular resistance, and certain treatment techniques may improve blood flow through one system while decreasing it through another. A common example of this is the effect of induced hypocapnia on the cerebral circulation. While controlled ventilation may improve arterial oxygen content, inadvertent hyperventilation may produce hypocapnia, leading to an increase in cerebral vascular tone and a decrease in cerebral blood flow. Arteriosclerosis may prevent peripheral vascular beds from dilating in response to generalized hypotension, so that blood flow in shock becomes closely related to perfusion pressure in many organ systems.

Cerebral Circulation

The cerebral circulation is unique in that it is relatively insensitive to changes in arterial blood pressure or to adrenergic stimulation, but extremely sensitive to changes in both arterial oxygen and carbon dioxide tension. In fact, it is the only vascular bed in the body exhibiting such marked dependence upon arterial carbon dioxide tension.[37] Schmidt[38] and Kety and Schmidt[39] demonstrated that voluntary hyperventilation reduced total cerebral flow from 750 to 473 ml/min, while hypercapnia increased it to 1,293 ml/min. Hypoxemia increased cerebral blood flow to 1,015 ml/min, while high arterial oxygen tensions reduced it to 625 ml/min. In contrast, locally applied epinephrine or stimulation of the cervical sympathetic trunks has only a mild vasoconstrictor effect compared to that observed in other organ systems.

There is a curvilinear relationship between arterial carbon dioxide tension and cerebral blood flow (Fig 4–16).[40] Another study from Wollmann et al.[41] showed that extreme hyperventilation with progressive reduction of arterial carbon dioxide tension from 37 to 19 mm Hg and then to 10 mm Hg reduced cerebral blood flow from 44.1 to 25.3 and 21.0 ml/100g/min.

The interrelated effects of hypoxemia and hypocapnia were studied in a unique

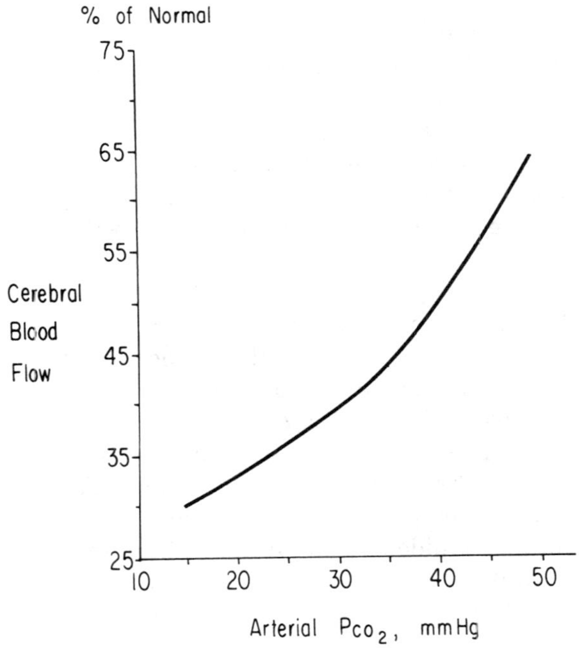

FIG 4–16.
Curvilinear relationship between arterial dioxide tension and cerebral blood flow (Adapted from Alexander SC, Wollman H, Cohen PJ, Chase PE, Behar M: Cerebrovascular response to PA_{CO_2} during halothane anesthesia in man. *J Appl Physiol* 1964; 19:561.)

series of experiments performed by Severinghaus et al.[42] on seven healthy volunteers living for 5 days at an altitude of 4,000 meters. Carbon dioxide tension initially decreased to an average of 35 mm Hg, oxygen tension to 44 mm Hg. By 3 to 5 days, chronic hyperventilation dropped carbon dioxide tension from 30 mm Hg and raised oxygen tension to 51 mm Hg. Cerebral blood flow increased 24% initially but fell to 13% above control levels by 3 to 5 days. Of great interest is that when oxygen administration restored arterial oxygen tension to normal, cerebral blood flow was normal even though arterial carbon dioxide tension was 30 mm Hg. These studies demonstrated that cerebral blood flow returns to normal in chronic hypocapnia, presumably because cerebrospinal fluid and extracellular fluid bicarbonate concentrations slowly decrease, maintaining extracellular hydrogen ion concentration in the normal range.

The relationships between cerebral blood flow and oxygen and carbon dioxide tensions have great importance in clinical medicine. Mechanical hyperventilation with a sudden decrease in arterial carbon dioxide tension and an elevation in oxygen tension may produce cerebral vasoconstriction with diminished cerebral blood flow. While the patient may become acclimatized to this environmental assault within several days, irreversible mental changes may have already occurred. The importance of cerebrospinal fluid bicarbonate concentration in regulating brain hydrogen ion concentration and blood flow have suggested the use of a carbonic anhydrase inhibitor, acetazolamide, as a cerebral vasodilator. Kronenberg and Cain[43] demonstrated that acclimatization progressed more rapidly when acetazolamide was administered, mainly because of a decrease in plasma bicarbonate concentration. The importance of bicarbonate and hydrogen ion concentration was emphasized by Cotev, Lee, and Severinghaus[44] who demonstrated that cerebral blood flow was higher for equivalent carbon dioxide tensions when acetazolamide was administered.

The unique dependence of cerebral blood flow upon carbon dioxide tension is presumably related to the nature of cerebral function. The brain initiates and maintains the entire continuum of bodily activities and is the prime regulator of function in other organ systems. Metabolic activity of neuronal groups initiates a variety of local and remote responses and must be supported by local increases of blood flow. Sokoloff and Kety[45] used radioautographic techniques to measure blood flow in various regions of the central nervous system. General anesthesia reduced cerebral blood flow in sensorimotor, visual, and auditory areas of the cerebral cortex compared to the unanesthetized state, but did not change blood flow in 16 of the 28 areas involved. Anesthesia presumably depressed certain aspects of cortical function, leading to decreases in oxygen requirements and blood flow in those areas. Increased neuronal activity, in contrast, increases oxygen consumption and carbon dioxide production. Local vessels dilate, and increased oxygen requirements are met by increasing blood flow. Such an arrangement makes teleologic sense since there could be no advantage to a general increase in cerebral blood flow during exercise or anxiety.

Coronary Blood Flow

Regulation of the coronary circulation stands in marked contrast to that of the brain. The heart is forced to respond to demands imposed on it by the whims and caprices of the brain as well as to conditions of the external environment. Whether an individual is sleeping, jogging, mountain climbing at high altitudes, or engaging in sexual activity, the coronary circulation must provide enough oxygen to the myocardium to allow it to generate sufficient wall tension for maintenance of an adequate stroke output.

Resting coronary blood flow is 70 to 90 ml/100 g/min of left ventricular tissue. Increased myocardial oxygen requirements are met by increasing coronary blood flow up to five times basal levels. Myocardial oxygen extraction remains relatively fixed at 65 to 70%, so that cellular oxygen tension and coronary sinus oxygen content are unchanged in the face of marked increases in total oxygen consumption.[46] Both extrinsic sympathetic activity and intrinsic autoregulatory activity closely match coronary blood flow with metabolic need.

A number of parameters have been correlated with myocardial oxygen consumption, and may operate both through the sympathetic nervous system and through intrinsic autoregulatory mechanisms. Heart rate and blood pressure are the most obvious determinants of myocardial oxygen consumption, but less apparent factors such as the contractile state of myocardial fibers, rate of fiber shortening, and myocardial wall tension (related to ventricular dimensions) are probably equally important. The cardiac output itself has little relationship to oxygen requirements.

Aortic pressure is an important determinant of coronary blood flow, particularly in patients with coronary arterial disease. The normal coronary vascular bed dilates in response to decreasing perfusion pressure, maintaining coronary blood flow. In coronary arterial disease (particularly in the patient in coronary shock), diseased vessels lose their autoregulatory capacity and the vascular bed becomes increasingly flow dependent. A detailed discussion of the coronary circulation in coronary shock is found in Chapter 5.

Coronary blood flow in most instances is regulated by changes in arteriolar resistance. While metabolic and neurohumoral effects are major determinants of coronary vascular resistance, certain mechanical effects are also important. Wall tension, particularly during systole, contributes to coronary resistance. Since intracavitary pressure is low in the right ventricle, significant coronary blood flow occurs throughout the cardiac cycle in this chamber, while in the left ventricle the major portion of coronary blood flow occurs during diastole. Other things being equal, both diastolic pressure and diastolic filling time are important determinants of left ventricular perfusion. In the presence of aortic insufficiency a low diastolic perfusion pressure associated with increased myocardial oxygen requirements (due to the dilated ventricular chamber and increase in systolic pressure) may lead to coronary insufficiency. Tachycardia, on the other hand, results in decreased diastolic coronary filling time and increased oxygen requirements, placing the myocardium at a disadvantage. While changes in arteriolar resistance may compensate for these factors by increasing flow appropriately, underlying coronary arterial disease may limit the response.

The other major factors (referred to above) that affect coronary resistance include level of catecholamine activity and adequacy of blood oxygenation. The cardiac effect of sympathetic nerve stimulation or administration of catecholamines (norepinephrine, epinephrine, isoproterenol) is complex. The overall effect of the catecholamines is to increase coronary blood flow, either by direct action on the coronary bed (primary vasodilation) or secondarily due to changes in heart rate, blood pressure, and cardiac work.[47] Norepinephrine is though to exert a diphasic effect, consisting of initial vasoconstriction probably due to alpha receptor stimulation followed by coronary vasodilation. The latter may be due to direct coronary beta receptor stimulation or to the myocardial effects of hypoxia. In contrast, isoproterenol is a primary coronary vasodilator and effects striking increases in coronary blood flow that are out of proportion to the increase in oxygen requirement, resulting in a decrease in oxygen extraction. While all of these agents increase coronary blood flow, their varying effects on heart rate and perfusion pressure should be appreciated for proper therapeutic application.

Arterial hypoxemia induces a profound increase in coronary blood flow—as much as 200–300% in the normal coronary bed. Studies in normal human subjects have shown that compensation for arterial oxygen saturation as low as 40% occurs by an appropriate increase in coronary blood flow, so that myocardial oxygen consumption remains adequate.[48] Maximal coronary dilatation occurs when the arterial oxygen saturation falls to about 20%. However, with this degree of arterial hypoxia, the increase in coronary blood flow alone is not sufficient for adequate oxygen delivery to the heart muscle, and myocardial oxygen extraction increases. Extraction of as much as 85–90% across the coronary bed has been reported and is associated with unusually low coronary sinus oxygen contents.

The adaptation of the coronary bed in chronic anemia is similar to that in arterial hypoxia. In the presence of a normal coronary bed and hemoglobin values of 10 g/100 ml or more, the decreased arterial oxygen content is compensated for by an increase in coronary blood flow, whereas myocardial oxygen uptake and systemic circulation remain essentially unchanged. When hemoglobin values reach 6–8 g/100 ml, however, coronary blood flow is maximally increased (300% and more) and is associated with an increase in myocardial oxygen extraction to maintain an adequate oxygen supply.

Pulmonary Blood Flow

The pulmonary vascular bed normally is highly distensible and has a low resistance to blood flow. While a pressure drop of 90–100 mm Hg is necessary to perfuse the systemic circulation at a normal rate of blood flow, a pressure drop of but 10 mm Hg suffices to perfuse the pulmonary circulation. Pulmonary vascular resistance is only 100 dynes-second-cm^{-5}, while systemic vascular resistance ranges between 1,300 and 1,500 dynes-second-cm^{-5}. The anatomic basis for this distensible vascular bed lies in pulmonary vessels containing little smooth muscle and with relatively thin walls compared to the size of their lumens. Pre- and postcapillary vessels have almost no identifiable muscle tissue. Proximal to these vessels are larger arterioles containing definite muscular layers which appear to be the sites of active vasoconstriction.

Flow through vascular tubes is directly related to the pressure drop through the tubes and inversely proportional to the resistance (Figs 4–12, 4–13). A variety of passive mechanical and active vasomotor changes profoundly influence both pressure gradient and resistance in the pulmonary vascular bed, and complicate interpretation of pulmonary arterial pressure. Pulmonary arterial pressure monitoring is an extremely useful technique, but serial changes in pressure must be interpreted with care.

Figure 4–17 summarizes some of these passive and active influences. The upper part of the figure describes the influence of the transmural pressure gradient on vascular size and resistance. A decrease in alveolar pressure or an increase in intravascular pressure dilates pulmonary vessels, while the reverse situation tends

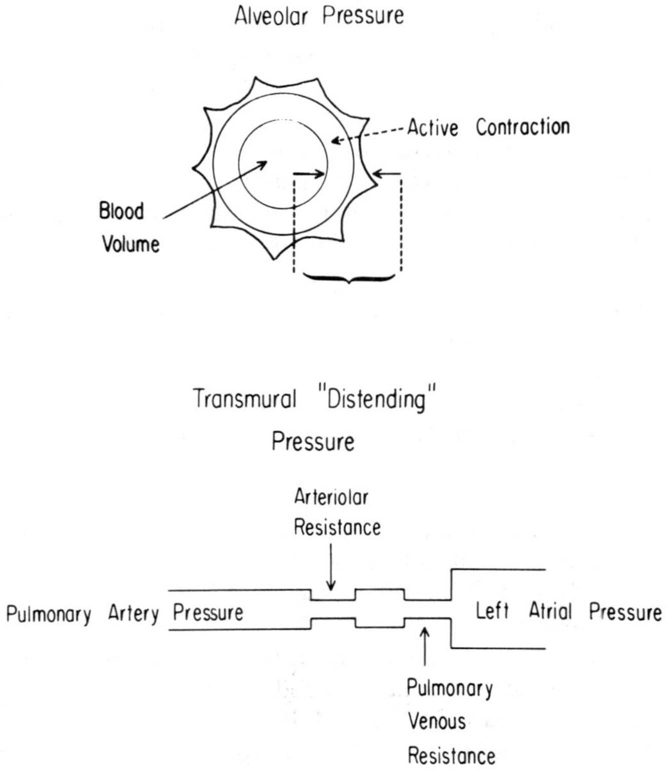

FIG 4–17.
Determinants of pulmonary blood flow. A. Cross-sectional view of a pulmonary arteriole. The caliber of the blood vessel is determined by the degree of smooth muscle contraction, the blood volume, and by the transmural distending pressure. The transmural distending pressure is the difference between intravascular and alveolar pressures. All of these factors determine the overall pulmonary vascular resistance. Note the dependency of vascular resistance on transmural and alveolar pressure; increasing alveolar pressure decreases transmural pressure and reduces the diameter of the vascular bed. B. The driving pressure—pulmonary arterial pressure—is opposed by the arteriolar vascular resistance, the pulmonary venous resistance, and the left atrial pressure.

to narrow them. Active contraction of vascular smooth muscle reduces vascular diameter and increases vascular resistance. The lower part of the figure shows that an increase in left atrial pressure or pulmonary venous constriction can also cause an increase in pulmonary arterial pressure. In this situation pulmonary resistance may actually decrease since the increased pulmonary vascular pressure tends to distend the vascular bed. Thus, an increase in pulmonary arterial pressure does not always mean an increase in pulmonary vascular resistance.

Cardiac output and pulmonary blood flow directly influence pulmonary arterial pressure and vascular resistance. Early investigations into the distensibility of the pulmonary vascular bed suggested that pulmonary pressure did not rise until pulmonary blood flow exceeded 3.5 times resting levels. More recent studies, reviewed by Fowler,[49] reveal a linear relationship between pressure and flow and suggest that pressure increases at lower flow rates than previously indicated. While increasing pulmonary blood flow may increase pressure, it might simultaneously decrease vascular resistance by distending the vascular bed. Increases in pulmonary blood volume decrease resistance at low volumes by dilating the bed; at higher volumes further increases rapidly fill the bed, making it rigid and producing disproportionately greater increases in pulmonary arterial pressure.

Effects of Respiration on Pulmonary Blood Flow

Respiratory changes in transmural pressure and vascular resistance produce cyclic changes in intrathoracic blood flow.

The right ventricle plays a key role in adjusting blood flow to changes in intrathoracic pressure so that systemic blood flow remains normal in spite of wide swings in intrathoracic pressure. During inspiration, intrathoracic and right atrial pressures fall, increasing the gradient from the periphery and increasing venous return.[50] The increase in venous return increases right ventricular output in accordance with Starling's law and increases pulmonary blood flow. Pulmonary venous flow appears to increase slightly, but systemic blood flow decreases, suggesting pooling of blood in the left ventricle. In the normal individual, the increase in pulmonary blood flow balances any change in pulmonary vascular capacity and left ventricular pooling, so that only minimal decreases in left ventricular output occur.[51]

The effect of changing intrathoracic pressure on pulmonary blood flow and resistance explains the fall in blood pressure frequently seen with positive-pressure ventilation. Increased intrathoracic pressure decreases venous return and pulmonary blood flow while increasing transmural pressure and increasing pulmonary vascular resistance. The early studies of Cournand, Motley, and Richards[52] demonstrated that a respirator pressure profile with inspiration lasting about one-third of the entire respiratory cycle had minimal effect on cardiac output. Increasing the duration of inspiration increased the mean intrathoracic pressure and led to decreases in cardiac output. Continuous positive-pressure breathing (positive pressure in both inspiration and expiration) discussed in chapter 7 tends to decrease cardiac output more than intermittent positive-pressure breathing. Fortunately, however, the intrathoracic pressure is poorly transmitted to the pulmonary vascular bed in patients with marked decreases in pulmonary compliance so that circulatory effects are frequently minimal in these patients. The reciprocal nature of systemic vascular resistance and pulmonary blood volume was shown in a study by Braunwald et al.[53] These investigators demonstrated that administration of metaraminol during positive-pressure ventilation reversed the observed decreases in pulmonary blood volume and flow. While the agent may have improved myocardial contractility, a major effect appeared to be related to a shift of blood volume from periphery to lung.

Active Vasomotion in Pulmonary Vessels

The shift in blood volume from periphery to lung (Fig 4–18) discussed above is due to the fact that peripheral vessels are more sensitive than pulmonary vessels to adrenergic stimulation. This observation forms the basis for Sarnoff's neurogenic theory of pulmonary edema. Increased adrenergic activity with peripheral vasoconstriction and increased pul-

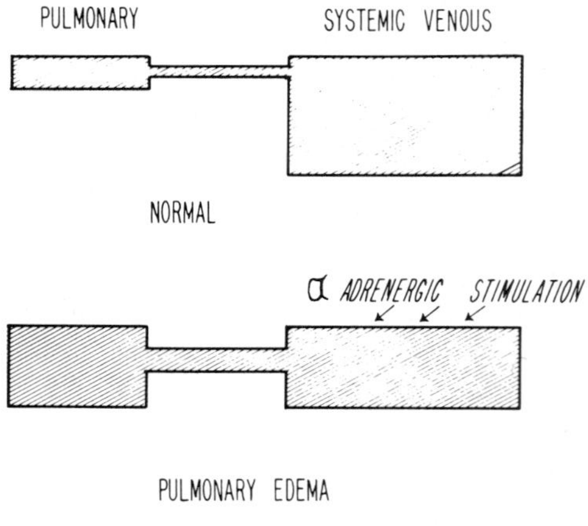

FIG 4–18.
The systemic venous and pulmonary vascular systems are the two primary vascular reservoirs of the body. The systemic reservoir is under active adrenergic control while the pulmonary reservoir is relatively passive. Alpha-adrenergic stimulation produces venoconstriction and shifts blood from the periphery to the lungs, producing pulmonary edema.

monary blood volume is suggested as a major causal factor in acute pulmonary edema. Of great interest is that spinal anesthesia, which blocks adrenergic outflow, improves clinical pulmonary edema, presumably by its effect on increasing peripheral pooling of blood. Alpha blocking agents (such as Dibenzyline) and intermittent positive-pressure improve pulmonary edema by a similar mechanism.

Pulmonary vessels are weakly reactive to adrenergic stimuli except in the presence of hypoxia and other metabolic-abnormalities. Alpha-adrenergic stimulation with dopamine increases pulmonary vascular resistance in the hypoxic lung to a much greater degree than in the noroxic situation. Beta-adrenergic stimulating with isoproterenol or dobutamin leads to vasodilatation, particularly in the hypoxic lung.[54]

Hypoxia and acidosis acting independently are much more vasoconstrictive than alpha-adrenergic stimulation alone. A number of studies have shown that both of these stimuli elevate pulmonary arterial pressure, particularly in patients with preexisting pulmonary disease. Liljestrand[55] suggests that increased hydrogen ion concentration is the chemical stimulus for vasoconstriction, and that hypoxia probably acts by promoting release of lactic acid. This hypothesis is strengthened by the study of Enson et al.,[56] who demonstrated that pulmonary arterial mean pressure in patients with chronic pulmonary disease could be mathematically related to both arterial oxygen saturation and to pH (Fig 4–19). Note that alkalosis appears to protect against the vasoconstrictive effects of hypoxia. A patient with a pH of 7.53 might be expected to have a normal pulmonary arterial mean pressure even though his arterial hemoglobin was only 70% saturated. Mean pulmonary arterial pressure would rise to 45 mm Hg in the presence of a normal pH and to 60 mm Hg with a pH of 7.35.

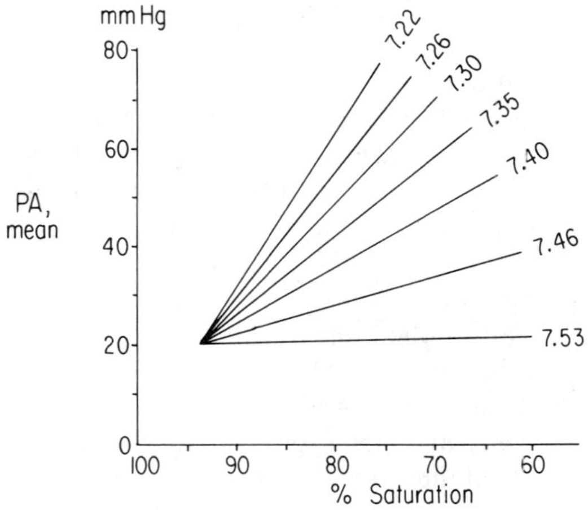

FIG 4–19.
Both hypoxemia and acidosis are potent pulmonary vasoconstrictors. The two factors are additive; for any level of hypoxemia, pulmonary arterial pressure rises as pH falls. (Adapted from Enson Y, Guintini C, Lewis L, et al: The influence of hydrogen ion concentration and hypoxemia on the pulmonary circulation. *J Clin Invest* 1964; 43:1146.)

Renal and Splanchnic Circulation

The function and control of the renal and splanchnic circulation contrasts with that of previously described vascular beds. While cessation of blood flow to brain, heart, and lung produces death within minutes, the organism can survive for considerable periods of time following cessation of renal or splanchnic blood flow. Both of these organ systems are well supplied with sympathetic nerve fibers, allowing them to function as a primary defense system.[57] In times of stress generalized vasoconstriction redistributes blood flow from these less vital regions to brain, heart, and lung. The kidney and liver are particularly well suited to be primary defense organs since they collectively receive almost 50% of the cardiac output and can be expected to contribute 2,500 to 3,000 ml of blood flow per minute to the rest of the body during stressful situations.

Renal arteries ascend to the cortex from the hilus, bending around the renal pyramids as arciform arteries. The latter give rise to cortical interlobular arteries, which supply each glomerulus via short lateral branches. The glomerulus is interposed between both afferent and efferent arterioles, each containing smooth muscle fibers richly supplied with sympathetic nerve endings. Normally, the afferent arterioles offer little resistance to blood flow so that glomerular vascular pressure is only slightly below arterial pressure. The efferent arterioles have a much greater resistance to blood flow, so that vascular pressure drops to 15 to 20 mm Hg as blood enters the peritubular capillaries. The capillary network of cortical tubules differs markedly from that of juxtamedullary tubules. Straight capillaries, following the course of the loop of Henle, descend into the medulla and are necessary for operation of the countercurrent multiplier system. Almost 90% of renal blood flow perfuses the cortex, 8–10% the medulla, and only 1–2% the renal papillae.

Pitts[58] pointed out that fright, pain, syncope, cold, severe exercise, deep anesthesia, and hemorrhage are serious emergencies which lead to alterations in the caliber of afferent and efferent arterioles, sacrificing glomerular filtration in order to perfuse more vital organs. He presented a patient who became anxious during the performance of experimental studies and decreased his renal blood flow from 700 to less than 400 ml/min (renal plasma flow measured as Diodrast clearance).[59] Renal blood flow and glomerular filtration rate are stable over the range 100 to 200 mm Hg mean pressure. Below 100 mm Hg, renal blood flow falls linearly with decreases in blood pressure. In one study renal blood flow dropped by half as perfusion pressure decreased from 80 to 40 mm Hg. Hypoxemia and hypercapnia also trigger reflex vasoconstriction, markedly decreasing renal blood flow. As might be expected from the abundant nervous supply of renal vascular tissue, epinephrine, norepinephrine, vasopressin, and renin all decrease renal blood flow.

Recent data point to the belief that the kidney plays a major role in regulating arterial blood pressure by functioning as an endocrine organ. Juxtaglomerular cells just proximal to the glomerulus act as pressure-sensitive detectors, liberating renin in response to hypotension. Renin is a proteolytic enzyme which converts an α_2 globulin found in plasma into angiotensin I. A single passage through the lung then converts the inactive compound, angiotensin I, to the vasoactive material, angiotensin II.[60] Even more recent studies suggest that the kidney may also liberate a newly discovered class of vasoactive substances—the prostaglandins—in various stress situations. A number of prostaglandins have been identified; some are vasodilators, others vasoconstrictors.

The enteric-portal-hepatic vascular bed also serves as an emergency reservoir. Normally, the portal circulation serves to facilitate the absorption and digestion of food material. During periods of stress sympathetic nervous stimulation constricts mesenteric arterioles, decreasing portal blood flow and making extra blood available for use elsewhere. The amount of blood available for such redistribution is considerable; Bradley et al. estimated the average hepatic venous flow to be about 1.5 liters/min.[61] Hepatic arterial flow is thought to constitute 20–35% of total hepatic blood flow; portal blood flow makes up the rest.

The discussion thus far has centered on the value of renal and splanchnic vasoconstriction in defending the body against decreases in total or effective blood volume. While useful as an emergency response, continued visceral and renal vasoconstriction produces profound changes in these organs. Acute renal failure with tubular necrosis and stress ulceration of the gastrointestinal tract are two serious complications occurring in the wake of prolonged vascular constriction. Patients may survive periods of prolonged shock but succumb later to renal, respiratory, or hepatic failure.

PHYSIOLOGY AND PHARMACOLOGY OF THE AUTONOMIC NERVOUS SYSTEM

The oxygen requirements of an active human vary from 200 to 2000 ml/min depending upon whether the individual is resting or engaging in vigorous physical activity. Oxygen delivery is neatly matched to oxygen requirements by intrinsic autoregulatory mechanisms, by the autonomic nervous system, and by the secretion of a group of regulatory humoral substances. The rate of blood flow to the individual organ systems is controlled by the adjustment of the volume of blood pumped by the heart each minute and by the resistance to blood flow in each vascular bed. Sympathetic fibers are generously supplied to the myocardium and to the smooth muscles of blood vessels. Discharge of these nerves produces an increase in cardiac output and either vascular constriction or dilatation.

The autonomic nervous system regulates such functions as respiration, circulation, digestion, body temperature, metabolism, sweating, and endocrine secretion, which are not under voluntary or conscious control. Both the sympathetic and parasympathetic nervous systems regulate the internal environment, but have contrasting functions. Animals can develop normally and lead a reasonably normal existence in the absence of the sympathetic (adrenergic) nervous system, but cannot respond to stressful situations. Stress in the animal with an adequate sympathetic nervous system provokes increased adrenergic discharge, mediating the well known fight or flight response. The parasympathetic (cholinergic) system, in contrast, is concerned with localized responses such as bradycardia, hypotension, and gastrointestinal stimulation that appear to conserve or restore body energy stores.

The Parasympathetic (Cholinergic) Nervous System

Acetylcholine serves as the neurotransmitter for many cerebral neurons, autonomic ganglia synapses, the somatic myoneural junction, a few sympathetic postganglionic junctions, and parasympathetic postganglionic junctions. The final step in the synthesis of acetylcholine is the transfer of an acetyl group from acetyl coenzyme-A to choline, a reaction mediated by the enzyme choline acetylase. Since peripheral nerve transmission is intermittent, acetylcholine must be quickly removed following discharge. Acetylcholinesterase performs that function, and many cholinergic activating agents actually decrease the activity of that inactivating enzyme.

The pharmacology of acetylcholine is divided into nicotinic and muscarinic effects. Muscarinic effects are similar to those produced by the action of the alkaloid muscarine, including bradycardia, heart block, vasodilatation, increased gastrointestinal secretion and motility, bronchoconstriction, and pupillary constriction. Nicotinic effects are similar to those of nicotine. Small doses stimulate autonomic ganglia and neuromuscular junctions while larger doses block both sites. Atropine blocks the muscarinic effects of acetylcholine, while the various ganglionic blocking agents and high doses of nicotine block the ganglionic and neuromuscular effects of the drug.

Both divisions of the autonomic nervous system maintain tonic activity with the parasympathetic inhibitory tone opposing the sympathetic facilitatory tone.[62] For example, the effect of increased sympathetic stimulation on heart rate becomes reduced as vagal stimulation is increased. Such interaction is not seen with AV nodal conduction, however; increased sympathetic tone increases AV nodal conduction while increased vagal tone decreases conduction rates. The effects of sympathetic stimulation are not affected by the level of vagal activity. Effects on myocardial contractility are biphasic and of great clinical importance. Hollenberg, Carriere, and Barger[63] showed that acetylcholine infused directly into a coronary artery in the open chest of the dog produced little decrease in contractility. If sympathetic tone were increased by sympathetic nerve stimulation or infusion of norepinephrine, however, acetylcholine infusion produced a marked decrease in contractile force. Combined sympathetic and vagal hyperactivity may coexist in the same patient, and can be expected to have an adverse effect on cardiac performance.

Muscarinic responses are much slower than nicotinic actions, suggesting a complex series of intermediate steps. The binding of acetylcholine to cardiac muscarinic receptors produces increased potassium permeability, a decrease in the slow inward calcium current, decreased cyclic AMP (cAMP) generation, and increased cylic guanine monophosphate (cGMP) generation.[64] Muscarinic stimulation produces increased hydrolysis of the membrane phospholipids, phosphoinositol. This response is similar to that seen with alpha-1 stimulation and is another example of the phosphoinositol-calmodulin cascade (see chapter 1, p. 13).

Vagal hyperactivity may complicate certain clinical situations. Activation of vagal afferents appears to be responsible for the striking parasympathetic hyperactivity seen within the first 30 minutes of acute myocardial infarction, particularly in patients with inferior or posterior wall ischemia.[65] Occlusion of the circumflex artery and, to a lesser degree, of the left descending coronary artery in the aorto-sinus denervated dog activated receptors producing bradycardia, hypotension, and a decrease in renal sympathetic nerve activity.[66]

Sympathetic (Adrenergic) Nervous System

The stress response described by Cannon and Selye has been discussed in Chapter 1 and Chapter 2. The simplest example of enhanced sympathetic activity is the baroreceptor response to hypotension or shock. If blood pressure is not rapidly restored to normal, a more generalized stress response may occur. ACTH release has long been recognized as an important part of the stress response, and recent studies suggest the central role of hypothalamic corticotropin releasing factor (CRF) in its genesis.[67] Epinephrine, norepinephrine, vasopressin, angiotensin II, vasoactive intestinal polypeptide, and direct neural stimulation from higher centers all increase CRF activity. Thus, different insults presumably initiate the stress response from different leverage points in the body defense system. Other levels are rapidly recruited, and within a short time, the generalized stress response with high circulating levels of catecholamines, ACTH, cortisol, and glucagon is observed. The sympathetic nervous system is key in the initial stages of this response.

Sympathetic neural activity arises in neurons located in the reticular formation of the pontomedullary region. Dorsal and lateral regions mediate vasoconstriction and cardiac acceleration; ventral areas mediate vasodepressor activities. Connections from these neurons descend into the spinal cord, reaching to the preganglionic neuronal bodies which, in turn, send fibers to the paraspinal sympathetic ganglia. Postganglionic fibers from these ganglia terminate in specialized nerve endings containing performed norepinephrine. Both epinephrine and norepinephrine are synthesized by the chromaffin cells located in the adrenal medulla. The relationship among nerve endings, granules and receptor sites is shown in Figure 4–20. Sympathetic neural activity leads to release of norepinephrine into the synaptic cleft and makes it available for binding to a group of peripheral sympathetic receptors. Afferent impulses from the vagus, the carotid sinus chemoreceptors, and baroreceptors project into the nucleus solitarius and influence the activity of the reticular effector neurons. Additional neural connections running between the pontomedullary region and the hypothalamus,limbic system, and cerebral cortex permit integration of conscious and unconscious activities. These interconnections are responsible for the classic Kocher-Cushing reflex, where a rise in intracranial pressure produces hypertension and bradycardia, presumably due to stimulation of areas near the floor of the fourth ventricle.

The biosynthesis of norepinephrine was described by Udenfriend[68] and is shown in Figure 4–21. Tyrosine (3 hydroxyphenylalanine) is enzymatically hydroxylated to dihydroxyphenylalanine or DOPA by an enzyme, tyrosine 3-monooxygenase. This step appears to be rate-limiting. DOPA is then decarboxylated to dishydroxyphenylethylamine or dopamine. Oxidation of the beta carbon in the phenylethylamine chain by a specific beta oxidase produces norepinephrine.

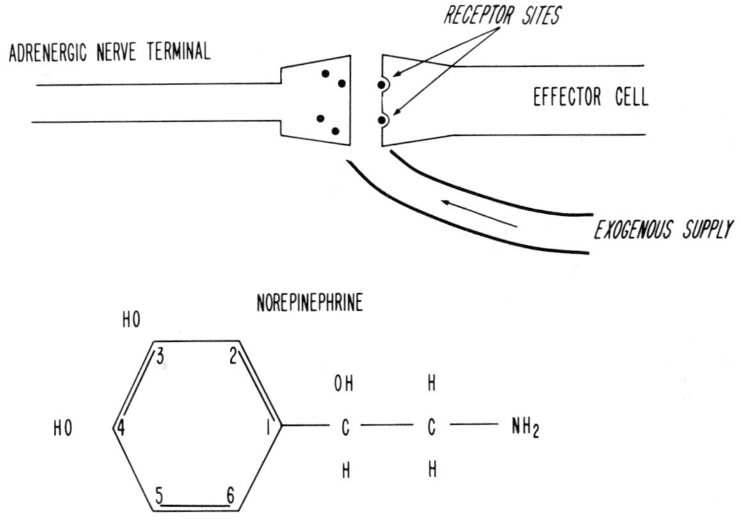

FIG 4–20.
Current concepts of adrenergic activation. Norepinephrine is synthesized in the adrenergic nerve terminal (1) and stored in specific granules (2). An action potential releases norepinephrine from the granules, which then combines with a specific receptor (3) on the effector cell. An exogenous supply of norepinephrine brought by the bloodstream can combine with receptor sites in the same manner (4). The structural formula of norepinephrine is shown at the bottom. All catecholamines have 3-4 hydroxy substitutes on the benzene ring. Various substitutions in the structural formula of nonepinephrine modify the physiologic action—e.g., epinephrine from the addition of a methyl group to the terminal amine, isoproterenol from the substitution of an isopropyl group.

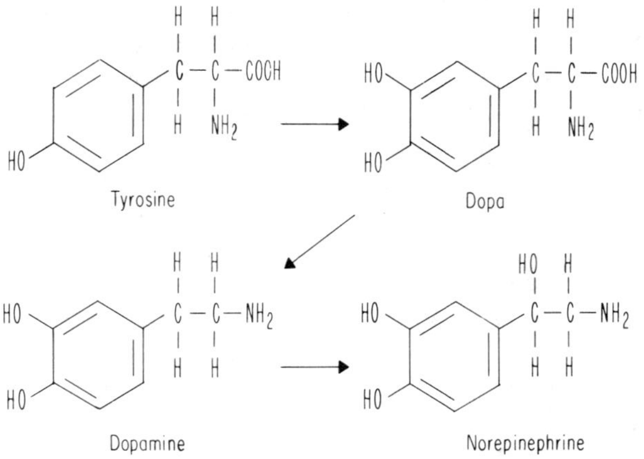

FIG 4–21.
Biosynthesis of norepinephrine. Tyrosine is hydroxylated in the two position to form dopa, which is subsequently dicarboxylated to form dopamine. Beta-hydroxylation of dopamine produces norepinephrine. Epinephrine develops from the subsequent end methylation of norepinephrine. (Adapted from Udenfriend S: Biosynthesis of the sympathetic neurotransmitter, norepinephrine. *Harvey Lectures* 1964–1965; 60:57.)

Methylation of the amino group by another specific enzyme restricted to the adrenal medulla converts norepinephrine to epinephrine. An influx of calcium into the adrenergic nerve terminal stimulates synthesis and release of neurotransmitter; ATP, magnesium and calcium are required for the reaction. Both a cyclic AMP dependent protein kinase and a specific calmodulin-dependent protein kinase (kinase II) can activate the rate-limiting enzyme, and coordinated action of both kinases probably plays an important regulatory role.

Norepinephrine is degraded in two ways. In one reaction the amine is oxidized by monoamine oxidase. The other reaction is initiated by a catechol-O-methyl transferase. Both oxidative deamination and O-methylation occur in normal man, but the relative activities of the two systems may vary from individual to individual. The end products of the two degradation systems are vanillic acid and 3-methoxy-4-hydroxymandelic acid, which are excreted in the urine and are useful indicators of the norepinephrine secretion rate.

Yamaguchi, de Champlain, and Nadeau[69] have shown experimentally that circulating catecholamine concentrations are closely related to the rate of sympathetic neural stimulation with a plateau at 8–10 Hz. Norepinephrine is released from adrenergic nerve endings and enters the synaptic cleft, where it binds to adrenergic receptors. The effects of neural stimulation are short lived, however, because active recapture (reuptake) of norepinephrine by the terminal ends occurs. Reuptake is less prominent in synaptic clefts associated with blood vessels because of rapid enzymatic breakdown and diffusion.

The existence of specific receptors was first proposed by Langley in 1905[70] to explain the actions of nicotine. The present-day availability of agonist radioligands have made possible the identification, localization, and characterization of many of these receptor sites. Receptors are now known to be specific molecules which react with a neurotransmitter on the outside of the plasmalemma and with an enzyme system inside the cell that generates an effector material or "second messenger" when the receptor is occupied by the neurotransmitter or "first messenger."

Dale showed that ergot blocked the pressor response of injected epinephrine, and Ahlquist postulated that at least two adrenergic receptors must be present to explain the observed responses to different catecholamines. The following responses were considered by Ahlquist to be typical of either alpha or beta receptors.

- Alpha receptor responses
  - Vascular smooth muscle contraction (vasoconstriction)
  - Iris dilator contraction (mydriasis)
  - Nictitating membrane smooth muscle contraction
  - Orbital smooth muscle contraction
  - Splenic smooth muscle contraction
  - Myometrial contraction
  - Retractor penis contraction
  - Seminal vesicle contraction
  - Philomotor muscle contraction
  - Intestinal smooth muscle relaxation
- Beta receptor responses
  - Vascular smooth muscle relaxation (vasodilation)
  - Bronchial smooth muscle relaxation
  - Myometrial relaxation
  - Intestinal smooth muscle relaxation
  - Myocardial positive inotropic response
  - Cardiac positive chronotropic response (sinus node)
  - Adenyl cyclase augmentation
  - Phosphorylase augmentation
  - Protein lipase augmentation
- Probable alpha type
  - Release of ACTH
  - Transient ganglionic blockade

Specific receptor blocking agents have confirmed Ahlquist's[72] postulation of two separate receptor sites, and improved analytic techniques have identified receptor-linked intracellular mediators. Relationships among adrenergic receptors, membrane channels, biochemical pumps, and intracellular events are shown in Figure 4–22. Sutherland and Rall[73] demonstrated that beta-adrenergic stimulation activates adenylate cyclase, which increases cyclic AMP synthesis. Cyclic AMP, in turn, phosphorylates a protein kinase that initiates smooth muscle relaxation. Calmodulin is an important and ubiquitous calcium-binding protein that modulates the activity of intracellular Ca^2. Alpha receptor stimulation either increases the influx of Ca^2 into the cell from extracellular sources, or increases the release of calcium from cytosolic stores, permitting binding and activation of calmodulin. An alpha-adrenergic mediated hydrolysis of phospholipids by specific phospholipase initiates calcium release. This linkage of calcium to alpha agonist activity explains the actions of alpha-adrenergic stimulation to increase myocardial contractility or constrict vascular tissues. The action of the two second messengers, Ca^{++} and cAMP, is described in Chapter 1.

The contrasting action of the beta agonist isoproterenol on smooth and cardiac muscle led Lands et al.[74] to suggest that two types of beta receptors existed. Beta-1 receptors were suggested to mediate stimulation of cardiac muscle and sinus node activity, inhibition of intestinal smooth muscle, and stimulation of lipolysis; beta-2 receptors to mediate inhibition of smooth muscle in the bronchioles, arterioles, and uterus, and to promote glycogenolysis.

A better understanding of membrane receptors soon led to the identification of presynaptic as well as postsynaptic adrenergic receptors. The classic alpha and beta receptors envisioned by Ahlquist[72] were postsynaptic receptors on cell membranes that were stimulated by neurotransmitter release into the synaptic cleft. Additional receptors on adrenergic nerve endings regulate adrenergic activity and are presynaptic in location. Alpha-adrenergic presynaptic receptors are termed alpha-2 receptors. Stimulation of these presynaptic alpha receptors causes negative feedback, decreasing norepinephrine secretion. Presynaptic beta receptors also have been identified, but stimulation of these enhances norepinephrine release producing positive feedback. Presynaptic alpha and beta receptors are also found in

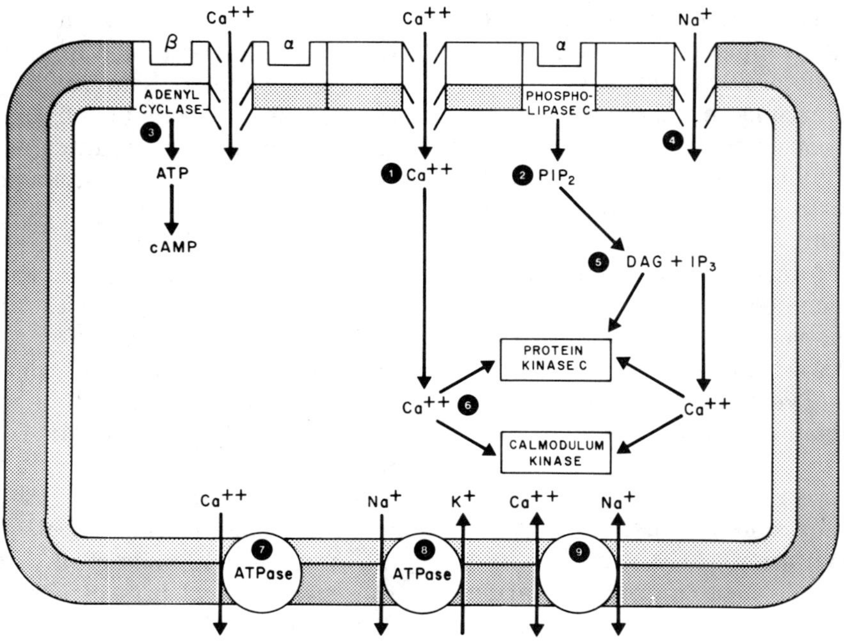

FIG 4–22.

Specialized organelles within the phospholipid bimolecular phospholipid cell membrane communicate with the environment and control cell function. Voltage-dependent-calcium gates allow calcium to enter the cell down a concentration gradient generating the slow calcium current (1). Calcium is mobilized within the cell by stimulation of alpha-1 receptors which activate phospholipase C to hydrolyze membrane phospholipids releasing phosphytidylinositol 4,5 biphosphate (PIP_2)(2). PIP_2 is hydrolyzed to diacylglycerol (DAG) and inosital 1,4,5 triphosphate (IP_3) Beta-adrenergic receptors are coupled to adenyl cyclase which generates cylic AMP (cAMP) and also opens other beta-adrenergic controlled calcium channels, particularly in myocardial cells. Voltage-dependent sodium channels open during depolarization in certain tissues and allow sodium influx into the cell (4). DAG directly activates protein kinase C by increasing the affinity of the kinase for calcium. IP_3 acts as an inophore and mobilizes intracellular calcium (5). Calcium entering through calcium channels performs many intracellular messenger functions as well as activating protein C kinases and calmodulin kinase (6). At least three pumping systems maintain intracellular ionic concentration. An energy-dependent calcium ATPase pump extrudes calcium from the cell (7). Cell polarization is maintained by a sodium-potassium ATPase pump which exchanges sodium and potassium across the cell membrane. Inactivation of this pump by digitalis leads to an increase in intracellular sodium concentration, which is subsequently exchanged for calcium by a calcium-sodium exchange mechanism driven by the inward movement of calcium from the exterior.

the central nervous system and appear to be important regulators of central sympathetic activity.

Continued study of adrenergic receptors provides sometimes unexpected findings that may be useful in the care of critically ill patients. Alpha-2 receptors are not only presynaptic, but also may be located on blood vessels (postsynaptic). There is good evidence that the alpha-1 postsynaptic receptor is located near an adrenergic nerve terminal. The alpha-2 postsynaptic receptors, in contrast, appear to be extrajunctional and are located some distance from the synaptic cleft where they are in a position to be directly exposed to the circulation. Stimulation of alpha-2 receptors increases the influx of calcium from the exterior, suggesting a direct effect on calcium channels. Indeed, calcium channel blockade with nifedipine or verapamil inhibits alpha-2 mediated vasoconstriction. In contrast, alpha-1 receptor stimulation produces vasoconstriction by release of calcium from intracellular pools.[75]

The synthesis of adrenergic receptors may be increased (up-regulated) or decreased (down-regulated). When tissues are deprived of their sympathetic input, for example, an increased uesponsiveness of the adenylate cyclase receptor is noted; a decreased responsiveness is seen when tissues are overexposed to norepinephrine. The down-regulation of alpha-adrenergic receptors in critically ill patients may explain their lack of responsiveness to exogenously administered catecholamines.

A recent symposium on the effects of aging on adrenergic receptors[76] pointed out that both baroreceptor and chronotropic responses were diminished in elderly individuals. Evidence suggesting a decreased density of alpha and beta receptors in both the periphery and the brain of older animals were presented. Elderly patients exhibit decreased homeostatic cardiovascular responses in a variety of clinical situations, and a down-regulation of adrenergic receptors may be an important reason for these blunted responses to stress. Adrenergic blockade might have unexpectedly adverse consequences in patients with down-regulated receptors.

The differential effects of alpha-1 and alpha-2 receptor stimulation may be exploited in certain clinical situations. Phenoxybenzamine is an alpha-1 blocking agent that has been used in vasoconstrictor states. Clonidine may accomplish a similar effect by stimulating alpha-2 receptors and decreasing the release of norepinephrine from nerve terminals. Prazosin has a high affinity for alpha-1 receptors and a low affinity for alpha-2 receptors. Unlike phentolamine and tolazoline, it is an effective antihypertensive agent because it blocks the postsynaptic norepinephrine receptor but does not interfere with the action of the presynaptic receptor to limit norepinephrine release.

A third class of receptor, the dopamine (DA-1) receptor, mediates vasodilatation in the renal, mesenteric, coronary and cerebral vascular beds. Like beta receptor agonists, DA-1 agonists stimulate adenylate cyclase to synthesize cyclic AMP. DA-2 receptors act as alpha-2 receptors and inhibit the release of norepinephrine for adrenergic terminals. They either decrease or have no effect on the formation of cyclic AMP. To date, DA-2 receptors have not been localized in vascular muscle.

Sympathomimetic Amines in Shock and Ventricular Failure

Both beta-1 and alpha-adrenergic stimulation increase myocardial contractility, and sympathomimetic amines long have been used to support the heart and circulation. These agents are molecules that mimic the action of sympathetic neural stimulation. The neurotransmitter norepinephrine, when administered exogenously, becomes "sympathomimetic." Sympathomimetic amines may also be called adrenergic agonists because their physiologic effect is derived from occupancy of adrenergic receptors. They are substituted phenylethylamines; when hydroxy groups are present at the 3 and 4 positions of the benzene ring, they are termed catecholamines. Not all inotropic substances are sympathomimetic, and not all sympathomimetic drugs are catecholamines. Some drugs, like theophylline for example, increase cyclic AMP by preventing its destruction by phosphodiesterases rather than by functioning as adrenergic agonists.

Ephedrine was first used by the Chinese as a general tonic 5,000 years ago. It directly stimulates alpha and beta receptors and also releases norepinephrine. Its cardiovascular effects, in general, resemble those seen after administration of a dilute solution of epinephrine, although its onset of action is slower and its effects more prolonged. The effects of the drug decline after repeated use (tachyphylaxis), in part due to depletion of norepinephrine from nerve endings. The physiologic catecholamines, epinephrine, norepinephrine, and dopamine, have different and specific effects on vascular and cardiac smooth muscle, on the airway, on certain neuronal receptors, and on certain metabolic pathways. Chemical manipulation of these naturally occurring molecules has produced new agents such as isoproterenol and dobutamine, which have been created for specific pharmacologic effects (Table 4–5).

Almost all catecholamines possess substantial inotropic activity; choice of a specific agent is based on its associated

TABLE 4–5.
Absolute Changes in Hemodynamics and Myocardial Metabolism Produced by L-Norepinephrine (NE), Dopamine (DOPA), and Isoproterenol (ISO)

MEASUREMENT (MEAN VALUES)	NE (4.5 μ MINUTE)	DOPA (0.43 MG/MINUTE)	ISO (2.14 μ/MINUTE)
Ventricular rate (beats/minute)	+ 12[a,b]	+ 22[c]	+ 24[d]
Arterial pressure			
Systolic	+ 38[a,d]	+ 18[cd]	− 2.00
Diastolic	+ 19[a,b,d]	+ 3.0	− 2.11
Mean	+ 23[a,b,d]	+ 7.0[c,d]	− 7.12
Cardiac index (liters/minute/meter^2)	+ 0.20[a,b]	+ 1.11[d]	+ 0.98[d]
Systemic vascular resistance (dynes-second-cm^{-5})	+384[a,b,d]	−472[d]	−580[d]
Left ventricular work index (kg meter/minute/meter^2)	+ 1.21[d]	+ 1.87[c,d]	+ 0.70
Time-tension index (mm Hg second/minute)	+656[bd]	+625[d]	+152
Systolic ejection rate (ml/second/meter^2)	+ 4.10[a,b]	+ 35	+ 24
Coronary blood flow (ml/100 g/minute)	+ 13[b,d]	+ 23[c,d]	+ 53[d]
Myocardial oxygen consumption (ml/100 g/minute)	+ 1.68[b,d]	+ 2.04[d]	+ 4.05[d]
Myocardial oxygen extraction (%)	+ 2.03[b]	+ 3.12[c]	− 6.12
Myocardial lactate extraction (%)	− 6.12	− 3.02	− 2.10
Myocardial pyruvate extraction (%)	− 4.13	− 4.10	− 3.10
Urine (cc/hour)	− 8.00	+ 75[a,d]	ND[e]

Change is significant at a level $p < .05$ or less
[a]L-Norepinephrine-dopamine.
[b]L-Norepinephrine-isoproterenol.
[c]Dopamine-isoproterenol.
[d]Control-drug.
[e]No data.

peripheral vascular effects. Dobutamine appears to be useful in patients with ventricular dysfunction or failure because it is a pulmonary and systemic vasodilator as well as an inotrope. Indeed, dobutamine occasionally produces hypotension, especially if volume contraction is present. When systemic hypotension is profound and it has been determined that volume loading is optimal, peripheral vascular resistance should be increased with either l-norepinephrine or dopamine. L-norepinephrine is generally preferred because it usually does not increase heart rate. An increase in perfusion pressure may improve myocardial oxygenation in patients with ischemic heart disease but the increasing afterload produced by vasoconstriction increases pulmonary capillary wedge pressure and may lead to further myocardial deterioration. In addition the use of vasoconstrictors may further intensify the effect of endogenous catecholamines and further reduce perfusion to the renal and splanchnic vascular beds, especially in the presence of hypovolemia. Where possible, blood pressure in patients with ventricular failure should be elevated by improving stroke output with an inotrope rather than by increasing peripheral resistance.

L-Norepinephrine (Levophed)

The effect of exogenously administered norepinephrine is identical to that following stimulation of the sympathetic nervous system. It acts primarily on alpha receptors in peripheral arterioles and beta receptors in the heart, causing an increase in peripheral vascular resistance and an increased force of myocardial contraction. The former effect is responsible for the increase in arterial blood pressure. Cardiac output and rate do not increase significantly because of reflex vagal inhibition triggered by the rise in arterial blood pressure. Norepinephrine causes a rise in cardiac output in isolated heart preparations, in persons with hypotension, and in those in whom the vagal regulatory reflexes are suppressed by atropine.

Myocardial work, myocardial oxygen consumption, and coronary flow are all increased. With low concentrations of the drug, the increase in coronary flow appears to be adequate for the increased oxygen requirement. High concentrations of norepinephrine, however, increase myocardial work and oxygen consumption to a much greater degree than coronary flow, leading to a deterioration in cardiac nutrition.

Peripheral blood flow is decreased in all vascular beds. This is most marked in the splanchnic and renal circulations. Renal blood flow may fall to zero with high concentrations of Levophed. Splanchnic vasoconstriction explains the ulcerations occasionally seen in the gastrointestinal tract following norepinephrine infusion in shock patients.

Epinephrine (Adrenalin)

Epinephrine differs from norepinephrine only by the presence of a methyl group on the terminal amine. While norepinephrine raises blood pressure by increasing peripheral vascular resistance, there is good evidence that epinephrine raises blood pressure primarily by increasing cardiac output. The overall peripheral vascular resistance falls, indicating that the stimulation of beta receptors exceeds that of alpha receptors. Skeletal muscle, coronary, cerebral, and splanchnic blood flow increase, while renal and cutaneous blood flow decrease.

The increase in cardiac output is due to an increase both in the force of myocardial contraction and the heart rate. Myocardial oxygen consumption is markedly increased and may actually exceed the increase in coronary flow, leading to a net decrease in myocardial nutrition. Epinephrine appears to be a useful agent for the treatment of cardiogenic shock except for shock following acute myocardial infarction. In the latter kind of shock, maintenance of aortic and thus coronary perfusion pressure is of more importance than improvement of cardiac output (chapter 5).

Isoproterenol (Isuprel)

The substitution of an isopropyl group for the methyl group on the terminal amine of norepinephrine produces an active compound that is an almost pure beta stimulator. Isoproterenol stimulates beta-1 adrenergic receptors, increasing myocardial contractility and heart rate, and stimulates beta-2 receptors, producing marked vasodilatation which may shunt blood preferentially to skeletal muscle. It also lowers the diastolic aortic pressure. Isoproterenol rarely is used to support the failing heart because of its adverse effects on oxygen balance. Increased heart rate and myocardial contractility increase oxygen demand while a fall in diastolic pressure decreases the coronary perfusion. The stage is set for uneven distribution of coronary blood flow as flow increases in dilated normal segments, while the low end-diastolic arterial pressure deprives atheromatous segments of adequate perfusion.

Dopamine and Dobutamine

Dopamine became widely used in the late 1960s because it appeared to have mixed alpha and beta adrenergic agonist activities that closely resembled epinephrine in its pharmacologic activity. It was later found that dopamine, unlike epinephrine, had selective vasodilating effects on certain vascular beds because of its action on specific dopamine receptors. Since norepinephrine decreased peripheral perfusion even though it increased coronary blood flow, and since isoproterenol increased myocardial oxygen requirements inordinately, dopamine was used widely as a compromise agent. Dopamine has significant beta agonist activity, however, and Mueller, Evans, and Ayres[77] showed that while dopamine improved cardiac performance, it also decreased myocardial oxygenation in the ischemic myocardium.

Dobutamine was specifically synthesized as an inotrope.[78] The two enantiomers that make up the commercially available racemic mixture have dramatically different receptor affinities. Levo-dobutamine is an alpha-1 agonist with weak beta activity, while dextro-dobutamine is a selective beta agonist with greater beta-1 than beta-2 activity. The net effect is a strong positive inotropic effect due to stimulation of both alpha-1 and beta-1 receptors in the heart. The expected beta-2 chronotropic effect is blunted by the parallel effects on alpha-1 receptors. An integrated effect on the peripheral vasculature is also a consequence of combined alpha-1 and beta-2 stimulation; the effect on peripheral resistance and blood pressure depends upon the balance between alpha-adrenergic constrictor and beta-adrenergic dilator actions. In many clinical situations, mild vasodilatation is observed.

The dose-related positive intropic effect of dobutamine was demonstrated by Vatner, McRitchie, and Braunwald[79] in conscious and in anesthetized dogs. Peak dP/dt more than doubled when 40 ug/kg/min were administered. Left ventricular end-diastolic volume or pressure did not change in these normal ventricles, but end-systolic diameter decreased 18%, reflecting an increase in myocardial fiber shortening. The same investigators noted that coronary and iliac blood flow increased at doses of 8 and 20 ug/kg/min while at 40 ug/kg/min mesenteric flow also was increased. Robie and Goldberg[80] found that dobutamine produced a preferential distribution of blood flow to muscle, while dopamine increased renal and mesenteric flow. An important difference in pulmonary vascular tone was observed by Furman et al.[81] in a perfused pig lung preparation. Dopamine at doses of 20 ug/kg/min produced pulmonary vasoconstriction. Dobutamine did not change pulmonary vascular resistance during normoxic perfusion but decreased pulmonary vasoconstriction during hypoxic ventilation in a dose-dependent manner. Akhtar et al.,[82] working in Cohn's laboratory, demonstrated that dobutamine increased stroke output and decreased pulmonary capillary pressure in patients with severe ventricular failure. A group of studies published in 1977 and 1978 compared the effects of dopamine and dobutamine. (Table 4-6) The study of Leier et al.[83] of patients with cardiomyopathy is representative of these publications. Dobutamine increased stroke output in a linear manner as dosage was increased in increments to 10.0 ug/kg/min. In contrast, stroke output reached a peak with doses of 4.0 ug/kg/min and fell almost to control levels at doses of 8 ug/kg/min. Systolic pressure rose almost linearly with dopamine; with dobutamine it rose modestly and then levelled off at 7.5 ug/kg/min. Both pulmonary and systemic vascular resistance decreased linearly with increasing doses of dobutamine, but not with dopamine. Pulmonary capillary pressure decreased by 20% with dobutamine, but rose in an almost linear manner as the dose of dopamine was increased. The increase in pulmonary capillary pressure and return of stroke output to control levels demonstrates the damaging effect of increased afterload on ventricular function. Dopamine produced somewhat more tachycardia than dobutamine at higher doses and also produced more ventricular premature contractions than dobutamine ($p \leq 0.05$). Interestingly, urine flow and creatinine clearance increased with dobutamine at doses of 7.5 ug/kg/min but not with dopamine at doses of 3.85 ug/kg/min. Mean hepatic blood flow measured by indocyanine green clearance did not change significantly with either drug, but mean upper limb blood flow measured by venous-occlusive plethysmography increased significantly with dobutamine but not with dopamine.

The availability of two inotropic molecules with differing effects on the peripheral vasculature provides the intensivist with considerably flexibility. Dobutamine increases stroke output and decreases systemic vascular resistance while maintaining blood pressure in most individuals. Dopamine, in low doses, increases renal and splanchnic blood flow by specific action on dopaminergic receptors. At higher doses, however,

TABLE 4–6.
The Hemodynamic Actions of Dobutamine and Dopamine

	SHOCK		NO SHOCK	
	DOPAMINE	DOBUTAMINE	DOPAMINE	DOBUITAMINE
Stroke Output	+27%	+19	+23	+96
Arterial Pressure	+33	+ 2	+18	+ 5
Pulmonary Wedge	+64	−17	+32	−18
Heart Rate	+14%	+ 6%	+38%	+ 4

Dopamine: 15ug/kg/min in both groups ()
Dobutamine: 15ug/kg/min in shock; 10 ug/kg/min in no shock

Adapted from Leier CV, Heban PT, Huss P, Bush CA, Lewis RP: Comparative systemic and regional hemodynamic effects of dopamine and dobutamine in patients with cardiomyopathic heart failure. *Circulation* 1978; 58:466-475; and Francis GS, Sharma B, Hodges M: Comparative hemodynamic effects of dopamine and dibutamine in patients with acute cardiogenic circulatory collapse. *Am Heart J* 1982; 103: 995-1000.

alpha-adrenergic activity dominates and produces systemic vasoconstriction with an increase in pulmonary capillary pressure. Combining the two agents in varying proportions may be useful in certain clinical situations. Richard et al.[84] found that a mixture of 7.5 ug/kg/min of each drug produced the same effect on cardiac output as either agent alone, significantly increased mean arterial pressure compared to dobutamine alone, and maintained that pulmonary capillary wedge pressure within normal limits compared to the increase seen when dopamine was used as a single drug.

The ability to manipulate the catecholamine molecule theoretically could lead to a spectrum of agents specifically tailored to individual clinical situations. Many clinicians believe that a small concentration of dopamine is almost always indicated in seriously ill patients because of its effect on renal blood flow. Since the alpha and beta-1 adrenergic properties of dopamine may not always be desired, a new molecule which stimulates, DA-1, DA-2, and beta-2 receptors has been synthesized (dopexamine).[85] Renal blood flow and peripheral vasodilatation results and DA-2 receptor occupancy reduces norepinephrine secretion. Its role in critical care medicine remains to be evaluated.

Phosphodiesterase Inhibitors as Inotropes

Cyclic AMP is degraded by enzymes called phosphodiesterases (Fig 4–23); inhibition of these enzymes leads to an increase in cAMP and a consequent increase in myocardial contractility. Methylxanthines such as aminophylline (theophylline) have long been used for the emergency treatment of acute pulmonary edema or acute bronchoconstriction but have a variety of effects in addition to their inhibition of phosphodiesterase. These additional effects include direct blockade of adenosine, inhibition of calcium uptake by the sarcoplasmic reticulum, enhancement of the affinity of troponin for calcium, and increased synthesis and release of catecholamines. The actions of the newer inotropes such as amrinone appear related to the inhibition of phosphodiesterase F-III, the cyclic AMP specific cardiac phosphodiesterase. The inhibition is selective so that many of the additional effects seen with theophylline are avoided. Amrinone is both an inotrope and vasodilator; both of these actions probably account for its ability to raise cardiac output and decrease filling pressures. It produces a group of side effects including thrombocytopenia, and has been suspected, but not proven, to enhance ventricular dysfunction.[86] The oral preparation was withdrawn, but an intravenous preparation is now available for hospital use. Franciosa[87] recently has reviewed studies suggesting that it is a vasodilator rather than an inotrope and concluded that it should be used only as a "last resort after careful documentation that other available agents such as dobu-

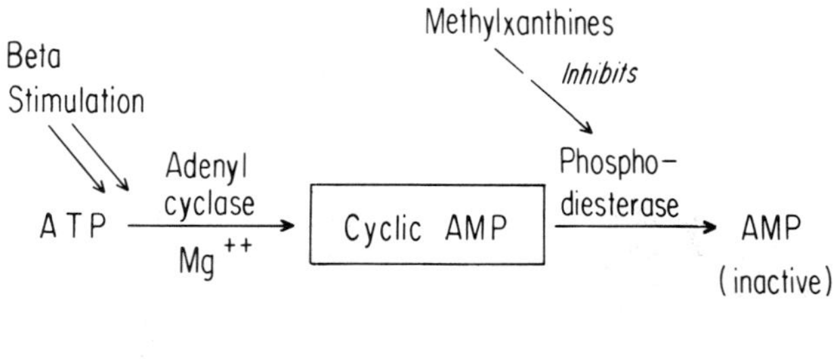

FIG 4–23.
Adrenergic action. Beta-adrenergic agonists are believed to bind to a specific receptor and activate adenyl cyclase. The adenyl cyclase converts adenosine triphosphate (ATP) to cylic AMP. This important compound is believed to activate a variety of protein kinases, which then perform a variety of cellular functions. Cyclic AMP is inactivated by the enzyme phosphodiesterase. Phosphodiesterase is inhibited by methylxanthines.

tamine, dopamine, and nitroprusside have been properly tried first without success." Sudden hypotension may be observed with its use, particularly in volume depleted patients. Saltiel, Adelman, and Rubin[88] have recently pointed out that a long half-life of up to 12 hours in patients with heart failure makes titration of effect difficult.

In general it seems preferable to begin treatment with sympathomimetic agents such as norepinephrine, dobutamine, or dopamine. Amrinone activity is not mediated through the adrenergic receptor, and the agent may be useful in situations where high concentrations of catecholamines have occupied all available adrenergic receptors. A related compound, milrinone, appears much less toxic than amrinone and could play an important role in the ambulatory care of individuals with poor ventricular function.

REFERENCES

1. Harvey W: De Motu Cordis, 1628. (Transl. by C. D. Leake, Springfield, 1928, C. C. Thomas.)

2. Frank O: Die Grundform des arteriellen Pulses. *Z Biol* 1890; 37:483.

3. Patterson SW, Piper H, Starling EH: The regulation of the heart beat. *J Physiol* (Lond) 1914; 48:465.

4. Braunwald E, Ross J, Sonnenblick EH: *Mechanisms of Contraction of the Normal and Failing Heart.* Boston, Little, Brown, 1968; 56.

5. Hill AV: Heat of shortening and dynamic constants of muscle. *Proc R Soc Lond [Biol]* 1938; 126:136.

6. Fawcett DW: Sarcoplasmic reticulum of skeletal and cardiac muscle. *Circulation* 1961; 24:336.

7. Katz AM: *Physiology of the Heart.* New York, Raven Press, 1977.

8. Scheuer J, Bhan AK: Cardiac contractile proteins: Adenosine triphosphate activity and physiologic function. *Circ Res* 1979; 45:1.

9. Drummond GI, Severson DL: Cyclic nucleotides and cardiac function. *Circ Res* 1979; 44:145.

10. Sonnenblick EH, Spiro D, Spotnitz HM: Ultrastructural basis of Starling's law of heart: Role of sarcomere in determining ventricular size and stroke volume. *Am Heart J* 1964; 68:336.

11. Frank O: On the dynamics of cardiac muscle. (Translated by Chapman CB, Wasserman E.) *Am Heart J* 1959; 58:282, 467.

12. Starling EH: *The Linacre Lecture on the Law of the Heart.* London, Longmans, Green, 1918.

13. Sarnoff SJ, Berglund E: Ventricular function. I. Starling's law of the heart studied by means of simultaneous right and left ventricular function curves in the dog. *Circulation* 1954; 9:706.

14. Lewis BM, Houssay HE, Haynes FW, et al: Dynamics of both right and left ventricles at rest and during exercise in patients with heart failure. *Circ Res* 1953; 1:312.

15. Dodge HT, Sandler H, Ballew DW, et al: Use of biplane angiocardiography for the measurement of left ventricular volume in man. *Am Heart J* 1960; 60:762.

16. Kennedy JW, Baxley WA, Figley MM, et al: Quantitative angiocardiography. I. The normal left ventricle in man. *Circulation* 1966; 34:272.

17. Sanmarco ME, Bartle SH: Left ventricular volume determinations: Comparison of angiocardiographic and thermal washout techniques. *Circulation* 1964; 30(suppl III): 151.

18. Gault JH, Ross J Jr, Braunwald E: Contractile state of the left ventricle in man. *Circ Res* 1968; 22:451.

19. Sonnenblick EH: Force-velocity relations in mammalian heart muscle. *Am J Physiol* 1962; 202:931.

20. Wiggers CJ: *Physiology of Shock.* New York, The Commonwealth Fund, 1950.

21. Sibbald WJ, Calvin J, Driedger AA: Right and left ventricular preload and diastolic ventricular compliance: Implications for therapy in critically ill patients, in Shoemaker WC, Thompson WL, Holbrook PR (eds): *Textbook of*

Critical Care. Philadelphia, WB Saunders Co, 1984.

22. Calvin J, Driedger A, Sibbald W: The effect of phentolamine in low cardiac output syndrome as assessed by radionuclide angiography. *Crit Care Med* 1980; 8:240.

23. Calvin JE, Driedger AA, Sibbald WJ: The hemodynamic effect of rapid fluid infusion in critically ill patients. *Surgery* 1981; 90:61.

24. Sutherland GR, Calvin JE, Driedger AA, et al: Anatomic and cardiopulmonary responses to trauma with associated blunt chest injury. *J Trauma* 1981; 21:1.

25. Johnson PC (ed.): Autoregulation of blood flow. *Circ Res* 1964; 15(Suppl. I):1.

26. Warner HR: Control of the circulation as studied with analog computer technics. In *Handbook of Physiology*, Section 2. Washington, DC, American Physiological Society, 1965, vol 3, chap 50, p 1825.

27. Rushmer RF: Postural effects on the baselines of ventricular performance. *Circulation* 1959; 20:897.

28. Damato AN, Galante JG, Smith WM: Hemodynamic response to treadmill exercise in normal patients. *J Appl Physiol* 1966; 21:959.

29. Robinson S, Pearcy M, Brueckman FR, et al: Effects of atropine on heart rate and oxygen intake in working man. *J Appl Physiol* 1953; 5:508.

30. Bowditch HP: Über die Eigenthümlichkeiten der Reizarkeit, welche die Muskelfasern des Herzens zeigen. *Berichte Köngl Sächs Ges Wissen* 1871; 23:652.

31. Guyton AC: Circulation. In *Handbook of Physiology*, Section 2. Washington, DC, American Physiological Society, 1963, vol 2, chap 32, p 1099.

32. Burton AC: *Physiology and Biophysics of the Circulation*. Chicago, Year Book Publishers, 1965.

33. Burton AC, Yamada S: Relation between blood pressure and flow in the human forearm. *J Appl Physiol* 1951; 4:329.

34. Levy MN: Relative influence of variations in arterial and venous pressure on resistance to flow. *Am J Physiol* 1958; 192:164.

35. Zweifach BW: Basic mechanisms in peripheral vascular hemostasis, in *Third Conference on Factors Regulating Blood Pressure*. New York, Josiah Macy Jr Foundation, 1950.

36. Krogh, A: *The Anatomy and Physiology of Capillaries*. New Haven, Conn, Yale Univ Press, 1929.

37. Smith AL, Neufeld GR, Ominsky AJ, et al: Effect of arterial CO_2 tension on cerebral blood flow, mean transit time, and vascular volume. *J Appl Physiol* 1971; 31:701.

38. Schmidt CF: *The Cerebral Circulation in Health and Disease*. Springfield, Ill, Charles C Thomas, 1950.

39. Kety SS, Schmidt CF: The effects of altered arterial tensions of carbon dioxide and oxygen on cerebral blood flow and cerebral oxygen consumption of normal young men. *J Clin Invest* 1948; 27:484.

40. Alexander SC, Wollman H, Cohen PJ, et al: Cerebrovascular response to Pa_{CO_2} during halothane anesthesia in man. *J Appl Physiol* 1964; 19:561.

41. Wollmann H, Smith T, Stephen GW, et al: Effects of extremes of respiratory and metabolic alkalosis on cerebral blood flow in man. *J Appl Physiol* 1968; 24:60.

42. Severinghaus JW, Chiodi H, Eger EI, et al: Cerebral blood flow in man at high altitude. *Circ Res* 1966; 19:274.

43. Kronenberg RS, Cain SM: Effect of acetazolamide and hypoxia on cerebrospinal fluid bicarbonate. *J Appl Physiol* 1968; 24:17.

44. Cotev S, Lee J, Severinghaus JW: The effects of acetazolamide on cerebral blood flow and cerebral tissue P_{O_2}. *Anesthesiology* 1968; 29:471.

45. Sokoloff L, Kety SS: Regulation of cerebral circulation. *Physiol Rev* 1960; 40 (suppl 4):38.

46. Messer JV, Wagman RJ, Levine HJ, et al: Patterns of human myocardial oxygen extraction during rest and exercise. *J Clin Invest* 1962; 41:725.

47. Berne RM: Effect of epinephrine and norepinephrine on coronary circulation. *Circ Res* 1958; 6:644.

48. Neill WA: Effects of arterial hypox-

emia and hyperoxia on oxygen availability for myocardial metabolism. *Am J Cardiol* 1969; 24:166.

49. Fowler NO: The normal pulmonary arterial pressure-flow relationship during exercise. *Am J Med* 1969; 47:1.

50. Golinko RJ, Kaplan N, Rudolph AM: The mechanism of pulsus paradoxus during acute pericardial tamponade. *J Clin Invest* 1963; 42:249.

51. Morgan BC, Dillard DH, Guntheroth WG: Effect of cardiac and respiratory cycle on pulmonary vein flow, pressure, and diameter. *J Appl Physiol* 1966; 21:1276.

52. Cournand A, Motley HL, Richards DW Jr: Physiologic studies of the effects of IPPB on cardiac output. *Am J Physiol* 1948; 152:162.

53. Braunwald E, Binton JT, Morgan WL, et al: Alterations in central blood volume and cardiac output induced by positive pressure breathing and counteracted by metaraminol (Aramine). *Circ Res* 1957; 5:670.

54. Patel DJ, Burton AC: Active constriction of small pulmonary arteries in rabbits. *Circ Res* 1957; 5:620.

55. Liljestrand G: Chemical control of the distribution of the pulmonary blood flow. *Acta Physiol Scand* 1958; 44:216.

56. Enson Y, Guintini C, Lewis L, et al: The influence of hydrogen ion concentration and hypoxemia on the pulmonary circulation. *J Clin Invest* 1964; 43:1146.

57. Takeuchi J, Aoki S, Nomura G, et al: Nervous control of renal circulation—On the existence of sympathetic cholinergic fibers. *J Appl Physiol* 1971; 31:686.

58. Pitts RF: *Physiology of the Kidney and Body Fluids*, 2nd ed. Chicago, Year Book Medical Publishers, 1968.

59. Smith HW: Physiology of the renal circulation. *Harvey Lect* 1939—1940; 35:166.

60. Laragh JH: Renin, angiotensin, aldosterone, and hormonal regulation of blood pressure and salt balance. *Fed Proc* 1967; 26:39.

61. Bradley SE, Ingelfinger FJ, Bradley GP, et al: The estimation of hepatic blood flow in man. *J Clin Invest* 1945; 24:890.

62. Levy MN: Cardiac sympathetic-parasympathetic interactions. *Fed Proc* 1984; 43:2598.

63. Hollenberg M, Carriere S, Barger AC: Biphasic action of acetylcholine on ventricular myocardium. *Circ Res* 1965; 16:527–536.

64. Brown JH, Masters SB: Muscarinic regulation of phosphatidylinositol turnover and cyclic nucleotide metabolism in the heart. *Fed Proc* 1984; 43:2613.

65. Webb SW, Adgey AAJ, Pantridge JF: Autonomic disturbance at onset of acute myocardial infarction. *Br Med J* 1972; 3:89–92.

66. Thames MD, Abboud FM: Reflex inhibition of renal sympathetic nerve activity during myocardial ischemia mediated by left ventricular receptors with vagal afferents in dogs. *J Clin Invest* 1979; 63:395–402.

67. Makara GB: Mechanisms by which stressful stimuli activate the pituitary–adrenal system. *Fed Proc* 1985; 44:149.

68. Udenfriend S: Biosynthesis of the sympathetic neurotransmitter, norepinephrine. *Harvey Lect* 1964–65; 60:57.

69. Yamaguchi N, de Champlain J, Nadeau R: Correlation between the response of the heart to sympathetic stimulation and the release of endogenous catecholamines into the coronary sinus of the dog. *Circ Res* 1975; 36:662–668.

70. Langley JN: On the reaction of nerve endings to certain poisons chiefly as regards the reaction of striated muscles to nicotine and to curare. *J Physiol (Lond)* 1905; 33:374–413.

71. Dale HH: On some physiological action of ergot. *J Physiol* 1906; 34:163.

72. Ahlquist RP: A study of the adrenotropic receptors. *Am J Physiol* 1948; 153:586.

73. Sutherland EW, Rall TW: The relation of adenosine- 3′,5′ phosphate and phosphorylase to the action of catecholamines and other hormones. *Pharmacol Rev* 1960; 12:265.

74. Lands AM, Arnold A, McAuliff JP, et al: Differentiation of receptor systems activated by sympathomimetic amines. *Nature (Lond)* 1967; 214:597.

75. Matthews WD, Kim KF, Hieble JP, et al: Postsynaptic alpha adrenoceptors on vascular

smooth muscle. *Fed Proc* 1984; 43:2923.

76. Roberts J, Steinberg GM: Effects of aging on adrenergic receptors. Introduction. *Fed Proc* 1986; 45:40.

77. Mueller HS, Evans R, Ayres SM: Effect of dopamine on hemodynamics and myocardial metabolism in shock following acute myocardial infarction in man. *Circulation* 1978; 57:361.

78. Tuttle RR, Mills J: Dobutamine: Development of a new catecholamine to selectively increase cardiac contractility. *Circ Res* 1975; 38:185–196.

79. Vatner SF, McRitchie RJ, Braunwald E: Effects of dobutamine on left ventricular performance, coronary dynamics, and distribution of cardiac output in conscious dogs. *J Clin Invest* 1974; 53:1265–1273.

80. Robie NW, Goldberg LI: Comparative systemic and regional hemodynamic effects of dopamine and dobutamine. *Am Heart J* 1975; 90(3):340–345.

81. Furman WR, Summer WR, Kennedy TP, et al: Comparison of the effects of dobutamine, dopamine, and isoproterenol on hypoxic pulmonary vasoconstriction in the pig. *Crit Care Med* 1982; 10(6):371–374.

82. Akhtar N, Mikulic E, Cohn JN, et al: Hemodynamic effect of dobutamine in patients with severe heart failure. *Am J Cardiol* 1975; 36:202–205.

83. Leier CV, Heban PT, Huss P, et al: Comparative systemic and regional hemodynamic effects of dopamine and dobutamine in patients with cardiomyopathic heart failure. *Circulation* 1978; 58:466–475.

84. Richard C, Ricome JL, Rimailho A, et al: Combined hemodynamic effects of dopamine and dobutamine in cardiogenic shock. *Circulation* 1983; 67:620–626.

85. Brown RA, Farmer JB, Hall JC, et al: The effects of dopexamine on the cardiovascular system of the dog. *Br J Pharmacol,* 1985; 85:609.

86. Colucci WS, Wright RF, Braunwald E: New positive inotropic agents in the treatment of congestive heart failure. *N Engl J Med* 1986; 314:290–299.

87. Franciosa JA: Intravenous amrinone: an advance or a wrong step? *Ann Intern Med* 1985; 102:399.

88. Saltiel E, Adelman DC, Rubin SA: New positive inotropic agents for congestive heart failure (letter). *N Engl J Med* 1986; 315:397.

5 CARDIOVASCULAR DYSFUNCTION, FAILURE, AND SHOCK

The function of the heart is to pump blood to the peripheral tissues and lungs. Blood flow to each organ system is determined by the mean arterial pressure generated by the heart and by the resistance to blood flow imposed by that organ system. Heart failure implies inadequacy of that function so that the heart is unable to pump blood at a rate sufficient to meet the metabolic requirements of the body tissues. The rate of pumping (cardiac output) is usually diminished in heart failure, but may be normal or even elevated when peripheral demands are great. Thus, the precise level of cardiac output is less important than its relationship to peripheral needs. In the hypothyroid state, for example, cardiac output may be reduced, yet heart failure may not be present since the metabolic requirements are very low. In contrast, beriberi, hyperthyroidism, and sepsis are characterized by a marked increase in cardiac output that may, nevertheless, be inadequate to meet the tissue needs so that heart failure, by definition, exists. Heart failure, then, is associated with inadequate cardiac output due to a defect in myocardial contraction and is best labelled as *contractile failure*.

The classic manifestations of heart failure due to defects in myocardial contractility are a consequence of inadequate delivery of blood to metabolizing tissues (*circulatory insufficiency or forward failure*) and to a back-up of blood in the lungs and peripheral tissues (*circulatory congestion or backward failure*).[1] Although early writers argued whether forward or backward failure was the major problem, it is difficult to see how one could occur without the other, since the cardiovascular system is a relatively closed loop. In hemodynamic terms, circulatory insufficiency is suspected when cardiac output is reduced, and circulatory congestion is suspected when ventricular end-diastolic volumes or pressures are increased. At either end of the spectrum are the clinical syndromes of acute circulatory insufficiency (cardiogenic shock) and acute circulatory congestion (acute pulmonary edema), but even here insufficiency and congestion appear to coexist.

Circulatory insufficiency or congestion may result from causes other than contractile failure. A cardiac output lower than necessary for metabolic requirements may be due to increased metabolic need, hypovolemia with decreased preload, increased afterload, or peripheral circulatory failure. Sepsis, in its earlier stages, is characterized by an increased cardiac output that may become inadequate for metabolic needs; later, peripheral circulatory collapse may lead to decreased peripheral perfusion even though left ventricular output is greater than normal. Systolic overload may occur with systemic or pulmonary hypertension, or with outflow obstruction of either ventricle. Diastolic overload may occur with valvular insufficiency, left to right shunts, and high output states. Restriction of ventricular filling may be due to a variety of valvular abnormalities and pericardial constriction. Overtransfusion in oliguric states, acute nephritic and nephrotic syndromes, and excessive steroid therapy may cause circulatory congestion without circulatory insufficiency.

Contractile failure may be global or segmental. Global contractile failure occurs with the cardiomyopathies, hearts overloaded by either hypertension or valvular abnormalities, and in critically ill patients with shock or multiple injury. Ischemic heart disease is the most common cause of segmental ventricular dysfunction.

The initial response to decreased contractility appears to be an increase in preload due to ventricular dilatation; less commonly a reduction in afterload may occur. If these adjustments are effective, stroke output may be maintained within normal limits. When contractility is impaired but stroke volume is close to normal, the ventricle is *dysfunctional*. When adaptive responses are overwhelmed and stroke output falls, the ventricle has *failed*. Mild levels of ventricular dysfunction may be identified by a sudden increase in afterload following angiotensin or during exercise. Angiotensin increases pulmonary wedge pressure and decreases stroke output when contractility is impaired. Ventricular dysfunction may also be assumed if acute pressure or volume loads seriously depress stroke output. Acidosis, hypocalcemia, hypophosphatemia, and hypoxia may intensify the deterioration in ventricular failure. Ventricular dysfunction decreases the velocity and duration of ejection and the stroke volume, and increases the residual volume.[2] Since the volume of diastolic inflow remains essentially the same, there is a net volume increase during diastole. The greater diastolic distention improves stroke volume, and ejection velocity may return to normal.[3]

An animal model developed by Meerson[4] demonstrates the stages of dysfunction that follow aortic constriction. Similar sequential events occur with other forms of global contractile failure. In the initial stage, increased resistance to ejection produces ventricular dilatation with depletion of high energy phosphates as the dilated ventricle consumes more oxygen (see LaPlace relationship, page 74). An acute afterload mismatch decreases ejection fraction dramatically, but stroke output is maintained by ventricular dilatation and utilization of the preload reserve. The second, or hypertrophic, stage follows initiation of protein synthesis. Increasing muscle increases the number of fibers able to contract, improving the contractile state, and allowing a reduction in preload. In the final stage, cell death in the overloaded heart leads to progressive fibrosis and ventricular dilatation. Once again, preload reserve must augment stroke output. Ultimately, both contractile and preload reserves are exhausted and the ventricle fails.

THE SHOCK SYNDROME

A falling blood pressure and the development of the shock syndrome is an all too common "early" indicator of serious illness. The arterial blood pressure is but one facet of the integrated cardiopulmonary system. Unfortunately, the arterial blood pressure measurement per se has mesmerized the medical profession—clinician and investigator alike. It is only in recent years that proper emphasis has been assigned to the realization that shock may be present with normal arterial blood pressure and, conversely, that adequate circulation may occur with unusually low blood pressure. Figure 5–1 presents the three components of the Pouiseille equation (see page 86), and emphasizes that a drop in blood pressure may be due either to a decrease in stroke output or to a decrease in systemic vascular resistance. Hypotension in cardiogenic shock is due to decreased stroke output; sympathetic neural stimulation provides a compensatory increase in systemic vascular resistance and blunts the fall in stroke output. Perfusion pressure to vital vascular beds is maintained, but at the expense of an increase in afterload (see page 79), which further decreases stroke output. Vasodilators like nitroprusside attempt to increase stroke output by decreasing afterload, while inotropes achieve this by increasing myocardial contractility.

Figure 5-1 emphasizes the importance of both vascular resistance and preload in determining arterial pressure. A decrease in vascular resistance or a decrease in preload decreases arterial pressure. Sepsis is an example of a condition that reduces both preload and vascular resistance. Vigorous fluid replacement is necessary to restore preload and, sometimes, vasopressor agents are necessary to increase vascular resistance.

Vasopressor agents may be necessary to maintain vital organ perfusion pressure in a variety of clinical situations. They must only be used for short periods of time and after volume contraction has been ruled-out by hemodynamic monitoring. These agents raise blood pressure by producing vasoconstriction, however, and may actually decrease perfusion to many organs. In addition, they increase ventricular afterload and may actually decrease stroke output. Vasopressor agents produce venous constriction as well as arteriolar constriction. Venoconstriction reduces venous capacitance and raises venous pressure and may lead to a misleading appraisal of vascular volume. The use of vasopressor agents in hypovolemic shock is particularly dangerous. Arterial constriction raises arterial blood pressure and venoconstriction raises central venous pressure but the increased venous tone decreases vascular volume. Irreversible shock may develop if

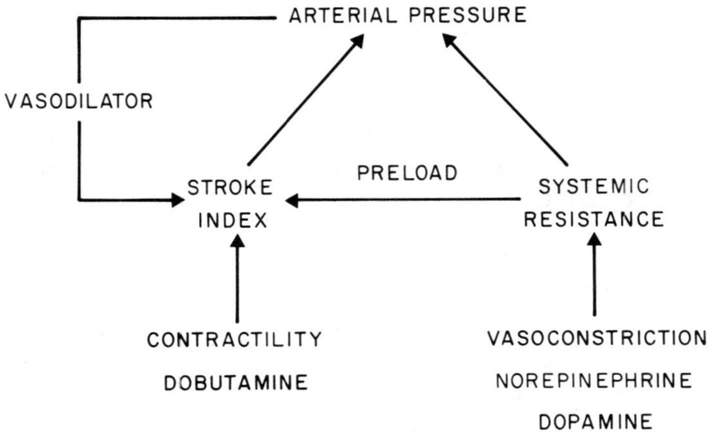

FIG 5–1.
A rearrangement of the Pouiseille equation demonstrates that arterial pressure is determined by stroke output and systemic vascular resistance. Arterial pressure can be increased by increasing contractility and stroke volume or by increasing systemic vascular resistance. Increasing arterial pressure by increasing resistance leads to increased afterload and reduced stroke output. The use of an inotrope with vasodilator properties increases stroke output by increasing contractility and decreasing afterload. Increased venous resistance mediated by vasopressor agents increases preload and stroke output.

the volume deficit is not recognized and corrected.

Vasopressor agents increase vascular resistance but may have a variable effect on left ventricular afterload. Afterload reflects the combined effects of arterial blood pressure, ventricular volume, and wall thickness. Lang et al.[5] have shown that various pharmacologic agents have different effects on the relationship between systemic vascular resistance and left ventricular afterload. A pure vasoconstrictor like methoxamine increases afterload much more than systemic vascular resistance. Norepinephrine actually reduces afterload, even though it increases resistance because it decreases ventricular dimensions and increases wall thickness. Dobutamine, a vasodilator inotrope, decreases afterload even more than it decreases vascular resistance.

Identification of Ventricular Dysfunction and Failure in the Critically Ill

The terms *decreased myocardial contractility* or *contractile failure* must be used with some precision in order to develop adequate therapeutic approaches. Although a reduced stroke output is good clinical evidence for ventricular failure, it cannot distinguish contractile failure from hypovolemic or mechanical causes, and it cannot separate right ventricular failure from left ventricular failure. Moreover, as emphasized above, a normal stroke output may reflect inadequate ventricular reserve if it occurs in a setting such as sepsis. Similarly, an elevated pulmonary capillary wedge pressure suggests ventricular failure, but it could represent fluid overload, mechanical obstruction, or increased ventricular stiffness. A normal pulmonary capillary wedge pressure could be found in a poorly functional ventricle if ventricular compliance were increased (a "flaccid" or floppy dilated ventricle).

Measurement of events occurring during ejection (ejection fraction, fractional shortening, velocity of circumferential shortening) do not directly measure contractility since they are sensitive to changes in preload and afterload, as well as contractility. They are, however, useful in assessing the basal state in conditions producing chronic ventricular dysfunction, and can assess inotropic and other therapeutic interventions *if the other determinants of stroke output are held constant.* The importance of preload reserve as an immediate response to contractile failure makes the measurement of ventricular volume a sensitive indicator of ventricular failure. Indeed, Braunwald has stated[6] that "When ventricular end-diastolic volume is clearly elevated (greater than 108 ml/M^2), and total stroke volume and/or cardiac index and work are either reduced or within normal limits, while heart rate and afterload are normal, *cardiac contractility is depressed*" (emphasis added). Despite potential problems with the use of ejection fraction, fractional shortening, or the velocity of circumferential fiber shortening, the measurements are simple and provide rapid differentiation between normally and abnormally functioning hearts. The major disadvantage of these variables is their inability to separate potential responders from nonresponders to afterload reduction. Very little difference in these indices is generally observed in critically ill patients, despite major changes in hemodynamic status.[7,8]

A number of recent studies have shown that the contractile state of the heart can be assessed best by its force-velocity relationships.[9] Suga and Sagawa[10] exploited the observation that the extent of systolic shortening declines as afterload increases. They demonstrated in isolated hearts that the relationship between end-systolic pressure and volume is relatively insensitive to end-diastolic volume or ejection resistance. The linearity of the end-systolic pressure-volume relationship has been repeatedly confirmed, and its sensitivity to change in the contractile state has been demonstrated.[11,12] No measurement of contractile state can be perfect, however, and must always be interpreted in light of the clinical situation. Table 5–1 shows the differing responses of four indices to an increase in afterload (angiotensin), increase in volume (dextran), and increase in contractility with decrease in afterload (dobutamine).[13]

It is even more difficult to evaluate the contractile state in patients with segmental ventricular dysfunction due to coronary artery disease. The ischemic or fibrotic segments show decreased rates of systolic shortening, and may even bulge paradoxically with systole. Sympathetic neural activity increases the contractile state of the uninvolved myocardium so that global ejection rates and ventricular volumes remain within normal limits. (Failure to increase ventricular ejection rates with exercise or identification of large noncontractile segments by radionuclide ventriculography or echocardiography is necessary to identify ventricular dysfunction in this situation.)

Neurohumoral Responses to the Failing Heart

Blood pressure is maintained in the face of a falling cardiac output by a neurohumorally mediated increase in systemic vascular resistance. Acute withdrawal of 500 ml of blood from a normal individual, for example, evokes a sympathetic response that maintains pressure by arterial and venous constriction, even though stroke output is reduced. A similar vasoconstrictor response is elicited when venous return is acutely reduced by positive pressure ventilation.

Several types of afferent receptors initiate the neurohumoral stress response by transmitting neural information to the central nervous system (CNS). Aortic baroreceptors are sensitive to small decreases in aortic blood pressure; their stimulation by hypotension evokes an immediate constrictor response. Peripheral chemoreceptors responding to acidosis, hypoxia, and other stimuli announce a decrease in peripheral blood flow to the CNS. Generalized sympathetic efferent nerve stimulation produces arterial and venous constriction in skin, muscles, kidney, and splanchnic circulation, thus increasing aortic pressure and redistributing blood flow to the brain and heart.

The humoral response to stress can

TABLE 5–1.
Percent Change in Stroke Volume (SV), Slope (m), Ejection Fraction (EF), and dP/dt with Various Interventions in Conscious Dogs*

	PROPRANOLOL	ANGIOTENSIN	DEXTRAN	DOBUTAMINE
SV	0%	0	+33	+ 24
Slope	− 13	− 9	− 8	+ 38
EF	− 8	− 9	+11	+ 24
dP/dt_{max}	− 27	+14	+27	+110

*Adapted from Sodums MT, Badke FR, Starling MR, et al: Evaluation of left ventricular contractile performance utilizing end-systolic pressure-volume relationships in conscious dogs. *Circ Res* 1984; 54:731.

amplify or dampen the response of an organ to neural stimulation. Both epinephrine and norepinephrine are released from the adrenal medulla, and norepinephrine diffuses into the blood following its release from sympathetic nerve endings. Angiotensin is produced from renin, and both bradykinin and a variety of prostaglandins are produced locally.[14,15]

L-norepinephrine itself may trigger a positive or negative feedback mechanism that regulates its further release. Presynaptic receptors described earlier may either reduce or increase its release, and $alpha_1$ blocking agents may increase plasma norepinephrine by blocking alpha receptors. These neurohumoral imbalances may initiate a self-propelling cycle of myocardial deterioration, so that their early correction is necessary. For example, renin produced by the kidney in response to neural stimulation significantly augments vascular resistance. Captopril, a synthetic angiotensin-converting enzyme inhibitor, decreases systemic vascular resistance, increases stroke output, and reduces pulmonary wedge pressure, thus demonstrating the important role of the stress response on left ventricular function.[16]

Clinical Expression of the Shock Syndrome

Severe ventricular failure with marked impairment of cardiac output from any cause ultimately leads to peripheral circulatory collapse. This syndrome, the shock syndrome, is the expression of severe oxidative failure. Oxygen delivery to the peripheral tissues decreases, mitochondrial oxidation of substrate diminishes markedly, unmetabolized acid intermediates accumulate, and cellular stores of creatine phosphate and adenosine triphosphate are exhausted. Cellular death develops inexorably unless casual factors are removed.

Shock is traditionally considered in three broad subdivisions. *Hypovolemic* (hemorrhagic) shock is produced by a decrease in circulating blood volume, either externally or into an internal body compartment. It is usually produced by injury, hemorrhage, burns, operative trauma, salt and water depletion, and peritoneal inflammation. *Cardiogenic* or central shock is produced by ventricular dysfunction caused by coronary artery disease, cardiomyopathy, severe hypertension, acute valvular dysfunction, acute pulmonary embolism, or pericardial constriction. Differential diagnosis is facilitated by considering myocardial, coronary arterial, valvular, pericardial, and afterload-increasing processes. *Septic shock* occurs frequently in older patients with sepsis and is usually caused by gram negative organisms, although other organisms may also be implicated (see chapter 2).

Although the division of the shock syndrome into separate etiologic groups is helpful in the understanding of the shock syndrome, clinical shock is frequently caused by two or more of the basic mechanisms described above. For example, an elderly patient with acute gastrointestinal bleeding may develop shock because of a decrease in circulating blood volume and also because the decrease in coronary blood flow associated with this unmasks subclinical coronary artery disease. Another patient with obvious coronary shock may develop a stress ulcer or become dehydrated, so that hypovolemic shock is superimposed on the original coronary shock.

The clinical picture of shock is dominated by evidence of poor tissue perfusion. Blood pressure is generally low, but a better evaluation of cardiac output and the peripheral circulation may be obtained by the quality of radial and pedal pulses, the temperature of the hands and feet, and the color of the nailbeds. The quality of the peripheral pulsations is a very important indicator of cardiac output. With satisfactory cardiac output and normal flow distribution, the radial and pedal pulses are palpable and possess a certain quality of "fullness." In this situation, the systolic and diastolic arterial blood pressures are easily measured by auscultation. Generally, the hands and feet are warm and the nail beds pink. Occasionally, there may be some vasoconstriction in response to either cold or an emotional stimulus; then the hands and feet may be cool and some nail bed cyanosis present. However, if the pulses are strong and the blood pressure easily determined by auscultation, then the cardiac output probably is satisfactory despite these changes.

If the amount of blood flow through the brachial and lower extremity arteries diminishes, there is a corresponding diminution in the amplitude of the pulses—and instead of being full, they are "thready." There are several variations in the type of deterioration of pulse quality. The pulse may become less easily palpable, along with an associated fall in the systolic and diastolic pressures. This type of pulse contour is given in Figure 5–2 (curve B). The blood pressure becomes less easily measured by auscultation, and in fact it may be possible to obtain the systolic pressure by palpation only. With another type of abnormal pulse, the arterial blood pressure is less easily measured by auscultation; but, if obtainable, it may be that the systolic and diastolic pressures are still in the normal range. The reason for this is apparent in Figure 5–2 (curve C), where the recorded pulse tracing is shown to consist of a very rapid systolic upstroke and then a very sharp fall toward diastolic pressure. Mean arterial pressure in this instance is not very much above the diastolic level. This type of pressure contour, associated with a thready pulse, is a reflection of diminished cardiac output being ejected into an arterial system that is constricted. If the arterial blood pressure can be heard only with difficulty, irrespective of the values obtained (which may be normal), then it is almost certain that cardiac output is seriously diminished. *Mean arterial blood pressure can be low with normal systolic and diastolic values.* Reliance should never be placed upon the recorded blood pressure values on the hospital chart. Personal examination should be made by the physician, and it should include blood pressure as only one part of an overall analysis of the state of the circulatory system. Also included should be the nature of the pulses, the temperature of the skin, and the color of the nail beds.

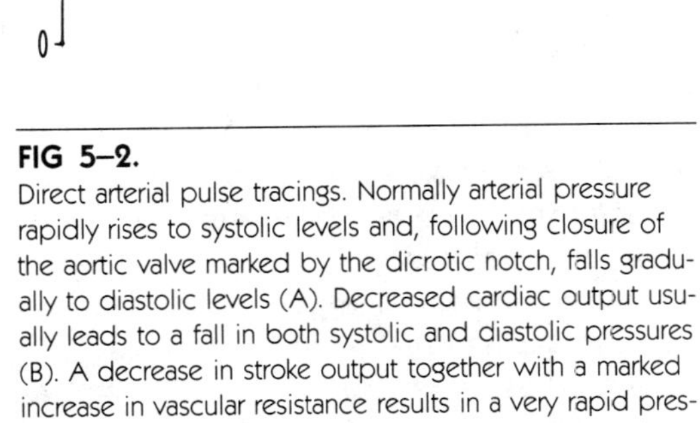

FIG 5–2.
Direct arterial pulse tracings. Normally arterial pressure rapidly rises to systolic levels and, following closure of the aortic valve marked by the dicrotic notch, falls gradually to diastolic levels (A). Decreased cardiac output usually leads to a fall in both systolic and diastolic pressures (B). A decrease in stroke output together with a marked increase in vascular resistance results in a very rapid pressure rise in systole followed by a rapid fall to diastolic levels. Mean arterial blood pressure is very close to diastolic blood pressure (C).

The cutaneous changes are related to intense adrenergic activity and may be a striking sign of early shock. A fall in cardiac output stimulates aortic and carotid baroreceptors and initiates adrenergic activity in attempts to restore blood pressure. Constriction of cutaneous arterioles and stimulation of sweat glands produces the characteristic cold, pale, clammy skin.

Cyanosis

Cyanosis is produced by an increase in the absolute amount of reduced hemoglobin in mucocutaneous capillary beds and generally signals serious trouble. We have become less and less confident of our ability to recognize cyanosis. When present, it means severe tissue hypoxia in the vascular beds under observation. Its absence, however, does not mean the absence of hypoxia. Recognition of cyanosis may be obscured by lighting conditions, anemia, and deep skin pigmentation. (It is very difficult to recognize in blacks.) A classic experiment pointed out that several observers could not agree on the presence of cyanosis in the same patient. *Every critically ill patient should have an arterial blood sample analyzed.*

Normally, venous blood is approximately 75% saturated and contains about 2.5 g of reduced hemoglobin per 100 ml of blood. Either inadequate oxygenation of arterial blood in the lung or increased extraction of oxygen from capillary blood increases the amount of reduced hemoglobin circulating through the capillaries of the skin and mucous membranes. Cyanosis is discernible when reduced hemoglobin is present at a concentration higher than 5 g/100 ml. For this reason, it becomes apparent much earlier in a patient with polycythemia than in a patient with extreme anemia.

The term central cyanosis applies to those situations in which the blood leaving the lung is not fully saturated with oxygen. The absence of cyanosis in a patient with lung disease should not be considered reassuring because the flat upper segment of the oxyhemoglobin dissociation curve prevents oxygen saturation from falling significantly until oxygen tension drops below 40 mm Hg. Most observers cannot perceive cyanosis until oxyhemoglobin saturation has dropped to 80–85% with the hemoglobin level at 15 g/100 ml, or 70–75% with hemoglobin at 10 g/100 ml.

Arterial desaturation in respiratory center depression is due to inadequate alveolar ventilation. Cyanosis in emphysema, atelectasis, and pulmonary edema is due to an uneven distribution of inspired air relative to perfusion (both distribution and true shunt effect). In congenital heart disease, cyanosis is due to the presence of a large venoarterial shunt.

A decrease in organ blood flow decreases the available supply of oxygen to that organ unless oxygen is more completely extracted from capillary blood. Compensation for decreased flow by increasing extraction increases the amount of reduced hemoglobin in capillary blood and causes peripheral cyanosis. This mechanism accounts for the blue lips and nailbeds seen in normal individuals after a cold swim. The presence of cyanosis in a sick patient with normal arterial oxygen tension is a valuable sign of early shock, because the shifting of extremity and cutaneous blood flow to more vital organs is an early defensive maneuver.

The important distinction between these two types of cyanosis—central and peripheral—may be made by considering the clinical setting, by measuring arterial oxygen tension, and by observing the response of cyanosis to the breathing of 100% oxygen (Table 5–2). Arterial oxygen tension is always ab-

TABLE 5–2.
Differential Diagnosis of Cyanosis

	CENTRAL CYANOSIS	PERIPHERAL CYANOSIS
Arterial saturation	Low	Normal
Distribution	Generalized	Extremities, nose, etc.
Response to 100% oxygen	Reverses	Unchanged
Associated conditions	Pulmonary disease	Shock

normally low in central cyanosis (by definition) and normal in peripheral cyanosis. Breathing 100% oxygen fully saturates arterial blood in patients with alveolar hypoventilation or diffusion defects, and in patients with true venoarterial shunts of less than 40% of the cardiac output. It does not correct peripheral cyanosis. An elevated carbon dioxide tension is indirect evidence of central cyanosis, but a normal carbon dioxide tension does not rule out central cyanosis. Although an attempted distinction between central and peripheral cyanosis is essential for rational therapy, many patients have a mixture of these two types of cyanosis. The patient with pulmonary edema, for example, has central cyanosis due to venoarterial shunting through fluid-filled alveoli, and peripheral cyanosis due to poor cutaneous blood flow.

Alterations in Cerebral Function

Often the first signs of impaired oxygen delivery to the tissues are alterations in cerebral function. Either diminished cerebral blood flow or oxygen content of the perfusing blood can cause inadequate brain oxygenation. Restlessness, agitation, and disorientation can result. These signs usually appear under circumstances that make it possible to ascribe them to a number of causes. The patient may be in a postoperative state, and restlessness could be ascribed to incisional pain. The unfamiliar and emotionally disturbing atmosphere of an intensive care unit could also be cited as the cause of patient apprehension. *Unless the physician considers cerebral anoxia as a prime suspect in all situations of altered cerebral function, this valuable early warning sign is missed.* Furthermore, injudicious sedation may quiet the patient, mask the true state of affairs, and lull the physician and nursing personnel into an unwarranted sense of security.

The drowsy and comatose patient with respiratory failure contrasts with the agitated, anxious patient in shock. The former symptoms are due to the anesthetic nature of high arterial carbon dioxide tensions. In addition, there is an increased cerebral blood flow in these patients due to the vasodilator action of carbon dioxide on cerebral vessels. This may lead to cerebral edema and increased intracranial pressure. Papilledema occasionally occurs, and may further confuse the picture. If a patient has renal or hepatic disease, alterations in cerebral function may be attributed to one of these processes, and cerebral hypoxia of hypercapnia can easily be overlooked.

An orderly and periodic assessment of mental function is necessary to detect early evidence of abnormal cerebral function. The mnemonic MOD reminds the physician or nurse to evaluate *M*emory (past, recent, and very recent), *O*rientation (time, place, person), and evidence of *D*elusion (paranoid ideation, visual or auditory hallucination). Subtle abnormalities in these functions suggest a toxic delerium that may be due to functional or organic causes. Recent experience in the intensive care unit has emphasized that sensory deprivation and the injudicious use of sedatives are major factors in the development of toxic delerium.

Urinary Output

A decrease in urinary output to below 20–30 ml/hour is a valuable sign of early shock. Blood is shunted from the kidneys in a similar manner as it is shunted away from the skin. This decrease in renal blood flow decreases glomerular filtration. In severe shock, renal flow may fall to zero and precipitate acute renal failure.

Anaerobic Metabolism and Lactic Acidosis in the Shock Syndrome Chapter 1 described how decreased cellular oxygen delivery led to anaerobic metabolism with the production of lactic acid. The addition of lactic acid to the tissues decreases body buffer stores, and can be identified by a falling plasma bicarbonate concentration. The metabolic acidosis associated with anaerobic metabolism decreases cardiac output and systemic vascular resistance, increases pulmonary vascular resistance, alters the response to exogenous catecholamines, and may produce serious cardiac arrhythmias. Patients with shock frequently hyperventilate, so that the pH may not be as low as it would be if the patient were ventilating at a normal level (see page 304). A sudden decrease in ventilation could produce a cataclysmic fall in pH that might produce fatal ventricular tachyrhythmias. Rapid restoration of bicarbonate levels is vital in patients with shock and lactic acidosis.

Many physicians hesitate to replace deficits rapidly because of recent literature that suggests that bicarbonate replacement in diabetic ketoacidosis may produce CNS symptoms,[17] or because the American Heart Association guidelines for cardiopulmonary resuscitation caution against the routine use of bicarbonate solutions. It is certainly true that bicarbonate administration in a diabetic may produce side effects. Bicarbonate ion does not readily cross the blood-brain barrier while carbon dioxide is freely diffusable. Administration of bicarbonate raises plasma bicarbonate and decreases the hydrogen ion stimulus to hyperventilation. Since bicarbonate concentration does not change in the cerebrospinal fluid but carbon dioxide tissue rises towards normal, brain pH falls as a result of metabolic acidosis. It is also true that excessive use of bicarbonate in cardiopulmonary collapse with subsequent restoration of cardiac output may produce a metabolic alkalosis that may lead to ventricular arrhythmias. The situation with the patient in shock is far different, however. The life-limiting condition is the metabolic acidosis, and prompt restoration towards normal is necessary.

Figure 5–3 shows the acidosis, hyperventilation, and shift of potassium from cell to extracellular space that accompanies metabolic acidosis in a patient with acute myocardial infarction, shock, and ventricular fibrillation. Repeated attempts at defibrillation were unsuccessful until bicarbonate was infused. Following bicarbonate therapy, the patient was readily defibrillated, and the potassium concentration returned towards normal. Figure 5–4 shows that alkalosis associated with mechanical hyperventilation is as arrhythmogenic as acidosis.

Rapid restoration of plasma bicarbonate levels to normal is facilitated by calculating the estimated base deficit. The volume of extracellular fluid (about 20% of body weight) is multiplied by the existing deficit in each liter of blood. For example, a patient weighing 80 kg has 0.20 times 80, of 16 liters of extracellular water. If his plasma bicarbonate is 16 mEq/L, he

SHOCK & METABOLIC ACIDOSIS

Prior to conversion

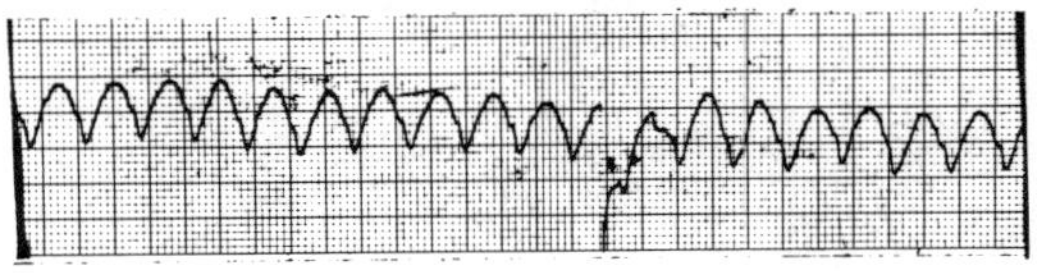

5-10-67	10 am	12 N
pH	7.217 units	7.24
P_{CO_2}	31.7 mm Hg	13.9
P_{O_2}	39.6 mm Hg	179.6
Sat.	65 %	98.8
BHCO	12 meq/L	5.5
K^+	8.0 meq/L	

A

AFTER TREATMENT

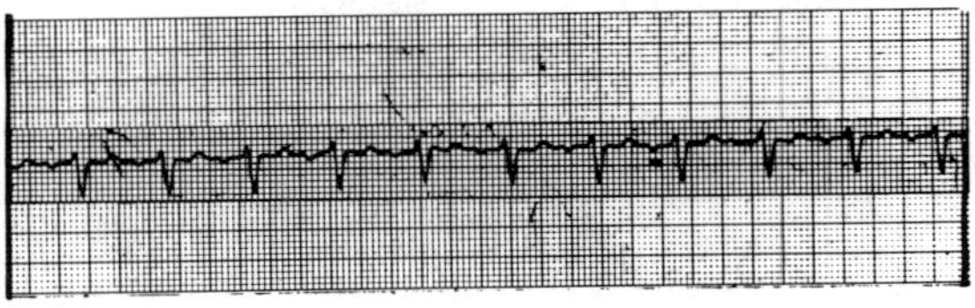

	5-10-67 3pm	5-11-67 10 am
pH	7.35 units	7.48
P_{CO_2}	20 mm Hg	35.3
P_{O_2}	99.7 mm Hg	162.7
Sat.	96.7 %	99.2
$BHCO_3$	10.8 meq/L	29.8
K^+	6.3 meq/L	5.1

B

FIG 5–3.
A. Ventricular fibrillation in a patient with severe metabolic acidosis and shock. Note the elevated potassium of 8.0 milliequivalents per liter which is secondary to the acidosis itself. It was impossible to defibrillate the patient in the presence of this severe acidosis.

B. Following bicarbonate therapy, the patient is readily defibrillated, plasma bicarbonate rises to normal, and potassium concentration falls.

has a deficit of 24 minus 16 or 8 mEq/L. His total bicarbonate deficit would be 8 mEq/L times 16 liters or 128 mEq. Since the plasma bicarbonate deficit represents only part of the total body buffer deficit, some authors recommend a factor of 0.30 for the volume of equilibrium. A more conservative approach is to use the factor of 0.20 and replace to a concentration of 20 mEq/L, rather than the normal level of 24. In either case, frequent measurements of bicarbonate concentration facilitate the adequate correction of the buffer deficit.

SHOCK ASSOCIATED WITH ACUTE MYOCARDIAL INFARCTION

For many years the relationship between the symptom of angina and coronary obstruction was not clear. It is now generally accepted that acute myocardial infarction (AMI) is almost always due to severe coronary artery disease, although coronary thrombosis without significant atherosclerosis has been observed in some situations, particularly in women who smoke and use oral contraceptives. Injection of radio-opaque medium into the coronary arteries during post-mortem examination has shown that the hearts of patients with angina pectoris usually had experienced one or more occlusions of coronary arteries with a rich development of collateral circulation. Subsequent post-mortem studies have emphasized that severe coronary arterial occlusive disease can be expressed as angina pectoris, acute myocardial infarction, congestive heart failure, or sudden ischemic death. More

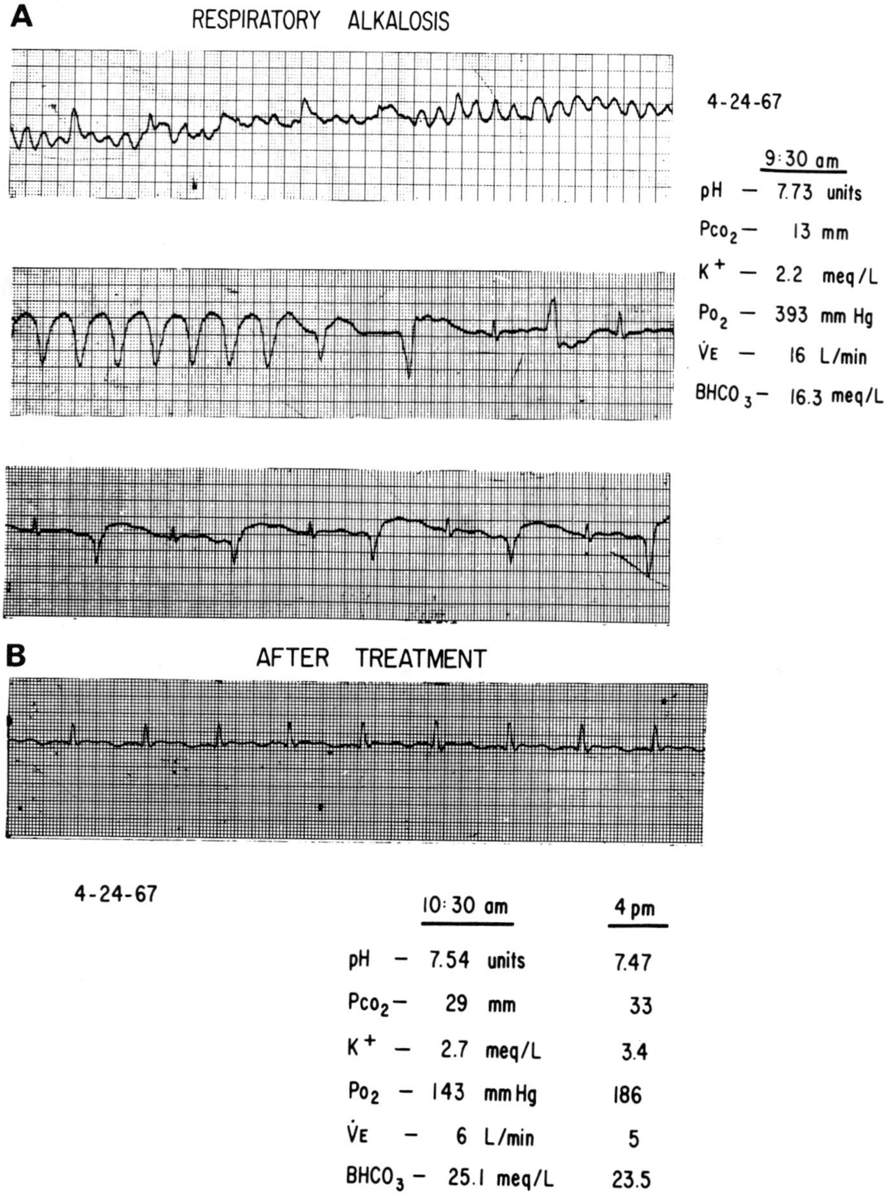

FIG 5–4.
A. Repeated ventricular arrhythmias in an intubated patient hyperventilated with a pressure cycled respirator. The arrhythmias persisted despite repeated electrical countershock. Arterial blood gas analysis obtained several hours later revealed the pattern of severe respiratory alkalosis. The hypokalemia represents a transcellular shift and is due to the alkalosis. B. Following proper adjustment of the ventilator, the patient spontaneously reverted to normal sinus rhythm as carbon dioxide tension and potassium concentration changed toward normal.

than one third of all deaths in the United States are due to ischemic heart disease; half of these deaths are due to acute myocardial infarction, but the death rate understates the actual incidence of coronary atherosclerosis. Routine autopsies at the Mayo Clinic in Rochester, Minnesota[18] demonstrated the presence of significant coronary artery disease in 74% of unselected autopsies. Chest pain was reported in only 32% of the patients studied in Rochester. Asymptomatic coronary disease is obviously quite common, and the intensivist must not only be skilled in the treatment of patients with acute myocardial infarction, but also those with subclinical coronary artery disease who experience critical illness or injury. In these patients, the outcome may be more dependent upon the underlying coronary disease than upon the immediate cause of sudden illness. Hypotension, hypoxemia, acidosis, sepsis, and endogenous or exogenous catecholamines may increase myocardial oxygen requirements beyond the capacity of a diseased vascular bed or may lead to local coronary thrombosis.

The treatment of shock associated with acute myocardial infarction has become increasingly more important. Mortality rates above 90% for the syndrome in the 1970s fell significantly with the advent of intra-aortic balloon counterpulsation and coronary artery bypass surgery. Mortality rates remained greater than 50% for many years, but the recent discovery that many acute ischemic episodes are due to coronary thrombosis suggests that acute revascularization might salvage myocardial tissue. The general use of thrombolytic therapy and angioplasty may lead to substantial declines in the incidence of coronary shock and of mortality from acute myocardial infarction.

Although the disease was once called coronary thrombosis, early pathologic studies failed to reveal evidence of clot, and it was generally believed that transient increases in myocardial oxygen consumption in the face of fixed coronary obstruction was responsible for both infarction and unstable angina. This less-than-satisfactory explanation was shattered in 1980, when DeWood et al.[19] found thrombotic occlusion of coronary arteries during the early hours of infarction, and again in 1985, when Falk[20] presented evidence that dynamic coronary thrombosis led to infarction or sudden death in patients with unstable angina. Recent studies by Fitzgerald et al.[21] suggest that plaque rupture with thrombosis and liberation of the vasoconstrictor thromboxane A_2 may produce rythmic coronary vasoconstriction. Studies by Sobel[22], using tissue-type plasminogen activator manufactured by recombinant DNA techniques, have shown that coronary thrombolysis with intravenous administration is possible in the early hours of infarction. Support of the failing ventricle and maintenance of coronary flow during thrombolysis and angioplasty now become more important than ever before.

Ventricular Geometry in Ischemic Heart Disease

Ventricular dysfunction in ischemic heart disease is usually caused by regional abnormalities in wall motion rather than by global malfunction of the ventricle. Herman et al.[23] demonstrated that regional abnormalities of contractility (asynergy) were commonplace in patients with ischemic heart disease. They identified four distinct patterns of dysfunction: *akinesis*, or total lack of motion of a wall segment; *dyskinesis*, or paradoxical systolic expansion of a segment; *asyneresis*, or diminished wall motion; and *asynchrony*, or disturbed temporal sequence of contraction. Patients with asynergy had substantially lower stroke indices than those with normal contractile patterns had, and ventricular end-diastolic pressures were somewhat higher in those with asynergy compared with those having a normal pattern of contraction. Herman et al. noted that abnormalities in regional lactate metabolism frequently occurred without asynergy, suggesting that the metabolic abnormality might precede the contractile one. Their study emphasized the importance of ventricular dimensions as a prognostic index of therapeutic response; isoproterenol improved ventricular function in 13 of 16 patients with end-diastolic volumes of more than 110 ml/M^2, but seemed to have a neutral or deleterious effect with smaller ventricles.

Chamber size is an important determinant of prognosis and response to treatment. Afterload reducing agents such as hydralazine increase stroke output with large hearts, but may actually decrease stroke output with normal sized hearts.[24] A similar difference related to ventricular function was noted by Pozen et al.[25] Lactate metabolism was unchanged in 14 patients with acute myocardial infarction with demonstrated significant improvements with dobutamine. Four patients with higher pretreatment cardiac indices (3.34 compared to 2.60 L/min/M^2) exhibited increasingly abnormal lactate metabolism, and three experienced angina pectoris. Kazamias, Gander, and Ross[26] showed that all patients with a normal spine to left heart border survived, while 9 of 12 with an increased dimension died. Bulkley[27] made a major contribution to the understanding of ventricular geometry during acute myocardial infarction by measuring abnormal wall motion by sequential echocardiography. Her group noted that one of the causes of cardiac dilatation after acute myocardial infarction was regional expansion with disproportionate dilatation and progressive bulging (dyskinesis) of the infarcted area. Patients exhibiting dyskinesis usually had more than 10% of the left ventricle infarcted and were at high risk for the development of ventricular aneurysm.

Pathogenesis of Shock Associated with AMI

Detailed pathologic studies of patients hospitalized in coronary care units revealed that those dying in shock had infarction of 35–70% of the left ventricular surface.[28] The volume of infarcted myocardium, rather than location of the infarction, determined ventricular function and the development of the shock syndrome.[29] Most studies of patients dying with coronary shock have demonstrated extremely severe coronary artery disease with extensive disease of the left coronary artery. In one study, 68% of patients dying with cardiogenic shock had three vessel disease compared to 35% dying with severe heart failure; 80% of both groups had more than 75% occlusion of the left anterior descending coronary artery.[30] Patients dying from AMI without shock in one study exhibited well-demarcated infarct zones that comprised less than 30% of the left ventricle, while those dying with shock had a ragged edge and contained many damaged cells, suggesting continuation of the ischemic process. These patients and those dying with shock in the absence of AMI had scattered islands of necrosis in both ventricles.[31]

Bedside measurements in patients with cardiogenic shock compared to those with acute myocardial infarction without shock showed striking differences.[32] Cardiac index averaged 1.38 and 2.41 L/min/M^2 and mean arterial pressures were 54 and 93 mm Hg in patients with shock and those without shock, respectively. While the mean values were significantly different, some patients with cardiac indices between 1.5–2.0 L/min/M^2 exhibited shock while others did not. The left ventricular work index, a calculation including both flow and pressure, uniformly separated the two groups; all patients with indices less than 1.5kg–/min/M^2 were in shock. Considerable overlap in systemic vascular resistance was noted, but the mean value for the patients in shock was significantly lower than in patients without shock. Mortality in studies of coronary shock ranged from 73 to 100%; Scheidt, Axcheim, and Killip[29] noted that "sinus tachycardia, atrioventricular block, late onset of shock, cool moist skin, coma, oliguria, and over pulmonary edema were associated with mortality of more than 90%." They also noted that neither norepinephrine nor isoproterenol seemed to influence survival.

Many groups attempted to predict subsequent mortality from hemodynamic data in shock patients. Weber et al.[28] noted that the stroke index in nonsurvivors was half that in survivors, and that the left ventricular end-diastolic pressure in nonsurvivors was almost double that in survivors. Ratshin, Rackley, and Russell[33] found that the combination of a stroke index below 2.3 L/min/M^2 and a left ventricular end-diastolic pressure greater than 15 mm Hg was associated with 100% mortality. Left ventricular end-diastolic pressures are related to ventricular compliance (stiffness) as well as to ventricular size. End-diastolic pressures may be normal in patients with low cardiac outputs and dilated ventricles, but elevated in those with acute myocardial infarction and noncompliant ventricles. Diamond and Forrester[34] found that left ventricular compliance was reduced in patients with coronary artery disease, and further reduced in those with acute myocardial infarction. High values of end-diastolic pressure predict a poor prognosis because they reflect either decreased compliance, increased diastolic volume or both.

The studies described above and others allow a general understanding of the pathogenesis of coronary atherosclerosis and its consequences: angina, unstable angina, acute myocardial infarction, chronic congestive heart failure, and shock. Most infarctions involve the full thickness of the myocardial wall and are termed "transmural infarcts." Since blood flow is most dynamic in the subendocardial layers, some infarcts are limited to the subendocardium and part of the intramural myocardium, and are termed "subendocardial infarcts." The size and location of the ultimate infarct is related to the severity of coronary atherosclerosis, the amount of myocardium perfused by the affected vascular bed, the presence of thrombi or vascular spasm, the character of the collateral circulation, and the oxygen requirements of the myocardium. Clinical experimental evidence suggests that these factors lead to the establishment of at least three zones in acute myocardial infarction: a central necrotic zone beginning near the subendocardium, an ischemic or jeopardized zone that should be the focus of therapeutic intervention, and large noninfarcted zones of the remaining myocardium. An understanding of the oxygen delivery and oxygen requirements of the myocardium explains the inhomogeneity of myocardial oxygenation in patients with coronary artery disease.

Myocardial Oxygenation and Metabolism in AMI

The oxygen consumption of any organ is calculated by its rate of blood flow and by the fraction of oxygen extracted by that tissue from the perfusing blood. Myocardial oxygen consumption ($M\dot{V}O_2$)

is the product of coronary blood flow (CBF) and the arterial-coronary sinus oxygen difference $(A\text{-}CS)O_2$. Unlike other organ systems which extract less oxygen, the heart extracts 60–65% of the oxygen from the perfusing blood so that the oxygen tension of the coronary sinus blood averages 25 mm Hg. Changes in oxygen demand must be regulated by changes in coronary blood flow, since increased oxygen extraction would reduce oxygen tension in the coronary sinus blood to dangerously low levels. If the ability of coronary blood flow to adjust to metabolic needs is impaired, oxygen extraction must rise in order to meet the oxygen requirements of the myocardium. An oxygen extraction above 70% is considered abnormal, suggesting myocardial hypoxia and anaerobic metabolism.

In the normal heart coronary blood flow (CBF) is mainly regulated by changes in coronary vascular resistance (CVR), while coronary perfusion pressure (aortic pressure, AP) is of secondary importance:

$$\mathrm{CBF} = \frac{\mathrm{AP}}{\mathrm{CVR}}$$

In severe coronary arterial disease, however, coronary vasodilation is impaired, coronary vascular resistance is relatively fixed, and perfusion pressure becomes a primary determinant of coronary blood flow.[35–38] Since coronary blood flow is the major determinant of myocardial oxygen consumption, the importance of aortic pressure for myocardial oxygenation in the presence of impaired coronary vasodilatation is obvious (Fig. 5–5).

This dependency of coronary blood flow upon perfusion pressure in human coronary shock is demonstrated in Figure 5–6. Coronary blood flow (milliliters per 100 g per minute) of 23 patients in severe shock following acute myocardial infarction is plotted against mean aortic pressure.[38] During shock coronary blood flow is low—mean, 68 ml/100g/minute (normal 88±10, 1 S.D.)—and the mean aortic pressure is decreased to an average of 55 mm Hg. If mean aortic pressure is elevated, either by *l*-norepinephrine or by cardiac assist (intra-aortic balloon counterpulsation),[39] coronary blood flow increases an average of 27 and 23 ml/100 g/minute, respectively. The curve is relatively flat above 65 mm Hg and becomes steeper below this point, emphasizing that mean arterial pressures below 60 mm Hg are associated with a precipitous drop of coronary blood flow. Extrapolation of the curve beyond the observed data intercepts the point of no flow at a mean arterial pressure of about 30 mm Hg, which is similar to the critical closing pressure for the canine myocardial vascular bed.[40]

In addition to myocardial perfusion and oxygen extraction, lactate utilization by the heart is a helpful indicator of the state of myocardial oxygenation. Under normal conditions, the heart functions as an aerobic organ. Among other substrates, lactate is extracted from the blood by the myocardial cell and oxidized to pyruvate (Fig. 5–7). If oxygen is freely available, pyruvate is catabolized in the Kreb's cycle, and adenosine triphosphate (ATP) is generated, the ultimate energy source for cardiac contraction. In myocardial hypoxia, intracellular glucose is metabolized

$$MV_{O_2} = \mathrm{CBF} \times (A-CS)_{O_2}$$

$$\mathrm{CBF} = \frac{\mathrm{AP}}{\mathrm{CVR}}$$

FIG 5–5.
Oxygen supply (MV_{O_2}) to the myocardium in coronary shock. Coronary blood flow (CBF) as the major determinant of MV_{O_2} becomes dependent upon aortic pressure (AP) in coronary shock. Therefore, MV_{O_2} also becomes dependent upon perfusion pressure. CVR, coronary vascular resistance.

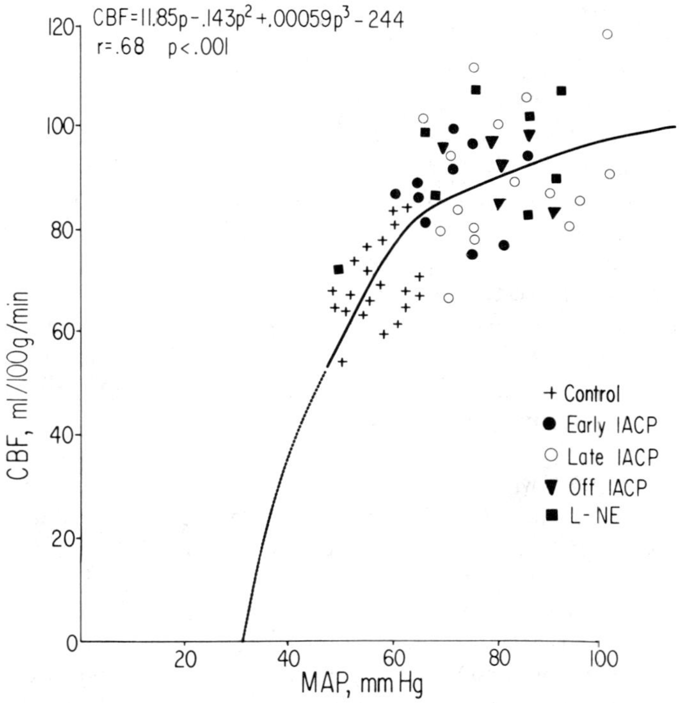

FIG 5–6.
Pressure dependency of coronary blood flow in the severely diseased coronary bed in man. Coronary blood flow (CBF) improves regardless of whether mean aortic pressure (MAP) is increased by l-norepinephrine (L-NE) in intraaortic counterpulsation (IACP). Pressure-flow points during isoproterenol (ISO) therapy fall to the left of the curve, suggesting coronary vasodilatation in less diseased myocardium (coronary steal syndrome). (From Mueller H, *Circulation* 1972; 45:346. Used by permission.)

without oxygen to pyruvate and finally to lactate, generating small amounts of adenosine triphosphate. Therefore in myocardial hypoxia, lactate accumulates in the myocardial cell, and lactate extraction from the blood decreases. In severe myocardial hypoxia, the lactate content in the myocardial cell exceeds that of the coronary blood, and lactate diffuses out of the cell; thus lactate is produced by the myocardium. Normally 20–30% of the arterial lactate content is extracted by the myocardium (Ex_L). A lactate extraction ratio below 10% or production of lactate suggest anerobic metabolism.

Myocardial oxygen requirements and coronary flow are directly related to heart rate, tension developed by the ventric-

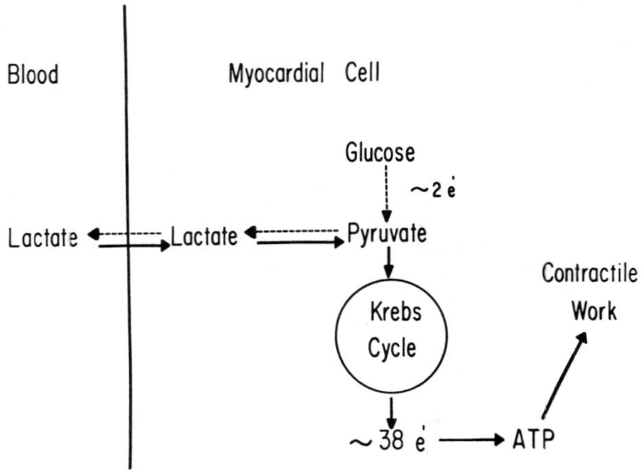

FIG 5–7.
Myocardial lactate metabolism. In aerobic myocardial metabolism (dotted arrow), lactate is extracted from the blood by the myocardial cell and metabolized in the Krebs cycle, generating adenosine triphosphate (ATP). In myocardial hypoxia intracellular glucose is metabolized anaerobically to lactate, and only a small amount of ATP is generated (solid arrow). Lactate accumulates within the myocardial cell. (From Mueller H, et al: *Crit Care Med* 1973; 1:1–29. Used by permission.)

ular wall in ejecting blood and developing arterial pressure, and the rate of myocardial fiber shortening. The tension required to achieve a given systolic pressure depends upon ventricular diameter because of the LaPlace relationship. Factors that increase heart rate, arterial pressure, or myocardial contractility require increased coronary blood flow. It is easy to understand how the failure to adequately increase coronary flow can produce myocardial ischemia, which could decrease cardiac output, lower blood pressure, and further decrease coronary blood flow.

In 1970, Mueller et al.[41] reported studies of coronary blood flow and myocardial metabolism in coronary shock. Catheters were placed in the coronary sinus and used for the collection of blood for calculation of extraction ratios and measurement of coronary blood flow by a radioactive iodo-antipyrine method. Coronary sinus blood represents the flow-weighted averages of contributions from all regions of the myocardium. Ischemic segments produce great amounts of lactate and extract up to 90% of the oxygen from arterial blood, but are underrepresented in coronary sinus blood because of reduced coronary perfusion to these segments. Variations from normal thus reflect the size of the ischemic portions of the myocardium. Figures 5–8 and 5–9 show hemodynamic and metabolic function in patients with shock due to AMI. Heart rate, systemic vascular resistance, and mean arterial pressure are increased while cardiac index and the left ventricular work index are low. Coronary blood flow, coronary sinus oxygen tension, and lactate extraction are low while oxygen extraction is increased.

The same investigators used the coronary sinus sampling method to study the effects of various therapeutic approaches on myocardial metabolism. Figures 5–10 and 5–11 show strikingly different effects on myocardial metabolism with isoproterenol, l-norepinephrine and intra-aortic balloon counterpulsation. Isoproterenol markedly increases the cardiac index but does not increase mean arterial pressure; myocardial oxygen extraction de-

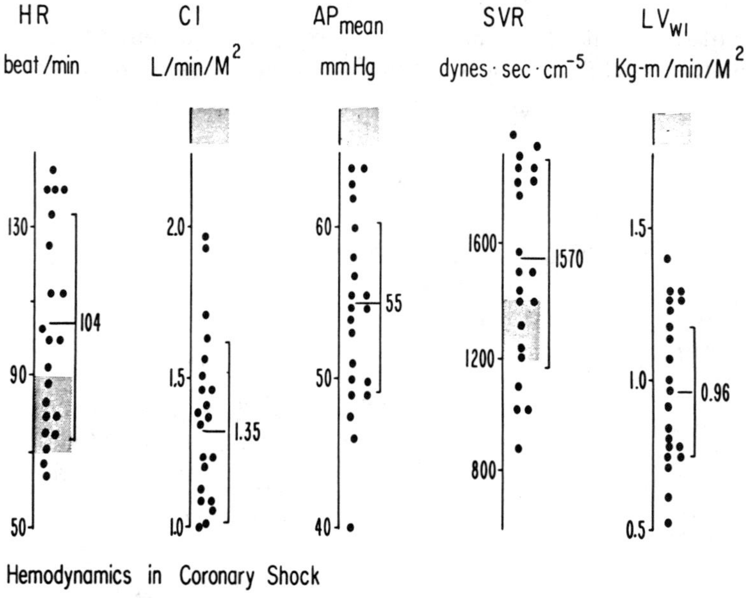

FIG 5–8.
Hemodynamic changes in coronary shock in man. Cardiac index (CI), mean aortic pressure (AP_{mean}), and left ventricular work index (LV_{WI}) are markedly reduced. Systemic vascular resistance (SVR) varies, suggesting an inadequate response of the peripheral vascular bed to the low cardiac output state. Normal values are indicated by the hatched areas. HR, heart rate. (From Mueller H, et al: *Circulation* 1972; 45:340. Used by permission.)

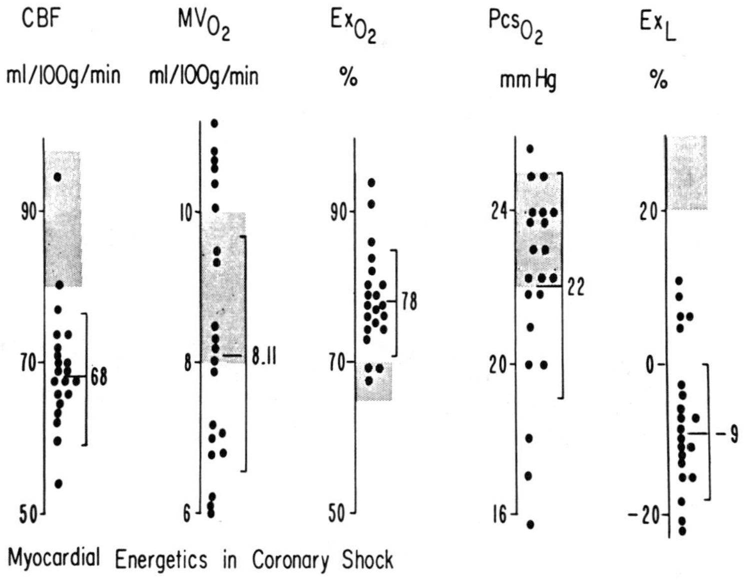

FIG 5–9.
Cardiac energetics in coronary shock in man. Coronary blood flow (CBF) is reduced. Myocardial oxygen consumption (MV_{O_2}) varies but is inadequate in all patients, as indicated by abnormally high extraction of oxygen (Ex_{O_2}) and production of lactate (Ex_L) by the myocardium. Normal values are indicated by the hatched areas. Pcs_{O_2}, coronary sinus oxygen tension. From Mueller H, et al: *Circulation* 1972; 45:345.)

creases slightly because it is a general vasodilator, but lactate extraction is decreased. Isoproterenol intensifies myocardial hypoxia because it increases heart rate and myocardial contractility while decreasing aortic diastolic pressure. Oxygen demands outstrip oxygen delivery. In contrast, administration of norepinephrine increases arterial blood pressure, has little effect on cardiac index, leads to a slight decrease in myocardial oxygen extraction, and produces a pronounced improvement in myocardial lactate extraction. Intra-aortic balloon counterpulsation is even better. It raises blood pressure, increases cardiac index, markedly decreases oxygen extraction, and improves lactate extraction.

The studies with IACP provide an unusual opportunity to generate *in vivo* pressure-flow curves in humans with severely diseased coronary arterial beds. Figure 5–6 shows that coronary blood flow is relatively well maintained until the

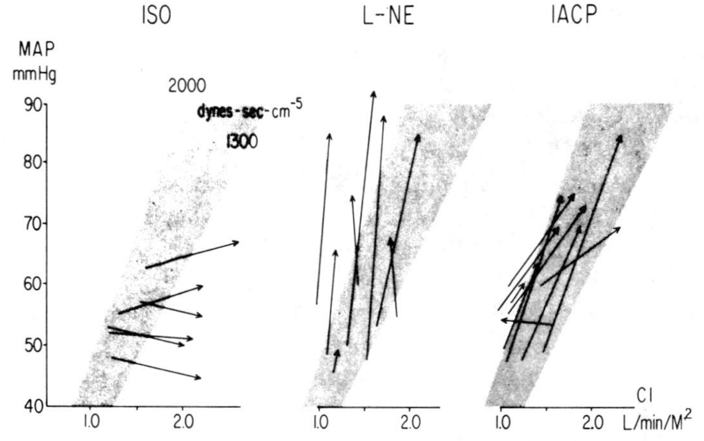

FIG 5–10.
Systemic flow-pressure relationships in coronary shock and the response to therapeutic interventions. Isopleths are drawn for 1,300 and 2,000 dynes-sec-cm^{-5}. Systemic vascular resistance decreases uniformly with isoproterenol (ISO), increases with l-norepinephrine (L-NE), and varies during intra-aortic counterpulsation (IACP), MAP, mean aortic pressure. (From Mueller H, et al: *Circulation* 1972; 45:345. Used by permission.)

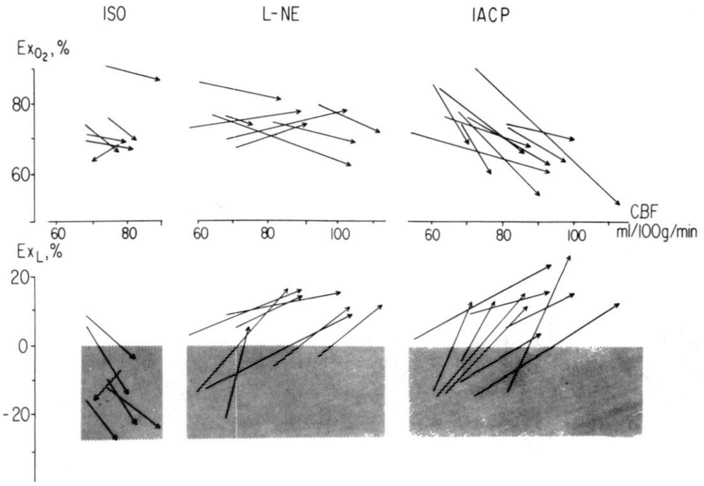

FIG 5–11.
Interrelationship of coronary blood flow (CBF) and myocardial metabolism. Isoproterenol (ISO) increases coronary blood flow inadequately to the need. Myocardial lactate extraction (Ex_L) shifts to production, or the rate of lactate production increases. L-norepinephrine (L-NE) and intra-aortic counterpulsation (IACP) both improve coronary blood flow and myocardial lactate metabolism. Myocardial oxygen extraction (Ex_{O_2}) changes toward normal during counterpulsation but remains abnormally high with l-norepinephrine. (From Mueller H, et al: *Circulation* 1972; 45:347. Used by permission.)

mean arterial pressure falls below 70 mm Hg. Below that point, flow drops precipitously; extrapolation to zero flow suggests that a critical closing pressure is reached at 30–35 mm Hg. Clearly, the importance of maintaining perfusion pressure in the patient with shock associated with AMI is demonstrated. *Hypotension must be treated vigorously in any patient who could have clinical or subclinical artery disease.*

Preventing Shock by Salvaging Myocardium

The high mortality of the shock syndrome, and our realization that evidence of extensive myocardial ischemia could be identified by coronary sinus sampling *before* the development of shock, led us to emphasize a "preshock state" in acute myocardial infarction.[42] Supraventricular tachycardia, arterial hypoxemia, acidosis, and an unstable blood pressure suggested a potentially reversible situation that, if untreated, led inexorably to cardiogenic shock. Maroko et al.,[43] from Brauwald's group, performed a series of animal experiments which refined this concept, and opened their landmark paper on salvaging myocardial tissue with the following prescient comment:

> The classical treatment of power failure of the heart consequent upon myocardial infarction is relatively ineffective. Considering that the infarct's size is an important determinant of power failure, a possible therapeutic approach to this syndrome would be an attempt to limit the size of the infarction. Accordingly, the purpose of the present investigation was the examination of the hemodynamic conditions and pharmacologic interventions that might alter the size of an infarct by *changing the balance between oxygen supply and demand in the area of myocardium supplied by the occluded vessel.*[43]

The group used a method of precordial ECG mapping and calculated infarct size from the summed S-T segment elevation in the open-chested group. Agents that increased myocardial contractility, such as isoproterenol, ouabain, glucagon, and bretylium, increased the area of infarction. Hemorrhagic hypotension also increased infarct size, while elevation of arterial pressure with methoxamine decreased it. Mueller and associates from our group[44] found that propranolol decreased lactate production by the human ischemic myocardium, even though it also decreased cardiac output.

These observations laid the groundwork for the use of beta blockade in ischemic heart disease and also supported the idea that myocardial salvage might have to be achieved at the expense of moderately reduced peripheral perfusion.

The clinical ideas of a "preshock" state and of myocardial salvage were given experimental validity by the studies of Reimer and Jennings,[45] who demonstrated stepwise transmural progression of necrosis in experimental animals, and by Gutovitz, Sobel, and Roberts,[46] who showed that cardiogenic shock in many was associated with progressive myocardial damage with continuing release of creatine kinase-MB into the circulation.

Admittedly, reducing myocardial oxygen consumption is difficult, but increased demands caused by tachycardia could be controlled. The interest shifted to the supply side in 1978, when Maseri et al.[47] published results in patients with unstable angina entitled "Coronary vasospasm as a possible cause of myocardial infarction." Vetrovec et al.[48] rekindled interest in coronary thrombosis as an explanation for decreased oxygen delivery, and the concept of myocardial salvage was redefined with an emphasis on increasing supply.

Treatment of Ventricular Dysfunction and Shock in AMI

The treatment and prevention of ventricular dysfunction in AMI is evolving rapidly because of the availability of revascularization techniques. The studies summarized above led to a focus on pharmacologic agents such as propranolol and nitroprusside. While beta blockade appeared to improve survival after AMI,[49] it was difficult to demonstrate significant improvement in hospital mortality with either beta blockade or nitroprusside. The accumulating knowledge base of the 1970s, however, underscored the importance of left ventricular function to prognosis after AMI.[50]

The philosophic advantage of increasing supply, rather than the more fatalistic approach of reducing oxygen demands by various approaches to organ hibernation, have important implications for other realms of critical care medicine and should be studied in some detail. Wright, Marple, and Beck,[51] had presented data in 1954 that oral coumarin derivatives (warfarin) improved survivorship in AMI. As a result of Wright's influence, heparin and warfarin were widely used throughout the 1960s, even though randomized studies had failed to demonstrate a significant effect of anticoagulant therapy.[52] Pathologic and physiologic studies in the early 1970s played down the importance of coronary thrombi[53] and emphasized the importance of the pharmacologic reduction of myocardial oxygen requirements.[43,54] The inadequacy of these approaches has led to the mid-1980s concept of early revascularization and is consistent with the "golden hour" approach to critically ill individuals discussed elsewhere in this text.

Unfortunately, the rapidly changing approach to limiting infarct size has led to considerable controversy and an unevenness of treatment standards on a national level. Eugene Braunwald, in a 1985 editorial,[55] emphasized the two approaches to therapy: "conventional and aggressive; in this discussion, the latter refers to efforts designed to achieve immediate reperfusion of the infarcting myocardium." This distinguished author carefully chose the word "infarcting" rather than "infarcted." Three basic principles were presented: (1) limiting the size of the initial infarct determines survival; (2) interventions to reduce infarct size must be applied within the first four hours after symptoms; and (3) revascularization techniques should be considered in patients after infarction who are at high risk for reinfarction or sudden death.

Clinical and physiologic classification of patients with AMI is essential in order to understand when aggressive therapy is necessary. Three approaches to staging AMI are shown in Table 5–3. Killip and Kimball[56] emphasized the importance of ventricular dysfunction in determining mortality in a study of 250 patients. Mortality was 8% in individuals without evidence of pump failure, rose to 30% with clinical evidence of ventricular failure, was 44% with acute pulmonary edema, and was 80–100% with shock. Up to 50% of patients were considered to be Class II. Some of the patients in this group require little pharmacologic treatment, while others require vigorous therapy to prevent the evolution of ventricular damage. Forrester et al.[57] used physiologic staging. Mortality was lowest with normal hemodynamics, rose to 10% with an elevated pulmonary capillary wedge pressure, rose to 22% with a decrease in cardiac output, and jumped to 55.5% when both abnormalities were present. Subsequent studies showed that mortality could also be related to ejection fractions during acute myocardial infarction. A pulmonary catheter should be inserted whenever patients begin moving through Killip stage II status. Clinical and hemodynamic observations form the basis for clinical decisions (see Figure 5–12).

Treatment of AMI must begin as early as possible. Pantridge and Gaddes[58] showed that most deaths associated with AMI were due to ventricular fibrillation and occurred in the first hour after infarction. The availability of highly trained mobile coronary care units with trained paramedical personnel able to initiate resuscitation and prevent subsequent ventricular fibrillation has had a major impact on overall mortality. Ventricular arrhythmias should be treated with beta blockade when evidence of sympathetic hyperactivity is obvious; prophylactic lidocaine is indicated in many other situations. It is also likely that intravenous thrombolytic therapy with tissue-type plasminogen activator will be administered either in the coronary ambulance or in the hospital emergency room.

Therapy in the hospital depends upon a clinical and hemodynamic evaluation of left ventricular function. Patients without evidence of ventricular dysfunction (Killip Class I) should be treated with bed rest and morphine for chest pain. Beta blockers are useful in certain patients. Routine oxygen is indicated if arterial hypoxemia is present. A single arterial analysis is useful for both diagnostic and treatment purposes. A reduced oxygen tension suggests the presence of left ventricular dysfunction, places the patient in Killip class II, and signals the need for oxygen and other therapeutic agents. Additional reas-

TABLE 5–3.
Classification of Patients with Acute Myocardial Infarction

CLINICAL CLASS	MORTALITY	EJECTION FRACTION
I No failure	8%	0.47
II Mild failure	30%	0.36
III Pulmonary Edema	44%	0.31
IV Shock	80–100%	0.12

*Adapted from Killip T, Kimball JT: Treatment of myocardial infarction in a coronary care unit. A two-year experience with 250 patients. *Am. J. Cardiol* 1967; 20:457.

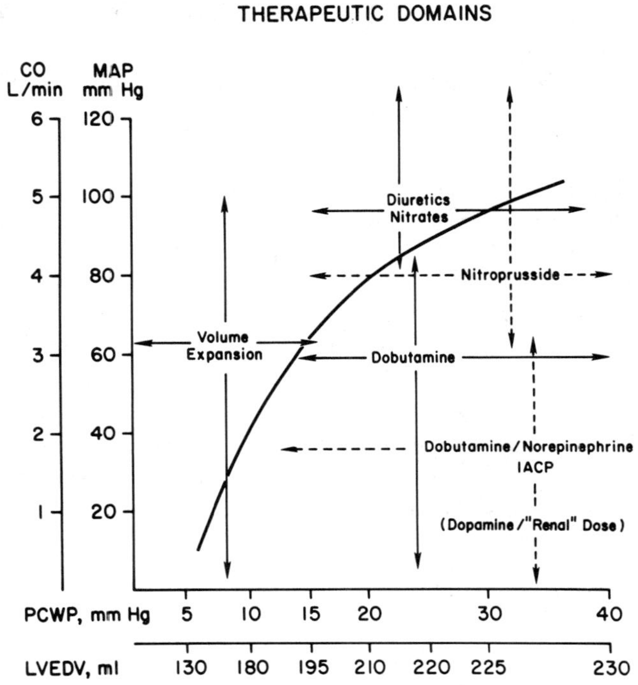

FIG 5–12.
The Starling relationship, plotting mean aortic pressure of stroke output on the ordinate against pulmonary artery wedge pressure on the abscissa, provides an important conceptual basis for the use of pharmacologic agents in patients with ventricular dysfunction. The expression *domains* is used to suggest regions where a specific agent might be implied. The borderline of the various domains obviously overlap with one another. Volume expansion is indicated when a fall in blood pressure or stroke volume is associated with a low wedge pressure. Diuretics, intravenous nitroglycerine, and nitroprusside are indicated when an elevated wedge pressure is associated with reasonably well maintained arterial blood pressure. Dobutamine should be administered when stroke output begins to fall and wedge pressure continues to rise. Hypotension decreases coronary blood flow and is particularly harmful in patients with coronary artery disease. When blood pressure falls below a mean pressure of 65–75 mm Hg, a group of options should be considered. Low dose dopamine may be added to dobutamine. Norepinephrine may be added to dobutamine or used with dopamine (see text). Intra-aortic balloon counterpulsation should be considered if hypotension persists for more than several hours in patients with coronary artery disease.

surance that ventricular function is close to normal may be obtained by noninvasive techniques, such as echocardiography or radionuclide ventriculography.

A pulmonary artery catheter should be inserted whenever the patient appears to be at increased risk. Sobel and Braunwald[59] present sensible guidelines for the use of hemodynamic monitoring in AMI, which closely reflect the thinking of most intensivists. Table 5–4 is modified from their recommendations and those of others.

Hypovolemia in AMI

Wags have occasionally observed that surgical patients are generally overhydrated, while medical patients are frequently allowed to remain volume contracted. Hemodynamic monitoring demonstrated that hypovolemia was responsible for hypotension in a significant number of patients with AMI, and failure to assess volume status adequately may lead to the confusion of hypovolemic shock and cardiogenic shock.

In 1969, Loeb et al.[60] gave low molecular weight dextran to 12 patients with the features of shock after acute myocardial infarction. Two had high central venous pressures and did not improve with volume expansion; ten had central venous pressures below 7 mm Hg. Five of these improved with dextran infusion and survived; the other five did not improve and ultimately died. Vagal hyperactivity in inferior wall myocardial infarction may enhance diuresis and sweating; the prior use of diuretics and lack of adequate oral

TABLE 5–4.
Indications for Hemodynamic Monitoring in AMI

(1)	Hypotension unresponsive to simple measures such as atropine in individuals with bradycardia
(2)	Evidence of left ventricular dysfunction evidenced by physical examination, radiographic evidence of pulmonary congestions, tachypnea, arterial hypoxemia, cyanosis, or lactic acidosis.
(3)	Unexplained sinus tachycardia or other tachyarrhythmias
(4)	Evidence of mitral regurgitation, ventricular septal defect, or pericardial effusion.

fluids may also lead to volume deficits. Crexells et al.[61] used diuretics and fluid infusion, and determined that the optimal filling pressure of the left ventricle in acute myocardial infarction was 14–18 mm Hg. These studies demonstrate optimal values for cardiac output, but ignore the effect of increased ventricular dimensions on myocardial oxygen requirements. Since changes in ventricular compliance prevent an accurate assessment of volume from filling pressures in acute myocardial infarction (see pages 75 and 80), direct volume measurements may be necessary.

Preload and Afterload Reduction in AMI

Venous distention and increased ventricular preload in patients with ventricular dysfunction and AMI have classically been treated with diuretics and vasodilators (see Figure 4–9). Furosemide, 40 mg, at intervals of 3–4 hours is indicated if filling pressures are elevated. The agent acts by producing peripheral vasodilatation within 15 minutes and a later diuresis. Vigorous diuresis without monitoring of filling pressures may convert a congested patient into a hypovolemic and hypotensive individual. Nitroglycerine is a powerful venodilator, and many of its effects are related to the resultant decrease in preload.

A reduction in systemic vascular resistance with rapidly acting vasodilators such as nitroprusside, nitroglycerine, and other agents increases cardiac output and decreases pulmonary capillary wedge pressures. Nitroprusside, in initial doses of 5.0 μg/kg/min followed by maintenance doses of 10 μg/kg/min or more, improves both segmental and global function in AMI.[62,63] It is important to recognize that afterload is not the same as systemic vascular resistance, but is the total force opposing ventricular fiber shortening during left ventricular ejection. The external resistance to ejection can be approximated by calculating systemic vascular resistance but this calculation ignores the contribution of left ventricular wall stress to internal resistance to ejection. The LaPlace principle indicates that wall stress is directly related to chamber dimension and pressure and is inversely related to wall thickness. Thus, an agent which reduces ventricular dimensions, decreases chamber size, and increases wall thickness leading to a substantial decrease in this internal resistance or geometric factor.

The effects of vasodilators on afterload and coronary blood flow are complex. Nitroprusside and dobutamine decrease afterload as well as systemic vascular resistance; norepinephrine increases systemic vascular resistance but may actually decrease afterload by decreasing chamber size. The effects of vasodilators on coronary blood flow depend, in part, upon the reduction of coronary perfusion pressure and the decrease in subendocardial vascular resistance due to decreases in left ventricular end-diastolic pressure. In general, vasodilator therapy should be discontinued if aortic diastolic pressures fall below 60 mm Hg.

The availability of intravenous nitroglycerine has led to a major reassessment of its use in AMI. At one time nitroglycerine was considered to be contraindicated, because it produced venodilatation and decreased cardiac output. Intravenous nitroglycerine is generally administered in doses of 10–15 μg/min with increasing 5 μg/min increments every five minutes. It may improve the perfusion of ischemic myocardium either by reducing preload and end-diastolic pressure or by a direct effect on coronary vessels. Relief of chest pain is a useful indicator of therapeutic effects; doses should be reduced if blood pressure is significantly reduced.

Inotropic Support in Acute Myocardial Infarction

Support of the failing ischemic heart has been a major therapeutic challenge. Catecholamine and digitalis glycosides generally have been thought to affect the determinants of myocardial oxygen demands—wall tension, heart rate, and velocity of contraction—in an adverse manner. By definition, an inotrope increases the velocity of contraction, and catecholamine inotropes uniformly increase heart rate at some dose. The effect of an inotrope on wall tension is more complex, since tension is related to intraventricular pressure and ventricular diameter by the LaPlace relationship. Digitalis and catecholamines that stimulate alpha-adrenergic receptors increase arteriolar resistance and thus intraventricular pressure. Catecholamines with beta-adrenergic properties may decrease ventricular dimensions and thus decrease myocardial wall tension. The effects of catecholamine inotropes also have different effects on myocardial blood flow. Those stimulating beta-2 adrenergic receptors have direct vasodilating action on the coronary vascular bed. Even more significant, however, is the effect of decreasing diastolic pressures on decreasing transmural subendocardial coronary vascular resistance and thereby increasing blood flow. Isoproterenol, with its strong beta-2 dilating effect, decreases aortic diastolic pressure and thereby decreases the diastolic pressure head available for coronary perfusion. Tachycardia is a two-edged sword; it increases myocardial oxygen consumption, and at the same time decreases coronary perfusion by decreasing the time of diastole.

Decreasing ventricular size is of paramount importance for patients with failing hearts. A smaller heart consumes less oxygen, contracts more efficiently, and protects the lungs by contracting at lower end-diastolic pressures. Fortunately, certain inotropes administered to individuals with dilated hearts improve myocardial oxygen dynamics and may reduce myocardial ischemic damage. Watanabe et al.[64] studied the effects of inotropes and vasopressors on infarct size measured by epicardial mapping. They raised arterial pressure by administering phenylephrine to dogs with normal hearts and with pharmacologically induced cardiac depression. Elevation of arterial pressure decreased infarct size in dogs with normal sized hearts. The same intervention increased left atrial pressure from 10 to 23 mm Hg in the depressed heart and increased infarct size. Ouabain, in contrast, lowered mean atrial pressure from 25 mm Hg to 11 mm Hg in the failing heart and decreased infarct size. Isoproterenol increased infarct size at higher doses; doses of 0.05 μg/kg/min decreased left atrial pressure and infarct size.

It is likely that inotropes may have different effects on normal and ischemic myocardial segments in the same heart. Vatner and Baig[65] studied the responses of various myocardial segments in the conscious dog by producing transient coronary occlusion. Occlusion did not affect the normal regions of the heart, but decreased the velocity of contraction by 97% and produced bulging instead of shortening in the severely ischemic zone. Dopamine, 4 μg/kg, and dobutamine, 4 μg/kg, increased the extent and rate of shortening, but not to the degree observed in the normal zone. Both dobutamine and dopamine increased regional blood flow in the moderately ischemic zone, but the increase was greater with dobutamine. Neither agent increased regional blood flow to the severely ischemic zone. When doses were increased to 10 μg/kg/min, about half of the animals developed a significant tachycardia with either drug. Dobutamine produced a significant increase in the extent of myocardial shortening in those animals who did not exhibit tachycardia, but not in those who did. There were no changes in systolic shortening with either drug in the severely ischemic zone in those animals without tachycardia, and both drugs increased paradoxical bulging in those animals with tachycardia. The comparison of changes in segment shortening from all ischemic zones with changes in heart rate demonstrated the extremely important conclusion that drug-induced increases in heart rate produced decreases in segment shortening. Their studies emphasize the importance of the nature of the catecholamine, its dose, the underlying status of the myocardium, and the effect on heart rate in determining myocardial performance and regional blood flow in experimental myocardial infarction.

Maekawa, Liang, and Hood,[66] using a similar conscious dog model but applying the coronary occluder distal to the first diagonal branch of the anterior descending coronary artery so that a smaller infarction may have been produced, observed that dobutamine, 10 μg/kg/min, decreased infarct size by 24%; there was no change in infarct size with dopamine. They also demonstrated that dopamine infusion increased coronary sinus norepinephrine concentration by 140%, while the increase produced by dobutamine was not much higher than those observed with the saline controls. Dopamine, of course, has the physiologic function of releasing norepinephrine from sympathetic nerve endings within the myocardium. Such local release may increase myocardial irritability and unfavorably affect infarct size by increasing myocardial oxygen consumption and producing local vasoconstriction.

These experimental observations support the clinical observations that dobutamine is useful for inotropic support in certain patients with acute myocardial infarction. Gillespie et al.[67] showed that dobutamine, given in doses of 1–40 μg/kg/min for 24 hours, increased cardiac output from 4.9 to 6.0 l/min and decreased pulmonary artery occlusive pressure from 21.5 to 16.7 mm Hg. Heart rate or systemic arterial pressure were not affected, and infarct size, measured by hourly creatine kinase measurements, was not increased compared to predicted values. Investigators from the same laboratory[68] compared dobutamine with intravenous digoxin in six patients with acute myocardial infarction and cardiac failure. Dobutamine decreased pulmonary artery occlusion pressure from 22.3 mm Hg to 9.8 mm Hg, and increased cardiac index from 2.4 to 3.2 L/min/M^2. In contrast, digoxin had a minimal effect on cardiac output (2.2 to 2.4 l/min) and did not affect pulmonary artery occlusion pressure.

Francis, Sharma, and Hodges[69] compared dobutamine with dopamine in 13 patients with acute cardiogenic circulatory collapse due to either acute myocardial infarction (9 patients) or acute decompensation of a previously stable ischemic cardiomyopathy. The patients were extremely ill; cardiac index averaged 1.6 L/min/M^2, mean arterial pressure 72 mm. Hg and pulmonary occlusive pressure were 19 mm Hg. Dobutamine, 5 μg/kg/min, increased stroke index and cardiac index significantly more than did dopamine at the same dose. The pulmonary artery occlusion pressure increased 37% with dopamine, but only 5% with dobutamine when doses of 10 μg/kg/min for both drugs were used. The authors concluded that it appears "patients go through a phase of 'pre-shock' or moderate hypotension, where early intervention with dobutamine seems more prudent that using an intense vasoconstrictor such as norepinephrine or high dose dopamine."

Dobutamine is particularly useful when cardiac output is substantially reduced. Pozen et al.[25] administered the agent to 18 patients with ventricular failure associated with ischemic heart disease. Lactate metabolism was unchanged in 14 patients who demonstrated significant hemodynamic improvement with dobutamine. Four patients exhibited abnormal lactate metabolism with dobutamine, and three of these experienced angina pectoris. These individuals with adverse effects had higher pretreatment cardiac indices (3.34 compared to 2.60 L/min/M^2) and lower systemic vascular resistances than the other patients studied. Pulmonary occlusion pressures were the same in both groups. Dopamine may be added to dobutamine if arterial pressure falls.[70]

Early Revascularization in the Treatment of Acute Myocardial Infarction

Thrombolytic therapy with streptokinase has been shown to improve ventricular function in AMI, but randomized studies analyzing survivorship have not yet been reported.[22] A recent multicenter cooperative trial using tissue plasminogen activator produced by recombinant techniques demonstrated recanalization within 60 minutes of administration in 75% of patients with angiographically documented coronary artery thrombi. Fibrinogen was not significantly reduced, demonstrating that the agent could produce clot lysis without creating a general systemic lytic state.[71]

Until recently, the role of tissue factors in regulating coagulation was not particularly well understood. The evolution of a clot stimulates endothelial cells to produce a plasminogen activator, which ultimately aims to contain the coagulation process. The activator binds to fibrin along with plasminogen and converts it into the lytic enzyme plasmin. Since the conversion occurs in relationship to fibrin, the reaction is contained and does not lead to a systemic lytic state. Urokinase or streptokinase, in contrast, act directly on plasminogen throughout the vascular volume and produce plasmin, which in turn degrades fibrinogen as well as fibrin. These fibrinogen degradation products themselves have anticoagulant and antiplatelet effects, so that a general hemorrhagic diathesis may be elicited.[72]

Mechanical techniques for revascularization have also been successful. Primary percutaneous transluminal coronary angioplasty (PCTA) can rapidly open occluded vessels without producing hemorrhagic complications.[73] The skills of individual groups and the inherent risk associated with interventions undertaken during active ischemia suggest that the various revascularization techniques may be used as sequential steps in the aggressive management of AMI. Early administration of TPA may produce enough clot lysis to improve myocardial oxygenation.

O'Neill et al.[74] randomized 56 patients treated an average of 3–4 hours after the onset of symptoms with either coronary angioplasty or intracoronary streptokinase. Recanalization was achieved in 83% and 85% of the two groups, respectively; residual luminal stenosis of 70% or more was present in 4% of the patients treated with angioplasty and in 83% of those treated with streptokinase. Increases in global ejection fraction were greater for the group treated with angioplasty. Most of the patients were classified as Killip class I; one patient died in the hospital. Thus acute intervention by experienced cardiologists appears safe and effective.

Reperfusion is not an unalloyed benefit. The sudden restoration of blood flow to the ischemic heart does not immediately restore full function. Loss of regulatory enzymes and nucleotides, depletion of protein matrices, loss of membrane function, and other abnormalities lead to what Braunwald and Kloner called the "stunned myocardium."[75] Accumulation of superoxide anion and calcium within cells decreases cell function even when oxygenation is restored. Pharmacologic agents, such as free-radical scavengers and calcium channel blockers, have been shown to improve function in ischemic organs, and might be used in conjunction with techniques that produce revascularization. At some point, revascularization is ineffective as cellular swelling and destruction produce a no-reflow phenomenon.[76]

Intra-aortic Balloon Counterpulsation (IACP)

The intra-aortic balloon pump was first used in patients with cardiogenic shock by Adrian Kantrowitz et al. in 1968.[77] A balloon is placed into the descending thoracic aorta just below the left subclavian artery. Balloon inflation during diastole increases diastolic pressure at the aortic root. Deflation of the balloon during early systole (before opening of the aortic valve) decreases aortic pressure and left ventricular outflow resistance. The remarkable increase in diastolic perfusion pressure aids revascularization and might be considered to be a mechanical forerunner of the more direct techniques used today. Mueller et al.[78] demonstrated that during the initial 4–6 hours of IACP, systolic pressure and left ventricular outflow resistance decreased by 18% and 24%, respectively, while cardiac index improved by 38%. Diastolic arterial pressure rose 98%, and coronary blood flow increased from 68 to 91 ml/100g per minute. The increase in flow was significantly correlated with mean arterial pressure, and was best expressed as a third order curve shown in Figure 5–6. Myocardial oxygen extraction decreased from 79% to a normal level of 61%, and lactate metabolism approached normal. Systemic perfusion improved dramatically as arterial lactate dropped from 5.08 to 2.98 mmoles/liter, and urine output increased an average of 18–60 ml/hour. Mental status improved dramatically, peripheral pulses improved in quality, and the skin became warmer and dry.

IACP has been used for the management of patients with unstable angina, before and after bypass surgery, and for the treatment of shock associated with AMI. It is a powerful method for maintaining myocardial oxygenation while more definitive techniques are under consideration. Early use is important to prevent the development of progressive myocardial necrosis. Alcan et al.,[79] for example, in a study of consecutive patients with cardiogenic shock, showed that mortality rates with IACP were 33% when used within the first 24 hours, and 89% when used later. Mortality was 17% when IACP was linked to early surgery; it was 80% when surgical techniques were not appropriate. Its use with thrombolytic therapy or primary angioplasty depends upon the general status of the patient.

The Conquest of Coronary Shock

The application of revascularization techniques such as IACP, early coronary bypass surgery, thrombolytic therapy and angioplasty have reduced the mortality from shock associated with acute myocardial infarction. Mortality rates were 90-95% in the early nineteen seventies and now may be lowered to 10-15%. Each attempt at reperfusion led to a modest reduction in overall mortality but the results of percutaneous coronary reperfusion with angioplasty suggest that this technique is most likely to rapidly improve oxygen delivery to ischemic myocardial segments. Rutherford et al[80] performed angioplasty in 43 severely compromised patients within 1-6 hours of infarction; 33 required support with IACP. Hospital mortality was 37% for the entire group, 12% in patients supported with IACP and 46% in patients with ejection fractions less than 0.30. An overall hospital mortality of 38% in anterior AMI and 20% in inferior AMI was observed by O'Neill et al[81] in 27 patients with cardiogenic shock. The patients were treated an average of 17 hours after AMI and successful revascularization was achieved in 24 of 27 patients.

Right Ventricular AMI

Cohn et al.[82] defined the syndrome of right ventricular infarction in 1974. Patients with this syndrome usually have electrocardiographic evidence of diaphragmatic wall infarction and some degree of heart block. Distended neck veins and hypotension were the predominant clinical findings. Early recognition and treatment of RV infarction as a cause of cardiogenic shock is essential because this form of coronary shock is partially amenable to medical therapy. RV infarction is suspected when right atrial pressures are higher than left atrial pressures which tend to be normal or even low. Echocardiography can confirm the involvement of RV free wall, septum, and left ventricle.[83]

Volume expansion that raises right atrial pressures to as high as 25–30 mm Hg have been suggested. Addition of an inotrope-vasodilator like dobutamine may increase right ventricular output by its effect on the right ventricular myocardium and its direct vascular action to decrease pulmonary vascular resistance. Volume replacement is a two-edged sword, because increasing right ventricular cavity size increases its oxygen requirements and may lead to additional ischemia. The combined use of fluid and dobutamine increases stroke output without the marked increases in right atrial pressure observed with fluid therapy alone.

Complications of AMI Requiring Immediate Surgical Correction

Three mechanical complications must be corrected by immediate surgery. *Rupture of the ventricular septum*[84] may be recognized by the appearance of a parasternal murmur, circulatory instability, and increased oxygenation of pulmonary arterial blood due to the left to right ventricular shunt. *Rupture of papillary muscles* causing mitral insufficiency may be recognized by the appearance of an apical systolic murmur and the finding of a large regurgitant V (or R) wave in the pulmonary capillary wedge pressure tracing. Inferior wall infarction leads to postromedial papillary muscle rupture; rupture of the anterolateral muscle with anterolateral AMI is less common.[85] The diagnosis of *pericardial tamponade* is discussed in the section on thoracic trauma (page 366). While cardiac rupture may produce tamponade in AMI, death is almost immediate, so that surgical correction, even if possible, cannot be accomplished in the time available.

Treatment of Ventricular Dysfunction in AMI: Summary and Synthesis

The Starling diagram present in Figure 5–12 provides a framework for the treatment of ventricular dysfunction based on physiologic principles. Hypovolemia with low filling pressures should be treated with volume replacement. Early revascularization procedures should be considered in patients with either increased pulmonary artery wedge pressure or reduced cardiac output. If revascularization is unavailable or not indicated, nitrates or diuretics might be considered, if cardiac index is not below 2.5 to 3.0 L/min/M^2 and diastolic blood pressure is not below 60 mm Hg. Intravenous nitroglycerine is rapidly replacing nitroprusside. When wedge pressure rises or cardiac index falls below 2.5 to 3.0 L/min/M^2, dobutamine in increasing concentrations (beginning with 5 μg/kg/min) is indicated. If the diastolic blood pressure falls below 60 mm Hg, an inotrope with vasopressor activity should be added to dobutamine. Dopamine frequently has been considered the vasopressor of choice in AMI. Dopamine, however, is a two-edged sword because of its combined alpha, beta and dopaminergic properties (see page 108). Mueller, Evans, and Ayres[86] demonstrated that titration of dopamine to achieve a mean arterial pressure of 65–70 mm Hg increased urine output to greater than 40 ml/hr, but heart rate increased from 95 to 118 beats/min. Pulmonary wedge pressure and right atrial pressure decreased from 23 to 18 and from 10 to 8 mm Hg, respectively. Improvement of hemodynamic status by dopamine was associated with deterioration of myocardial metabolism. Myocardial oxygen extraction ratios increased from 73% to 75%, and lactate production by the myocardium increased. For these reasons, we and others prefer to add l-norepinephrine at 2–8 μg/min to the infusion of dobutamine. If the patient has been in shock for more than 12 hours with decreased renal blood flow and urine output, low dosages of dopamine (under 5 μg/kg/min) should be added.

Since cardiogenic shock in AMI usually occurs as a result of a continuous wave-like extension of necrotic myocardial regions, early revascularization must be considered in all patients who are hemodynamically unstable on admission. Mortality rates of greater than 70% for cardiogenic shock with conservative medical treatment can be substantially reduced with revascularization techniques. The early use of revascularization techniques is essential if maximum volumes of myocardium are to be salvaged. While stabilization and thrombolytic therapy can be instituted at most institutions, transfer within 6-12 hours of the onset of symptoms to comprehensive medical centers able to perform balloon angioplasty is essential.

NON-CORONARY CARDIOGENIC SHOCK

Ventricular dysfunction and cardiogenic shock may occur in patients with normal coronary blood flow and myocardial metabolism. Either right or left ventricular overload, constrictive pericarditis or pericardial tamponade, or primary myofibrillar failure in spite of adequate oxygenation may be responsible. In general, inotropes may be used without fear of producing myocardial ischemia in these patients, and balloon counterpulsation is less effective because the increased coronary flow due to diastolic augmentation is not necessary. Cardiomyopathies exemplify chronic ventricular dysfunction with ultimate deterioration and shock; ventricular dysfunction associated with sepsis is probably a more common problem in most critical care units.

Cardiac Dysfunction Associated with Sepsis

An earlier section (page 40) detailed the abnormalities observed in septic shock and emphasized that both hyperdynamic and hypodynamic stages characterized the syndrome. Inadequate fluid resuscitation is a prominent cause of hypodynamic ventricular function in sepsis; in other patients, myocardial depression appears to be present. A number of groups have identified myocardial depressant factors in sepsis, but the most convincing demonstration is probably the recent study of Parillo et al., [87] which found a humoral factor in patients with sepsis that depressed newborn rat myocardial cell contractility in tissue culture. Similar activity was not found in other critically ill patients and was absent from serum obtained during the recovery phase from survivors of septic shock.

Radionuclide and thermal conductivity studies[88] demonstrate decreased ejection fractions and increased end-diastolic volumes in patients with septic shock. Reductions in ejection fraction correlated with increases in myocardial depressant factor. The same group[89] confirmed the presence of increased ventricular compliance in dogs with gram negative bacteremia. These studies assist in the interpretation of right atrial and pulmonary capillary wedge pressures in sepsis. Filling pressures are low early, but rise with adequate volume replacement. As ventricular dysfunction develops, filling pressures rise, but ventricular relaxation or flabbiness prevents the elevations in pressure that would be seen with normal or decreased ventricular compliance. Changes in filling pressures might be quite misleading in this situation, where adequate diastolic volumes are necessary for optimal stroke output.

Coronary flow and myocardial metabolism appear to be normal in most patients with septic shock,[90] but may become abnormal in hypodynamic patients. Mueller[91] compared coronary hemodynamics in septic patients with increased cardiac indices and another group with cardiac indices that were markedly reduced. Clinical shock with elevated arterial lactate concentration and markedly reduced arterial blood pressures were present in both groups. Coronary blood flow was lower, and myocardial lactate production was observed in the group with low cardiac indices. The management of septic shock is detailed on pages 357–358.

Ventricular Dysfunction in the Cardiomyopathies

Primary cardiac muscle dysfunction is termed cardiomyopathy. For many years the cardiomyopathies were considered "idiopathic" in nature because precise causes had not been delineated. Three forms are distinguished on hemodynamic study: dilated cardiomyopathies are characterized by dilated ventricles with decreased ejection fractions and reduced stroke output. Restrictive cardiomyopathy is a much less common form characterized by a relatively normal heart size, still (noncompliant) ventricles, and relatively normal ejection fraction. This form must be distinguished from constrictive pericarditis. Hypertrophic cardiomyopathy is similar physiologically to the restrictive form, but the ventricular stiffness is due to ventricular hypertrophy, producing a "muscle-bound" state. Outflow obstruction was once thought to be the major abnormality, and the disorder was termed hypertrophic aortic stenosis. Global ventricular dysfunction, however, due to decreased compliance appears to be the central pathogenetic problem in most patients. Experience with endomyocardial biopsy is rapidly growing, in part because of its use to evaluate rejection of the transplanted heart. A substantial number of patients exhibit an inflammatory infiltrate which might respond to anti-inflammatory treatment.

Approximately 50% of patients with dilated cardiomyopathy die within the first two years, and 20% are alive at eight years.[92] The chronic course exhibited by these patients ensures their appearance in critical care units at frequent intervals. Long term care with salt restriction, afterload reduction, and digitalis is necessary, although it is not clear how much inotropic support is beneficial. New oral inotropes more effective than digitalis may well overstimulate the myocardium, and could actually increase ventricular dysfunction. Fluids, inotropes, afterload reduction, and pressors must be carefully balanced during hospital admissions. Fluid therapy is complicated because of wide variation in ventricular compliance. A relatively small volume in a patient with restrictive cardiomyopathy may produce a major increase in pulmonary capillary wedge pressure without markedly increasing end-diastolic volume. Since volume, not pressure, determines preload, the elevated wedge pressure would have been achieved without an adequate increase in stroke output. The reverse situation may be seen in dilated cardiomyopathies where large volumes of fluid may increase stroke output without prohibitive increases in wedge pressures.

Cardiac arrhythmias are common in cardiomyopathy, and present major therapeutic problems. Conversion to normal sinus rhythm is frequently desirable, since loss of atrial systole may hasten the progression of ventricular dysfunction. Use of quinine or procainamide following conversion to maintain sinus rhythm, however, may lead to drug-related decrements in myocardial contractility.

The major improvement in survivorship after cardiac transplantation makes this option an important one for many patients. If transplantation is contemplated, maintenance of adequate pulmonary and systemic blood flow is necessary to allow adequate recovery following transplantation.

Mechanical Support of the Failing Heart

Akutsu and Kolff[93] observed a 90-minute survival in a dog given a total artificial heart. Almost 20 years later, Devries et al.[94] demonstrated the possibility of prolonged human survival (112 days) in a cardiomyopathy patient who died following a postoperative course complicated by recurrent pulmonary insufficiency, recurrent acute renal failure, fever of undetermined etiology, and hemorrhagic complications of anticoagulation. The demonstration that total support for prolonged periods was possible has provided new impetus to the use of partial mechanical assistance for patients with pharmacologically unresponsive ventricular failure in critical care units.

The Saint Louis University cardiovascular surgery group[95] has reported an experience in the use of IACP in cardiac surgical patients that parallels that of other groups. IACP was used in three hundred and seventy eight (6.8%) of 5,546 patients undergoing cardiac operations between March, 1973 and April, 1982. The survival rate was: preoperatively in patients with angina pectoris, 82%; preoperatively in patients with cardiogenic shock, 42%; intraoperatively, 55%; postoperatively, 43.6%. There were eight IACP related deaths (2.1%). Survival was higher in patients with insertion by percutaneous femoral puncture (99/161; 62%) compared to femoral arteriotomy (99/201; 49%), but major IACP complications were more common with percutaneous insertion (9.9% versus 3.5%). Similar studies in medical patients suggest that the overall mortality from cardiogenic shock associated with acute myocardial infarction can be reduced from 90–95% to below 50% when combined with angiocardiography and either angioplasty or bypass surgery. Early insertion to preserve myocardial integrity appears to be associated with reduced mortality rates compared to insertion after 24 hours.

Extracorporeal Membrane Oxygenation (ECMO)

ECMO for patients with severe acute respiratory failure was judged disappointing in a collaborative randomized prospective study sponsored by the NHLBI in the mid-1970s. Since the trial was organized by the Lung Division, patients with chronic heart failure or markedly elevated wedge pressures were excluded. Pennington et al.,[96] from the Saint Louis University surgical group, studied its application in 14 patients with severe heart failure from a variety of causes. Total time on ECMO ranged from 8 to 216 hours (mean, 58 hours), and seven were successfully weaned. Three were weaned with inotropic support, two by ventricular assist devices, and two by cardiac transplantation. Cardiac output and systemic arterial pressures increased, and right atrial pressures decreased in all patients immediately after the institution of ECMO. Within twelve hours, hemodynamic deterioration was observed in those who could not be ultimately weaned.

A number of groups have attempted to develop left heart bypass support for postoperative cardiogenic shock following the initial successful use of these techniques by Spencer et al. in 1964[97] and DeBakey in 1966.[98] The Saint Louis group[99] has used a nonpulsatile centrifugal blood pump (CPVAD) and the newer Pierce-Donachy ventricular assist device (VAD) in 18 and 13 patients, respectively. The Pierce-Donachy VAD is a paracorporeal pneumatic sac-type device with Bjork-Shiley inlet and outlet valves. It has a stroke volume of 65 ml and a dynamic ejection fraction of approximately 0.75. The primacy of IACP over VAD for most patients is shown by the use of IACP in 7% and VAD in 0.6% of patients in the treatment of postoperative cardiogenic shock during the same time period. Preoperative hemodynamic function did not appear to influence the frequency of postoperative ventricular failure, which seemed to be associated with the incidence of perioperative acute myocardial infarction. The presence of biventricular failure greatly influenced outcome. Five of twenty-one patients receiving left ventricular assistance had isolated left ventricular failure, and four of these were weaned. None of the sixteen with biventricular failure and only LV assistance could be weaned. Five of ten patients with biventricular failure who received biventricular support could be weaned, and three of these are long-term survivors. An unusual observation was the biphasic effect of inotropic support during left ventricular assistance. Initially, isoproterenol produced an increase in cardiac output, but increasing doses led to a decline in cardiac output, an increase in right atrial and pulmonary artery diastolic pressure, and a decrease in left atrial pressure. In the absence of pulmonary hypertension, the right ventricle appeared to recover before the left, but the isoproterenol-induced increases in pulmonary vascular resistance are not easily explained.

Complications with ventricular assist devices are related to the severe shock and to the device itself. Excessive bleeding was observed in 28 of 31 patients, and 14 required re-exploration. Bleeding occurred, even though intraoperative heparin had been fully reversed with protamine, and heparin was not restarted for the first 48 hours after insertion of the VAD. Multiple organ failure was common, and hemolysis *prior* to the insertion of VAD was observed in ten patients.

Thrombi arising in pump cannulae and VAD sacs were noted in five patients, but emboli were seen only in the two with thrombi in the cannulae.

HYPERTENSIVE EMERGENCIES

An elevated blood pressure in a critically ill patient may be the primary reason for admission, or may be secondary to other primary causal factors. Left ventricular failure, for example, may cause hypertension or be a result of it. Hypertension is observed in up to one-third of patients with acute myocardial infarction, but usually falls to normal within several hours. Primary hypertension affects 25–30% of the American population, but hypertensive crises occur in only a small number of hypertensive patients. Progression to malignant hypertension is highest in young and middle-aged black men and in patients with hypertension due to renal vascular or parenchymal disease.

Hypertensive crises are termed accelerated hypertension if papilledema is not present. The syndrome of malignant hypertension includes papilledema and may have hypertensive encephalopathy, characterized by confusion, somnolence, seizures, and focal neurological signs. Hematuria, proteinuria, and reduced creatinine clearance are common.

An elevated blood pressure is obviously harmful to vascular structures, but is also important evidence of severe vasoconstriction. Cardiac output is almost always lower than normal in patients with primary hypertension, and systemic vascular resistance may be 25% greater than normal.[100] Fibrinoid changes in the vascular endothelium in malignant hypertension causes a structural increase in systemic vascular resistance; increase in vasoconstriction commonly produces an additional functional increase in vascular resistance. Since organ blood flow is reduced by the decreased flow and increased resistance, pharmacologic therapy must be aimed at reducing vascular resistance.

Hypertensive crises are customarily divided into hypertensive emergencies and hypertensive urgencies.[101] A hypertensive emergency requires admission, and usually presents with a diastolic blood pressure in excess of 120 mm Hg and at least one of the following: cerebral vascular accident, subarachnoid bleed, hypertensive encephalopathy, acute aortic dissection, left ventricular failure or pulmonary edema, toxemia of pregnancy, pheochromocytoma crisis, grade 3 or 4 Keith-Wagener retinopathy, acute renal insufficiency, myocardial ischemia, antihypertensive withdrawal syndromes, head injuries, burns, or drug interactions. If evidence for end-organ failure without any of the above abnormalities is present, the crisis may be called an "urgency" rather than an "emergency." Patients with hypertensive emergencies should be admitted, and the blood pressure reduced to a safe level within one hour.

Hypotensive therapy must avoid major decrements in blood flow to the brain, heart, and kidneys. Autoregulation normally maintains flow to these organs, even with wide blood pressure fluctuations. Houston[101] has reviewed autoregulation in cerebral vessels and emphasized that flow in a normotensive patient remains unchanged between a mean arterial pressure of 60 to 120 mm Hg. In hypertensive patients, in contrast, it remains unchanged between 120–160 mm Hg. A reduction below the lower limit in hypertensive patients can lead to a reduction in brain blood flow, while pressure above the upper limit produces a pressure-dependent vasodilatation. Cerebral autoregulation is impaired in elderly individuals, so that much smaller shifts in blood pressure can produce significant CNS disturbances.[102] Oral hypertensive agents are selected for hypertensive urgencies, while intravenous therapy is usually advisable for patients with hypertensive emergencies. The intravenous agents with rapid onset and shortest duration of action are sodium nitroprusside, trimethaphan, and phentolamine. They permit close control of blood pressure and prevent unacceptable hypertension or hypotension. Diazoxide, hydralazine, and labetalol have a rapid onset of action, making them difficult to control. Sodium nitroprusside is probably the most commonly used intravenous agent; intravenous nitroglycerine is useful for hypertension associated with ischemic heart disease, but it may produce wide swings in blood pressure that require careful monitoring. Nifedipine and clonidine are excellent oral agents for the treatment of hypertensive urgencies.

Leigh Thompson, a clinical pharmacologist with extensive experience caring for the critically ill, suggests the use of nitroprusside (200 μg/ml) beginning with 5 μg/min and rarely exceeding 500 μg/ml. He concluded his review of hypertensive emergencies with the following analysis:[103]

> Nitroprusside is a potent, reliable, and safe vasodilator that works immediately and has a short duration of action. It is perfect for a close-loop control system that may maintain mean arterial pressure at any set point with great precision. This therapy will remain quite useful for patients with highly labile arterial pressures and for short term therapy.
>
> Nifedipine is, in my opinion, the most exciting of the newer forms of therapy. It acts quickly when given sublingually,it has few hemodynamic effects other than arterial dilation, it is highly reliable, and moderately potent. Concomitant therapy may not be needed in many patients, but nifedipine may be combined with diuretics, beta-adrenergic receptor agonists, and other vasodilators. The intravenous form of nifedipine, now in clinical trials, may provide a challenge to nitroprusside when heart failure is not a major factor in hypertension.

CARDIAC ARRHYTHMIAS IN THE CRITICALLY ILL

Probably the greatest single step forward in the treatment of critically ill patients was the demonstration that previously fatal ventricular arrhythmias could be quickly terminated by electrical means. Lown, Amarasingham, and Neuman[104] developed direct current countershock for terminating ventricular arrhythmias in 1962, and Brown et al.,[105] Day,[106] Meltzer and Kitchell[107] and Grace[108] introduced the concept of continuous electrocardiographic monitoring in coronary care units in 1963. Indeed, refinement of these pioneering concepts dominated medical thought in the decade following, and it has only been recently that attention has shifted to ventricular failure as a parallel problem. When patients regularly died almost immediately during ischemic episodes, subsequent ventricular dysfunction was not a problem. As is so often the case, therapeutic techniques antedated the understanding of pathophysiology.

Electrophysiologic Considerations

Neither myocardial fiber shortening nor the development of a propagated action potential is possible unless myocardial cells are both surrounded by and contain optimal concentrations of inorganic ions. Many ions play a role in the regulation of cardiac function, but potassium, sodium, and calcium exert such an important influence that their functions should be understood in detail.

The myocardial cell, like cells in general, possesses a potassium concentration approximately 30 times greater than that of the surrounding extracellular fluid. The presence of a concentration gradient across the relatively impermeable cell membrane permits the cell to act as a capacitor and to store electrical energy. In the resting state, the cell is polarized with negative charges in the interior and positive charges on the exterior. Microelectrode studies from single cells have shown that the resting myocardial cell maintains a potential difference of about 90 mV across the cell membrane—the resting potential.

A recording from a single myocardial cell is shown in Figure 5–13. A sudden decrease in resting potential which falls to zero and then changes polarity, with the interior becoming positive relative to the exterior, is characteristic of the action potential. The action potential, termed phase 0, coincides with the R wave of the surface electocardiogram. As sodium is actively pumped out of the cell, the transmembrane potential returns to the resting state in three distinct phases. Phase 1 is rapid, early repolarization; phase 2 is slow, early repolarization; and phase 3 is rapid, late depolarization. Phase 3 coincides with the T wave of the surface electrocardiogram.[109]

The cell shown in Figure 5–13 is not capable of developing an action potential unless stimulated. Figure 5–14 shows another type of cell which has the additional property of *automaticity*. Stage 4 is not flat (as in the cell shown in Figure 5–13), but gradually rises toward the thresh-

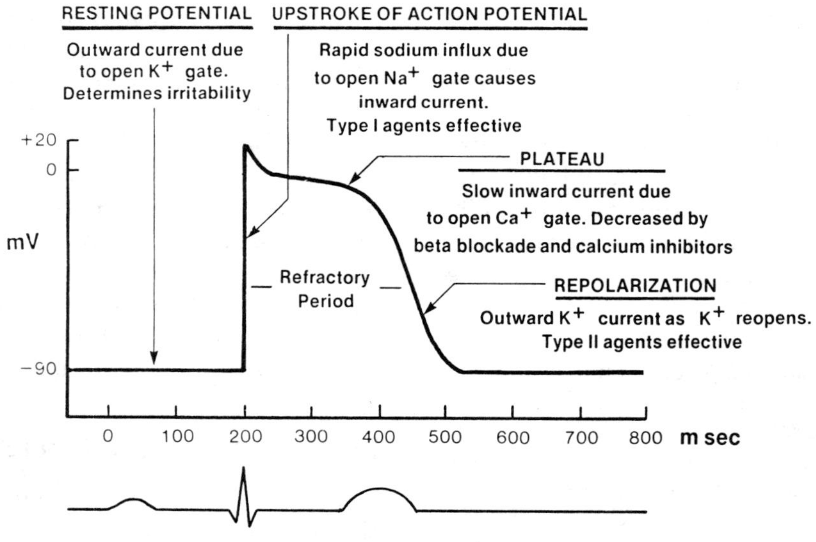

FIG 5–13.

Recording from a single cell. A resting potential of minus 90 millivolts is recorded by the microelectrode. Following an appropriate stimulus the cell rapidly depolarizes becoming less negative and then positive with respect to the external electrode. This rapid depolarization is responsible for the QRS complex of the surface electrode. Depolarization is then followed by a phase of early rapid replarization termed phase one followed by a prolonged phase of slow replarization termed phase two and a terminal phase of rapid repolarization termed phase three. The ionic evens responsible for these potential changes are shown . Type I agents (older classification) alter the rapid inward current and the action potential while Type II agents alter repolarization. Beta adrenergic blocking agents and calcium channel blocking agents alter the slow inward calcium current.

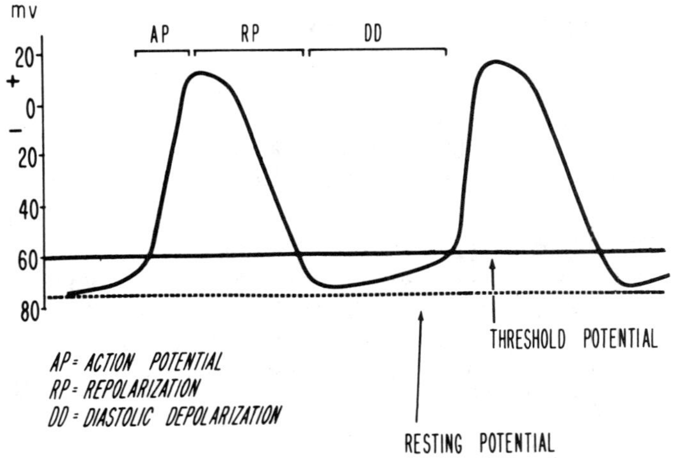

FIG 5–14.
Recording from a single automatic cell with pacemaker potential. The resting potential is not constant as in Figure 1, but gradually decreases. This phase of diastolic depolarization (DD) continues until the threshold potential is reached. The entire cell then depolarizes, generating an action potential. In this illustration, the action potential is labelled AP, and the three phases of repolarization are labelled RP. (After Hoffman EF, Cranefield FF. *Electrophysiology of the Heart.* New York, McGraw-Hill, 1960.)

old potential. The diastolic depolarization continues until the threshold potential is reached. At that point, an action potential is generated. Diastolic depolarization is responsible for the rhythmicity of cardiac tissue. Cells in the sinoatrial node, atrial conduction pathways, parts of the atrioventricular node, and His-Purkinje system may all demonstrate diastolic depolarization. Ordinarily, the rate of diastolic depolarization in cells other than those found in the sinoatrial node is so slow that automaticity in these cells is suppressed by the propagated impulse arising from the sinus node.

The ability of a myocardial cell to respond to an electrical stimulus is termed *excitability*. The cell loses its ability to respond following depolarization and cannot respond again until repolarization has occurred. The cell is completely refractory until the transmembrane potential has been restored to −55 mV. At this point the cell responds, but high voltage stimuli are required, and the response is of low amplitude and is not propagated. This period of low responsiveness, together with the absolute refractory period, is termed the effective refractory period. Antiarrhythmic drugs are believed to abate arrhythmias because they increase the duration of the effective refractory period relative to the speed of impulse conduction. Complete responsiveness is restored when the transmembrane potential returns to the resting level.

Impulse Conduction

The rate of rise and amplitude of the action potential is directly related to the level of transmembrane potential.[110] The most rapid rate of rise occurs when the stimulus is delivered at a transmembrane potential close to the resting potential. If the resting potential is reduced by drugs or disease, the resultant action potential is reduced in amplitude and rate of rise. Since the ability to stimulate adjacent cells and thus *conduct* the impulse throughout the heart is closely related to the slope of the action potential, it is clear that the velocity of conduction is related to the magnitude of the resting potential.[111]

The rate of conduction is not the same in all regions of the heart. It is rapid in the atrium (800 to 1,000 mm/second), slows abruptly to 20–200 mm/second in the atrioventricular junction, and speeds up to 4,000 mm/second in the Purkinje fibers.

Alterations in conductivity produce local or general heart block. Block is particularly common in the atrioventricular node because of the slowness of conduction through that area. Two important physiologic mechanisms, the presence of *refractory tissue* and the phenomenon of *decremental conduction*, account for many of the conduction disturbances seen in the critically ill.

An impulse cannot be transmitted by refractory cells. If impulses are generated at high rates they may reach tissue that has not yet repolarized and thus are blocked. This is particularly common in the right bundle because of its long refractory period. In general, the refractory period lengthens from the sinoatrial node to the Purkinje fibers.

Normal conduction is dependent upon each action potential eliciting an adequate response in adjacent cells. In decremental conduction, a weaker than normal stimulus elicits progressively weaker responses from adjacent cells.[112] The impulse is propagated slowly, and eventually depolarization may fail. Myocardial fiber stretch, hypoxia, administration of potassium, antiarrhythmic drugs, or digitalis may all lead to decremental conduction.

Atrioventricular Junction

Recent studies have examined the behavior of the atrioventricular (AV) junction and have provided data which may be helpful in the management of conduction disturbances in the critically ill patient. The impulse travels at a rapid rate until it reaches the central cells of the junction. The action potential generated by these cells exhibits a low rate of rise, explaining the slow rate of conduction through this region.[113] As the impulse leaves the central junction, it rapidly increases its velocity and traverses the His-Purkinje system to reach the ventricular muscle. This behavior may be seen in His bundle recordings obtained in the intact individual. Figure 5–15 shows a normal His electrocardiogram. Note that almost 90 milliseconds are required to travel from the lower atrium to the His

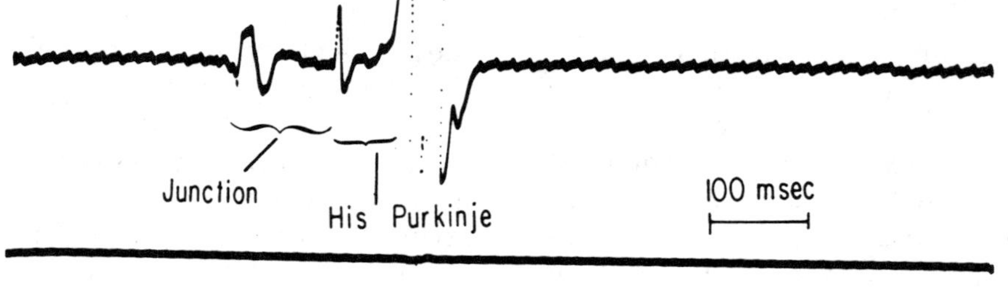

FIG 5–15.
Electrical recording from the interior of the right heart reveals three distinct depolarizations, which may be compared with the surface electrocardiogram: Atrial depolarization (A), His bundle depolarization (H), and ventricular depolarization (V). This His bundle recording technique actually permits division of the PR interval into two components. The A–H time represents conduction from the beginning of atrial repolarization through the A–V junction to a bundle of His. The H–V time represents conduction down the bundle of His; the QRS time indicates actual intraventricular conduction and reflects both Purkinje fibre and myocardial fibre conduction.

bundle (AV junction transit time) while the greater distance from the His bundle to the ventricular musculature is traversed in 40 milliseconds.

The atrioventricular junction may be regarded as the achilles heel of the heart. Since it is the only conduit between the atrial and ventricular conduction systems, a small lesion may have catastrophic consequences, while a lesion of similar size in another location might be silent or produce at most a few ectopic beats. Another reason for its vulnerability is the slow action potential and rate of conduction of junctional cells. Conduction is normally sluggish throughout the junction, and any change in external environment may produce serious disturbances in conduction. Hypoxia, vagal stimulation, and administration of digitalis, quinidine, or procaine amide decrease atrioventricular conduction and are particularly prone to produce atrioventricular abnormality in the critically ill patient. The effects are additive so that a little digitalis, for example, might produce heart block in a hypoxic heart.

Decreases in atrioventricular conduction commonly lead to heart block. Abnormalities of the Wenckebach variety may occur first and be followed by the Mobitz type of complete block of atrial impulses. The automaticity of cells distal to areas of decreased conduction gives rise to junctional escape rhythm, junctional tachycardia, and atrioventricular dissociation.

The Ionic Basis for Cardiac Rhythmicity

The electrophysiologic events described above are regulated by the cell membrane or sarcolemma, which may be viewed as a cell insulator preventing leakage of electrical charge and electrocution of adjacent tissues. Openings or "gates" in the insulating sarcolemma open in response to changes in electrical current and allow the movement of ions. Their subsequent closure renders the sarcolemma impermeable to ion traffic. These channels or gates are composed of protein or protein-lipid complexes positioned within the phospholipid sarcolemma.

Other proteins within the sarcolemma have energy requiring pumping functions. The Na-K (sodium-potassium) ATPase pump activates ATP and moves sodium out of the cell and potassium into the cell against concentration gradients. They are called "pumps" because they move ions uphill, much as a garden pump moves water to the surface.

The cellular quietude of the resting stage is broken when an electrical stimulus reduces the resting transmembrane potential to threshold (−70 to −60 mV) and opens the sodium channels. Sodium rushes into the low-sodium cell interior and further depolarizes the cell membrane. Zipes[114] have lucidly described the gated system model based on studies on the squid giant axon. In this model, both activation and inactivation gates are envisioned. During the resting phase, the activation gate is closed, the inactivation gate open, and the channel functionally blocked to the passage of sodium. Depolarization opens the activation channel and allows a short moment of sodium ingress because the inactivation channel is slow in closing. The sudden depolarization produced by opening the sodium channel produces action potentials with extremely rapid upstrokes in normal atrial, ventricular, and His-Purkinje tissues. Calcium channels have similar activation and inactivation gates. These channels open and close much more slowly than sodium gates and produce a lower amplitude slow upstroke current in normal sinus and atrio-ventricular nodes. Slow response channels are also found in ischemic and other diseased regions of the myocardium. Agents that increase cyclic AMP increase the slow inward current while beta blockers decrease it. Beta adrenergic receptors within the sarcolemma may play a physiologic role in regulating the permeability of the slow channel. The slow inward current probably is responsible for the upstroke of the action potential in sinus and AV nodes, accounting for their physiologic properties. Potassium channels open during repolarization and lead to a restoration of the resting potential. Vaughn Williams[115] has proposed a classification of antiarrhythmic drugs based on their actions on transmembrane ionic exchange (see page 157).

Development of Arrhythmias in the Critically Ill

Cardiac arrhythmias may be produced by alterations in impulse formation or by disturbance of conduction. Ectopic rhythms result when a subsidiary focus replaces the normal sinus mechanism. Secondary automatic foci emerge either because sinus node automaticity is suppressed, or because the automaticity of secondary foci is greater than that of the sinus node.[116] The former mechanism is generally termed suppression, the latter, usurpation. A number of factors may influence automaticity (Table 5–5). The selection of a treatment program may depend on whether an ectopic focus has arisen from suppression or usurpation. If a ventricular pacemaker has arisen because all higher centers are depressed, use of conventional suppressive therapy might suppress the last remaining automatic tissue in the heart. In contrast, if a rapid ectopic focus usurped the function of the normal pacemaker, suppressive therapy might allow restoration of sinus activity. Unfortunately, many arrhythmias in the critically ill patient develop when higher centers are suppressed, and antiarrhythmic agents must be administered with considerable caution.

Conduction disturbances lead to arrhythmias because they invite reentry phenomenon.[117] Two parallel circuits—one with normal conduction and the other with unidirectional conduction block—comprise a classic situation for the development of such reentrant arrhythmias.[118] The impulse traverses the normal pathway, depolarizing a region of myocardium, but the block prevents other areas from depolarizing; these areas remain excitable. The conducted impulse then "turns around," enters the excitable tissue, is transmitted retrogradely up the blocked conduction pathways, and is once again transmitted down the normally conducting pathways. Antiarrhythmic agents that slow conduction or increase refractoriness may actually perpetuate the events predisposing to such reentrant

TABLE 5–5.
Environmental Influences Affecting Electrophysical Properties of Heart Muscle

INFLUENCE	AUTOMATICITY	EXCITABILITY CONDUCTIVITY
Vagal stimulation	Decrease	Decrease
Hyperkalemia	Decrease	Decrease
Hypokalemia	Increase	Increase
Catecholamines	Increase	Increase
Hypercapnia and acidosis	Increase	Decrease
Hypoxia	Increase	Decrease
Increased temperature	Increase	Decrease
Myocardial fiber stretch	Increase	Decrease

arrhythmias. Factors affecting excitability and conductivity are shown in Table 5–5.

Hypoxia is an extremely important cause of cardiac arrhythmias in the critically ill patient. While hypoxia produces adrenergic stimulation in the normal individual with elevation of pulse and blood pressure, this response is frequently attenuated in the critically ill patient. Vagal stimulation in the presence of hypoxia is particularly dangerous and may lead to bradycardia or complete inhibition of impulse formation.[119]

Respiratory acidosis due to sudden ventilatory failure may also provoke arrhythmias.[120] While chronic hypercapnia is associated with minimal shifts in pH, acute increase in carbon dioxide tension in the previously normal individual leads to precipitous decreases in pH with increases in myocardial irritability (chapter 7). The combined effect of hypercapnia and hypoxia account for many of the fatal arrhythmias observed in the critically ill. Together, acute pulmonary hypertension and cor pulmonale further impair cardiac impulse formation.[121]

Metabolic acidosis leads to hyperkalemia, which may precipitate ventricular arrhythmias. Figure 5–3 shows the electrocardiogram of a patient with shock and severe metabolic acidosis. Correction of the acidosis by the rapid administration of large quantities of bicarbonate led to a decrease in plasma potassium and a prompt cessation of ventricular fibrillation. Acidosis renders the heart insensitive to the effects of catecholamines, decreases myocardial contractility, and leads to arrhythmias which cannot be terminated by electrical countershock.

Hyperventilation with respiratory alkalosis and hypokalemia may also provoke cardiac arrhythmias.[122] Figure 5–4 shows a series of electrocardiograms from a patient who was unwittingly mechanically hyperventilated following successful cardiac resuscitation. The ventricular arrhythmias could be controlled only when the carbon dioxide and potassium concentrations were restored to normal.

PHYSIOLOGIC CONSEQUENCES OF ARRHYTHMIAS

An increase in heart rate is the normal physiologic response to exercise. Adrenergic stimulation increases the firing rate of the sinoatrial node and, at the same time, enhances myocardial contractility so that the same or a greater fraction of total diastolic blood volume is ejected with each systole. Stroke volume may be unchanged or may slightly increase, but the fact that the same volume is ejected in a shorter period of time indicates enhanced myocardial contractility.

Laboratory studies have shown that tachycardia induced by electrical pacemaking increases cardiac output, coronary blood flow, and myocardial oxygen consumption. Anaerobic metabolism and myocardial hypoxia are prevented, since increased oxygen is supplied to accomplish the increased mechanical work performed at the rapid heart rate. The relationship is so constant that Katz and Feinberg[123] were able to predict oxygen consumption in the heart-lung preparation from an empirical index obtained by multiplying heart rate times mean arterial pressure. For example, doubling heart rate doubles oxygen consumption.

Heart disease of many types has been shown to interfere with this neat relationship between heart rate and cardiac output. Stroke volume may decrease along with heart rate because the myocardium is unable to increase its force and velocity of contraction. In consequence, a modest tachycardia may fail to increase cardiac output, whereas a rapid tachycardia may produce a decrease in cardiac output.

Furthermore, increasing heart rate in

patients with heart disease has profound implications for myocardial energetics. Unlike most vascular beds, increased oxygen delivery to the coronary bed is accomplished by increasing the rate of coronary blood flow, since oxygen is normally extracted almost maximally from coronary blood flow. Increasing heart rate increases mechanical work per minute (as indicated by the blood pressure multiplied by heart rate index), but coronary flow and oxygen consumption in the diseased heart are unable to keep pace. This situation is magnified in the patient with coronary arterial disease in whom rigid coronary vessels additionally conspire to block the expected increase in oxygen consumption with tachycardia. Anaerobic metabolism develops, myocardial cellular oxygen tension drops, and irreversible structural changes soon develop unless the arrhythmia is rapidly terminated.

Atrial systole normally augments cardiac output, and its relationship to ventricular systole determines, in part, the effect of an arrhythmia on cardiac output.[124] A properly timed atrial systole raises end-diastolic pressure and volume, increasing the force of the subsequent ventricular contraction. Systolic pressure is significantly lower with prolongation of the P-R interval or delay of atrial contraction, so that it falls during ventricular systole.

The value of a forceful and properly timed atrial contraction provides an argument for the attempted conversion of arrhythmias to regular sinus rhythm. A number of carefully designed studies have shown a 30–40% increase in cardiac output following electrical conversion in most patients. Other studies have shown that cardiac output is significantly lower with atrial fibrillation compared to sinus rhythm, even if ventricular rates are identical. Unfortunately, certain critically ill patients cannot muster forceful atrial contractions, even if atrial systole is properly timed. In this group, reversion to sinus rhythm would not increase cardiac output above that obtained by slowing the ventricular rate with digitalis, although it would eliminate the symptom of palpitations and probably decrease the chance of atrial thrombus formation.

Pharmacologic Treatment of Cardiac Arrhythmias

Zipes[125] has recently pointed out that it is not really possible to develop useful classifications of antiarrhythmic drugs that can be used to design therapy. Studies in whole animals or with isolated cellular preparations are extremely useful, but tissue damage, heart rate, ionic and osmotic concentration, state of acid-base balance, and nutritional and energy status dramatically change the effects of various agents. As Zipes stated: "Lidocaine exerts little effect on a normal Purkinje fiber action potential upstroke at a pacing cycle of 1,000 msec, but can profoundly depress it when the cell becomes depolarized and discharges at a rapid rate, such as might occur during ischemia-induced tachycardia." Once a specific mechanism for terminating an arrhythmia has been elucidated by electrophysiologic testing, however, it frequently is possible to predict the response of a similar arrhythmia to therapy. A number of new antiarrhythmic drugs have been developed and are extremely useful in critically ill patients.

While many mechanisms may underlie drug action, the effects on increased automaticity or reentry serve as models. If increased automaticity is due to a decrease in threshold or increased rates of diastolic depolarization, agents which increase threshold or decrease diastolic depolarization are useful. The situation is a little more complicated with arrhythmias due to reentry. Decreased conduction allows a normally propogated impulse to return to an area that is not refractory because of unilateral block. Either decreased conduction or decreased duration of refractoriness favor the development of reentrant arrhythmias. Most drugs in use *decrease* conduction rates and *increase* refractoriness so that it is the *relationship* or *ratio* between the change in each that determines therapeutic efficacy. An agent that slows conduction and action potential duration without adequate prolongation of the refractory period may promote reentry. Such a perverse effect of a presumed antiarrhythmic agent can occur with any agent; "proarrhythmic effects" are seen in procaine amide in the treatment of ventricular arrhythmias, for example[126] (Table 5–6).

Antiarrhythmics act at a variety of intracellular regulatory steps, and it would be useful if specific pathophysiologic abnormalities could be treated by specific agents. An earlier electrophysiologic classification emphasized effects on automaticity, conduction, and the refractory periods. Group I included procaine amide and quinidine. These drugs decreased automaticity and conduction, but increased the duration of the refractory period. Group II drugs, exemplified by lidocaine, decreased automaticity and refractoriness, but either increased or had no change on conduction. Propranolol decreased automaticity, conduction, and refractoriness. A classification based on locus of action has been proposed by Vaughn Williams.[115] In this classification, Group I agents are sodium channel blockers and include both Groups I and II of the earlier classification. Group II agents are beta blockers, Group III agents are molecules such as amiodarone and bretylium that prolong the action potential duration, and Group IV are calcium channel blockers that decrease the slow inward calcium dependent current. Table 5–6 shows *in vitro* electrophysiologic effects of some of these agents. The effects may be far different *in vivo* because of modifying environmental influences. They do demonstrate, however, the different actions of different types of antiarrhythmic drugs. If a member of one group is unsuccessful, it would be unlikely for another molecule from the same group to have a beneficial effect.

Dramatic effects on conduction are not uncommon with quinidine and make it less useful in critically ill patients than other Type I agents. Prolonged QRS and Q-T duration as well as SA or AV nodal

TABLE 5–6.
In-vitro Electrophysiologic Effects of Anti-Arrhythmic Drugs

DRUG ACTION	DURATION AP	CONDUCTION VELOCITY	REFRACTORY PERIOD	VENT FIB THRESHOLD	EXCITABILITY THRESHOLD
Na Channel Blocker					
Quinidine	↑	↓	↑	↑	↑
Procainamide	↑	↓	↑	↑	↑
Lidocaine	↓	0 ↓	↑	↑	0 ↑
Beta Blocker					
Propranolol	0 ↓	0	↓	0 ↑	0
Prolongs Action Potential					
Amiodarone	↑	↓	↑		
Bretylium	↑	0	↑	↑	0
Calcium Channel Blocker					
Verapamil	↓	0	0	0	0

conduction delay may occur. An unusual arrhythmia with the memorable name *torsade de pointes* (from the French, meaning literally a twisted fringe of points) demonstrates the proarrhythmic action of agents that produce excessive decrease in conduction rates. A prolonged Q-T interval sets the stage for the abnormal rhythm. Widened QRS complexes at a rate of 200–250/min of changing amplitude (polymorphic) seem to twist around the isoelectric line in an undulating manner. The use of quinidine, procaine amide or other Class I agents obviously make the arrhythmia worse; increasing heart rate with either ventricular pacing or isoproterenol suppresses the arrhythmia. While isoproterenol is effective, its use must be limited to short periods prior to electrical management because of increases in myocardial oxygen requirements. Other causes of *torsade de pointes* are hypokalemia, hypomagnesemia, bradycardia, and phenothiazine administration.

The use of specific antiarrhythmic drugs is discussed below. The electrophysiologic classification system described above forms an effective conceptual network, even though it is not necessarily useful in the care of individual patients.

Quinidine

Quinidine produces six major pharmacologic effects: (1) altered impulse formation, (2) depression of atrioventricular and intraventricular conduction, (3) increase in refractory period of the heart, (4) depression of myocardial contractility, (5) peripheral vasodilatation, and (6) vagal blockade.

Metabolic studies indicate that quinidine blocks both alpha- and beta-adrenergic receptors, perhaps by direct inhibition of an ATP system believed necessary for adrenergic response. Alpha blockade accounts for peripheral vasodilatation, while beta blockade antagonizes the myocardial effects of catecholamines and decreases contractility. This effect on energy systems presumably explains the action of quinidine on cardiac cell membrane and its efficacy as an antiarrhythmic drug. Quinidine slows the influx of sodium and calcium into, and the efflux of potassium out of, the myocardial cell, inhibiting or slowing diastolic depolarization in automatic cells and prolonging the action potential. High doses of quinidine maintain cellular polarization and resting potential, blocking the production of an action potential.[127]

The goal of therapy is to add enough quinidine to slow diastolic depolarization and thereby prevent ectopic automaticity without depressing myocardial contractility and blocking action potential production. Unfortunately, myocardial hypoxia, acidosis, and electrolyte imbalance alter the passage of sodium and potassium across cellular membranes. A therapeutic dose of quinidine in such a situation might markedly depress myocardial contractility without affecting the abnormal rhythm that served as an indication for its administration.

Quinidine may be used to convert supraventricular tachycardias to sinus rhythm, to prevent their recurrence, or to suppress lower ectopic foci. While electric conversion is generally preferable to that with quinidine, certain situations may favor conversion with quinidine and, therefore, one should be familiar with all aspects of quinidine therapy. In attempting conversion, quinidine may be given by mouth in 200–400 mg doses every four hours until success or symptoms or signs of toxicity occur. An alternative method is to administer the drug in five divided doses two hours apart on successive days, increasing the divided dose by 200 mg each day if the arrhythmia persists. It is not advisable to use a total daily dose greater than 3.0 g unless serum quinidine levels are available, since gastrointestinal absorption of the drug is unpredictable. Other considerations modifying effectiveness of a given dose include state of hepatic (detoxified in liver) and renal (excreted by kidney) function.

Furthermore, in critically ill patients serum levels bear little relationship to physiologic effects because of an altered response to quinidine by an abnormal myocardium. In these patients relatively small doses may cause fatal arrhythmias. Serum levels between 4 and 23 mg/liter have been reported necessary for conversion from chronic atrial fibrillation to sinus rhythm, and a level between 4 and 7 mg/liter is usually adequate to maintain sinus rhythm after conversion. On the other hand, some individuals may be very difficult to maintain in sinus rhythm regardless of blood level.

Nausea, vomiting, diarrhea, and tinnitus are manifestations of toxicity. Electrocardiographic toxicity includes widening of the QRS complex by more than 50%, complete AV block, and ventricular tachyarrhythmia. Another danger is a sudden increase in ventricular response to atrial flutter due to a change in atrioventricular conduction, usually associated with slowing of the atrial rate. This may be avoided by digitalization prior to conversion, and this is particularly advisable in cases with borderline or overt heart failure. Myocardial toxicity is rarely seen at serum levels less than 6 mg/liter. True hypersensitivity manifested by fever, purpura, skin rash, or marked hypotension is rare and can be identified by an initial small test dose of 0.2 g.

It is sometimes difficult to distinguish between quinidine and digitalis induced electrophysiologic abnormalities when both drugs are used together. Indeed sudden cardiovascular death has been reported with their combined use. Quinidine decreases the renal and nonrenal elimination of digoxin and a two-fold increase in digoxin blood levels may be observed when quinidine is given to a digitalized patient.

Procaine Amide

Procaine amide has electrophysiologic effects similar to those of quinidine and is generally used interchangeably[128] with it. It appears to exert less of a depressant effect on the myocardium than does quinidine. Early studies suggested it was particularly useful in ventricular arrhythmias, although it is also effective in atrial arrhythmias. It may be given orally or intramuscularly in doses of 250–500 mg. It may also be administered intravenously to convert or prevent ventricular arrhythmias. Hypotension can be avoided by never giving the drug at an intravenous rate greater than 25 mg/minute.

Lidocaine

This potent Group II local anesthetic is a sodium channel blocker and has been used widely in the treatment of ventricular arrhythmias associated with acute myocardial infarction, digitalis intoxication, and cardiac surgery.[129] It depresses automaticity in Purkinje fibers but not in the sinus node, and does not affect conduction rates under normal conditions. Its action changes in the presence of acidosis or hyperkalemia; the rate of rise of the action potential and the rate of conduction are decreased. These properties probably explain its efficacy in acute myocardial infarction. Decreased conduction rates are harmful if they result in unidirectional block, but helpful if they render an irritable segment of myocardium essentially inert by producing bidirection block.[130] Slow calcium channels are not affected by lidocaine.

It is the first drug of choice of ventricular arrhythmias associated with acute myocardial ischemia. It has a distribution half-life of 8–10 minutes so that a continuous infusion of 2 mg/min can be started at the time of initial intravenous boluses (slow injection of 1.5 mg/kg followed by 1 mg/kg in 10–15 minutes).[131] If arrhythmias persist, an additional bolus of 25–50 mg with an infusion rate of 3–4 mg/min may be indicated. Lidocaine is metabolized in the liver and administered doses should be reduced by at least one-third in patients with low cardiac output or liver dysfunction. Toxicity is usually evidenced by changes in mental status, seizures, or respiratory depression.

Verapamil

Verapamil is a calcium channel blocker that blocks the slow inward current and exhibits electrophysiologic effects quite different from other antiarrhythmic agents. It is the preferred agent for the treatment of supraventricular tachycardias, and has terminated more than 80% of paroxysmal arrhythmias of this type in several series.[132] It slows the ventricular rate in both atrial fibrillation and flutter, but does not terminate the arrhythmia.

Both electrophysiologic and hemodynamic actions are probably responsible for its antiarrhythmic activity. It prolongs the conduction time and refractory period of the AV node, but does not appear to affect these properties in other cardiac tissues. It produces coronary and systemic vasodilatation, which may improve ventricular function, although its effect on calcium channels usually leads to decreased contractility. It is hazardous to administer verapamil and beta blockers simultaneously in patients with reduced ventricular function, although rapid termination of an atrial arrhythmia may improve ventricular function.

The usual dose is 0.15 mg/kg intravenously over 1–2 minutes followed by an infusion of 0.005 mg/kg/min if necessary. Hypotension and decreased ventricular function are the major adverse effects.

Propranolol

The versatile beta blocker propranolol is an important antiarrhythmic drug in many circumstances.[133] Other beta blocking agents may also be used but most of the available information is based on studies performed with propranolol. Cardioselective beta-1 blockers may reduce certain side effects, and changes in pharmacokinetics may allow more precise dosing, but the greatest possibility for innovation may lie in blocking agents that possess some intrinsic sympathetic agonist activity. Patients with serious illness frequently exhibit sympathetic hyperactivity that may be harmful. Profound beta blockade eliminates a major part of beta agonist activity. A modest amount of sympathetic tone is probably desirable in most clinical situations so that agents which block excessive activity, while providing some controllable sympathetic tone, may be useful.

Beta blockade reduces heart rate and myocardial contractility. The consequent decrease in myocardial oxygen requirements frequently attenuates acute ischemia and reverses a variety of arrhythmias associated with ischemia. Sudden withdrawal of beta blockade aggravates ischemic symptoms including arrhythmias and testifies to the importance of that treatment in patients with myocardial ischemia.

Beta blockade is particularly useful for arrhythmias developing in patients with increased sympathetic neural activity. Conversely, beta blockade is not indicated when excessive vagal activity, sometimes seen in inferior wall myocardial infarction, for example, is present. Negative inotropy and sinus bradycardia are associated with vagal stimulation. Since beta blockade decreases the effect of sympathetic stimulation to increase the rate of diastolic depolarization, it slows automaticity in the SA node and Purkinje fibers. Propranolol does not produce a membrane-stabilizing "quinidine-like" effect at usually therapeutic doses. It is quite useful in the treatment of supraventricular tachyarrhythmias due either to increased automaticity or reentrant mechanisms. Propranolol is also useful in situations such as thyrotoxicosis, phenochromocytoma, and anesthesia with halothan or cyclopropane, where sympathetic hyperactivity is present. Many digitalis-related arrhythmias also respond to beta blockade.

Propranolol should be given in a bolus dose of 0.1–0.15 mg/kg. Since dose responses vary widely depending upon patient circumstances, no more than 1 mg/minute should be administered.

Bretylium Tosylate

Bretylium blocks the release of norepinephrine from sympathetic nerve terminals after first causing its release and producing a transient hypersympathetic state. Its effective antifibrillatory activity probably derives from prolongation of the ventricular refractory period and its increase of the fibrillation threshold.[134] It should be used for the treatment of recurrent ventricular arrhythmias when adequate doses of lidocaine or procaine amide have been unsuccessful. The usual initial dose is 5–10 mg/kg given over 10–20 minutes. The full effect may not be realized for 30 minutes to 2 hours, so additional doses of 5 mg/kg (not exceeding 30 mg/kg) should be delayed for 1–2 hours.[135] Bretylium does not affect myocardial contractility, but produces hypotension by blocking the baroreceptor reflex.

Diphenylhydantoin

The analeptic agent was suggested for the treatment of ventricular arrhythmias unresponsive to other medication before the development of many of the newer antiarrhythmic agents.[136] It is useful in the treatment of digitalis-induced arrhythmias, and some authorities have gone so far as to suggest that a response to the agent suggests digitalis toxicity. It appears to act centrally to decrease sympathetic neural activity. Direct administration centrally prevents the development of digitalis-induced ventricular arrhythmias.[137]

The agent is similar to quinidine in many respects, but several differences are striking. Diphenylhydantoin increases atrioventricular and His-Purkinje conduction. Quinidine increases while diphenylhydantoin lowers the threshold for stimulation. Diphenylhydantoin has less effect on automaticity than quinidine. Electrocardiographically, the agent does not prolong the QRS complex (as does quinidine) and shortens the QT interval.

Many reports have demonstrated that diphenylhydantoin is most effective in the treatment of digitalis-induced arrhythmias. Bellet suggested that almost two-thirds of digitalis-induced ventricular arrhythmias responded favorably, while only 40% of nondigitalis-related ventricular arrhythmias showed a favorable response.[138] Mercer and Osborne[139] had the best results when diphenylhydantoin was used for arrhythmias of short duration occurring during the induction of cardiac anesthesia, cardiac catheterization, cardiac surgery, and following cardiac conversion. These observations suggest that it may be an ideal drug to use in the treatment of acute ventricular arrhythmias in the critically ill patient. Like lidocaine, the agent has little effect on supraventricular arrhythmias.

The major obstacle to the use of digitalis in the critically ill patient has been the risk of serious ventricular arrhythmias. One approach to this problem might be the combination of digitalis with diphenylhydantoin in an attempt to take advantage of the inotropic properties of digitalis without risking its common electrophysiologic side effects.

Diphenylhydantoin may be given as a single intravenous bolus. It is convenient to administer 100 mg every 5 minutes until the desired effect is achieved or until a total of 1,000 mg has been given. The drug can also be administered orally, 100–200 mg several times daily to a total of 300–800 mg.

A number of extracardiac side effects have been reported. These include cerebellar signs, coma, megaloblastic anemia, lymphoma-like syndrome, giant urticaria, depression, arthralgia, gingival hypertrophy, and transient eosinophilia. Most of these are reversible following cessation of the drug.

Amiodarone

Amiodarone might be considered as a relatively toxic but broad spectrum antiarrhythmic agent. Although in use for more than 20 years elsewhere, it was released for oral use in 1986 and, at this writing, has not yet been released for intravenous use. The agent prolongs action potential duration and refractoriness in atrial, ventricular, and Purkinje fiber tissue. It depresses sinus node automaticity and prolongs the PR, QRS and Q-T intervals. It has been effective in more than 50% of patients with recurrent life-threatening ventricular arrhythmias where other agents had failed.[140] Leak[141] recently described the successful use of Amiodarone in 10 of 11 critically ill patients with recurrent ventricular fibrillation, ventricular tachycardia, or supraventricular tachycardia. The side effects of hypotension, ventricular failure, and bradycardia were not observed.

Unusual pharmacokinetics have suggested that the effects on cardiac electrical activity may relate to interference with the cellular effects of thyroid hormone. Plasma concentrations peak after several hours, but therapeutic effects may take 2 to 21 days to develop. Adverse effects include hypotension, negative inotropy, and AV blockade. *Torsade de pointes* has also been observed. General release has been delayed by a 2–7% prevalence of pulmonary fibrosis with a mortality rate of 10%. These effects were reversed, however, when the drug was discontinued.

Leak[141] administered 150 mg intravenously over five minutes using an infusion pump, and administered an additional 150 mg 15 minutes later if the arrhythmias were not controlled. The initial dose was then followed by 25 mg/hour for three to four days; at that time oral administration was begun.

Digitalis

Digitalis was introduced by Withering in 1785[142] and remains an important agent for the treatment of left ventricular failure. The sodium-potassium ATPase pump describes above is probably the membrane receptor for its action. Digitalis increases Na-K ATPase activity, allowing sodium to accumulate within the cell. By some related mechanism, calcium influx is transiently increased and produces a positive inotropic effect. Since sodium and potassium gradients maintain the transmembrane resting potential, changes in that potential might be expected with shifts in intracellular sodium concentration. The parallel effects of digitalis on calcium release and membrane potential explain why inotropy and arrhythmias may go hand in hand; the therapeutic ratio is low, and potentially lethal adverse effects are not uncommon. Digitalis slows the ventricular response in atrial fibrillation because it increases the refractory period and decreases the conduction velocity of AV nodal tissue and Purkinje fibers. A prolonged P-R interval with normal sinus rhythm reflects these effects. Dose-dependent changes in Purkinje fibers may be responsible for the production of ventricular arrhythmias. Purkinje fiber function is unchanged at lower doses of digitalis that produce positive inotropy. Increasing concentrations of digitalis, however, lead to reduction in resting potential and increased rate of diastolic depolarization (increased automaticity).

Digitalis is useful in the treatment of supraventricular tachyarrhythmias. It may prevent the recurrence of such arrhythmias after initial termination with verapamil. Since it may not decrease conduction through aberrant pathways in the Wolff-Parkinson-White Syndrome, it should probably not be used alone in this situation.

Digitalis is an effective inotrope when there is evidence of ventricular dysfunction, and many of its beneficial effects on cardiac rhythm may be due to improved hemodynamic status. Sinus tachycardia, for example, may improve when digitalis improves stroke output and decreases sympathetic hyperactivity. The inotropic effect is dose related, contrary to earlier views; maximum inotropy is probably associated with serum concentrations of 1.5–2.0 ng/ml.[143] Digitalis appears much more useful in ambulatory settings than in the critically ill. Verapamil is as useful as digitalis in treating atrial arrhythmias, and dobutamine is a more effective inotrope. The elimination half-life of verapamil is 3–8 hours and that of dobutamine is measured in minutes, while that of digoxin is 36–40 hours in patients with normal renal function. Much greater flexibility in the face of rapidly changing patient status is obviously possible using the two more specific agents instead of digitalis.

Digoxin should be administered in an initial intravenous dose of 0.5–1.0 mg over 5 minutes. Additional increments of 0.25 mg may be given every 2 hours to a maximum of 1.5 mg.

Electrical Termination of Cardiac Arrhythmias

A completely new mode of therapy was introduced when Bernard Lown[144] demonstrated the efficiency of direct current in terminating a variety of arrhythmias. Kouwenhoven, Jude, and Knickerbocker[145] previously had demonstrated that alternating current applied to the thorax could effectively defibrillate the heart. Experimental work led him to discard direct current and design an instrument which administered a 5 amp AC current at a voltage of either 220 or 440 volts for one-quarter of a second. The instrument was extremely effective in reversing ventricular fibrillation, but was not useful for the control of other arrhythmias because it frequently produced ventricular fibrillation and also damaged myocardial tissue. Lown developed a DC circuit with a capacitor discharge that lasted for 2.5 msec compared to the 250 msec of the Kouwenhoven AC unit. When delivered near the end of slow repolarization (just before the peak of the T wave in the surface electrocardiogram), DC discharge frequently produced ventricular fibrillation; when synchronized to the downstroke of the QRS complex, it "converted" a high percentage of arrhythmias without producing ventricular fibrillation.

When cardiac arrhythmias lead to hemodynamic deterioration, direct current cardioversion is frequently indicated. The synchronized shock depolarizes all excitable pathways, including a variety of reentrant circuits. For this reason, it is most useful in terminating arrhythmias due to reentry but is less useful in those due to increased automaticity. Depolarizing the reentry pathway deals with the mechanism causing the tachycardia, while an irritant focus may resume abnormal activity immediately after the direct current depolarization.

Cardiac conversion should be accomplished at the bedside using an agent such as diazepam, 2.5–5.0 mg up to 10 mg at 30 second intervals. Respiratory depression is possible, and individuals able to rapidly gain airway access should be at hand. Digoxin is usually not discontinued if toxicity has not been evident.[146] Paddles should be positioned over the right sternal border at the second interspace and the left fifth interspace in the anterior axillary line. The electrical energy needed for conversion may be as low as 10 joules in paroxysmal supraventricular tachycardias and 100 joules with atrial fibrillation. Given this range, it makes sense to begin with 25–50 joules and increase energy levels with successive shocks if the initial attempt is not successful.

Electrical Pacing

Pacing techniques can be used to raise heart rate in patients with bradycardia, prevent certain ventricular arrhythmias, and terminate both supraventricular and ventricular arrhythmias. Complete heart block with syncope was the original indication for transvenous pacemaking, and conduction disturbances will constitute the major reasons for its use. Varying degrees of heart block occur in acute myocardial infarction, acute myocarditis, severe electrolyte disturbances (especially hyperkalemia), digitalis toxicity, shock from any cause, hemodialysis, and other sudden illness. The ventricular rate in patients with complete atrioventricular block is usually slow when the pacemaker is located in the Purkinje system, or more nearly normal (40–60) if the pacemaker is in the His bundle. Heart block may be the only warning of cardiac arrest. For example, 30% of patients with acute myocardial infarction and bundle branch block develop complete heart block.[147] Since cardiac output and mean arterial pressure fall when the ventricular rate drops below 40, the primary aim of monitoring is to detect heart block quickly, to increase heart rate with electrical pacing, and to prevent asystole.

Since it is better to insert temporary transvenous pacemakers under favorable circumstances and not be forced into an invasive procedure in the midst of cardiac resuscitation, indications for early use become important. They are also somewhat controversial. Indications for pacemaker use in the critical care unit must be much more flexible than those for individuals with stable heart disease. The presence of acute ischemia warns of considerable instability and abnormalities of the conduction system that would not be life threatening in other situations and demand immediate attention. The precise nature of the conduction defect, the nature of the underlying problem, and the patient's status or likelihood of not surviving the acute illness must all be considered in deciding on the need for transvenous pacemaking. Conduction disturbances in anterolateral infarctions are of greater concern than those in inferior wall infarctions because of the proximity of the latter region to the conduction system. Patients with anterolateral infarction and impending shock might require a pacemaker in a situation where one would not even be considered in other situations. In general, the presence of a Mobitz type II 2nd degree AV block, a new left or right bundle branch block, alternating bundle branch block, or bifascicular block should lead to the strong consideration of temporary pacemaking.

Ventricular pacing at rates faster than the arrhythmic rate may terminate ventricular arrhythmias.[148] Rates of 90–120 beats per minute may be necessary. The ventricular arrhythmia tends to reduce coronary blood flow while increasing heart rate increases myocardial oxygen consumption, so careful observation during the period of pacing is essential. Rapid atrial pacing may terminate atrial flutter and AV reciprocating tachycardia.[151]

Cardiopulmonary Resuscitation

The twin techniques of direct current defibrillation and closed chest massage have revolutionized the treatment of sudden cardiac collapse and have salvaged many electrical disasters that could have led to sudden death.

William Grace, a pioneer in the development of coronary care units, described the importance of the treatment of cardiac arrest in the first edition of this book:

> Sudden death is a common occurrence in patients hospitalized with acute myocardial infarction, primary myocardial disease, pulmonary infarction, and other cardiorespiratory illnesses. Sudden cessation of effective heart beat and cardiac output may be due to either failure of impulse formation (cardiac standstill) or ineffective impulse formation (ventricular fibrillation).
>
> Experience has demonstrated that about three-fourths of the episodes of cardiac arrest in patients with myocardial infarction are due to ventricular fibrillation; approximately one-third of these patients may be resuscitated. The remaining fourth of the patients have cardiac arrest on the basis of cardiac standstill; none of these patients has been resuscitated at our hospital. This experience, together with the relative safety of electrical defibrillation, leads us to recommend that *cardiac arrest in myocardial infarction should be treated with immediate defibrillation before recording of the electrocardiogram.*
>
> The 3-minute "grace" period before the appearance of irreversible cerebral change applies to patients with normal circulatory systems. Considerably less time is available in patients with preexisting cardiorespiratory disease. For this reason, nurses as well as house staff in an intensive care unit should be thoroughly trained in the techniques of electrical defibrillation and closed chest massage.

He developed one of the first training programs for nurses using a single animal who lived for many years instead of the plastic models preferred today.

> ### A Note on Teaching of Cardiac Resuscitation
>
> Because of the urgency of therapy for cardiac arrest, it is imperative that all individuals working with the patients in an intensive care or coronary care unit be expert in the techniques of resuscitation, whether they are interns, residents, attending physicians, or nurses. It is frequently stated that the patient may survive cardiac arrest for as long as 3–4 minutes without circulation. Although this may be applicable to 18 year olds who have drowned, it is certainly not true for those who are in the atherosclerotic disease age group and who have had an acute coronary thrombosis. It is likely that such patients have less than 60 seconds without circulation before the situation becomes irreversible. Therefore, almost no harm can be done by anyone who attempts to restore the circulation in a patient with cardiac arrest.
>
> We personally instruct each of the nurses who works in the coronary care unit and in the intensive care unit in the technique of closed chest cardiac massage and supervise them during the actual attempt at resuscitation. The technique of electrical defibrillation is taught to the nurses, employing dogs in the animal experimental laboratory. These classes are held every week for approximately one and a half hours; every nurse who work on this service is taught to handle the electrical defibrillation equipment. She must handle this equipment over and over again until she is capable of doing this alone. We then inform the staff that the nurse on duty may carry out electrical defibrillation of the heart within 30 seconds of the detection of this event, if no doctor is present.

> It is a pleasant experience to see how quickly and efficiently the nurses can do this. It is likely that nursing personnel can learn to handle the equipment better than the physicians, since they participate in all of the cardiac resuscitations, whereas any one physician participates in only a few cases.

The success of in-hospital resuscitation led to its extension to out-of-hospital cardiac arrest. Pantridge and Geddes in Belfast,[150] introduced the concept of the "mobile coronary care unit" staffed by professionals in 1967 and Cobb et al advanced the concept further by training nonhealth professional "citizens" in the treatment of cardiac arrest.[151] More than 400 patients with ventricular fibrillation were resuscitated in an out-of-hospital setting; "citizens" played key roles in about one-third of resuscitations. William Grace had been diplomatically cautious in suggesting the "grace period" and suggesting that nurses might defibrillate patients after making certain physicians were not available. Cobb took it a giant step farther. Guidelines for cardiopulmonary resuscitation, building on the efforts of many, were first published in 1974. The guidelines were last updated in July of 1985.[152] In this latest revision, four quick breaths have been changed to two 1.5-second breaths and chest compressions increased from 60–80 per minute to 80-100. The use of agents such as intravenous nitroglycerine, amrinone, and verapamil are discussed in some detail; routine bicarbonate use is discouraged. The force of national committees and the printed word has sometimes led physicians to confuse "guidelines" with "rules." Rules may be necessary in the first few minutes of resuscitation, but must be quickly supplemented by careful clinical judgment.

Weisfeldt and Halperin[153] have recently reviewed their evidence that the major effect of closed chest massage is to rhythmically raise intrathoracic pressure, which in turn produces carotid blood flow. While it has generally been accepted that compression of the heart between sternum and vertebral column produces cardiac pumping action, these investigators have shown that increases in arterial pressure are correlated with increases in intrathoracic pressure. Intrathoracic pressure is transmitted directly to the carotid arteries, but not to the jugular veins because of venous valves at the thoracic inlet. Were these valves to be incompetent, intrathoracic pressure would also be transmitted to the jugular venous system and the arterial-venous gradient would be unchanged. In contrast, there is little blood flow to kidneys, liver, and intestines because the abdominal lack valves. Bowel ischemia with perforation following successful resuscitation emphasizes the lack of splanchnic perfusion during closed chest massage. Increased carotid arterial resistance prevents vascular collapse at the thoracic inlet and allows transmission to the extrathoracic carotid artery. The demonstrated value of norepinephrine infusion in cardiopulmonary resuscitation may be to further maintain the rigidity of the vessels leaving the thorax. Weisfeldt and Halperin[153] contend that the dependence of blood flow on the duration of compression rather than the rate of compression demonstrates the importance of increasing intrathoracic pressure. The fact that a rate of 80–90 compressions per minute brings the compression duration to 50% of the total cycle is the reason an increased compression rate is recommended in the recent guidelines.

Criley, Blaufuss, and Kissel[154] have shown that continuous coughing, a maneuver that also rhythmically increases intrathoracic pressure, maintains consciousness during developing cardiac arrest. This supports the possibility that the lungs could be used as a pressure generator to maintain blood flow.

Immediate restoration of sinus rhythm must be the immediate goal of cardiopulmonary resuscitation. Closed chest massage at best can only partially restore the peripheral circulation, and its effect on coronary blood flow and myocardial metabolism is not well understood. The patient should be immediately shocked with 200 joules followed by 400 joules if the first shock is not successful. If sinus rhythm is not restored, a bolus of lidocaine followed by 400 joules is indicated. If ventricular fibrillation persists or is recurrent, intravenous bretylium is indicated. A rapid search for correctible metabolic abnormalities should also be undertaken.

Arrhythmias in the Critical Ill: Synopsis and Synthesis

A paroxysmal arrhythmia in a patient with severe cardiorespiratory-renal disease may spell the difference between survival or death. Therapy must be immediate, and generally involves the use of intravenous agents, electrical countershock, or both.

Hypoxia, acidosis, electrolyte abnormalities, and perfusion deficits must be quickly corrected. Intubation and controlled ventilation may be necessary to reduce pulmonary congestion and improve alveolar gas exchange. Regional perfusion should be maintained with an agent like dobutamine; coronary perfusion pressure should be maintained at reasonably normal levels in patients with coronary artery disease by the use of norepinephrine or balloon counterpulsation.

Perhaps the most difficult decision facing the physician is the choice of initial specific therapy. An early choice between pharmacologic agent or countershock is essential, since the former may complicate the subsequent use of countershock. Pharmacologic agents may be administered rapidly and desired effects maintained by continuous infusion pumps. Unfortunately, some of these agents may depress myocardial contractility or produce electrical abnormalities.

Electrical countershock is indicated when an arrhythmia has produced circulatory collapse since it may be lifesaving. Countershock liberates catecholamines from the myocardium, however, and postshock arrhythmias may occur. Since the amount of catecholamines released is related to the energy delivered to the myocardium, the intensity of the countershock stimulus should be kept as low as possible. Even the low doses of sedation generally used with countershock may produce hypoventilation with hypoxemia and hypercapnia.

Supraventricular tachyarrhythmias should be initially treated with intravenous verapamil followed by countershock if necessary. An early decision whether to control or convert atrial flutter or fibrillation must be made. If poor ventricular function is evidenced, electrical conversion to gain the advantage of atrial systole is usually indicated. Preventing recurrent fibrillation or flutter is often difficult, but Zipes[125] has had success with low doses (200 mg/day or on alternate days) of amiodarone. Quinidine is the more traditional approach to preventing recurrent atrial fibrillation, but its effects on contractility make it less useful.

Ventricular arrhythmias present a special situation. Islands of ventricular muscle are presumably arrhythogenic, and Zipes has suggested that antiarrhythmic drugs complete the agonal process by "making 'sick cells sicker' and in some way uncoupling them electrically from the rest of the ventricle".[125]

Precise diagnosis of tachyarrhythmias with wide QRS complexes is vital. Accelerated idioventricular rhythm is usually within 10 beats of the sinus rate, and is probably due to two competing pacemakers. Treatment is frequently unnecessary, and may respond to measures that increase the sinus rate, such as atropine. Ventricular tachycardia may be treated pharmacologically if hemodynamic deterioration is present. Lidocaine should be tried first, followed by either procaine amide or bretylium if unsuccessful. Direct current countershock is indicated if pharmacologic approaches are ineffective. Countershock should be administered immediately if hemodynamic deterioration develops. Recurrent ventricular arrhythmias resistant to pharmacologic and electrical intervention should be treated with intravenous amiodarone.

REFERENCES

1. Harrison TR: *Failure of the Circulation*, ed 2, Baltimore, Williams & Wilkins Co, 1939.

2. Wiggers CJ: *Physiology of Shock*. New York, The Commonwealth Fund, 1950.

3. Dodge HT, Sandler H, Baxley WA, et al: Usefulness and limitations of radiographic methods for determining left ventricular volume. *Am J Cardiol* 1966; 18:10.

4. Meerson FZ: The myocardium in hyperfunction, hypertrophy, and heart failure. AHA Monograph No. 26. New York, American Heart Association.

5. Lang RM, Borow DM, Newmann A, et al: Systemic vascular resistance: an unreliable index of left ventricular afterload. *Circulation* 1986; 74:1114.

6. Braunwald E: *Heart Disease*, ed 2, Philadelphia, WB Saunders, 1984.

7. Mirsky I, Pasternac A, Ellison R: General index for the assessment of cardiac function. *Am J Cardiol* 1972; 30:483.

8. Nixon JV, Murray RG, Leonard PD, et al: Effect of large variations in preload on left ventricular performance characteristics in normal subjects. *Circulation* 1982; 62:698.

9. Sonnenblick EH, Parmley WW, Urschel CW: The contractile state of the heart as expressed by force-velocity relations. *Am J Cardiol* 1969; 23:488.

10. Suga H, Sagawa K: Instantaneous pressure-volume relationships and their ratio in the excised, supported canine left ventricle. *Circ Res* 1974; 35:117.

11. Grossman W, Braunwald F, Mann T, et al: Contractile state of the left ventricle in man as evaluated from end-systolic pressure-volume relations. *Circulation* 1977; 56:845.

12. Mehmel HC, Stockins B, Ruffman K, et al: The linearity of the end-systolic pressure-volume relationship in man and its sensitivity for assessment of left ventricular function. *Circulation* 1981; 63:1216.

13. Sodums MT, Badke FR, Starling MR, et al: Evaluation of left ventricular contractile performance utilizing end-systolic pressure-volume relationships in conscious dogs. *Circ Res* 1984; 54:731.

14. Zimmerman BG: Actions of angiotensin on adrenergic nerve endings. *Fed Proc* 1978; 37:199.

15. Malik KU: Prostaglandins—modulation of adrenergic nervous system. *Fed Proc* 1978; 37:203.

16. Davis R, Ribner HS, Keung E, et al: Treatment of chronic congestive heart failure with captopril, an oral inhibitor of angiotensin-converting enzyme. *N Engl J Med* 1979; 301:117.

17. Posner J, Plum F: Spinal fluid pH and neurological symptoms in systemic acidosis. *N Engl J Med* 1967; 277:605–13.

18. Spiekerman RE, Brandenburg JT, Achor RWP, et al: The spectrum of coronary heart disease in a community of 30,000. A clinicopathologic study. *Circulation* 1962; 25:57–65.

19. DeWood MA, Spores J, Notske MD, et al: Prevalence of oral coronary occlusion during the early hours of transmural myocardial infarction. *N Engl J Med* 1980; 303:897–902.

20. Falk E: Unstable angina with fatal outcome: dynamic coronary thrombosis leading to infarction and/or sudden death: autopsy evidence of recurrent mural thrombosis with peripheral embolization culminating in total vascular occlusion. *Circulation* 1985; 71:699–708.

21. Fitzgerald DJ, Roy L, Catella F, et al: Platelet activation in unstable coronary

disease. *N Engl J Med* 1986; 315:983.

22. Sobel BE: Coronary thrombolysis with tissue-type plasminogen activator (t-PA): Emerging strategies. *J Am Coll Cardiol* 1986; 8:1220–1225.

23. Herman MV, Heinle RA, Klein MD, et al: Localized disorders in myocardial contraction. Asynergy and its role in congestive heart failure. *N Engl J Med* 1967; 277:222.

24. Parmley WW, Chatterjee K: Vasodilator therapy, in Harvey WP (ed): *Current Problems in Cardiology*, vol 2, no 12. Chicago, Year Book Medical Publishers, 1978, p 23.

25. Pozen RG, DiBianco R, Katz RJ, et al: Myocardial metabolic and hemodynamic effects of dobutamine in heart failure complicating coronary artery disease. *Circulation* 1981; 63(6):1279–1285.

26. Kazamias TM, Gander MP, Rose JR Jr: The prognostic significance of left ventricular size after acute myocardial infarction (AMI). *Am J Cardiol* 1970; 26:642.

27. Bulkley BH: Pathophysiology of coronary heart disease, in McIntosh HD (ed): *Baylor College of Medicine Cardiology Series*, vol 6. Princeton, NJ, Cardiology Series Inc, 1983.

28. Weber KT, Ratshin RA, Janicki JS, et al: Left ventricular dysfunction following acute myocardial infarction. A clinicopathologic and hemodynamic profile of shock and failure. *Am J Med* 1973; 54:697.

29. Scheidt S, Ascheim R, Killip T: Shock after acute myocardial infarction. *Am J Cardiol* 1970; 26:556.

30. Wackers FJ, Lie KI, Becker AE, et al: Coronary artery disease in patients dying from cardiogenic shock or congestive heart failure in the setting of acute myocardial infarction. *Br Heart J* 1976; 38:906.

31. Page DL, Caulfield JB, Kastor JA, et al: Myocardial changes associated with cardiogenic shock. *N Engl J Med* 1971; 285:133.

32. Mueller H, Ayres SM: Myocardial metabolism in shock following acute myocardial infarction, in Gunnar RM, Loeb HS, Rahimtoola SH (eds): *Shock in Myocardial Infarction*. New York, Grune & Stratton, 1974, p 173–207.

33. Ratshin RA, Rackley CE, Russell RO: Hemodynamic evaluation of left ventricular function in shock complicating myocardial infarction. *Circulation* 1972; 45:127.

34. Diamond G, Forrester JS: Effect of coronary artery disease and acute myocardial infarction on left ventricular compliance in man. *Circulation* 1972; 45:11.

35. Maroko PR, Kjekshus JK, Sobel BE, et al: Factors influencing infarct size following experimental coronary artery occlusion. *Circulation* 1971; 43:67.

36. Corday E, Williams JH, De Vera LB, et al: Effects of systemic blood pressure and vasopressor drugs on coronary blood flow and the electrocardiogram. *Am J Cardiol* 1959; 3:626.

37. Mosher P, Ross J, McFate A, et al: Control of coronary blood flow by an autoregulatory mechanism. *Circ Res* 1964; 14:250.

38. Mueller H, Ayres SM, Giannelli S Jr, et al: Effect of isoproterenol, l-norepinephrine and intra-aortic counterpulsation on hemodynamics and myocardial metabolism in shock following acute myocardial infarction. *Circulation* 1972; 45:335.

39. Mueller H, Ayres SM, Conklin EF, et al: The effects of intra-aortic counterpulsation on cardiac performance and metabolism in shock associated with acute myocardial infarction. *J Clin Invest* 1971; 50:1885.

40. Braunwald E: Topics in clinical medicine: The pathogenesis and treatment of shock in acute myocardial infarction. *Johns Hopkins Med J* 1967; 121:421.

41. Mueller H, Ayres SM, Gregory JJ, et al: Hemodynamics, coronary blood flow and myocardial metabolism in coronary shock: response to l-norepinephrine and isoproteronol. *J Clin Invest* 1970; 49:1885.

42. Mueller HS, Ayres SM, Giannelli S Jr, et al: Cardiac performance and metabolism in shock due to acute myocardial infarction in man: Response to catecholamines and mechanical cardiac assist. *Trans NY Acad Sci* 1972; 34:309–333.

43. Maroko PR, Kjekshus JK, Sobel BE, et al: Factors influencing infarct size follow-

ing experimental coronary artery occlusions. *Circulation* 1971; 43:67.

44. Mueller HS, Ayres SM, Religa A, et al: Propranolol in the treatment of acute myocardial infarction. Effect on myocardial oxygenation and hemodynamics. *Circulation* 1974; 49:1078–1087.

45. Reimer KA, Jennings RB: The "wavefront phenomenon" of myocardial ischemic cell death. II. Transmural progression of necrosis within the framework of ischemic bed size (myocardium at risk) and collateral flow. *Lab Invest* 1979; 40:633.

46. Gutovitz AL, Sobel BE, Roberts R: Progressive nature of myocardial injury in selected patients with cardiogenic shock. *Am J Cardiol* 1978;41:469.

47. Maseri A, L'Abbate A, Baroldi G, et al: Coronary vasospasms as a possible cause of myocardial infarction: A conclusion derived from the study of "preinfarction" angina. *N Engl J Med* 1978; 299:1271–1277.

48. Vetrovec GW, Leinbach RC, Gold HK, et al: Intracoronary thrombolysis in syndromes of unstable ischemia: angiographic and clinical results. *Am Heart J* 1982; 104:946–52.

49. Beta-blocker Heart Attack Trial Research Group: A randomized trial of propranolol in patients with acute myocardial infarction. *JAMA* 1982; 247:1707.

50. Rude RE, Muller JE, Braunwald E: Efforts to limit the size of myocardial infarcts. *Ann Intern Med* 1981; 95:736.

51. Wright IS, Marple CD, Beck DF: *Myocardial infarction: Its Clinical Manifestations and Treatment with Anticoagulants: A Study of 1,031 Cases.* New York, Grune & Stratton Inc, 1954.

52. Hilden T, Iversen K, Raaschou F, et al: Anticoagulants in acute myocardial infarction. *Lancet* 1961; 2:327.

53. Roberts WC: Coronary arteries in fatal acute myocardial infarction. *Circulation* 1972; 45:215.

54. Hood WB Jr: Salvage of myocardium in acute ischemia, editorial. *Circulation* 1971; 43:11.

55. Braunwald E: The aggressive treatment of acute myocardial infarction. *Circulation* 1985; 71:1087–1092.

56. Killip T, Kimball JT: Treatment of myocardial infarction in a coronary care unit. A two year experience with 250 patients. *Am J Cardiol* 1967; 20:457.

57. Forrester JS, Diamond G, Chatterjee K, et al: Medical therapy of acute myocardial infarction by application of hemodynamic subsets. *N Engl J Med* 1976; 295:1356, 1404.

58. Pantridge, JR, Geddes JS: Diseases of the cardiovascular system—Management of acute myocardial infarction. *Br Med J* 1976; 2:168.

59. Sobel BE, Braunwald E: The management of acute myocardial infarction, in Braunwald E (ed): *Heart Disease.* Philadelphia, WB Saunders Company, 1984.

60. Loeb HS, Pietras RJ, Tobin JR Jr, et al: Hypovolemia in shock due to acute myocardial infarction. *Circulation* 1969; 40:653.

61. Crexells C, Chatterjee K, Forrester JS, et al: Optimal level of filling pressure in the left side of the heart in acute myocardial infarction. *N Engl J Med* 1973; 289:1263.

62. Franciosa JA, Guiha NJ, Limas CJ, et al: Improved left ventricular function during nitroprusside infusion in acute myocardial infarction. *Lancet* 1972; 1:650.

63. Bodenheimer MM, Ramanathan K, Banka VS, et al: Effect of progressive pressure reduction with nitroprusside on acute myocardial infarction in humans: Determination of optimal afterload. *Ann Intern Med* 1981; 94:435.

64. Watanabe I, Covell JW, Maroko PR, et al: Effects of increased arterial pressure and positive inotropic agents on the severity of myocardial ischemia in the acutely depressed heart. *Am J Cardiol* 1972; 30:371–377.

65. Vatner SF, Baig H: Importance of heart rate in determining the effects of sympathomimetic amines on regional myocardial function and blood flow in conscious dogs with acute myocardial ischemia. *Circ Res* 1979; 45(6):793–803.

66. Maekawa K, Liang C, Hood WB: Comparison of dobutamine and dopamine in acute

myocardial infarction. Effects of systemic hemodynamics, plasma catecholamines, blood flows and infarct size. *Circulation* 1983; 67(4):750–759.

67. Gillespie TA, Ambos HD, Sobel BE, et al: Effects of dobutamine in patients with acute myocardial infarction. *Am J Cardiol* 1977; 39:588–594.

68. Goldstein RA, Passamani ER, Roberts R: A comparison of digoxin and dobutamine in patients with acute infarction and cardiac failure. *N Engl J Med* 1980; 303:846–850.

69. Francis GS, Sharma B, Hodges M: Comparative hemodynamic effects of dopamine and dobutamine in patients with acute cardiogenic circulatory collapse. *Am Heart J* 1982; 103:995–1000.

70. Richard C, Ricome JL, Rimailho A, et al: Combined hemodynamic effects of dopamine and dobutamine in cardiogenic shock. *Circulation* 1983; 67:620–626.

71. Collen D, Topol EJ, Tiefenbrunn AJ, et al: Coronary thrombolysis with recombinant human tissue-type plasminogen activator: A prospective, randomized, placebo-controlled trial. *Circulation* 1984; 70:1012–1017.

72. Collen D, Verstraete M: Systemic thrombolytic therapy of acute myocardial infarction. *Circulation* 1983; 68:462–465.

73. Pepine CJ, Prida X, Hill JA, et al: Percutaneous transluminal coronary angioplasty in acute myocardial infarction. *Am Heart J* 1984; 107:820.

74. O'Neill WO, Timmis GC, Bourdillon PD: A Prospective Randomized Clinical Study Of Intracoronary Streptokinase Versus Coronary Angioplasty For Acute Myocardial Infarction. *N Engl J Med* 1986; 314:812.

75. Braunwald E, and Koner RA: The stunned myocardium: Prolonged, postischemic ventricular dysfunction. *Circulation* 66:1146. 1982.

76. Kontos HA: Oxygen radicals in cerebral vascular injury. *Circ Res* 1985; 57:508.

77. Kantrowitz A, Tjonneland S, Krakauer JS, et al: Mechanical intra-aortic cardiac assistance in cardiogenic shock. Hemodynamic effects. *Arch Surg* 1968; 97:1000.

78. Mueller H, Ayres SM, Conklin EF, et al: The effects of intra-aortic counterpulsation on cardiac performance and metabolism in shock associated with acute myocardial infarction. *J Clin Invest* 1971; 50:1885.

79. Alcan KE, Stertzer SH, Wallsh E, et al: Current status of intra-aortic balloon counterpulsation in critical care cardiology. *Crit Care Med* 1984; 12:489.

80. Rutherford BD, Hartzler GO, McConahay DR, et al: Direct balloon angioplasty during acute myocardial infarction in patients with severely compromised hemodynamics. *Circulation* 1985;72 Supp III: 308.

81. O'Neill W, Erbel R, Laufer N et al: Coronary angioplasty therapy of cardiogenic shock complicating acute myocardial infarction. *Circulation* 1985; 72 Supp III: 309.

82. Cohn JN, Guiha NH, Broder MI, et al: Right ventricular infarction. Clinical and hemodynamic features. *Am J Cardiol* 1974; 33:209.

83. Jugdutt BI, Sussex BA, Sivaram CA, et al: Right ventricular infarction: Two-dimensional echocardiographic evaluation. *Am Heart J* 1984; 107:505.

84. Radford MJ, Johnson RA, Daggett WM, et al: Ventricular septal rupture: A review of clinical and physiologic features and an analysis of survival. *Circulation* 1981; 64:545.

85. Ryden L, Anniego R, Arnman K, et al: A double-blind trial of metoprolol in acute myocardial infarction. Effects on ventricular tachyarrhythmias. *N Engl J Med* 1983; 308:614.

86. Mueller HS, Evans RG, Ayres SM: Effect of dopamine on hemodynamics and myocardial metabolism and shock following acute myocardial infarction in man. *Circulation* 1978; 57 (II):361–356.

87. Parrillo JE, Burch C, Shelhamer JH, et al: A circulating myocardial substance in humans with septic shock. *J Clin Invest* 1985; 76:4:1539–1553.

88. Parker MM, Shelhamer JH, Bacharach SL, et al: Profound but reversible myocardial

depression in patients with septic shock. *Ann Intern Med* 1984; 100:483–490

89. Natanson C, Fink MP, Ballantyne HK, et al: Gram-negative bacteremia produces both severe systolic and diastolic cardiac dysfunction in a canine model that simulates human septic shock. *J Clin Invest* 1986; 78:259–270.

90. Cunnion RE, Schaer GL, Parker MM, et al: The coronary circulation in human septic shock. *Circulation* 1986; 73:4:637–644.

91. Mueller H: Unpublished observations.

92. Fuster V, Gersh BJ, Giuliani ER, et al: The natural history of idiopathic dilated cardiomyopathy. *Am J Cardiol* 1981; 47:525.

93. Akutsu T, Kolff WJ: Permanent substitutes for valves and hearts. *Trans Am Soc Artif Intern Organs* 1958; 4:230.

94. DeVries WC, Anderson JL, Joyce LD, et al: Clinical use of the total artificial heart. *N Engl J Med* 1984; 310:273–278.

95. Pennington DG, Swartz M, Codd JE, et al: Intra-aortic balloon pumping in cardiac surgical patients: A nine-year experience. *Ann Thorac Surg* 1983; 36:125–131.

96. Pennington DG, Merjavy JP, Codd JE, et al: Extracorporeal membrane oxygenation for patients with cardiogenic shock. *Circulation* 1984; 70:I130–I137.

97. Spencer FC, Eiseman NG, Trinkle JK, et al: Assisted circulation for cardiac failure following intracardiac surgery with cardiopulmonary bypass. *J Thorac Cardiovasc Surg* 1965; 49:56.

98. DeBakey ME: Left ventricular bypass for cardiac assistance: Clinical experience. *Am J Cardiol* 1971; 27:3.

99. Pennington DG, Merjavy JP, Swartz MT, et al: The importance of biventricular failure in patients with postoperative cardiogenic shock. *Ann Thorac Surg* 1985; 39:16–26.

100. Kaplan NM: *Clinical Hypertension*, ed 3. Baltimore, Williams & Wilkins, 1982.

101. Houston MC: Hypertensive urgencies and emergencies: Pathophysiology, clinical aspects and treatment, in Chernow B, Shoemaker WC (eds): *Critical Care—State of the Art.* Fullerton, CA, Society of Critical Care Medicine, 1986.

102. Wollner L, McCarthy ST, Soper NDW, et al: Failure of cerebral autoregulation as a cause of brain dysfunction in the elderly. *Br Med J* 1979; 1:1117–1118.

103. Thompson WL: Hypertensive crises in critical care, in Chernow B, Shoemaker WC (eds): *Critical Care—State of the Art.* Fullerton, CA, Society of Critical Care Medicine, 1985.

104. Lown B, Amarasingham R, Neuman J: New method for terminating cardiac arrhythmias: Use of synchronized capacitor discharge. *JAMA* 1962; 182:548.

105. Brown KWG, et al: Coronary unit: An intensive-care centre for acute myocardial infarction. *Lancet* 1963; 2:349.

106. Day HW: An intensive coronary care area. *Dis Chest* 1963; 44:423.

107. Meltzer LE, Kitchell JB: The incidence of arrhythmias associated with acute myocardial infarction. *Prog Cardiovas Dis* 1966; 9:50.

108. Grace WJ: The use of a coronary care unit for patients with acute myocardial infarction, in Bailey CP (ed): *Rheumatic and Coronary Heart Disease.* New York, JB Lippincott Co, 1967.

109. Hoffman BF, Cranefield PF: *Electrophysiology of the Heart.* New York, McGraw-Hill, 1960.

110. Weidmann S: Effects of calcium ions and local anesthetics on electrical properties of Purkinje fibers. *J Physiol* 1955; 129:568.

111. Hodgkin AL, Huxley AF: A quantitative description of membrane current and its application to conduction and excitation in nerve. *J Physiol* 1952; 117:500.

112. Singer DH, Lazzara R, Hoffman BF: Interrelationships between automaticity and conduction in Purkinje fibers. *Circ Res* 1967; 21:537.

113. Paes de Carvalho A: Excitation of the atrioventricular node during normal rhythm: Effects of acetylcholine, in Dreifus LS, Likoff W (eds): *Mechanisms and Therapy of Cardiac Arrhythmias. Fourteenth Hahnemann Symposium.* New York, Grune & Stratton, 1966, p 341.

114. Zipes DP: Genesis of cardiac arrhythmias: Electrophysiological considerations, in

Braunwald E (ed): *Heart Disease. A Textbook of CV Medicine*, vol 1. Philadelphia, WB Saunders, 1984.

115. Vaughn Williams EM: A classification of antiarrhythmic actions reassessed after a decade of new drugs. *J Clin Pharmacol* 1984; 24:129.

116. Hoffman BF, Cranefield PF: The physiological basis of cardiac arrhythmias. *Am J Med* 1964; 37:670.

117. Watanabe Y, Dreifus LS: Newer concepts in the genesis of cardiac arrhythmias. *Am Heart J* 1968; 76:114.

118. Watanabe Y, Dreifus LS: Inhomogeneous conduction of the A-V node: A model for re-entry. *Am Heart J* 1965; 70:505.

119. Sloan HE: The vagus nerve in cardiac arrest: The effect of hypercapnia, hypoxia and asphyxia on reflex inhibition of the heart. *Surg Gynecol Obstet* 1950; 91:257.

120. Chazan JA, Stenson R, Kurland GS: The acidosis of cardiac arrest. *N Engl J Med* 1968; 278:360.

121. Guzman SV, DeLeon AC Jr, West JW, et al: Cardiac effects of isoproterenol, norepinephrine, and epinephrine in complete A-V heart block during experimental acidosis and hyperkalemia. *Circ Res* 1959; 7:666.

122. Ayres SM, Grace WJ: Inappropriate ventilation and hypoxemia as causes of cardiac arrhythmias. *Am J Med* 1969; 46:495.

123. Katz LN, Feinberg H: The relation of cardiac effort to myocardial oxygen consumption and coronary flow. *Circ Res* 1958; 6:656.

124. Mitchell JH, Gilmore JP, Sarnoff J: The transport function of the atrium—Factors influencing the relation between left atrial pressure and left ventricular and diastolic pressure. *Am J Cardiol* 1962; 9:237.

125. Zipes DP: A consideration of antiarrhythmic therapy. *Circulation* 1985; 72:949–956.

126. Velebit V, Podrid PJ, Lown B, et al: Aggravation and provocation of ventricular arrhythmias by antiarrhythmic drugs. *Circulation* 1982; 65:886–894.

127. Conn HL Jr, Luchi RJ: Some cellular and metabolic considerations relating to the action of quinidine as a prototype antiarrhythmic agent. *Am J Med* 1964; 37:685.

128. Kayden JH, Brodie BB, Steele JM: Procaine amide: A review. *Circulation* 1957; 15:118.

129. Harrison DC, Sprouse JH, Morrow AG: The antiarrhythmic properties of lidocaine and procaine amide. *Circulation* 1963; 28:486.

130. Patterson E, Gibson JK, Lucchesi BR: Electrophysiologic actions of lidocaine in a canine model of chronic myocardial ischemic injury. Arrhythmogenic actions of lidocaine. *Circulation* 1981; 64(suppl IV):123.

131. Stargel WW, Shand DG, Routledge PA, et al: Clinical comparison of rapid infusion and multiple injection methods for lidocaine loading. *Am Heart J* 1981; 102:872–876.

132. Sung RJ, Elser B, and McAllister RG, Jr.: Intravenous verapamil for termination of reentrant supraventricular tachycardias. Intracardiac studies correlated with plasma verapamil concentrations. *Ann Intern Med* 93:682, 1980.

133. Nies AS, Shand DG: Clinical pharmacology of propranolol. *Circulation* 1974; 52:6.

134. Waxman MB, Wallace AG: Electrophysiological effects of bretylium tosylate on the heart. *J Pharmacol Exp Ther* 1972; 183:264–274.

135. Patterson E, Gibson JK, Lucchesi BR: Prevention of chronic canine ventricular tachyarrhythmias with bretylium tosylate. *Circulation* 1981; 64:1045.

136. Damato AN: Diphenylhydantoin: Pharmacological and clinical use. *Prog Cardiovasc Dis* 1969; 12:1.

137. Gillis RA, McClellan JR, Sauer TS, et al: Depression of cardiac sympathetic nerve activity by diphenylhydantoin. *J Pharmacol Exp Ther* 1971; 179:599.

138. Bellet S: *Clinical Disorders of the Heart Beat*, ed 3. Philadelphia, Lea & Febiger, 1971.

139. Mercer EN, Osborne JA: The current status of diphenylhydantoin in heart disease. *Ann Intern Med* 1967; 67:1084.

140. Marcus FT, Fontaine GH, Frank R, et al:

Clinical pharmacology and therapeutic applications of the antiarrhythmic agent, amiodarone. *Am Heart J* 1981; 101:480.

141. Leak D: Intravenous amiodarone in the treatment of refractory life-threatening cardiac arrhythmias in the critically ill patient. *Am Heart J* 1986; 111:456–462.

142. Withering W: An account of the Foxglove, and some of its medical uses with practical remarks on dropsy and other diseases. GGJ and J Robinson, London, 1785. Reprinted in *Cardiac Classics,* C. C. Mosby Co., St. Louis, 1941.

143. Smith TW: Medical treatment of advanced congestive heart failure: Digitalis and diuretics. In Braunwald E, Moch MB, and Watson JT (eds): *Congestive Heart Failure.* New York, Grune and Stratton, Inc., 1982, pp. 261–278.

144. Lown B, Amarasingham R, Neuman J: New method for terminating cardiac arrhythmias: Use of synchronized capacitor discharge. *JAMA* 1962; 182:548.

145. Kouwenhoven WB, Jude JR, Knickerbocker GG: Closed-chest cardiac massage. *JAMA* 1960; 173:1064.

146. Ditchey RV, Karliner JS: Safety of electrical cardioversion in patients without digitalis toxicity. *Ann Intern Med* 1981; 95:676.

147. Col JJ, Weinberg SL: The incidence and mortality of intraventricular conduction defects in acute myocardial infarction. *Am J Cardiol* 1972; 29:344.

148. Janse MJ, Van Capelle FJL, Morsink H, et al: Flow of "injury" current and patterns and excitation during early ventricular arrhythmias in acute regional myocardial ischemia in isolated procaine and canine hearts. Evidence for 2 different arrhythmogenic mechanisms. *Circ Res* 1980; 47:151–165.

149. Wells JL, MacLean WAH, James TN: Characterization of atrial flutter. Studies in man after open heart surgery using fixed atrial electrodes. *Circulation* 1974; 60:665– 673.

150. Pantridge JF, Geddes JS: A mobile intensive care unit in the management of myocardial infarction. *Lancet* 1967; 2:271.

151. Cobb LA, Baum RS, Alvarez H, et al: Resuscitation from out of hospital ventricular fibrillation: 4 years follow-up. *Circulation* 1975; 52:111–223.

152. Standards and guidelines for cardiopulmonary resuscitation (CPR) and emergency cardiac care (ECC). *JAMA* 1986; 255:21:2905–2989.

153. Weisfeldt ML, Halperin HR: Cardiopulmonary resuscitation: Beyond cardiac massage. *Circulation* 1986; 74:443.

154. Criley JM, Blaufuss AN, Kissel GL: Cough-induced cardiac resuscitation. *JAMA* 1976; 236:1246.

6 THE NORMAL RESPIRATORY SYSTEM

The vertebrate lung evolved to provide a rapidly available source of oxygen for the metabolic demands of the body described in Chapter One. Primitive gas-exchange surfaces were basically diffusing structures, airways without airspaces or air-water spaces without airways. While diffusion in air is 300,000 times more rapid than diffusion in water, it is effective only over short distances and cannot transport gas to respiring surfaces in any but the smallest animals. Combinations of airways and airspaces in an internalized and arborized arrangement that expands with the incoming tidal air and contracts with its ebb led to the vertebrate lung.

The lung transfers oxygen from atmosphere to blood, and carbon dioxide from blood to atmosphere. This transfer is accomplished by distributing the output of the right ventricle into a capillary network spread over the surface of the lung alveoli. This dispersion makes the distance between any region of the blood stream and the alveolar gas very small. Consequently, during the 0.75 second that the blood transits the capillary, there is adequate time for the gases to equilibrate between the liquid plasma phase and the gaseous alveolar phase.

GENERAL BEHAVIOR OF GASES

Life on earth is possible because of its atmosphere, a thin envelope of gases surrounding the planet. Man lives at the bottom of this ocean of air. Just as an ocean of water exerts pressure depending on its depth, the atmosphere exerts pressure depending on its distance from the earth's surface. At sea level, the weight of a 1 square inch column of air extending to the "top" of the atmosphere is 14.7 pounds. The huge forces exerted by atmospheric pressure may be demonstrated by the Magdeburg hemispheres, two iron half spheres 22 inches in diameter. When these hemispheres are placed together and evacuated of air, the force preventing their separation is about 5,600 pounds. Sixteen horses were unable to separate them in a classic demonstration staged 300 years ago.

While engineers customarily measure pressure in units of pounds per square inch, physiologists generally use the units millimeters of mercury or centimeters of water. This latter system is based upon Torricelli's* observation that the atmos-

*Evangelista Torricelli, Italian Physicist, 1608–47

pheric pressure is sufficient to hold a column of water 34 feet high in an evacuated tube. For this reason, it is impossible to raise water with a suction pump from a well deeper than 34 feet, since the pressure of the atmosphere is insufficient to force water to a height greater than that level. Torricelli reasoned that since mercury weighed 13.6 times more than water, a column of mercury could be supported only 30 inches by atmospheric pressure.

A column of mercury, water, or atmospheric gas measuring 1 square inch and extending 30 inches, 34 feet, or 30 miles, respectively, weighs 14.7 pounds (Fig 6–1).*

For this reason, a mercury column in an evacuated tube measuring 760 mm (30 inches) in height just balances the weight of the atmosphere. At sea level, the weight of the atmosphere supports a 760-mm column of mercury, regardless of the shape or diameter of the tube. The mercury barometer takes advantage of this; as atmospheric pressure falls, the height of the mercury column falls equivalently.

Atmospheric pressure is uniformly applied to all matter at the earth's surface. Properly speaking, the total systolic arterial blood pressure is 120 mm Hg plus 760 mm Hg. It is customary, however, to calibrate physiologic measuring instruments so that they read zero when exposed to the atmosphere. In this way the actual contribution of atmospheric pressure is neglected.

Practically the entire atmosphere is composed of molecules of nitrogen (78.09%) and oxygen (20.93%). In addition, variable amounts of water vapor, somewhat less than 1% of argon, extremely small amounts of carbon dioxide, and even smaller mounts of several other inert gases are present. The physiologic effects of a gas are proportional to the number of gas molecules present.

*Atmospheric gases are present for several hundred miles above the earth's surface, but the concentration of gas molecules at 30 miles is less than 1/1,000 the sea level value.

Individual gas molecules are in constant motion because of their kinetic energy. All gas molecules, regardless of species, have essentially the same kinetic energy. The bombardment by the constantly moving gas molecules against the wall of a container exerts a pressure on that wall proportional to the number of molecules present; in a mixture of different gases, each gas contributes to the total pressure in proportion to its fractional contribution to the total number of molecules. This relationship is expressed in Dalton's* law, which states that the "partial pressure" of a gas is proportional to its fractional composition. Thus, in a volume of atmospheric air, oxygen exerts a partial pressure of 0.2093 multiplied by 760 mm Hg or 159 mm Hg (Fig 6–2).

At a gas-liquid interface, gas molecules enter into solution because the kinetic energy of the molecules causes them to bombard the surface, and then to distribute themselves throughout the liquid. Gas molecules also are continually escaping from the fluid. The number of molecules that enter into solution is directly related to the partial pressure of molecules in the gas phase. At equilibrium the number of molecules leaving the liquid is equal to the number entering, and the partial pressure of gas in the liquid is equal to that in the gas phase.

Thus, the partial pressure of oxygen in a beaker of water exposed to room air is 159 mm Hg, the same as the partial pressure of oxygen in room air. The partial pressure of oxygen in the blood in a capillary leaving an alveolus is the same as that in alveolar air, 100 mm Hg. The partial pressure of a gas in a liquid is not dependent upon the nature of that

*John Dalton, English Scientist, 1766–1844

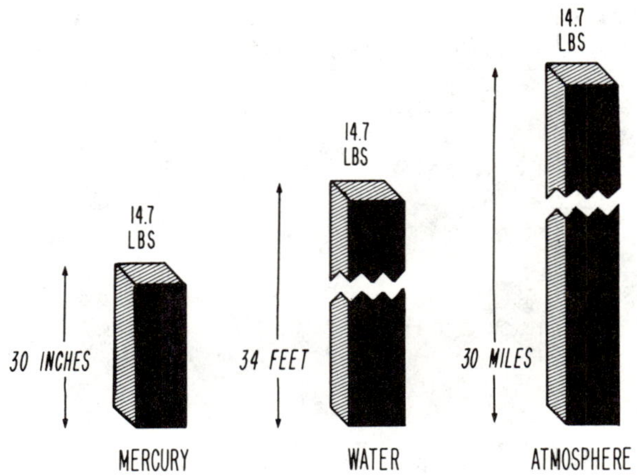

FIG 6–1.
A column of mercury, water, or atmospheric air measuring 1 square inch and extending 30 inches, 34 feet, or 30 miles, respectively, weights 14.7 pounds.

liquid. If the human circulatory system were filled with water, the water leaving the alveoli would still have an oxygen partial pressure of 100 mm Hg.

The amount of a gas dissolved in a liquid is directly proportional to the partial pressure of the gas existing in that liquid, and is also dependent upon the specific solubility of the gas in the liquid (Henry's Law*). If the partial pressure of the gas in contact with the fluid were to be doubled, there would be a twofold increase in the number of gas molecules in solution. At the same partial pressure, different amounts of the same gas are dissolved in different liquids. For practical purposes, body gases are dissolved in aqueous media, and the solubilities are similar in water, plasma, interstitial fluid, and intracellular fluid. Different gases, how ever, have markedly different solubilities in water; at the same partial pressure, more than 20 times as many carbon dioxide molecules as oxygen molecules go into aqueous solution. Nitrogen, in turn, is only about half as soluble as oxygen. The solubilities of gases are expressed as the Bunsen* coefficient, which is conventionally given the sign α (alpha). The α of a gas is the volume (in milliliters) of gas dissolved in 1 ml of the liquid at 1 atmosphere partial pressure, when the gas is at 0° C.

Table 6–1 shows the solubility coefficient and the total amount of gas contained in 100 ml of fluid at 100 mm Hg partial pressure for oxygen, nitrogen, and carbon dioxide, dissolved in whole blood

*William Henry, English Chemist, 1774–1836

*Robert Wilhelm Bunsen, German Scientist, 1811–1899

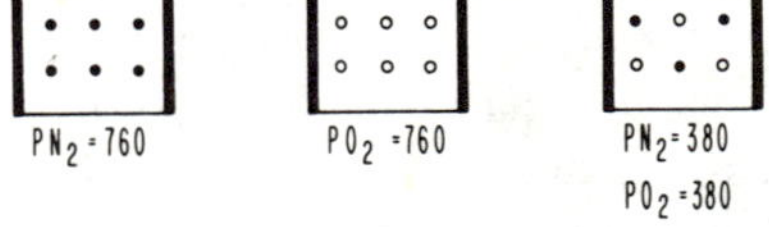

FIG 6–2.
The same number of molecules of either nitrogen or oxygen (or any other gas) exert the same pressure against the walls of a container. A mixture containing equal amounts of each gas would exert the same total pressure, but the partial pressure of each gas would be one-half the total pressure or 380 mm Hg.

TABLE 6–1.
Physical Solubility of Gases in Liquids

	OXYGEN	CARBON DIOXIDE	NITROGEN
Water			
Gas tension (mm Hg)	100	100	100
Solubility (α)	0.0232	0.545	0.0127
Amount (ml) in 100 ml	0.33	7.90	0.18
Blood			
Gas tension (mm Hg)	100	100	100
Solubility (α)	0.0230	0.490	0.0137
Amount (ml) in 100 ml	0.33	7.10	0.20

α = Bunsen coefficient, milliliters of gas STP per milliliter of liquid at 1 atmosphere partial pressure. Values given are for fluids at body temperature.

and water. The small amounts contained would not support complex mammalian life. To circumvent this, a fluid capable of holding considerably more oxygen and carbon dioxide than could be physically dissolved in aqueous solution was developed through evolution.

Diffusion refers to the net movement of molecules of a gas from one area to another by virtue of the random motion of the molecules imparted to them by their kinetic energy. The motion is so unordered that molecules in a mixture of gases distribute themselves throughout the entire volume of the system, just as differently colored marbles shaken in a container become randomly mixed. As a result, there is a net movement of molecules from a region of higher partial pressure to that of a lower partial pressure, from a region of higher concentration to a region of lower concentration, until an even distribution is achieved. This is not due to any "driving force" imparted to the individual molecules in the region of greater concentration, but is simply because the random motion of the molecules tends to distribute them equally.

The net rate of movement of gas molecules by diffusion is much slower in a liquid compared to a gas, and is related to both molecular weight and the solubility of that gas in the liquid. This explains why carbon dioxide is 20 times more diffusible across the alveolar membrane than is oxygen. Carbon dioxide is actually somewhat heavier than oxygen, but it is many times more soluble (Table 6–1) and hence many times more diffusible.

Two other gases besides oxygen and carbon dioxide are present in the body in large quantities: water vapor and nitrogen. Molecules of water are constantly escaping from the liquid into the gas phase, and equilibrium is reached when the rate of water molecules entering and leaving is the same. The gas in contact with the water is said to be saturated with water vapor when this equilibrium is reached, and the higher the temperature the greater the number of molecules in the gas phase at equilibrium. At body temperature (37°C), equilibrium is established when the number of molecules in the vapor phase exert a pressure of 47 mm Hg. The individual water molecules in this "vapor pressure" have the same kinetic energy as those molecules of oxygen and other gases, and therefore contribute to the total gas pressure to the same extent as the other molecules. All the gases in the body are fully saturated with water vapor, and their partial pressure of water vapor is 47 mm Hg.

Nitrogen is chemically inert. It serves no purpose, and the body can tolerate total lack of nitrogen in the atmosphere without apparent ill effects.

Although gas pressure may be compared to liquid pressure, individual gas molecules are much farther apart from one another than molecules in the liquid state. Temperature and pressure can affect the intermolecular distances in gas, but have little effect on molecular distances in fluids. Increasing atmospheric pressure pushes the gas molecules closer together, and at the same temperature the same number of molecules occupy a volume that is inversely proportional to pressure (Boyle's* law). Higher temperature increases the activity of the molecules, driving them farther apart and thus increasing the volume, which for the same Boyle, number of molecules and at the same pressure is proportional to the absolute temperature (Charles' law*). In reporting gas volumes, conditions of temperature and pressure must be specified because of these effects. It is customary to describe respiratory volume after correction to body temperature and pressure, assuming full saturation. In contrast, oxygen consumption, considered as a dry gas, is usually reported at standard pressure and temperature (760 mm Hg and 0°C).

Gas exchange in the lung may be considered as four separate and serial events: ventilation, distribution, diffusion and perfusion. *Ventilation* serves to replenish the gas in the lungs to maintain high oxygen and low carbon dioxide pressures, producing maximum gradients for diffusion. It is the mass movement of air in and out of the lung and is effective only to the extent that it adequately replenishes the gas mixture to the alveoli. *Distribution* is the delivery of ambient air to the separate gas exchange units and is accomplished by successively bifurcating the tracheobronchial system. *Diffusion* is the passive transfer of gas across the alveolar membrane from a region of higher concentration to that of a lower concentration. A diffusing membrane of over 90 square meters, in adult humans, is condensed in a lung volume of approximately 5 liters by the expedient of evagination into some 300 million alveoli. *Perfusion* is the means by which the outflow of the right ventricle is brought into intimate contact with the alveolar membrane.

The very nearness of the alveolar spaces to the outside environment makes the lung vulnerable to assault by inorganic and organic dusts, and by microorganisms; the intense perfusion of those spaces by almost the entire cardiac output makes the lung vulnerable to a group of blood-borne chemical, microbial, and immunologic enemies. More than 200,000 individuals in the United States, and countless millions worldwide, die each year from infectious, irritant, traumatic, and immunologic insults to the lung; many others die from the additive effects of these conditions and pulmonary congestion produced by left ventricular failure.

Lung diseases may develop over decades, with gradually increasing exertional dyspnea, cough and sputum production. They also may product disability rapidly over weeks or months, or may destroy the oxygen-transfer capacity of the lung in hours or days, producing acute respiratory failure and inevitable death.

STRUCTURE OF THE NORMAL LUNG

The lung's branching pattern, or tracheobronchial tree, is asymmetrically dichotamous so that each branch divides into two subbranches that need not be equal in diameter or length; 24 generations of branches reduce the 16 mm dia-

*Robert Boyle, Anglo-Irish Chemist, 1627–91

*Jacques Charles, French Physicist, 1746–1823

meter of the trachea to the 0.6 mm diameter of the terminal bronchiole.[1] The cartilages of the trachea and mainstem bronchi are horseshoe-shaped while those of the lobar and segmental bronchi are irregular. These cartilaginous plates become smaller as the bronchi become smaller; in bronchi 1–2 mm in diameter, they are found only at the origin of the bronchioles that arise from them. As the cartilage components decrease, smooth muscle begins to encircle the smaller airways, setting the stage for morphologic control of airway caliber. Patency of the cartilage-deficient bronchioles is probably maintained by radially disposed elastic fibers that are continuous with elastic fibers in the alveolar septa. Four types of epithelial cells—ciliated columnar cells, goblet cells, "brush" cells (microvilli but no cilia), and basal cells—compose most of the bronchial mucosa. Secretions from the goblet cells and from specialized mucous glands that extend into the lamina propria are probably identical. The conductive zone delivers the air to the diffusing surfaces of the lung. Although the airways become progressively smaller, their number increases more than their diameter decreases so that their overall resistance actually decreases. Small nonalveolated airways less than 2 mm in diameter constitute about 15% of the lung resistance and are frequently obstructed in the emphysematous lung.[2] After five or six additional branchings, these small airways terminate in the last nonalveolar bronchiole, the terminal bronchiole.

The ultimate terminal lung unit is difficult to define but, from a physiologic standpoint, might be a structure that functions and responds to various stimuli as a unit. The acinus, which is composed of the structures distal to the terminal bronchiole, is a likely choice for the fundamental lung unit, but it also may be an oversimplification, since respiratory bronchioles and even alveolar sacs may respond to extrinsic constrictor influences. Even smaller structures may autoregulate independently by reducing blood flow in response to hypoxia. The acinus has a skeleton of connective tissues which support a three-dimensional honeycomb of alveolar sacs, which are molded around the cylindrical alveolar duct to closely resemble packed bubbles of soap foam. The connective tissue skeleton also supports an envelope of alveolar epithelium, which contains a meshwork of alveolar capillaries.

Two morphologically different epithelial cell types line the alveolar wall. The flattened Type I cells have central nuclei surrounded by cytoplasm that stretches out in thin processes to form the alveolar wall. These thin wings are in contact with a thin basement membrane, which in turn is fused with the basement membrane of the capillaries; the diffusion path, therefore, consists only of the alveolar epithelium, capillary endothelium and fused basement membranes. The thicker side of each capillary contains an interstitium of collagen and elastin fibers, fibroblasts, macrophages, and proteoglycan-containing ground substance. This thick side holds the supporting framework and also provides a transient reservoir for filtered water prior to its removal by the pulmonary lymphatics. The Type II cell is a larger granular cell that actively synthesizes surfactant. Lamellar bodies are believed to produce or store surfactant for subsequent extrusion into the alveolar space.

Ventilation

Ventilation produces a successive fall in the oxygen tension in tracheal and alveolar air. It drops in tracheal air because the inspired air is warmed and humidified by the mucous membranes of nose and pharynx (Figure 6–3). The water vapor exerts a partial pressure which increases with the temperature and is 47 mm Hg at 37.5°C. The total volume of lung gas increases, and the partial pressure of oxygen is reduced to 144 mm Hg ((706 - 47)(0.209) = 144)).

A second fall in oxygen tension occurs as tracheal air enters the alveoli and oxygen is exchanged for carbon dioxide. Upon first consideration, the drop in oxygen tension in the alveoli would seem to follow this equation:

$$\frac{P_{A_{O_2}} = P_{T_{O_2}} - P_{A_{CO_2}}}{(104 = 144 - 40)}$$

where $P_{A_{O_2}}$ is the alveolar oxygen tension, $P_{T_{O_2}}$ the tracheal oxygen tension, and $P_{A_{CO_2}}$ alveolar carbon dioxide tension.

This equation is correct only when the respiratory exchange ratio (R)(volume of carbon dioxide produced divided by volume of oxygen consumed) is 1.0. With an exchange ratio of 0.8, 200 ml of oxygen leaves and 160 ml of carbon dioxide enters the alveoli each minute. Alveolar gas volume thus shrinks by 40 ml, increasing the concentration of its components. The true alveolar oxygen tension may be calculated from the alveolar equation,* which corrects for these changes in the respiratory exchange ratio.

$$P_{A_{O_2}} = P_{T_{O_2}} - \frac{P_{A_{CO_2}}}{R}$$

The mechanical properties of airway, lungs, and thorax determine both the mass movement and distribution of air within the thorax. Approximately 5% of the oxygen consumed by the body is used by the respiratory muscles (diaphragm, intercostal muscles, and accessory muscles of respiration) to convert good material into ATP. The efficiency of the respiratory muscles is believed to be quite low; only 5–15% of the energy produced is transformed into actual mechanical work. Pressure must be generated to overcome the resistance of the conducting airways to the flow of inspired air, to expand the elastic-like alveoli, and to stretch the tissues of the thorax and abdomen.

Distribution of an alveolar volume of 350 ml per breath (500 ml tidal volume minus 150 ml dead space) to the individual acinar units is accomplished by the conducting system described above and outlined in Figure 6–4. The conducting system is considered dead space since gas is not exchanged across its walls. Any increase in dead space must increase the total volume of ventilation required to

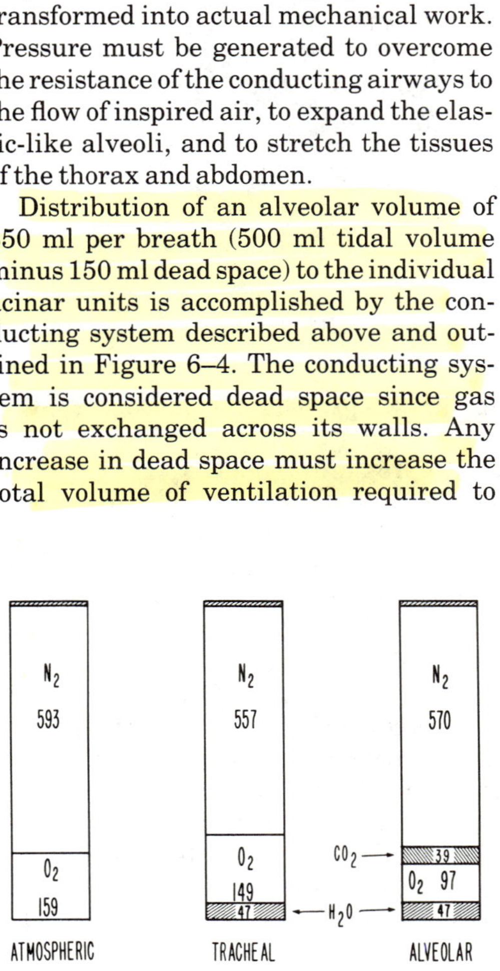

FIG 6–3.
Composition of atmospheric, tracheal, and alveolar air. Tracheal air has a lower oxygen tension than atmospheric air because it is diluted with water vapor. Alveolar oxygen tension is still lower as a result of exchange with carbon dioxide. The cross-hatching at the top of the bar graph represents argon and other inert gases, approximately 1% of the atmosphere.

*The form of the alveolar air equation given above is good enough for most clinical situations. For accurate calculation of physiologic data, however, the following more complicated equation is necessary:

$$P_{A_{O_2}} = P_{T_{O_2}} - P_{CO_2}\left[F_{I_{O_2}} + A\left(1 - \frac{F_{I_{O_2}}}{R}\right)\right]$$

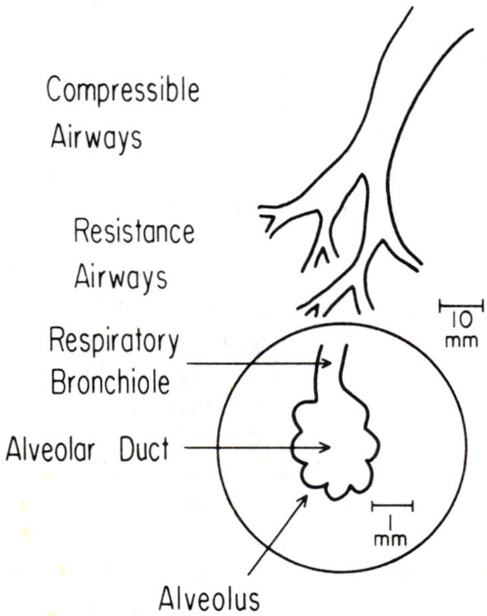

FIG 6–4.
Functional segments of the airway. Most of the airway resistance resides in airways averaging 2–3 mm in diameter. Larger airways contribute little to overall resistance but are compressible during expiration. Shown in the inset is a respiratory bronchiole and alveolar duct. Airway constriction or dilatation could involve any of the three functional levels of the conduction system: compressible airways, resistance airways, or respiratory bronchioles.

maintain a given level of alveolar ventilation.

A pressure gradient is necessary between mouth and alveolus in order to overcome the total resistance of the airways, and produce an average flow rate of inspired gas of 1 liter/second in normal individuals. This resistance is not uniformly distributed along the conducting airways, however. Figure 6–4 presents the three functionally different regions of the conducting system. Macklem and Mead[3] used intrabronchial pressure measurements to analyze the resistance of peripheral airways smaller than 2 mm in diameter and that of the larger central airways. These studies demonstrated that the peripheral airways constituted but 10% of the total airways resistance, and that most of the total pressure drop was due to resistance in the airways ranging in size from 3 to 8 mm in diameter.

Distal to the resistance airways described above are the terminal bronchioles, respiratory bronchioles, and alveolar ducts. While this segment of the conducting airways constitutes a small fraction of total airway resistance, recent evidence suggests that alveolar duct constriction may significantly decrease vital capacity and functional residual capacity. Proximal to the 3–8 mm resistance airways is an airway segment which may be compressed during expiration. Pressure within airway segments downstream (proximal) from the resistance segment decreases due to resistance losses. Whenever pleural pressure exceeds airway pressure dynamic compression is possible and may limit expiration airflow.[4]

Airway constriction, either reflexly or as a direct result of some disease process, may involve any level of the conducting system. Vagal stimulation produces constriction of the resistance segment and has little effect on alveolar ducts, while histamine and other humoral agents act primarily on alveolar ducts. Isoproterenol antagonizes both vagal-induced bronchospasm and histamine-produced alveolar duct constriction.

The conducting airway system is considered dead space because it does not participate in respiratory gas exchange. Since carbon dioxide is not added to gas during its residence in the conducting network, dead space air does not contain carbon dioxide and actually has the same composition as tracheal air. The carbon dioxide concentration of expired air results from the mixture of carbon dioxide-containing alveolar air and dead space air. The volume of the dead space may be readily calculated from alveolar and expired air carbon dioxide measurements using the Bohr relationship.

$$\text{dead space} = \frac{F_{A_{CO_2}} - F_{E_{CO_2}}}{F_{A_{CO_2}}}$$

where $F_{A_{CO_2}}$, and $F_{E_{CO_2}}$, are alveolar and expired air concentrations, respectively, and dead space is given as a percentage of either tidal volume or minute ventilation.

Pressure must also be developed in order to overcome the elastic resistance of thoracic tissue and to distend alveolar structures with air. An average pressure gradient of 2–3 cm H_2O is required for each 100 ml of air filling the thorax; approximately half of this is necessary to distend alveolar tissue. The remainder of the pressure generated is used to displace and stretch the tissues of chest wall and abdomen.[5]

The pressure necessary to overcome resistance to air flow is dissipated (it is frictional in nature). However, pressure utilized to stretch elastic tissue is stored as potential energy. Thus the energy requirements of breathing are markedly reduced by the elastic properties of the supporting structures, for pressure need normally be generated only during inspiration. Collagen and elastic tissue, vascular structures, and the surface-active material called surfactant (which lines the alveoli) collectively comprise the elastic resistance to deformation of the lung. They are stretched and store energy during inspiration. Expiration is normally passive and is accomplished by mobilization of this stored potential energy. In the process of airway obstructive disease, however, the stored potential energy is not sufficient, and additional active expiratory pressure must be generated in order to empty the alveoli.

The differences between frictional and elastic resistances are illustrated in Figure 6–5. The pressure required to overcome the elastic resistance of alveolar units and chest wall is directly proportional to the volume change and inversely proportional to the compliance of those structures. The pressure needed to overcome the elastic resistance of the lung equals the volume inspired divided by

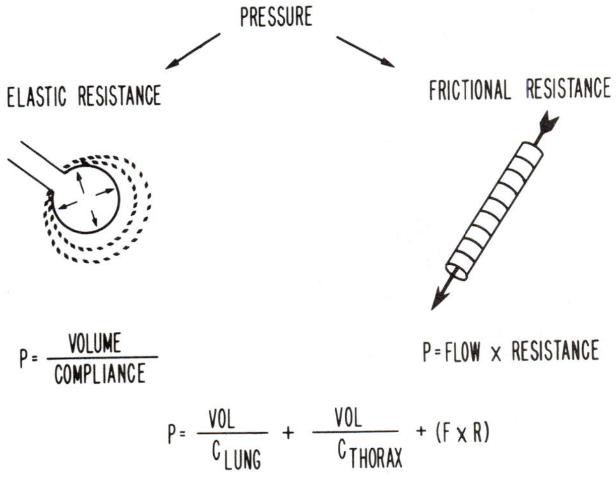

FIG 6–5.
Frictional and elastic resistances (R) impede the flow of air into the lung. The pressure (P) needed to overcome elastic resistance is directly proportional to the volume and inversely proportional to the compliance (C) or distensibility. The pressure needed to overcome frictional resistance is directly proportional to flow (F) and resistance. The total pressure generated by the respiratory muscles is the sum of the pressures required to overcome elastic resistance of the lung, elastic resistance of the thorax, and resistance of the tracheobronchial tree to air flow. The small fraction of pressure needed to overcome inertia has been disregarded.

lung compliance; that needed to overcome chest wall resistance equals volume divided by chest wall compliance. Compliance is conventionally represented as volume change in liters per centimeter of water pressure change. Pressure required to produce air flow
and overcome the frictional resistance of the airway is proportional to flow rate and resistance. These pressures may be summed to give the total pressure necessary for breathing (Table 6–2).

The fact that compliance is related to lung volume, whereas airway resistance is related to rate of air flow, explains why patients with pulmonary fibrosis take rapid shallow breaths and those with emphysema breathe slowly and deeply. Each group attempts to keep intrapleural pressure at a minimum. The patient with fibrosis breathes shallowly, since his low compliance would require prohibitively high pressures to maintain a normal tidal volume. A low flow rate is necessary for survival in the emphysematous patient because the high airway resistance would require prohibitively high pressures to maintain a normal flow rate.[6]

Ventilatory work may be analyzed by plotting pressure against volume. This product is equivalent to work since, conventionally, work is the product of force times distance. Thus:

$$\text{Work} = \text{force} \times \text{distance}$$

$$\text{Force} = \text{pressure} \times \text{area}$$

$$\text{Volume} = \text{area} \times \text{distance}$$

$$\text{Distance} = \frac{\text{volume}}{\text{area}}$$

$$\text{Work} = (\text{pressure} \times \text{area}) \times \frac{\text{volume}}{\text{area}}$$

$$\text{Work} = \text{pressure} \times \text{volume}$$

Two pressure-volume diagrams are shown in Figure 6–6. During normal inspiration intrathoracic pressure decreases from −2 to −5 cm H_2O while 500 ml of air is drawn into the lung. Potential energy is stored by the lung during inspiration and expended during expiration; in consequence, the entire expiratory cycle is passive. The darkened area represents pressure multiplied by volume and is the work of breathing. The lightly shaded area is the work required to overcome elastic forces, whereas the hatched area is the work required to overcome airway or frictional resistances. There is a marked increase in the airway resis-

TABLE 6–2.
Mechanics of Ventilation

	NORMAL	EMPHYSEMA	FIBROSIS
Volume (liters)	0.400	0.400	0.200
Lung compliance (liters/cm H_2O)	0.150	0.150	0.050
Thoracic compliance (liters/cm H_2O)	0.150	0.150	0.150
Flow (liters/second)	0.400	0.200	0.800
Resistance (cm H_2O/liter/second)	1.0	6.0	1.0
Pressure (cm H_2O) to overcome			
Lung elastic resistance	2.7	2.7	4.0
Thoracic elastic resistance	2.7	2.7	1.3
Airway frictional resistance	0.4	1.2	0.8
Total resistance	5.8	6.6	6.1
Respiratory rate (per minute)	15	15	30
Time of inspiration (seconds)	1	2	0.5
Ventilation (liters/minute)	6	6	6

FIG 6–6.
Volume is plotted against intrathoracic pressure in a pressure-volume diagram. During normal inspiration intrathoracic pressure becomes increasingly negative as lung volume increases. The total darkened area has the dimensions of pressure multiplied by volume and represents the total work of inspiration. The hatched area represents that fraction of total inspiratory work necessary to produce air flow. Total inspiratory work is markedly increased in a patient with emphysema because of the increase in the frictional work required to produce air flow. The elastic work, shown by the shaded triangle, is the same as in the normal. The hatched area to the left of the triangle represents active expiratory work necessary to overcome resistance to air flow during expiration. Expiration is passive in the normal subject because sufficient potential energy is stored during inspiration to produce expiratory air flow. Exp, expiration; Insp, inspiration.

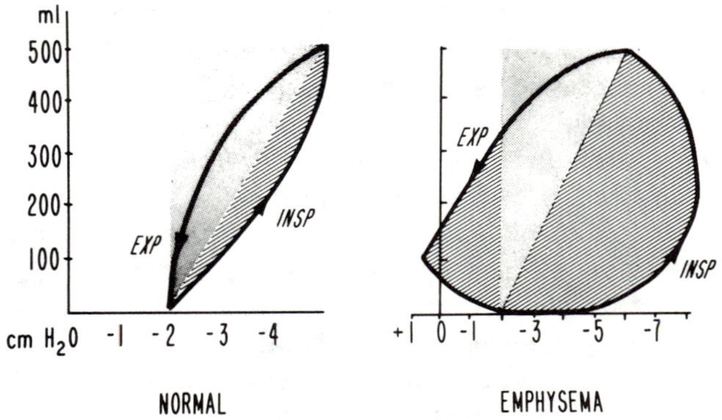

tive component of respiratory work in chronic obstructive lung disease (right hand panel). During expiration, only 150 ml of air leaves the lungs during the passive phase when intrathoracic pressure reaches the equilibrium value of −2 cm H_2O. Active effort, producing work, is required to force out the remaining 350 ml of air, and intrathoracic pressure actually becomes positive.

The symptom dyspnea is related to both the amount of pressure generated by the respiratory muscles and the total amount of work performed. The emphysematous patient in Figure 6–6 would experience dyspnea because of the increase in work. Respiratory work is generally related to the volume of ventilation it produces: kilogram-meters per liter of ventilation. A normal individual performs approximately 0.04 kg meters/liter of ventilatory work, which is the equivalent of 0.20 ml of oxygen uptake. In reality, because of the low efficiency of the respiratory muscles, he utilizes 5 ml of oxygen and produces 4 ml of carbon dioxide for each liter of ventilation. Conditions associated with increased respiratory work obviously require additional oxygen uptake and, in turn, produce more carbon dioxide.

Total ventilation, expressed as liters of air per minute, is related to the pressure generated by the respiratory muscles and also to the mechanical properties described above. Only about 75% of the total ventilation reaches the alveoli and is available for gas exchange. The remainder occupies the nonrespiratory tissues of the thorax—the pharynx, trachea, and bronchi—and is referred to as "dead space" ventilation. The pressure generated by the chest wall is uniformly applied to all regions of the lung. If all regions had identical mechanical properties, all would receive identical ventilation. The effects of ventilation on the constitution of blood gases are simplified by first describing an ideal lung in which all regions possess the same mechanical properties. This is probably not the case in the normal lung, and definitely not the case in the abnormal lung. The modifications of unequal distribution of ventilation are discussed in a subsequent section.

Alveolar and arterial blood gas tensions are closely related to the rate of alveolar ventilation. Figure 6–7 shows the important relationship between alveolar ventilation and blood carbon dioxide tension, oxygen tension, and oxyhemoglobin saturation. At this point in the discussion, it is assumed that arterial and alveolar gases are in perfect equilibrium, and therefore that arterial oxygen tension equals alveolar oxygen tension. Note that there is a gradual decrease in oxygen tension and an increase in carbon dioxide tension as alveolar ventilation decreases from 4 to 2 liters/minute. A greater alteration in blood gas tensions occurs as alveolar ventilation drops to 1 liter/minute; from this point, the curves become progressively steeper so that a small change in alveolar ventilation produces a profound change in blood gas tensions. Thus, in a critically ill patient, a small change in alveolar ventilation produced by the plugging of a single lobar segment could produce a sudden drop in oxygen tension sufficient to induce ventricular fibrillation. The sigmoid shape of the oxyhemoglobin dissociation curve maintains the saturation of hemoglobin until ventilation falls to a critical level. Note that carbon dioxide tension could rise to 77 mm Hg and oxygen tension fall to 62 mm Hg, while hemoglobin saturation would be 85%, and cyanosis would not be perceivable.

Diffusion

Oxygen passively diffuses from alveolar gas to the pulmonary capillary across a concentration gradient obeying the simple laws of diffusion.[7] The rate of diffusion of a gas across the alveolar-capillary membrane is given by the equation

$$\dot{V}O_2 = \frac{(P_A - Pa) \times D \times A}{\text{thickness}}$$

where $\dot{V}O_2$ is the amount of oxygen crossing the membrane in a unit time, D is the diffusibility of the particular gas across the membrane, A is the area of the membrane available for diffusion, $(P_A - Pa)$ is the difference between alveolar and pulmonary capillary oxygen tensions, and thickness is that of the alveolar-capillary membrane. A very large gradient exists as mixed venous blood enters the alveolus, since mixed venous oxygen tension is 40 mm Hg while alveolar oxygen tension is 100 mm Hg (Fig 6–8). Because of the large early gradient, 60 mm Hg, most of the diffusion of oxygen occurs during the first 25% of time that the erythrocyte is in the alveolar pulmonary capillary. As oxygen tension in the pulmonary capillary rises, the gradient falls and the amount of oxygen diffused also decreases. By the end of the pulmonary capillary,

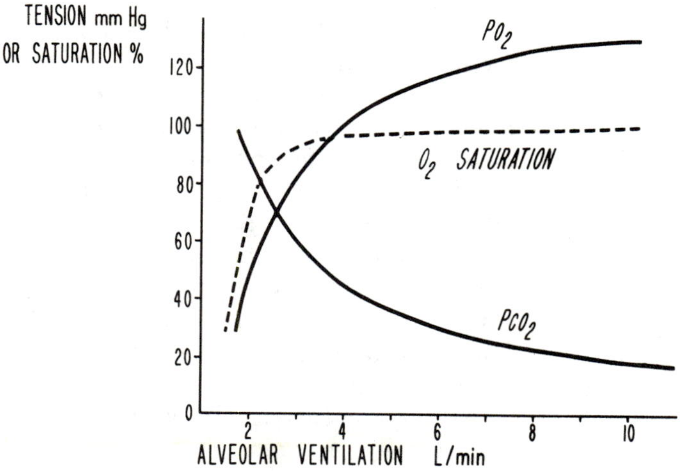

FIG 6–7.
Oxyhemoglobin saturation, oxygen tension, and carbon dioxide tension are related to alveolar ventilation. Note that oxyhemoglobin saturation does not fall significantly until carbon dioxide and oxygen tensions have become markedly abnormal.

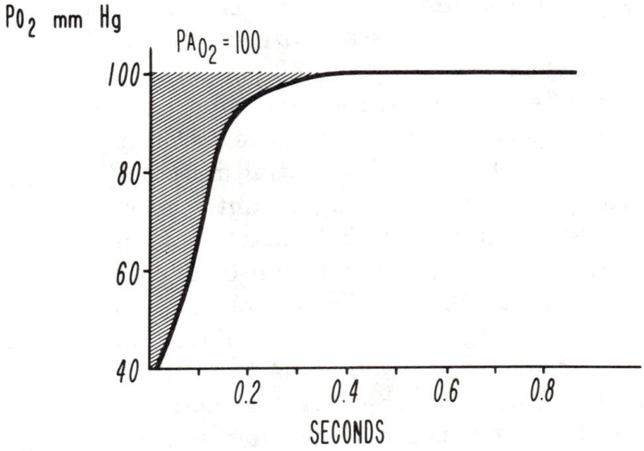

FIG 6–8.
Venous blood enters the pulmonary capillary with an oxygen tension of 40 mm Hg and reaches alveolar oxygen tension within 0.3 second. Hatched area demonstrates the large gradient existing initially between pulmonary capillary blood and alveolar air.

the oxygen tension within the erythrocyte equals that within the alveolus. Both the alveolar-capillary membrane and the finite time required for the chemical combination of oxygen with hemoglobin constitute the diffusion barrier which, if great enough, would prevent end-capillary oxygen tension from equaling alveolar oxygen tension.[8] Although diffusion blocks are frequently invoked to explain arterial desaturation, it is unusual for either the membrane to be thick enough or the reaction velocity slow enough to prevent complete equilibrium between pulmonary capillary and alveolar air.

The diffusion equation also demonstrates that a decrease in the total area available for diffusion can decrease the amount of oxygen diffused for any given gradient. Loss of alveolar surface area, rather than specific alteration in diffusing properties, may be important in the development of hypoxemia in emphysema.

One way of overcoming any true membrane diffusion barrier is to increase the diffusion gradient. This is easily done by breathing 100% oxygen. The initial gradient is then increased tenfold and sufficient oxygen diffuses across to saturate pulmonary capillary blood completely within 0.001 second in the normal lung. Since the blood cell is in the pulmonary capillary on the average of 0.75 second, there is sufficient time for complete saturation, even when diffusion is slowed down by an abnormal alveolar-capillary membrane. A diffusion block could never exist for carbon dioxide since the membrane would have to be so thickened that the patient would have died from hypoxemia long before carbon dioxide accumulation became a problem.[9–11]

Perfusion

Right ventricular output in normal man averages approximately five liters/minute, and alveolar ventilation averages approximately four liters/minute. The pulmonary vascular tree follows the bronchial tree as they both successively branch until they enter the acinus. Elastic arteries accompany the cartilage containing bronchi; vessels with complete internal and external lamina and certain muscular arteries accompany bronchioles and respiratory bronchioles. These arteries have a muscular medial layer that is much thinner than that in systemic muscular arteries, averaging three to five percent of vascular diameter. They appear much more distensible than systemic arteries, and probably are able to dilate substantially with increases in blood flow. Short vessels without muscular coats and less than 100 u long branch from these small arteries and supply the capillary bed. These vessels are probably arterioles, but any substantial muscular coat (and thereby any significant vasoactivity) is limited to their junction with the parent artery where the muscular coat increases to 10% of the parent artery's vascular diameter. Contractile fibers and cells identified as myofibroblasts continue as far distally as the alveolar septa, at which point it is not clear whether they regulate airway, vascular, or interstitial function.[12]

Precapillary and humoral regulation of vascular tone permits rapid adjustment to changing conditions, since many humoral regulators are inactivated by the pulmonary capillary endothelium during a single pass through the lungs.[13] Norepinephrine causes vasoconstriction, but its effect is limited by endothelial inactivation; isoproterenol causes vasodilation. Epinephrine appears to have a mixed effect, and it functions like a circulating hormone since it is not destroyed during lung perfusion. Recent pharmacologic studies have shown that beta-adrenergic agonists, alpha-adrenergic blockers, and smooth vessel dilators such as hydralazine and diazoxide reduce pulmonary vascular resistance and may be useful in the long-term management of primary pulmonary hypertension.

Serotonin, bradykinin, acetylcholine, and angiotensin II are also pulmonary vasaconstrictors. Histamine and bradykinin, like hypoxia and acidosis, constrict pulmonary vessels, but are dilators in most other vascular beds. PGE_2, $PGF_{2\alpha}$, and the thromboxanes are pulmonary vasoconstrictors. PGI_2 is an extremely potent vasodilator produced by the pulmonary endothelium and not degraded by passing through the lungs.[14]

Distribution of Ventilation and Perfusion

Thus far we have discussed a hypothetical lung in which the relationship between alveolar ventilation, diffusing capacity, and capillary perfusion is the same throughout. In such a lung, oxygen and carbon dioxide tension in arterial blood would equal that in alveolar air. Actually, the mechanical properties of the lung vary from region to region, so that alveolar ventilation varies from region to region.[15] Capillary perfusion is also unequally distributed throughout the lung. It is convenient to view the lung as containing an unspecified number of diffusion-ventilation-perfusion units. Each unit has its own ventilation/perfusion ratio, and the distribution of these ratios throughout the lung determines, in large part, the composition of arterial blood.[16,17]

Radioactive gas studies have revealed striking variations in the distribution of both ventilation and perfusion in normal man. Both increase from top to bottom in erect man, but the rate of blood flow increases about three times more rapidly than ventilation, so that the lower lobes have considerably lower ventilation/perfusion ratios than the upper lobes. Figure 6–9A shows the marked variation in ventilation, perfusion, and ventilation/perfusion ratios observed in normal man.[18] These differences are less marked in supine man, and ventilation/perfusion ratios are relatively uniform throughout the lung. In the lateral decubitus position, however, the upper lung presumably functions like the upper lobes while the lower lung exhibits the increased ventilation and perfusion typical of the lower lobes. This has major implications for positioning the critically ill patient, since positioning the diseased side down increases blood flow through poorly ventilated areas and increases the degree of hypoxemia.

Alveolar pressure, pulmonary arterial

FIG 6–9A.
Ventilation and perfusion in different lung regions. Levels of lung from base to apex are shown on a horizontal axis. Ventilation perfusion ratios with resultant oxygen and carbon dioxide tensions are shown on the right abscissa. Flow rate per unit volume is shown on the left abscissa. Both ventilation ($\dot{V}_A$) and blood flow ($\dot{Q}$) increase toward the base of the lung. The increase in blood flow is greater than the increase in ventilation, so the ventilation perfusion ratio ($\dot{V}_A/\dot{Q}$) decreases from apex to base. Blood draining the apex would have an oxygen tension of 141 mm Hg, while blood draining the base would have an oxygen tension of about 85 mm Hg. (Adapted from West JB: Regional differences in gas exchange in the lung of erect man. *J Appl Physiol* 1962; 17:893.)

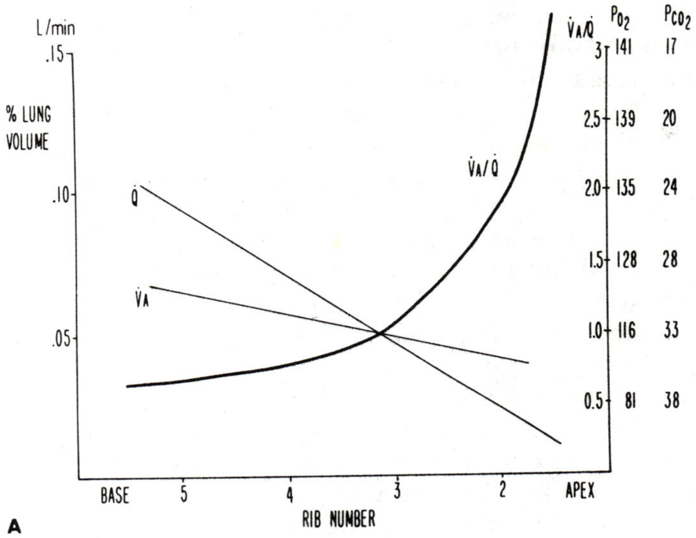

pressure, and pulmonary venous pressure all may determine the rate of pulmonary blood flow, but their relative influence depends upon the level of the lung involved (Fig 6–9B). West, Dollery, and Naimark[19] suggested that the lung may be divided into three segments. In the uppermost segment, alveolar pressure is greater than pulmonary arterial pressure, and flow does not occur. In the middle segment, pulmonary arterial pressure is greater than alveolar pressure, but alveolar pressure is greater than pulmonary venous pressure, so that a constriction develops somewhere in the venous system. This system has the hydraulic characteristics of a Starling resistor in which the pulmonary arterial-pulmonary alveolar pressure gradient, rather than the pulmonary arterial-pulmonary venous gradient, determines flow. In the lowest seg-

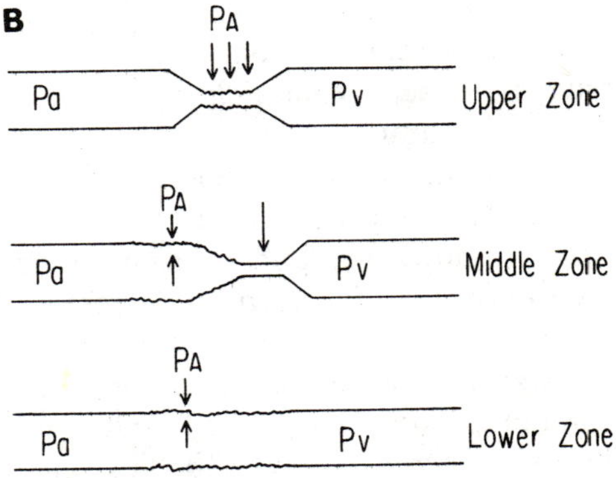

FIG 6–9B.
The lung may be viewed as containing three zones. In the upper zone alveolar pressure (PA) exceeds arterial pressure and there is no blood flow. In the middle zone arterial pressure is greater than alveolar pressure, but alveolar pressure remains greater than venous pressure (PV). In the lower segment alveolar pressure does not limit blood flow, which is governed by the usual hydraulic principles. See text for complete description.

ment, alveolar pressure does not limit blood flow, and flow is governed by the usual pulmonary arterial-pulmonary venous pressure gradient.

This regional variation in blood flow has several implications for the critically ill patient. (1) Intermittent positive-pressure breathing increases alveolar pressure and thus decreases blood flow, particularly in those segments above the left atrium. (2) Blood flow is greatest in the dependent segments of the lung (in any position) even during intermittent positive-pressure breathing. (3) Increased left atrial and pulmonary venous pressure may increase blood flow in the middle segment and counteract the effects of intermittent positive-pressure breathing. (4) Serious mismatching of ventilation and blood flow may occur in dependent segments; accumulation of interstitial and alveolar fluid decreases ventilation and leads to terminal airway closure, while dependency increases blood flow.

A variety of disease states produce marked abnormality in the distribution of ventilation and perfusion. Certain anatomic varieties of chronic airway obstructive disease (centrilobular emphysema, for example) are characterized by widespread areas of poorly ventilated lung tissue. Blood flow is relatively unaffected, however, and these regions develop extremely low ventilation/perfusion ratios. If an entire lung segment is destroyed, however, as in panlobular emphysema, both ventilation and perfusion are decreased and the ventilation/perfusion relationships may be close to normal. These differences explain why some patients with chronic lung disease have extremely abnormal arterial blood gas tensions (the "blue bloater"), while others have relatively normal oxygen and carbon dioxide tensions (the "pink puffer").

Many seemingly unrelated conditions—such as pulmonary congestion, the postoperative state, pulmonary inflammation, drug overdosage, trauma, and pulmonary embolization—produce another type of ventilation, perfusion maldistribution, in which alveolar units are completely collapsed and nonventilated while blood flow is maintained. The ventilation/perfusion ratios of these units approach zero, producing a true venoarterial shunt.

Effect of Ventilation-Perfusion Imbalance on Composition of Arterial Blood

The net effect of unequal distribution of ventilation and perfusion is to cause a fraction of the right ventricular outflow to pass through the lung without oxygenation, and to return unoxygenated to the left heart as venous admixture to the systemic circulation. Through usage, when a totally unventilated region of lung is perfused or when venous blood completely bypasses lung parenchyma, the term *true venoarterial shunt* is applied. The presence of some ventilation with proportionately greater perfusion is termed the *unequal ventilation-perfusion effect.* It is obvious that the former is merely a special case of the latter in which the ventilation/perfusion ratio is zero.[20,21]

The total venous admixture to the systemic circulation may be subdivided as follows:

- *True venoarterial shunt*
  - Anatomic shunt
    - Bronchial veins
    - Pleural veins
    - Thebesian veins
    - Arteriovenous communications
  - Physiologic shunt
    - Alveolar collapse (variable)
- *Unequal ventilation-perfusion effect*

The effect of a true venoarterial shunt on mixed arterial and alveolar gas tensions is seen in Figure 6–10. Circle A represents a normal alveolar unit with a

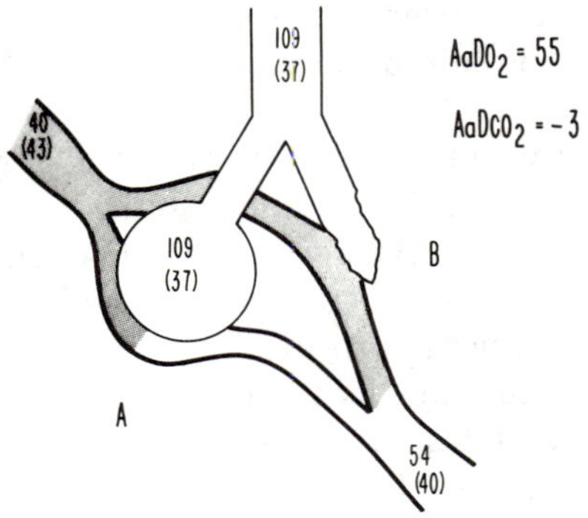

FIG 6–10.
Effect of true venoarterial shunt on mixed arterial and alveolar gas tensions. Alveolar unit B is totally collapsed, and the oxygen tension of capillary blood leaving that unit is the same as venous oxygen tension. An alveolar arterial oxygen difference ($AaDo_2$) of 55 mm Hg is produced. Carbon dioxide tensions are given in parentheses.

ventilation/perfusion ratio of 1.0. Alveolar oxygen and carbon dioxide tensions are 109 and 37 mm Hg, respectively; capillary blood leaving that unit has the same gas tensions. Alveolar unit B is totally collapsed. Capillary blood leaving that unit is actually unaltered mixed venous blood with oxygen and carbon dioxide tensions of 40 and 43 mm Hg, respectively. The oxyhemoglobin saturation of mixed arterial blood is, assuming equal blood flow to each unit, the average (87%) of that leaving unit A (98%) and that leaving unit B (75%). Carbon dioxide tension is only slightly higher than normal in mixed pulmonary venous blood.

Hypoxemia also results if one area of the lung is markedly underventilated, although not totally atelectatic. Figure 6–11 shows a model lung containing one normally ventilated segment (A) and another segment in which ventilation is only 20% of perfusion (ventilation/perfusion ratio equals 0.2), each receiving the same blood flow. Capillary blood leaving segment A has the same tensions as that in Figure 6–10. Oxygen and carbon dioxide tensions in the underventilated segment are 56 and 43 mm Hg, respectively. The oxyhemoglobin saturation of mixed arterial blood in this situation is the average (93%) of that leaving A (98%) and that leaving B (87.5%). The oxygen tension is 68 mm Hg.

The gas composition of pulmonary capillary blood leaving any alveolar unit is thus determined by the ventilation-perfusion relationships of that unit—not the absolute rate of either ventilation or blood flow. Figure 6–12 shows that alveolar oxygen, carbon dioxide, and nitrogen tensions resulting from various ventilation/perfusion ratios. Since capillary and alveolar gas tensions are identical unless a diffusion block is present, Figure 6–12 actually demonstrates the variety of capillary gas tensions theoretically possible within the lung. Note that capillary blood leaving a completely collapsed unit ($\dot{V}/\dot{Q} = 0$) is actually unchanged venous blood, while capillary blood tensions leav-

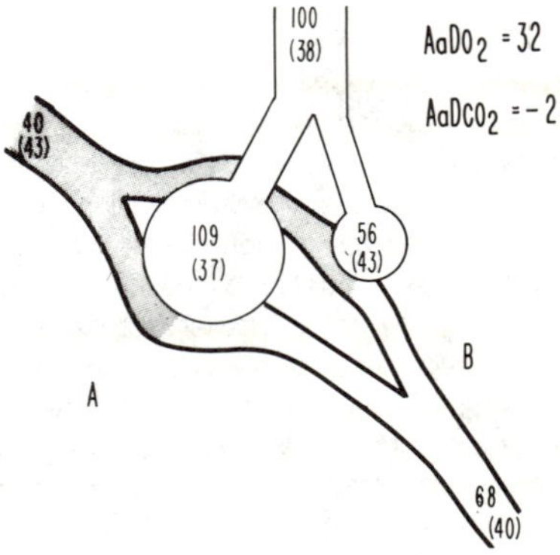

FIG 6–11.
Effect of unequal distribution of ventilation and perfusion on arterial gas tensions. Alveolar unit A is normally ventilated, and capillary blood leaving that unit has the same gas tension as alveolar air in that unit. Ventilation in unit B is reduced to 20% of perfusion; oxygen tension falls to 56 mm Hg. Mixed alveolar and arterial oxygen tensions are 100 and 68 mm Hg, respectively, producing alveolar arterial differences of 32 and −2 for oxygen and carbon dioxide.

ing units with greater $\dot{V}/\dot{Q}$ ratios are intermediate between venous blood and inspired gas tensions.

The position and shape of the $\dot{V}/\dot{Q}$ line is determined by mixed venous and inspired gas tension. Decrease in cardiac output and in mixed venous oxygen tension lowers the capillary oxygen tension for any given $\dot{V}/\dot{Q}$ ratio (Fig 6–13). Severe shock may produce arterial hypoxemia by this mechanism alone, even if gas exchange is relatively normal. Capillary oxygen saturation would be 96% in units with $\dot{V}/\dot{Q}$ ratios of 0.8, for example. In severe shock, saturation would drop to 86%, even if those units continued to have $\dot{V}/\dot{Q}$ ratios of 0.8.

Figures 6–10 and 6–11 also illustrate the creation of an alveolar-arterial oxygen difference ($AaDO_2$).*

If the entire lung were homogeneously ventilated and perfused as in segment A, mixed alveolar and mixed pulmonary venous blood would have identical gas tensions. Arterial blood oxygen tension would be slightly less owing to normal venous admixture. The existence of a totally nonventilated segment (Fig 6–10) and a markedly underventilated segment (Fig 6–11) lowers the arterial oxygen tension of mixed arterial blood and produces an alveolar-arterial oxygen difference. This difference develops because an underventilated but normally perfused alveolar unit contributes proportionately more of an oxygen tension decrease to mixed arterial blood than to mixed alveolar air.

Arterial carbon dioxide tension is slightly higher than alveolar carbon dioxide tension when certain segments are underventilated. This effect is intensified when one segment is ventilated but not perfused (Fig 6–14), as might occur with pulmonary embolization.[23] Segment A is normally ventilated and perfused, as in the preceding illustrations. Segment B is ventilated but not perfused and contains alveolar air with the same higher oxygen tensions as those present in dead space air. An alveolar-arterial oxygen difference results because mixed alveolar oxygen tension is higher than the oxygen tension in the blood leaving segment A. Of importance, however, is that the mixed alveolar carbon dioxide tension is significantly less than the mixed arterial carbon dioxide tension.

The measurement of alveolar and arterial carbon dioxide tensions was suggested by Robin et al.[23] as a useful method of recognizing pulmonary embolization. The technique has not been particularly useful clinically, however, because small carbon dioxide gradients may occur in other disease processes, and because ventilation usually decreases markedly in nonperfused segments. This latter phenomenon reduces the alveolar-arterial gradient for carbon dioxide by reducing the contribution of the embolized segment to mixed alveolar air.

*The alveolar-arterial oxygen difference ($AaDo_2$) is generally used to describe oxygen transfer in the lungs.[22] Physiologists during the early part of the twentieth century debated whether arterial oxygen tension was more or less than alveolar oxygen tension. The former hypothesis implied active oxygen secretion by the lung, the latter passive diffusion. August Krogh's belief that oxygen transfer was accomplished by diffusion was confirmed when sensitive measuring techniques demonstrated beyond doubt that arterial oxygen tension was always lower than alveolar oxygen tension. Recent studies have led to the fractionation of the overall alveolar-arterial oxygen difference into distribution venoarterial shunt and diffusion components, and have demonstrated the value of this measurement in the study of alveolar gas exchange.Arterial blood is easily sampled by direct arterial puncture, but no simple method exists for obtaining a sample of mean alveolar air. In fact, alveolar air varies in composition from region to region within the lungs so that "mean" alveolar air is actually a theoretical concept. In practice, alveolar air is sampled by collecting the last few milliliters of an expiration, using the early expirate to wash out the dead space air. Another technique, developed by Riley and Cournand,[16] assumes that alveolar and arterial carbon dioxide tensions are identical and calculates alveolar oxygen tension from the alveolar air equation.

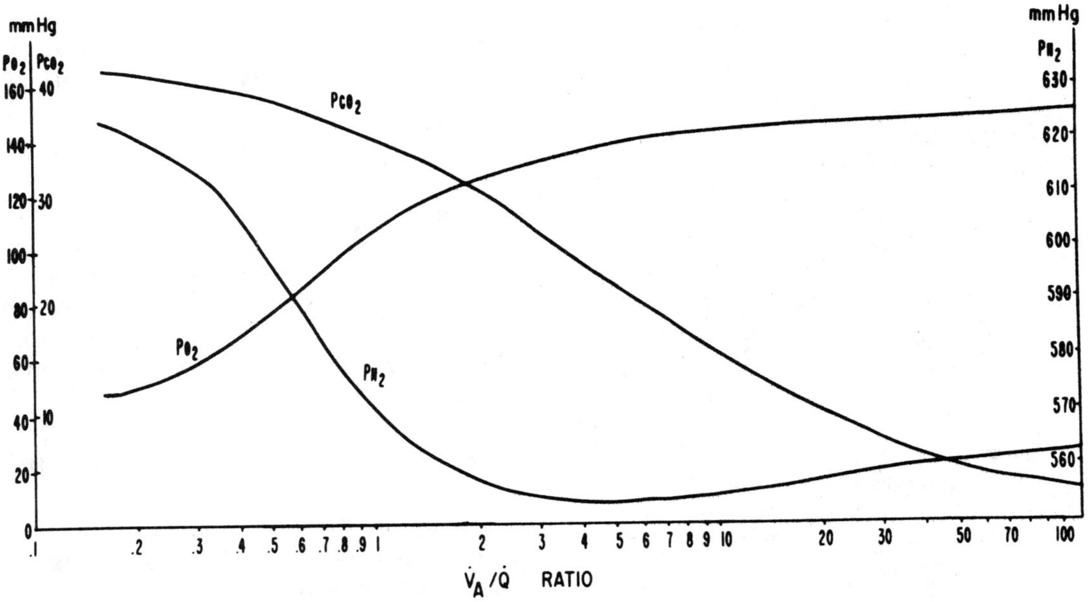

FIG 6–12.
The effect of changes in alveolar ventilation-perfusion ratios ($\dot{V}_A/\dot{Q}$ ratios) on oxygen, carbon dioxide, and nitrogen tensions. Note than P_{N_2} and P_{O_2} change rapidly with changes in $\dot{V}_A/\dot{Q}$ ratio in the lower ranges, while P_{CO_2} changes rapidly with changes in $\dot{V}_A/\dot{Q}$ ratio in the upper ranges. The $\dot{V}_A/\dot{Q}$ ratios are plotted on a semiologarithmic scale, since regions with ratios under 2.0 produce the greatest effect on blood gas tensions. [Adapted from Holman, Muschenheim: *Bronchopulmonary Diseases and Related Disorders.* Harper & Row, 1972.)

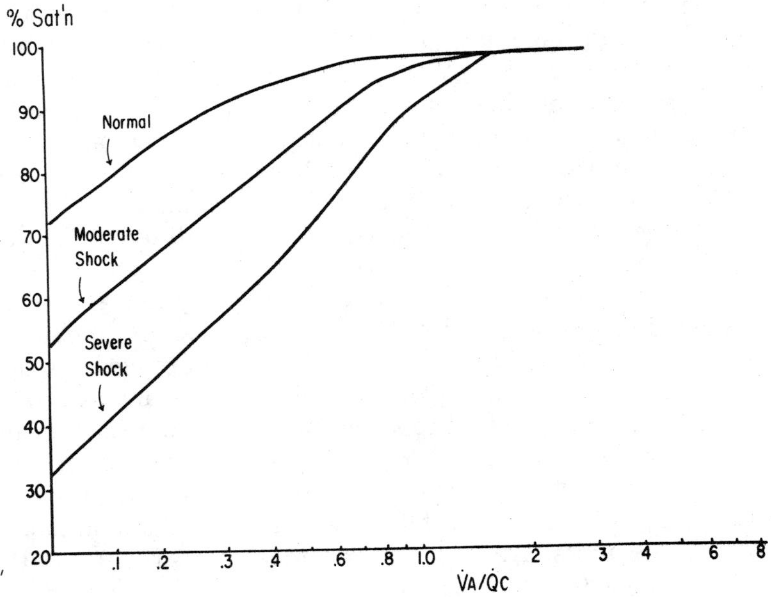

FIG 6–13.
Oxyhemoglobin saturation of blood leaving alveolar units with various $\dot{V}A/\dot{Q}c$ ratios. Relations for normal cardiac output and for moderate and severe shock are shown. The origin of each curve is the mixed venous point corresponding to a $\dot{V}A/\dot{Q}c$ ratio of zero. Saturation is lower for any ratio below 1.0 in patients with low cardiac output. (From Ayres SM, *Am J Cardiol* 1970, 26:588. Used by permission.)

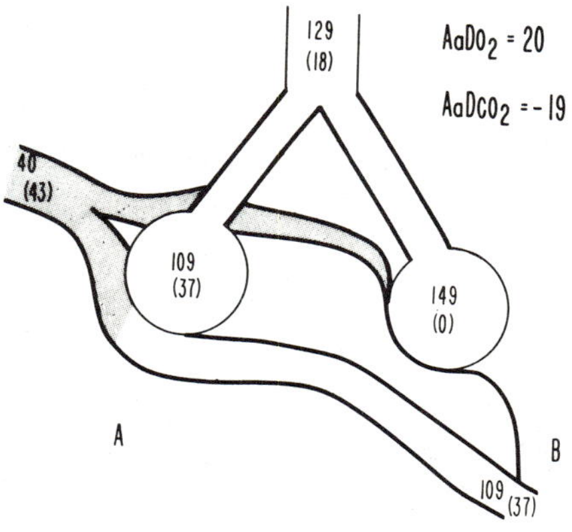

FIG 6–14.
Occlusion of the vascular supply to an alveolar unit increases the alveolar-arterial carbon dioxide gradient (AaD_{CO_2}). See text for complete description.

Ventilation-Perfusion Relationships and Oxygen Therapy

The relationships between ventilation and perfusion determine the effect of oxygen breathing on arterial blood oxygen tensions.[24] Three alveolar units with varying ventilation-perfusion relationships are shown in Figure 6–15A. The left hand unit has a $\dot{V}/\dot{Q}$ ratio of 0.85, the unit in the center has a $\dot{V}/\dot{Q}$ ratio of 0.20, and the right-hand unit is totally collapsed, resulting in a $\dot{V}/\dot{Q}$ ratio of 0. Saturation values shown for each capillary correspond to the oxygen tensions shown within each alveolar unit. Note that after breathing room air, blood leaving the well-ventilated unit has an oxyhemoglobin saturation of 97.5%; that leaving the poorly ventilated unit, 85.6%; and that leaving the completely collapsed unit, 72.6%, a saturation identical with that of venous blood. Blood leaving the latter unit is unaltered venous blood representing a venoarterial shunt.

Breathing 100% oxygen produces striking changes in capillary blood leaving two of the units. Alveolar oxygen tension rises to 677 and 672 in the well ventilated and poorly ventilated units (Fig 6–15B), so that blood draining those units is completely saturated with oxygen. The high oxygen concentration, in contrast, has no effect on the collapsed unit and its capillary drainage is unchanged. Low concentrations of oxygen almost completely saturate blood draining the well ventilated units (Figs 6–15C, D). Blood from the poorly ventilated units is 98.5% saturated while breathing 40% oxygen, 94.5% while breathing 30% oxygen. Blood draining the completely collapsed segment is unchanged and is obviously completely independent of the oxygen concentration of the breathing mixture.

These relationships explain the differing response to oxygen breathing of the hypoxemia due to the complete collapse and that due to unequal ventilation-perfusion relationships. With complete collapse, oxygen cannot gain access to capillary blood draining totally unventilated segments, and any improvement in arterial saturation must come from improved saturation in the still-ventilated portions of the lung. This effect together with an additional 1 ml of dissolved oxygen per 100 ml of blood (breathing 100% oxygen) permits the unaffected segments to compensate for the collapsed lung areas, maintaining an adequate arterial oxyhemoglobin saturation when as much as 30% of the lung is collapsed or filled with fluid. The situation with unequal distribution is obviously quite different, since even low concentrations of oxygen augment oxyhemoglobin saturation in poorly ventilated lung region-s.The implications of these observations are clear: Use low concentrations of oxygen when treating patients with chronic lung disease; and use high concentrations when treating patients with atelectasis, shock, pulmonary edema, or pulmonary inflammation.

Figures 6–16A, B show the three units of Figure 6–15 in a patient with low cardiac output and low venous oxygen

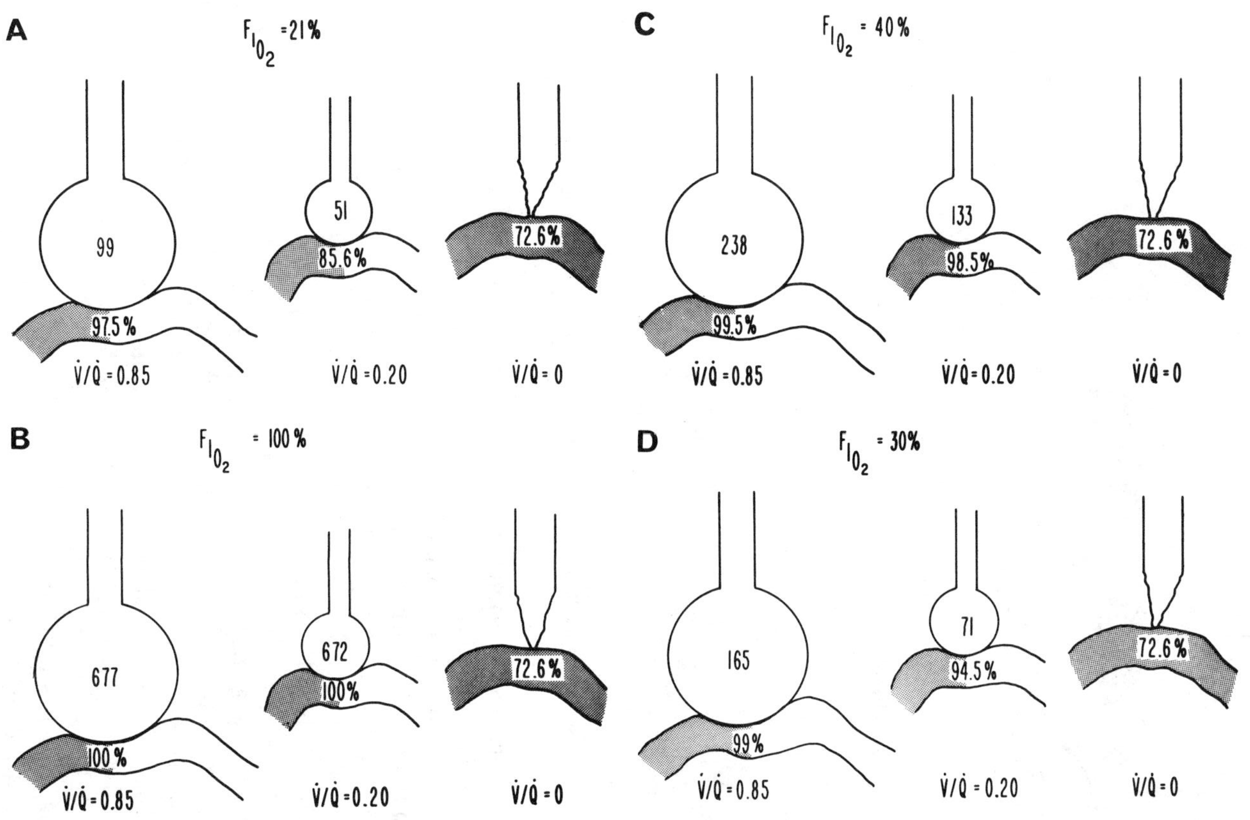

FIG 6–15.

Effect of increasing inspired oxygen concentration. At the left is a normally ventilated alveolar unit with a $\dot{V}/\dot{Q}$ ratio of 0.85. In the center is a poorly ventilated lung unit with a $\dot{V}/\dot{Q}$ ratio of 0.20. On the right is a completely collapsed alveolar unit with a $\dot{V}/\dot{Q}$ ratio of zero. A. Capillary saturation breathing room air. B. Breathing 100% oxygen. C. Breathing 40% oxygen. D. Breathing 30% oxygen.

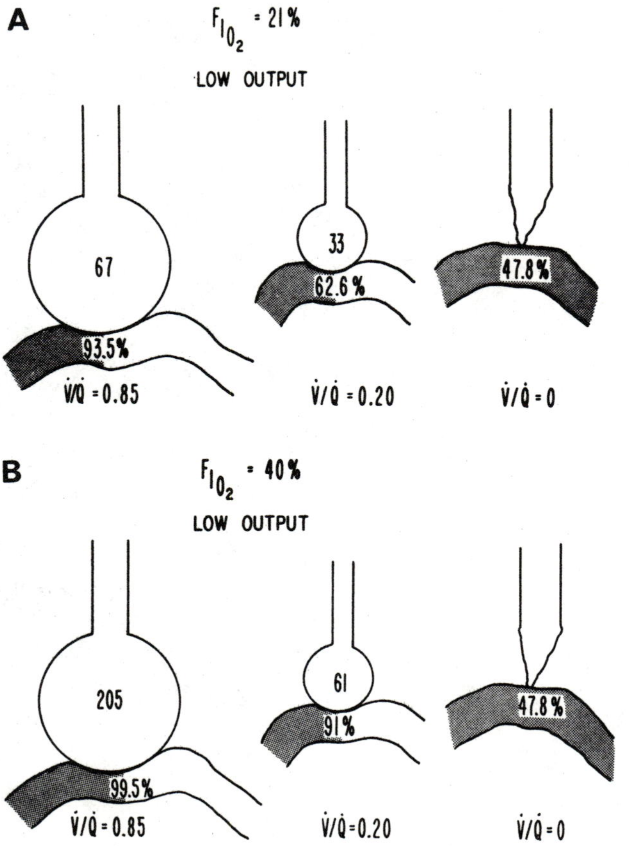

FIG 6–16.
Effect of low cardiac output on saturation of blood draining units shown in Figure 6–15. A. Saturation from each unit breathing room air. B. Breathing 40% oxygen.

tension. For each ventilation/perfusion ratio, capillary oxyhemoglobin saturation is significantly lower in the shock patient compared to the patient with normal cardiac output. Thus low cardiac output in a patient with chronic lung disease can dramatically lower arterial oxygen tension. Increased oxygen concentrations in the inspired air have the same effect as in the patient with a normal cardiac output, but higher concentrations are required.

The response of arterial blood to the breathing of 100% oxygen may be used to identify and measure true venoarterial shunting. If true shunting is absent, arterial oxygen tension would be close to alveolar oxygen tension, since even poorly ventilated alveolar units develop high oxygen tensions, as demonstrated above. The magnitude of the shunt may be calculated from the following equation:

$$\dot{Q}s/\dot{Q}t = \frac{(AaD_{O_2})(0.0031)}{(AaD_{O_2})(0.0031) + (a - v)_{O_2}}$$

where $\dot{Q}s/\dot{Q}t$ is the shunt expressed as a percentage of the cardiac output, AaD_{O_2} is the alveolar-arterial oxygen difference breathing 100% oxygen, $(a-v)_{O_2}$ the arterial-venous oxygen difference in milliliters per 100 ml, and 0.0031 the amount of oxygen dissolved in each 100 ml of blood for each unit (millimeter of mercury) of oxygen tension.

Alveolar Integrity; Prevention of Atelectasis

The first several breaths of life serve to expand the newborn lung, which was airless during intrauterine existence. Unless the lung becomes diseased, it remains in this expanded state until death. Both the surface lining of the alveoli and the pulmonary vascular framework serve an antiatelectasis function.

The lung may be likened to a fine foam in which the dispersed bubbles represent the alveoli, the bubble wall the alveolar lining, and the material between the bubbles the pulmonary stroma. Figure 6–17 shows the application of the LaPlace law to bubbles. As the radius of the bubble grows smaller, the pressure exerted within the cavity of the bubble by the membrane increases (pressure = 4 × surface tension/diameter). Ordinary bubbles are unstable for just this reason; as the bubble becomes smaller, its tendency to collapse tends to become greater. This would not present a liability to the mammalian lung during inspiration. However, during expiration, with a decrease in alveolar dimensions, a great deal of negative pressure would have to be generated in order to overcome the tendency to collapse produced by the wall of the small alveolus.

This problem is solved in the mammalian lung by the development of a surface-lining material (surfactant), a complex lipoprotein secreted by alveolar cells which has the fortunate property of changing its surface tension with a change in its dimensions.[25] As the layer thickens during expiration, the

tension. Stretching the surface lining substance during inspiration increases its surface tension, enabling it to store potential energy produced during inspiration. At least half of the potential energy available for expiration arises from stretching the elastic surfactant. The remain-

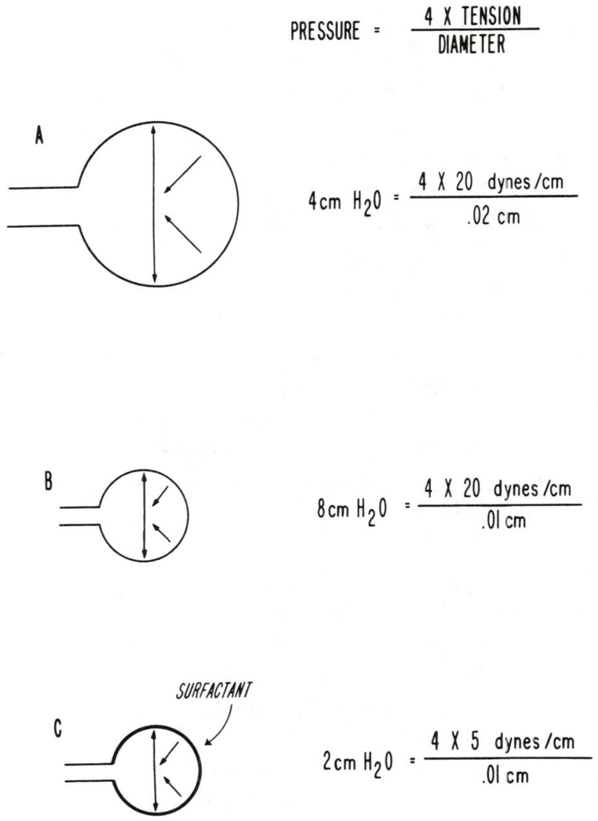

FIG 6–17.
The LaPlace law states that the pressure exerted by the membrane of an elastic sphere is directly proportional to the wall tension and inversely proportional to the diameter. If the diameter of a bubble is reduced by 50% (A to B) without change in the surface tension of the bubble wall, the pressure within the bubble doubles. In the lung the surface tension of the alveoli decreases as they deflate because the surface tension of the lipoprotein lining material, surfactant, decreases as its area decreases. Therefore, reducing the diameter by 50% may actually decrease the pressure exerted by the membrane. This reduces the pressure needed to keep alveoli open and minimizes the tendency toward alveolar collapse.

der presumably comes from a stretching of connective tissue and blood vessels. During expiration, as the alveolar radius decreases rapidly and high surface tension becomes a liability, the surfactant rapidly decreases its surface tension as its area decreases. In consequence, the pressure needed to maintain the alveolus open is kept at a minimum.

It was postulated many years ago that the turgid blood vessels of the lung have an erectile property that tends to keep the alveoli inflated. Recent studies in the isolated, perfused lung confirmed this, and demonstrated that the pulmonary vascular system provides a scaffold for the alveolar system. Clinical conditions associated with local or general decreased pulmonary blood flow may increase the tendency toward collapse.

In spite of these two defensive mechanisms, there remains a steady tendency toward alveolar collapse. If an anesthetized animal or human being is allowed to breathe at a constant tidal volume for several hours, there is a progressive collapse of certain alveoli.[26] The rate of collapse may be observed by measuring pulmonary compliance and arterial oxygen tension. Both of these measurements gradually decrease as alveolar units collapse and produce a venoarterial shunt. The same gradual collapse may be observed in a conscious human whose chest has been strapped with bandages either experimentally or postoperatively.[27,28] A sudden maximum inflation (Fig 6–18) however, reverses this tendency and opens the collapsed alveoli.

Normal individuals automatically interrupt this cycle of progressive collapse by sighing every 5–15 minutes. These brief, deep inspirations open collapsed alveoli. General anesthesia, sedation, the pain associated with recent surgery, general debility, and the shock state decrease the frequency of sighing.[29] Many of these same situations also decrease the antiatelectasis efficiency of surfactant and the vascular scaffold, increasing the need for frequent deep breaths. These two processes working together produce progressive alveolar collapse in most critically ill patients. Oxygen tension falls, secretions accumulate, and bronchopneumonia may develop. This chain of events may be interrupted and prevented by the administration of frequent deep inhalations by a respirator or by skillfully administered pulmonary physiotherapy.

Control of Ventilation

Total body oxygen consumption is closely matched to metabolic requirements by a central neural regulating mechanism, which responds to a variety of stimuli by adjusting the rate of ventilation. The mechanism is so effective that the varying metabolic states associated with sleep on one extreme and heavy exercise on the other do not result in significant alterations in blood oxygen or carbon dioxide tension. This is demonstrated in Figure 6–19, which shows a series of studies performed on a professional athlete doing treadmill exercise. The exercise

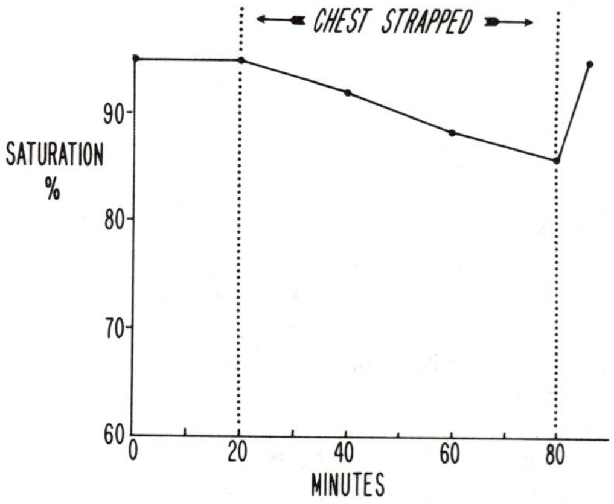

FIG 6–18.
Arterial oxyhemoglobin saturation progressively falls as alveolar collapse is produced in a normal individual by chest strapping. Sudden maximal inflation flowing release of the chest straps restores saturation to normal.

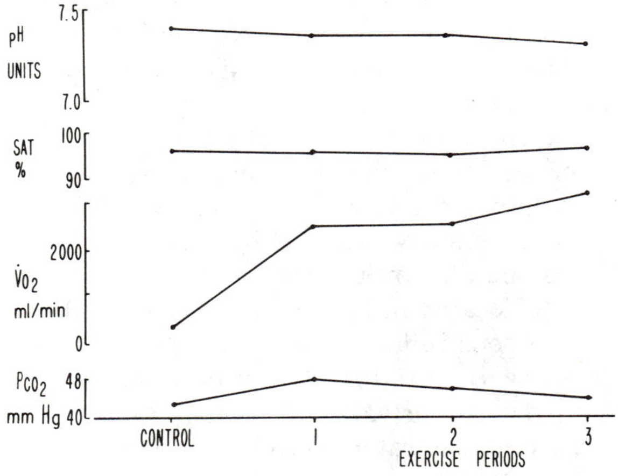

FIG 6–19.
Arterial blood gas tensions remain in the normal range despite three periods of treadmill exercise which produced a tenfold increase in oxygen consumption. An efficient central regulatory system closely matches the rate of alveolar ventilation to metabolic requirements.

resulted in a tenfold increase in oxygen consumption. An efficient central regulatory system produced a parallel increase in rate of ventilation and maintained arterial blood gases at a constant level.

This precise control system frequently malfunctions in the critically ill patient, leading to a ventilatory response inappropriate for the patient's metabolic needs. Either increased or decreased ventilatory responses, producing hypo- and hypercapnia, affect tissue hydrogen ion concentration and impair the function of critical organs. Table 6–3 gives data from a patient who had severe hyperventilation within 24 hours of an acute myocardial infarction associated with circulatory collapse. Arterial hypoxemia and acidosis were not present, and the striking hyperventilation which resulted in an arterial carbon dioxide tension of 11 mm Hg must have been due to other adaptive mechanisms. A discussion of the respiratory drive in this patient is given below

TABLE 6–3.
Hyperventilation in Acute Myocardial Infarction

Gas tensions		
PO_2	Arterial:	158 mm Hg[a]
	Venous:	24 mm Hg
PCO_2	Arterial:	11 mm Hg
	Venous:	30 mm Hg
pH	Arterial:	7.65 units
	Venous:	7.45 units
Plasma bicarbonate (venous)	12 mEq/liter	
Plasma lactate (venous)	59.6 mg/100 ml	
Minute ventilation	13.1 liters/minute BTPS	
Respiratory rate	30/minute	
Cardiac index	1.16 liters/minute/meter^2	
Erythrocyte pH (arterial)	7.29	

Normal values: lactate 10 mg/100 ml; cardiac index 3.0 to 3.5 liters/minute/meter^2; minute ventilation 5 to 7 liters/minute; erythrocyte pH 7.20.
[a]Breathing oxygen.

following a presentation of the several known levels of ventilatory control.

The alternate discharge of inspiratory and expiratory automatic or "pacemaker" cells located within the medulla is believed responsible for primary periodic ventilatory activity. This primary activity is constantly modified by a variety of extramedullar influences (Fig 6–20). Cell groups located in the cerebral cortex and in the pons influence the medullary respiratory center directly; stimulation of the pyriform cortex, for example, produces increased respiratory activity, while stimulation of the anterior cingulate gyrus appears to inhibit respiration.[30]

Reflex Stimulation of Medullary Centers

At least four sets of fibers associated with the vagus and glossopharyngeal nerves exert powerful effects on respiration. (1) The Hering-Breuer reflexes result in inhibition of inspiratory activity during inflation, and stimulation of inspiratory activity during lung collapse. Stretch receptors within lung tissue mediate the reflexes, and vagotomy completely abolishes them. (2) Irritation of bronchi, trachea, larynx, or nasopharynx produces cough or other ventilatory activity. (3) Stimulation of afferent fibers located in the aortic arch inhibits respiration and produces a decrease in blood pressure. (4) Stimulation of fibers leading from the aortic or carotid bodies produces hyperpnea and an increase in blood pressure.

The carotid body is a small reddish nodule that averages 1–2 mm in diameter, weighs about 2 mg, and is located at the bifurcation of the common carotid artery. Microscopic studies have shown that its arterial supply enters sinusoids, which are in close contact with large chemoreceptor cells. The blood flow of the carotid body averages 40 ml/minute; less than

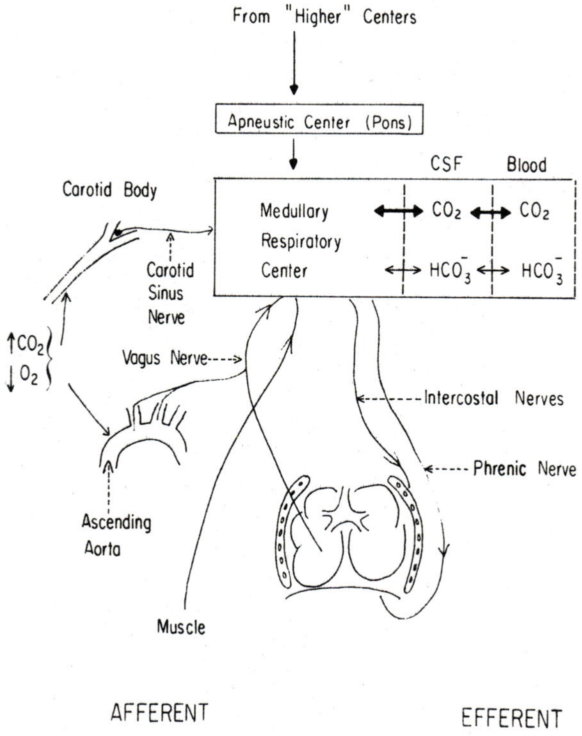

FIG 6–20.
The medullary respiratory center received afferent information from the apneustic center in the pons, higher centers, arteriole chemo- and baroreceptors, pulmonary stretch receptors, and stretch receptors located in muscle and joints. Carbon dioxide freely penetrates the blood-brain barrier and directly stimulates the respiratory center. The effect of carbon dioxide is believed related to the hydrogen ion concentration so that the effect of any given carbon dioxide level is related to the buffering capacity of the respiratory center. The blood-brain barrier is relatively impermeable to bicarbonate, so bicarbonate changes require several days for complete equilibrium. The high respiratory center bicarbonate concentrations in chronic lung disease are believed responsible for the diminished responsiveness to increasing carbon dioxide tensions. Efferent impulses leave the respiratory center and are transmitted by phrenic and intercostal nerves to the muscles of respiration.

0.2 ml of oxygen per 100 ml of blood is extracted so that venous blood leaving the body has about the same oxygen and carbon dioxide tensions and pH as the arterial blood entering.[31] Hypotension markedly reduces blood flow to the carotid sinus, increasing oxygen extraction and changing the oxygen and carbon dioxide concentrations of its venous effluent.[32] The aortic body presumably has a similar function, but its location deep in tissues close to the aortic arch complicates the performance of detailed studies.

A decrease in oxygen tension or increase in either carbon dioxide tension or hydrogen ion concentration in the arterial blood perfusing the carotid body increases the rate of neural impulse traffic through the carotid sinus nerve and stimulates respiration. Increases in carbon dioxide tension presumably increase the intracellular hydrogen ion concentration; hypoxemia may act in the same manner by provoking anaerobic metabolism with the production of intracellular hydrogen ions.

Severe hypoxemia produces reflex respiratory stimulation mediated by the carotid and aortic chemoreceptors even when the medullary respiratory center is unresponsive to the direct chemical stimulation. The chemoreceptors appear to be the final defense of the respiratory system, and continue to fire for 30 minutes or longer following circulatory or respiratory death. The hypoxemic drive becomes clinically important following respiratory center depression since the injudicious use of oxygen may shut off neural traffic from the chemoreceptors and interrupt reflex stimulation of the medullary center.[33] The relationship between arterial oxygen tension and carotid nerve impulse generation is shown in Figure 6–21. Note the rapid increase in impulse traffic as arterial hypoxemia develops and the still considerable impulse generation at oxygen tensions between 60 and 80 mm Hg. Low-flow oxygen therapy takes advantage of the fact that low concentrations of oxygen increase arterial oxyhemoglobin saturations to tolerable levels without completely obliterating peripheral chemoreceptor stimulation.

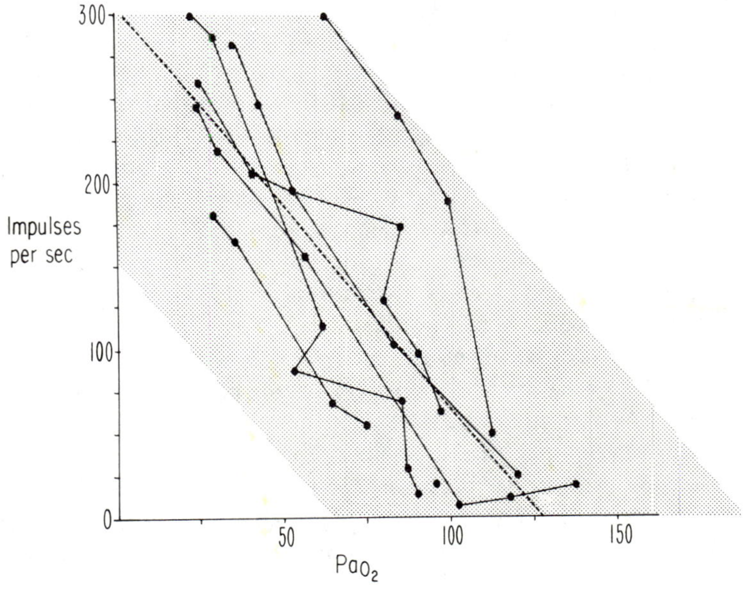

FIG 6–21.
Impulses per second recorded from carotid sinus nerve. Average response is shown by a dotted line; shaded area included ±2 standard deviations from the mean. Note that carotid sinus nerve activity is roughly a linear function of arterial-oxygen tension. Each increment in oxygen tension produces a change in nerve impulse generation and thus affects ventilation. (Adapted from Witzler EW: The excitation of chemoreceptors by arterial hypoxia and hypercapnia, in *Regulation of Human Respiration*. Philadelphia, FA Davis, 1963, pp 173–182.)

A number of respiratory stimulants—including nicotine, lobeline, acetylcholine, nikethamide (Coramine), and aminophylline—exert their effect by reflexly stimulating carotid and aortic chemoreceptor cells.

Direct Stimulation of Medullary Centers

Carbon dioxide and hydrogen ions have long been known to be potent central respiratory stimulants, while hypoxemia depresses central respiratory activity. Chemoreceptors are believed located both deep in medullary tissue and also superficially in the floor of the fourth ventricle where they may be stimulated directly by cerebrospinal fluid. Carbon dioxide inhalation produces striking hyperventilation that approaches the level of voluntary hyperventilation,[34,35] but most investigators believe that carbon dioxide produces its effect by changing the hydrogen ion concentration of chemoreceptor cells, both central as well as peripheral. In contrast to the peripheral chemoreceptors, however, central chemoreceptors are separated from capillary blood by a blood-brain barrier, which is relatively impermeable to fixed acids and bases. Molecular carbon dioxide diffuses freely, however, and raises intracellular hydrogen ion concentration, stimulating respiration.

The presence of a significant blood-brain barrier is of great importance, since it explains why the acid-base environment of central respiratory neurons may be quite different from that of the circulating blood.[36] Carbon dioxide-induced hyperventilation persists after the infusion of sodium bicarbonate returns arterial pH to normal, for example, because cerebrospinal fluid and brain tissue pH are unchanged. Chronic carbon dioxide retention gradually increases the bicarbonate concentration of central chemoreceptor cells, buffering their response to additional elevations in carbon dioxide tension. This is the presumed mechanism underlying the respiratory center depression associated with chronic hypercapnia, although associated chronic hypoxia is also responsible.[37] While reduction of blood bicarbonate levels should improve respiratory center responsiveness, central neuronal bicarbonate may lag several days behind blood changes. Carbonic anhydrate inhibitors, such as acetazolamide (Diamox), rapidly lower blood bicarbonate and presumably hasten the changes in central nervous system bicarbonate concentrations, restoring the central chemoreceptors' sensitivity to carbon dioxide.

Ventilatory Control in the Critically Ill Patient

A number of respiratory center abnormalities are observed in the critically ill patient. Shock, prolonged elevation of arterial carbon dioxide tension (hypercapnia), and sedation all decrease the activity of the central respiratory center. As little as 32 mg of phenobarbital decreases the ventilatory response to carbon dioxide in patients with emphysema. Greater depression is observed with 15 mg of morphine sulfate. Depression of the central respiratory center from any cause produces alveolar hypoventilation and hypercapnia.

Hyperventilation is extremely common in the critically ill patient. The central and reflex stimulatory drives summarized above may explain the striking hyperventilation exhibited by the patient presented in Table 6–3. Although arterial hydrogen ion concentration and oxygen tension were normal, venous hydrogen ion concentration and carbon dioxide tension were high and capable of stimulating both peripheral and central chemoreceptors. Erythrocyte pH, believed to be an indicator of tissue hydrogen ion concentration, was extremely low and suggests the environment that might have existed in the chemoreceptors.

The structure and function of the carotid body suggest that peripheral chemoreceptor stimulation may play an important role in the hyperventilation of hypotension. Hypotension decreases the rate of carotid body flow almost linearly, decreasing the oxidative metabolism and increasing the hydrogen ion concentration of carotid chemoreceptors. Well developed arteriovenous anastomoses have been identified in the carotid body and may provide an explanation of the extreme hyperventilation characteristic of septic shock. Hyperventilation is frequently the first physiologic event observed in experimental endotoxic shock; endotoxin may well promote carotid body arteriovenous shunting, decreasing the perfusion of chemoreceptor cells.

Kussmaul breathing—the deep and rapid respiratory pattern associated with metabolic acidosis—is due to stimulation of both central and peripheral chemoreceptors. Although the blood-brain barrier should prevent immediate direct stimulation by fixed acids, recent studies suggest that certain areas of the medulla (particularly the area postrema near the posterior part of the fourth ventricle) lack a blood-brain barrier, and may represent a site for direct stimulation of central chemoreceptors by fixed acids.

Cheyne-Stokes respiration is an unusual breathing pattern characterized by periods of hyperventilation and apnea. Typically, following a period of apnea the respiratory rate increases and then decreases in a crescendo-decrescendo pattern. Cheyne-Stokes respiration may exist for many years without obvious central nervous system disease, is usually not associated with cyanosis or polycythemia, and is most commonly seen in patients with heart disease. Certain of these patients are thought to have an abnormal central regulatory mechanism with alteration in the cyclic output to the respiratory muscles. Cheyne-Stokes respiration seen in conjunction with heart disease, however, probably is not due to an abnormal respiratory center but to the prolongation of circulation time. This is thought to cause the exposure of a normal respiratory center for relatively long periods of time to blood that contains either a higher or lower carbon dioxide tension. Blood passing through the pulmonary capillaries at the onset of inspiration normally has a carbon dioxide tension that is several millimeters of mercury lower than blood passing through just prior to renewal of alveolar air with the next inhalation. Presumably, the slow passage of carbon dioxide-rich blood through the respiratory center stimulates respiration, while that of blood low in carbon dioxide depresses respiration.

The Importance of the Diaphragm for Pulmonary Ventilation

A general understanding of the importance of diaphragmatic function to pulmonary ventilation has only recently been possible. Like the heart, the diaphragm must contract rhythmically against elastic and resistive forces and returns to a resting position after each contraction.[38] Most of the diaphragm's striated muscle fibers have good endurance characteristics; a transdiaphragmatic pressure of over 200 cm H_2O can be generated by the healthy individual during maximum effort. Both the force and duration of diaphragmatic contraction determine fatigue. Estimates of diaphragmatic contractile force may be made by tests which determine the onset of fatigue under a variety of ventilatory loads. Malnutrition, weight loss, and myopathy decrease ventilatory capacity and carbon dioxide tensions rise when muscle strength falls below 30% of normal. Decreased diaphragmatic blood flow, acidosis and hypercapnia reduce diaphragmatic function and may accelerate respiratory failure in critically ill patients. Recent efforts have shown that agents which increase cyclic AMP and are considered inotropes also improve diaphragmatic function. Aminophylline, caffeine, isoproterenol, and terbutaline have all been demonstrated to improve human diaphragmatic function.

REFERENCES

1. Cumming G, Horsfield K, Harding LK, et al: Biological branching systems with special reference to the lung airways. *Bull Physiopathol Respir* 1971; 7:31.

2. Hogg JC, Macklem PT, Thurlbeck WM: Site and nature of airway obstruction in chronic obstructive lung disease. *N Engl J Med* 1968; 278:1355.

3. Macklem PT, Mead J: Resistance of central and peripheral airways measured by a retrograde catheter. *J Appl Physiol* 1967; 22:395.

4. Head J, Turner JM, Macklem PT, Little JB: Significance of the relationship between lung recoil and maximum expiratory flow. *J Appl Physiol* 1967; 22:95.

5. Mead J: Mechanical properties of lungs. *Physiol Rev* 1961; 41:281.

6. Marshall R, Stone RW, Christie RV: The relationship of dyspnea to respiratory effort in normal subjects, mitral stenosis and emphysema. *Clin Sci* 1954; 13:625.

7. Forster RE: Exchange of gases between alveolar air and pulmonary capillary blood: Pulmonary diffusing capacity. *Physiol Rev* 1957; 37:391.

8. Roughton FJW, Forster RE: Relative importance of diffusion and chemical reaction rates in determining rate of exchange of gases in the human lung, with special reference to the true diffusing capacity of pulmonary membrane and volume of blood in the lung capillaries. *J Appl Physiol* 1957; 11:290.

9. Austrian R, McClement JH, Renzetti AD, et al: The syndromes of "alveolar-capillary block." *Am J Med* 1951; 11:667.

10. Finley TN, Swenson LW, Comroe JH: The cause of arterial hypoxemia at rest in patients with "alveolar-capillary block syndrome." *J Clin Invest* 1962; 41:618.

11. Arnot H, King TKC, Briscoe WA: Diffusing capacities and ventilation: Perfusion ratios in patients with clinical syndrome of alveolar-capillary block. *J Clin Invest* 1970; 49:408.

12. Ayres SM: The structural basis of pulmonary function, in Shoemaker WC, Thompson WL (eds): *Critical Care: State of the Art.* Fullerton, CA, Society of Critical Care Medicine, 1981.

13. Hyman AL, Spannhake WE, Kadowitz PI: Prostaglandins and the lung. *Am Rev Respir Dis* 1978; 117:111.

14. McGiff JC, Wong PY: Compartmentalization of prostaglandins and prostacyclin within the kidney: Implications for renal function. *Fed Proc* 1979; 38:89.

15. Otis AB, McKerrow CB, Bartlett RA, et al: Mechanical factors in distribution of pulmonary ventilation. *J Appl Physiol* 1956; 8:427.

16. Riley RL, Cournand A: Analysis of factors affecting partial pressures of O_2 and CO_2 in gas and blood of lungs: Theory. *J Appl Physiol* 1951; 4:77.

17. Farhi LE, Rahn H: A theoretical analysis of the alveolar-arterial oxygen difference with special reference to the distribution effect. *J Appl Physiol* 1955; 7:699.

18. West JB: Regional differences in gas exchange in the lung of erect man. *J Appl Physiol* 1962; 17:893.

19. West JB, Dollery CT, Naimark A: Distribution of blood flow in isolated lung: Relation to vascular and alveolar pressures. *J Appl Physiol* 1964; 19:713.

20. Finley TN, Lenfant C, Haab P, et al: Venous admixture in the pulmonary circulation of anesthetized dogs. *J Appl Physiol* 1960; 15:418.

21. Bristow GK, Kirk BW: Venous mixture

and lung water in healthy subjects over 50 years of age. *J Appl Physiol* 1971; 30:552.

22. Lenfant C: Measurement of ventilation perfusion distribution with alveolar-arterial differences. *J Appl Physiol* 1963; 18:1090.

23. Robin EO, Forkner CE Jr, Bromberg PA, et al: Alveolar gas exchange in clinical pulmonary embolism. *N Engl J Med* 1960; 262:283.

24. Clark JM, Lambertsen CJ: Alveolar-arterial O_2 differences in man at 0.2, 1.0, 2.0, and 3.5 Ata inspired Po_2. *J Appl Physiol* 1971; 30:753.

25. Morgan TE: Pulmonary surfactant. *N Engl J Med* 1971; 284:1185.

26. Mead J, Collier C: Relation of volume history of lungs to respiratory mechanics in anesthetized dogs. *J Appl Physiol* 1959; 14:669.

27. Caro CG, Butler J, DuBois AB: Some effects of restriction of chest cage expansion on pulmonary function in man: An experimental study. *J Clin Invest* 1960; 39:573.

28. Ferris BG Jr, Pollard DS: Effect of deep and quiet breathing on pulmonary compliance in man. *J Clin Invest* 1960; 39:143.

29. Marshall BE, Millar RA: Some factors influencing postoperative hypoxemia. *Anaesthesia* 1965; 20:408.

30. Pitts RF: Organization of the respiratory center. *Physiol Rev* 1946; 26:609.

31. Daly M de B, Lambertsen CJ, Schweitzer A: Observations on the volume of blood flow and oxygen utilization of the carotid body in the cat. *J Physiol* 1954; 125:67.

32. Hornbein TF, Roos A: Specificity of H ion concentration as a carotid chemoreceptor stimulus. *J Appl Physiol* 1963; 18:580.

33. Witzler EW: The excitation of chemoreceptors by arterial hypoxia and hypercapnia, in Cunningham DJC, Lloyd BB (eds): *Regulation of Human Respiration*. Philadelphia, FA Davis, 1963, pp 173–182.

34. Alexander JK, West JR, Wood JA, et al: Analysis of the respiratory response to carbon dioxide inhalation in varying clinical states of hypercapnia, anoxia, and acid-base derangement. *J Clin Invest* 1955; 34:511.

35. Brodovsky D, Macdonnel JA, Cherniack RM: The respiratory response to carbon dioxide in health and in emphysema. *J Clin Invest* 1960; 39:724.

36. Severinghaus JW, Mitchell RA, Richardson BW, et al: Respiratory control at high altitude suggesting active transport regulation of CSF pH. *J Appl Physiol* 1963; 18:1155.

37. Lee JE, Chu F, Posner JB, Plum F: Buffering capacity of cerebrospinal fluid in acute respiratory acidosis in dogs. *Am J Physiol* 1969; 217:1035.

38. Rochester DF: The diaphragm: Contractile properties and fatigue. *J Clin Invest* 1985; 75:1397–1402.

7 RESPIRATORY DYSFUNCTION AND FAILURE

The idea that failure to breathe was not synonymous with death began to gain credence with the wartime development of demand valves and positive pressure resuscitation equipment between 1941–45, and with the use of positive and negative pressure ventilators during the poliomyelitis epidemics of 1948–1952. McCann, Lovejoy, and Yu in 1952[1] developed the concept of the failing lung, pointing out that both intrapulmonary and extrapulmonary events could cause the lung to fail, and that either hypocapnia or hypercapnia could result. Between 1955 and 1965, the use of mechanical ventilation in patients with hypoxemia or hypercapnia secondary to severe airflow obstruction was described.[2] The tank respirator was used to treat severe staphylococcal pneumonia.[3] Acute pulmonary edema was treated with mechanical ventilation[4] and we, in 1968, treated acute respiratory acidosis complicating status asthmaticus with volume cycled ventilators.[5]

Successful treatment of respiratory failure requires the integrated use of a group of techniques collectively termed *respiratory therapy* and administered by respiratory therapists, physical therapists, registered nurses, physicians, and others. At one time, intermittent positive pressure breathing was considered the central technique of respiratory therapy. Better understanding of the physiologic effects of positive pressure ventilation and steadily improved ventilator design has led to improved support therapy with fewer complications. The use of intermittent positive pressure breathing as a panacea, or even placebo, for many respiratory disorders has all but disappeared. A randomized multi-institutional study of 3,218 patients with chronic obstructive lung disease failed to demonstrate improvement when IPPB was compared to bronchodilator therapy administered by air compressor.[6]

The use of respiratory therapeutic techniques should be based on the identification of specific pathophysiologic abnormalities; the treatment of patients with acute respiratory failure associated with chronic obstructive lung disease is quite different from the acute respiratory failure associated with diffuse pulmonary vascular leakage. Inhalation or aerosol therapy is indicated when airway obstruction is present. Oxygen therapy should be prescribed if hypoxemia is documented. Ventilatory therapy is indicated if hypercapnia or hypocapnia suggests that alveolar ventilation is inappropriate to metabolic needs. Physical techniques are used to remove airway secretions, improve the volume and distribution of alveolar ventilation, and maintain the function of the musculo-skeletal system.

The first edition of *Care of the Critically Ill* detailed experiences in a combined medical and surgical intensive care unit, and led to the identification of two groups of seriously ill patients with acute respiratory failure: those with hypoxemia and hypercapnia (respiratory failure associated with chronic obstructive lung disease, acute airways obstruction, and hypoventilation) and those with hypoxemia and normal or lower than normal carbon dioxide tensions. In 1969, Ashbaugh et al.[7] christened the latter syndrome the Adult Respiratory Distress Syndrome and provided important experimental evidence that positive end-expiratory pressure could prevent, as well as treat, this form of respiratory failure. Grouping all patients with acute respiratory failure developing after serious illness or injury into a new nosologic pigeonhole was a satisfying tour de force that focused attention on a group of situations that led to relatively similar structural and functional abnormalities. More recent studies have shown differences among patients with different etiologic events. Patients with respiratory failure associated with sepsis or pneumonitis, for example, appear more resistant to positive end-expiratory pressure than those with trauma and sustain a substantially higher mortality. The maturation of critical care practice requires much more emphasis on etiologic diagnosis and pathogenetic mechanism and much less reliance on stereotyped therapeutic responses. The mechanistic labels that served well in the formative years of respiratory care units should be discarded, perhaps, in favor of more informative diagnoses, such as acute respiratory failure associated with sepsis or acute respiratory failure with chronic airflow obstruction.

Precise nomenclature of *stages* of abnormal function are necessary for scientific communication and education. In general, organ dysfunction suggests a level of abnormality still consistent with the ability to meet metabolic needs during rest. Frequently, an individual may appear to be relatively normal at rest, but may exhibit physiologic abnormalities during exercise or other stress. Organ insufficiency or failure, in contrast, suggests that the organ is not performing adequately, and its output at rest is less than normal. Obviously, the level of deviation from normal is some evidence of the severity of the underlying malfunction.

Respiratory failure is generally diagnosed when the patient's arterial oxygen tension has fallen below 50 mm Hg while breathing ambient air. A classification system developed by the National Heart, Lung and Blood Institute,[8] and based on treatment rather than arterial oxygenation, has become a generally accepted approach for stratifying patients.

Mild: FIO_2 less than 50%. May or may not be intubated and require positive airway pressure.

Moderately Severe: FIO_2 more than 50% and intubated with positive airway pressure for more than 24 hours.

Severe: FIO_2 100% for eight hours or longer or more than 60% for 48 hours or longer. Intubated, controlled ventilation, and positive end-expiratory pressure.

These criteria were developed by groups emphasizing controlled ventilation and treating patients with the acute respiratory distress syndrome. While they may not apply to other diagnostic categories, they do demonstrate the importance of risk stratification.

PATHOPHYSIOLOGIC CONSIDERATIONS

Venoarterial Shunting

The effect of true venoarterial shunting on arterial oxygen tension was described earlier. While a number of anatomic venoarterial connections contribute to the right-to-left shunt observed in normal individuals, increased right-to-left shunting in disease states is primarily due to alveolar closure with persistence of capillary blood flow. Perhaps the most common cause of alveolar closure is atelectasis. The factors contributing to the development of atelectasis were also detailed earlier. Many of these are preventable and reversible with adequate programs of respiratory care. Another common cause of venoarterial shunting is the combination of pulmonary capillary congestion, interstitial edema, and atelectasis, known as congestive atelectasis. Sudden increases in pulmonary capillary pressure lead to obliteration of alveoli by pulmonary edema fluid. Bronchopneumonia with terminal airway obstruction, asthma with bronchospasm and mucus accumulation, and lobar consolidation are other causes of alveolar closure with venoarterial shunting.

It is important to recognize that administered oxygen cannot penetrate the obliterated alveoli and reach the pulmonary capillary blood (see Fig 6–15B). Any increase in mixed arterial oxygen saturation associated with oxygen enrichment of the inspired air is achieved by 100% saturation of blood draining well-ventilated alveoli. The simple expedient of breathing 100% oxygen produces an adequate arterial oxyhemoglobin concentration when as much as 30% of the lung is collapsed (Fig 7-1). A low cardiac output enhances the effect of the shunt on arterial oxygen tension, so that lower tensions result for the same percentage of collapse. The illustration also points out that hyperbaric oxygen at 2 atm can compensate for even larger shunts. The additional oxygen must all arrive in the pulmonary capillaries from normal alveoli; however, hyperbaric oxygen obviously does nothing for the obliterated alveoli, and indeed may speed the development of atelectasis in other borderline alveolar segments.

While oxygen therapy is the first line of defense in treating the hypoxemia of right-to-left shunting, definitive therapy involves the reexpansion of obliterated or congested alveoli. Most of the pathologic processes leading to collapse are reversible—reexpansion with relief of hypoxemia is frequently possible, if life can be supported by respiratory management while definitive measures are vigorously employed.

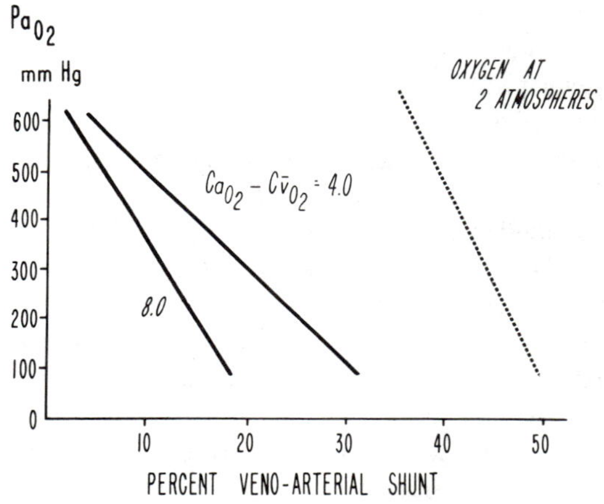

FIG 7–1.
Relationship between arterial oxygen during the breathing of 100% oxygen and venoarterial shunting. Values are plotted for normal arteriovenous oxygen content of 4.0 vol % and also for a CaO_2-$C\bar{v}O_2$ of 8.0 %. The latter value would be found with low cardiac output. Arterial oxygen tension progressively falls as the shunt increases. The lower oxygen tension is observed, for the same venoarterial shunt, in the patient with the abnormally large arteriovenous oxygen difference. Normal oxyhemoglobin saturation may be maintained in the patient with normal cardiac output and a venoarterial shunt comprising as much as 30 % of the cardiac output by the administration of 100% oxygen. Dashed line demonstrates that the breathing of oxygen at 2 atm pressure can maintain a normal oxyhemoglobin saturation in the presence of a venoarterial shunt, 50% of the cardiac output, and CaO_2-$C\bar{v}O_2$ of 4.0 vol.

Ventilation/Perfusion Abnormalities

The venoarterial shunt mechanism described above is commonly found in patients with nonobstructive (restrictive) acute respiratory failure—the so-called adult respiratory distress syndrome. In a sense, alveolar units in these patients are either open and ventilated or obliterated and nonventilated. In contrast to this are the alveolar units in patients with chronic obstructive lung disease. This disease process characteristically involves the lung in an irregular fashion, producing bronchial obstruction and alveolar destruction in some areas, bronchitis alone in others, and islands of perfectly normal lung tissue in between. Many of the diseased alveolar units are still capable of ventilation, but ventilate at extremely low rates. If perfusion through these segments is also reduced, the balance of ventilation/perfusion may be normal. If perfusion is maintained, extremely low ventilation/perfusion relationships result.

Low ventilation/perfusion ratios reduce mixed arterial oxygen tension. Of great importance for the design of oxygen therapy is the fact that even low concentrations of oxygen can penetrate poorly ventilated alveoli and increase mixed arterial oxygen tension (see Fig 6–15B). An important difference between the true venoarterial shunt pattern and the ventilation/perfusion inequality pattern is that, while the totally obliterated alveoli are useless for oxygen exchange, partially ventilated units are still capable of transferring oxygen to capillary blood. For this reason, high concentrations of oxygen are necessary to overcome the effects of true shunting, but relatively low concentrations of oxygen are adequate when hypoxemia is due to unequal distribution of ventilation/perfusion.

Obviously, both of these two abnormalities are examples of ventilation/perfusion imbalance. The true shunt is an extreme case where the ventilation/perfusion ratio is zero. Another extreme example of ventilation/perfusion imbalance arises when alveolar units are adequately ventilated but completely unperfused; their ventilation/perfusion ratio is actually infinity. These units constitute alveolar dead space and are useless for gas exchange. Alterations in pulmonary blood flow associated with decreases in cardiac output, rises in left arterial pressure, changes in pulmonary vascular resistance, or pulmonary embolization may all lead to the emergence of alveolar units with extremely high ventilation/perfusion ratios.

Diffusion Block

A diffusion block is an unusual cause of arterial hypoxemia. In the classically described alveolar capillary block syndrome, oxygen saturation was slightly lower than normal at rest, but fell markedly with exercise. It rose to normal following 100% oxygen intake.

DETERMINANTS OF ARTERIAL CARBON DIOXIDE TENSION

Arterial carbon dioxide tension is a curvilinear function of alveolar ventilation (see Fig 1–14). The mathematical relationship is:

$$P_{CO_2} = \frac{(0.863)\dot{V}_{CO_2})}{\dot{V}_A}$$

where $\dot{V}_{CO_2}$ is the carbon dioxide production, and $\dot{V}_A$ is the alveolar ventilation.

Carbon Dioxide Production

The above equation expresses the obvious fact that an increase in the volume of carbon dioxide produced by the tissues increases the arterial carbon dioxide tension unless balanced by an equivalent increase in alveolar ventilation. Patients with hypermetabolism due to fever, anxiety, hyperthyroidism, or the ingestion of certain drugs such as salicylates may develop hypercapnia in the face of an apparently normal alveolar ventilation. Patients with hypometabolism due to coma, heavy sedation, or hypothyroidism may become hypocapnic if ventilators are set for predicted levels of minute ventilation.

Alveolar Ventilation

The denominator of the equation, alveolar ventilation, is the major clinical determinant of arterial carbon dioxide tension, since carbon dioxide production is usually relatively constant. Although total alveolar ventilation is emphasized by the equation, the relationship of alveolar ventilation to capillary perfusion is actually the determinant of carbon dioxide clearance. This may be visualized by considering the fate of carbon dioxide brought to the pulmonary capillary bed by the venous circulation. If most of the pulmonary capillary blood is distributed to units which are adequately ventilated (another way of saying normal ventilation/perfusion ratios), carbon dioxide is cleared. If significant portions of pulmonary capillary blood are delivered to regions which are poorly ventilated, carbon dioxide is not cleared.

The amount of well-ventilated tissue relative to the amount of poorly ventilated tissue determine the actual carbon dioxide tension. Hyperventilation of normal areas can reduce capillary carbon dioxide tension to below 20 mm Hg and compensate for poorly ventilated areas with carbon dioxide tensions above 60 mm Hg. Since the carbon dioxide dissociation curve is relatively linear in this range, mixed arterial carbon dioxide may be close to normal. The effect of unequal distribution of ventilation/perfusion ratios on oxyhemoglobin saturation is quite different. Hyperventilation can obviously not increase saturation above 100%, so that hyperventilation of normal areas rarely corrects the hypoxemia produced by poorly ventilated areas. For this reason, arterial hypoxemia commonly occurs with normal carbon dioxide tensions.

Carbon Dioxide Tensions in the Critically Ill

Arterial carbon dioxide tension varies from normal levels whenever alveolar ventilation is inappropriate to metabolic needs.[9] The distribution of carbon dioxide tensions in 500 critically ill patients is shown in Figure 7–2. Note that while the modal value is close to 40 mm Hg, many extremely high and extremely low levels were observed. While the high-level tail of the distribution curve has long been known to represent serious respiratory malfunction, recent studies suggest that the low-level tail represents an equally damaging syndrome.

Hyperventilation in the critically ill patient was investigated in 19 consecutive patients with carbon dioxide tensions less than 15 mm Hg. Twelve of these patients were breathing without assistance; the remainder were mechanically ventilated. Shock was present in 92%; there was evidence of sepsis in 67%; and cardiac arrhythmias appeared in 42%. The pH was alkalotic, bicarbonate was low (average, 10.8 mEq/liter), potassium and chloride were normal (4.4 and 97.0 mEq/liter), and unidentified anions, presumably lactate, averaged 28.8 mEq/liter.

The mortality in these 19 patients was 89%. In contrast, mortality rates were 77, 74, and 28%, respectively, when carbon

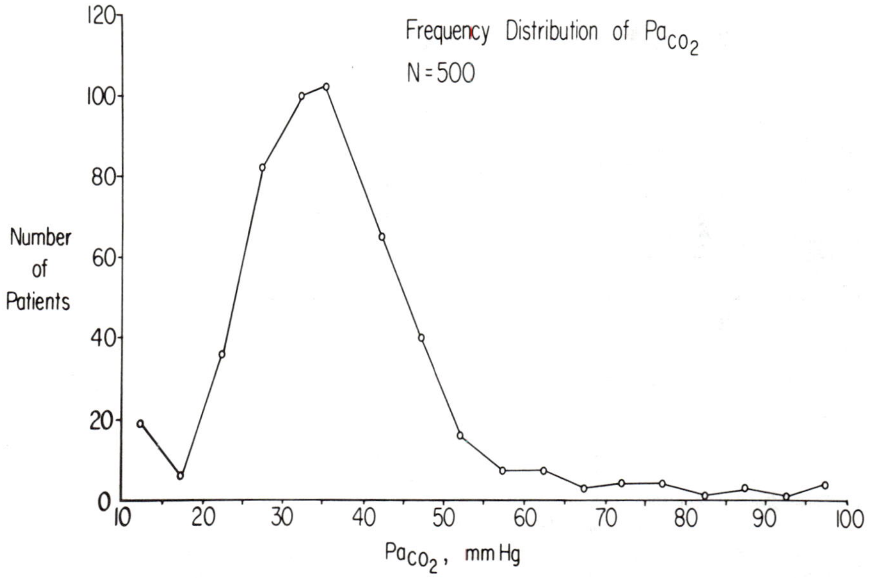

FIG 7–2.
Distribution of arterial carbon dioxide tension in 500 consecutive patients in an intensive care unit. Note that while most of the patients have relatively normal carbon dioxide tensions, many have hypo- and hypercapnia.

dioxide tensions ranged from 20 to 24, 25 to 30, and 35 to 45 mm Hg. Hypocapnia appears to be an important prognostic sign, but it is likely that the factors leading to massive hyperventilation (shock and sepsis) rather than the hypocapnia per se were responsible for the high death rate.

PHYSIOLOGIC EFFECTS OF HYPOXIA

Cardiovascular Responses to Hypoxemia

Oxygen delivery—the product of cardiac output and arterial oxygen content—could be maintained in the face of hypoxemia if cardiac output were increased. The cardiovascular response to sudden hypoxemia in a group of young subjects is shown in Table 7–1.[10] Arterial oxygen tension was decreased to 34 mm Hg, leading to significant increases in cardiac output, arterial blood pressure, and pulse rate. That these responses were due to stimulation of the sympathetic nervous system was shown by the observation that pretreatment with a beta blocking agent (pronethalol) almost completely eliminated the effect. The response is not completely abolished because hypoxemia also acts directly on vascular smooth muscle, producing vasodilatation. The resultant decrease in peripheral vascular resistance increases both cardiac output and regional blood flow. In most patients, hypertension and tachycardia are valuable signs of hypoxemia, as increased cardiac output attempts to maintain blood pressure in the face of hypoxia-mediated peripheral dilation. In certain critically ill patients and in patients who have taken sympatholytic drugs, the sympathetic nervous system response is inadequate, and hypotension, bradycardia, and circulatory arrest are observed.

While oxygen delivery may be maintained by increasing blood flow, a price

TABLE 7–1.
Circulatory Response to Acute Hypoxia[a]

PARAMETER	ROOM AIR	7.5% OXYGEN
Pa_{O_2} (mm Hg)	90	34
PCO_2 (mm Hg)	39	31
Cardiac index (liters/minute/meter^2)	2.8	4.3
Heart rate (beats/minute)	72	101
Forearm blood flow (ml/100 ml/minute)	2.4	3.2
AFTER SYMPATHETIC BLOCKADE WITH PRONETHALOL		
Pa_{O_2} (mm Hg)	90	33
PCO_2 (mm Hg)	39	31
Cardiac index (liters/minute/meter^2)	2.6	3.3
Heart rate (beats/minute)	70	91
Forearm blood flow (ml/100 ml/minute)	3.2	4.0

[a]Adapted from Richardson DW, Kontos HA, Raper AJ, Patterson JL Jr: Modification by beta-adrenergic blockade of the circulatory responses to acute hypoxia in man. *J Clin Invest* 1967; 46:77.
Hypoxic values are statistically different from control values for all measurements. Cardiac index and heart rate demonstrate statistically significant reduction in hypoxic effect following beta blockade with pronethalol. Pronethalol did not change hypoxic response of forearm flow.

is paid. The increased cardiac output and tachycardia increase cardiac work by as much as 50%, increasing myocardial oxygen demands. Such a response is possible in the healthy heart for short periods of time, but may be disastrous in the diseased heart. For this reason, cardiac output is usually normal or but slightly elevated in normal man living at high altitudes for prolonged periods of time. In these individuals, oxygen delivery is maintained by chronic hyperventilation (which elevates arterial oxygen tension and decreases carbon dioxide tension), plycythemia, and shifts in the hemoglobin dissociation curve.

Hypoxemia and Polycythemia

The oxygen delivery equation may also be balanced by increasing red cell mass, since each gram of hemoglobin binds approximately 1.34 ml of oxygen when completely saturated (see Fig 1–9). Polycythemia is commonly observed in individuals living at high altitudes and in chronically hypoxemic patients. Recent studies show that hypoxia stimulates the kidneys to produce erythropoietin, a substance which stimulates the bone marrow to increase its rate of red cell production. While an increase in hematocrit or hemoglobin concentration is the most obvious way to diagnose polycythemia, Filley[11] emphasized that associated expansions in blood volume may mask an increase in red blood cell mass.

Polycythemia is a useful adaptive response to chronic hypoxemia, particularly in patients with significant right-to-left shunts. Otis[12] calculated that an increase in oxygen capacity from 25 to 30 ml/100 ml in a patient with a right-to-left shunt and an arterial saturation of 75% would increase arterial oxygen tension by 9 mm Hg. Filley suggested that the increased plasma volume accompanying the polycythemia of hypoxemia may be a second adaptive mechanism, tending to maintain cardiac output in the face of increased viscosity.[11] With hematocrits in excess of 55–60, viscosity effects appear to overshadow the increased oxygen-carrying ability of polycythemia. Cardiac output is decreased by the increased vascular resistance produced by increased viscosity (see Poiseille equation, chapter 4), and oxygen delivery may fall. In this situation, phlebotomy is probably indicated.

Shifts in the Oxyhemoglobin Dissociation Curve

Rightward shifts of the oxyhemoglobin dissociation curve allow enhanced unloading of oxygen at higher venous oxygen tensions (see Fig 1–6). The important discovery of Benesch and Benesch,[13] that 2,3-diphosphoglyceric acid (2,3-DPG) regulates the position of the oxyhemoglobin dissociation curve, explains still another physiologic adaptation to hypoxemia. Hurtado[14] observed that the oxyhemoglobin dissociation curve is shifted to the right in natives living at high altitudes in the Chilean Andes, but could not explain this by either carbon dioxide or hydrogen ion changes. The explanation lies in an immediate increase in red cell 2,3-DPG, which shifts the oxyhemoglobin dissociation curve to the right. Lenfant and associates[15] took seven volunteers to an altitude of 15,000 feet and observed that the red blood cell 2,3-DPG increased from 90 to 142 μM phosphate per 100 ml packed cells while the P-50 (unloading tension) increased from 26.6 to 28.6 mm Hg, indicating a rightward shift of the curve (chapter 1).

Similar rightward shifts have been observed in patients with coronary arterial disease and in other conditions associated with hypoxia. A rightward shift in the oxyhemoglobin dissociation curve equivalent to a decrease in pH of 7.40–7.20 could maintain oxygen consumption and increase venous oxygen tension from 27 to 33 (see Fig 1–9).

Regional Oxygen Delivery in Hypoxemia

The examples given thus far have considered total oxygen delivery to the peripheral tissues. Since the overall aim of respiratory therapy is the delivery of adequate oxygen to all organ systems, an understanding of the factors influencing regional perfusion in the critically ill patient is important. Perfusion of various organ systems and the response of the regional beds to hypoxemia, hypercapnia, and sympathetic stimulation were discussed in Chapters 4 and 5. Several examples of regional oxygen delivery are given here to emphasize that oxygen delivery to one organ might decrease, even when total oxygen delivery is increased.

Figure 7–3 shows that cerebral oxygen delivery is decreased by the arterial hypoxemia demonstrated in Figure 1–

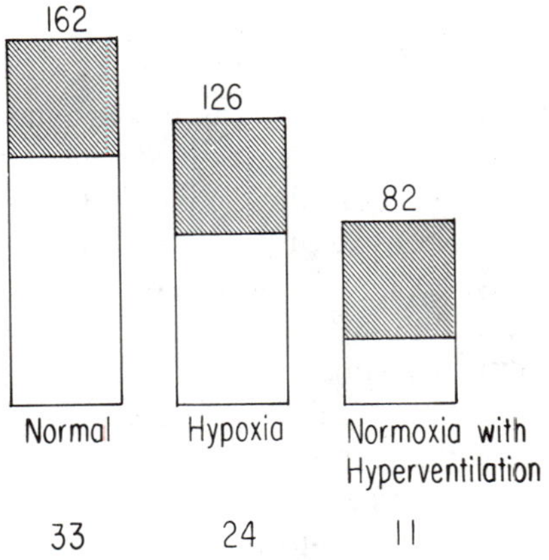

FIG 7–3.
Oxygen delivery in the cerebral circulation. The bars represent the same factors as in Figure 7–1. Arterial hypoxemia of the degree shown in Figure 7–1 reduces oxygen delivery to the brain. Hyperventilation with a respirator restores arterial oxygen tension to normal, but by dropping the carbon dioxide tension markedly reduces cerebral blood flow. Total oxygen delivery is actually lower than in the hypoxemic state, and mixed venous oxygen tension falls to 11 mm Hg.

9. If a patient is hyperventilated following intubation sufficiently to reduce carbon dioxide tension from 60 to 30 mm Hg, cerebral blood flow and oxygen delivery would significantly decrease. Renal oxygen delivery is also decreased by the general hypoxemia illustrated in Figure 1–9. A general sympathetic response of the type shown in Table 7–1 would increase cardiac output in an attempt to maintain total oxygen delivery, but would produce renal arteriolar constriction (chapter 4), reducing renal blood flow and oxygen delivery. These two examples reveal that hypocapnia and sympathetic stimulation are capable of reducing blood flow in certain vascular beds, and may actually decrease oxygen delivery.

PHYSIOLOGIC EFFECTS OF CHANGES IN CARBON DIOXIDE TENSION

Vascular Effects

Increased concentrations of carbon dioxide, like reduced concentrations of oxygen, increase peripheral blood flow and stimulate the sympathetic nervous system. The only exception to this general rule is the pulmonary vascular bed, which exhibits vasoconstriction in response to both hypoxia and hypercapnia. Carbon dioxide is an extremely potent cerebral vasodilator, explaining why hypercapnia may produce cerebral edema, increased intracranial pressure, headache, drowsiness, and coma. It may occasionally even produce papilledema leading to a brain tumorlike syndrome. Increased extremity blood flow produces cutaneous redness and increased sweating.

Carbon dioxide increases tissue hydrogen ion concentration and depresses most metabolic processes. It is not clear whether a decrease in oxygen availability or increased hydrogen ion concentration is the primary rate-limiting step in tissue energy production, but the combination of hypercapnia and hypoxia is clearly a major threat to the integrity of the organism.

Hydrogen Ion Responses to Hypocapnia and Hypercapnia

The changes in hydrogen and bicarbonate ion concentrations associated with acute or chronic changes in carbon dioxide tensions were discussed in Chapter 5. Much of these data were obtained on laboratory animals or in normal man. Hydrogen ion changes actually observed in patients with extreme alterations in carbon dioxide tension are shown in Figure 7–4. Hydrogen ion concentration is plotted against carbon dioxide tension, and the confidence limits of Brackett, Conen, and

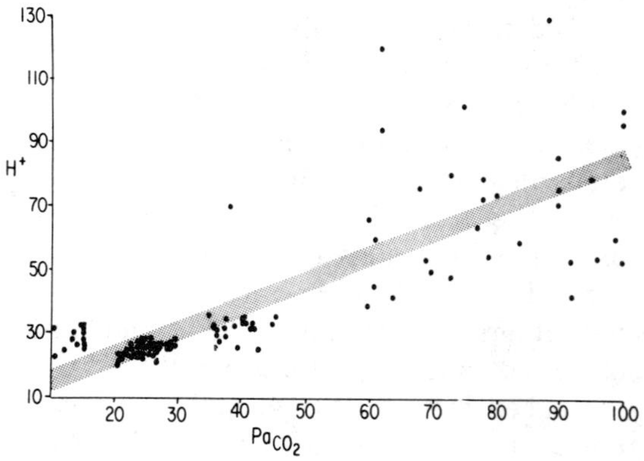

FIG 7–4.
Response of hydrogen ion concentration to alterations in arterial carbon dioxide tension in a group of patients in an intensive care unit. Shaded area shows the predicted change in hydrogen ion concentration associated with acute elevations of carbon dioxide tension. Points falling above the confidence limits indicate decreased buffering capacity, while points below the confidence limits represent increased buffering capacity. (Adapted from Brackett NC Jr, Cohen JJ, Schwartz WB: Carbon dioxide titration curve of normal man: effect of increasing degrees of acute hypercapnia on acid-base equilibrium. *N Engl J Med* 1965; 272:6.)

Schwartz[16] are shown for reference. Many of the patients with low carbon dioxide tensions have relatively high hydrogen ion concentrations, suggesting an associated bicarbonate or buffer base deficit. The effect of this simultaneous decrease in buffer base (probably not "compensation," but an associated metabolic abnormality) is to produce a pH in the 7.40–7.55 range. Only in several patients did the pH exceed 7.70.

The hydrogen ion response to high carbon dioxide tension varies widely depending upon the buffer stores of the patients. While in vitro blood equilibration and canine studies demonstrate the qualitative nature of total body buffering, studies on chronically hypercapnic patients are necessary to evaluate fully the relationship of body buffer stores to acute hypercapnia. Figure 7–5 shows a series of pH-carbon dioxide tension curves generated from data on patients with high carbon dioxide tensions. These patients had been intubated and ventilated with a volume-cycled ventilator. Carbon dioxide tension promptly fell to normal levels, allowing calculation of the change in pH associated with a rapid change in carbon dioxide tension. The slope (dH^+/dP_{CO_2}) averaged 1.24 with a normal bicarbonate concentration and fell to 0.16 when the plasma bicarbonate concentration was 40 mEq/liter. Figure 7–5 allows prediction of pH shift for any bicarbonate level, and demonstrates the importance of total body buffering in minimizing the increase in hydrogen ion associated with an acute increase in carbon dioxide tension. Chronic increases in buffer capacity protect the organism against sudden increases in carbon dioxide tension. Marked acidosis may develop if carbon dioxide tension rises acutely in patients with normal or decreased buffer stores (the shock patient, for example).

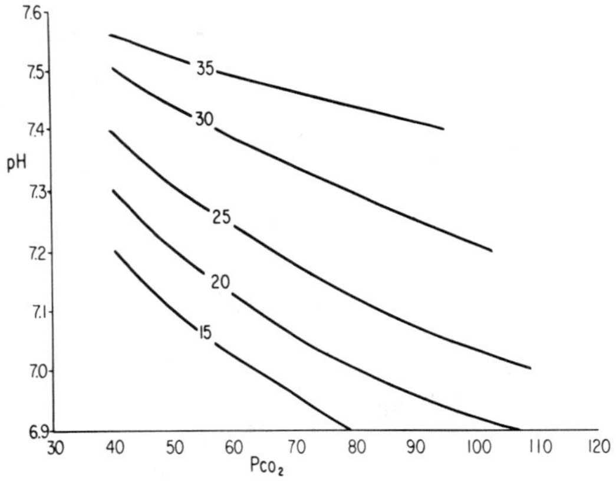

FIG 7–5.
pH responses to acute hypercapnia are shown for different plasma bicarbonate concentrations. Each curve represents the total body buffer effect to changes in carbon dioxide tension. Note the progressive flatness of the response curves with increasing plasma bicarbonate. Acute hypercapnia is obviously much more hazardous to a patient with normal or low plasma bicarbonate concentration.

Electrolyte Changes

Table 7–2 lists average plasma electrolyte changes for the patients presented in Figure 7–4. Hypochloremia is striking in the chronically hypercapnic patient and is reciprocal to the increase in bicarbonate concentration. Potassium concentrations are similar, on the average, in all three groups of patients, in spite of theoretical predictions of hypokalemia with hypocapnia and hyperkalemia with hypercapnia. Other factors such as glomerular filtration rate, mineralocorticoid secretion, potassium intake, and diuretic usage also affect potassium balance. Plasma potassium levels varied widely in these patients and could not be predicted from either carbon dioxide tension or bicarbonate concentration.

TABLE 7–2.
Electrolyte Changes Associated with Hypocapnia and Hypercapnia

PARAMETER	HYPOCAPNIA	HYPERCAPNIA ACUTE	HYPERCAPNIA CHRONIC
P_{CO_2} (mm Hg)	13	73	83
pH (units)	7.55	7.13	7.29
HCO_3 (mEq/liter)	10.8	23.1	38.4
Cl^- (mEq/liter)	97	99	89
Lactate (mEq/liter)	29	–	–
K^+ (mEq/liter)	4.4	4.2	4.2

SPECIFIC FORMS OF ACUTE RESPIRATORY FAILURE

Acute respiratory failure may occur in a number of clinical situations producing diffuse lung damage and may be associated with hypoventilation, normal ventilation, or hyperventilation. The pathophysiology and clinical manifestations are related to the presence of obstructive or restrictive defects, to the underlying status of lung function prior to the development of respiratory failure, and to etiology. Treatment is strikingly different for the patient with chronic obstructive lung disease and acute respiratory failure compared to one with acute diffuse lung damage in previously normal lungs (The Acute Respiratory Distress Syndrome). A classification of clinical varieties of respiratory failure follows:

1. **Airway obstructive diseases** (associated with ventilatory failure)
   a. Chronic obstructive lung disease with acute hypoventilation usually due to pulmonary infection or to injudicious use of sedation or oxygen.
   b. Acute obstructive lung disease due to bronchospasm or retained secretions (status asthmaticus).
2. **Restrictive lung disease** (usually associated with hyperventilation)
   a. Chronic restrictive disease such as pulmonary fibrosis, chronic inflammatory disease, kyphoscoliosis.
   b. Acute restrictive disease usually occurring with previously normal lungs: the "stiff lung syndrome" or adult respiratory distress syndrome occurs in a variety of situations: the postoperative state, pulmonary edema, shock, aspiration pneumonitis, trauma, viral pneumonitis, sepsis, and fat embolization.
3. **Acute ventilatory failure** due to respiratory center or neuromuscular dysfunction.

More than one variety of respiratory failure may occur in the same patient; a patient with chronic obstructive lung disease may have abnormal respiratory muscle function or may have an automobile accident producing the adult respiratory distress syndrome. In addition, ARDS is not a homogenous syndrome, and mortality may vary widely with its etiology.[17]

ARDS, acute respiratory failure associated with chronic airways obstruction, and acute respiratory failure due to bronchospasm are discussed in the following pages. Acute respiratory failure due to other causes such as trauma and drug overdosage are discussed in Chapter 11. Rather arbitrarily, the uses of mechanical ventilation, airway management, continuous positive airway pressure (CPAP), and techniques of airway management are considered in the section on ARDS, while oxygen enrichment of the inspired air and aerosol therapy are discussed in the section on chronic airway obstruction.

THE ADULT RESPIRATORY DISTRESS SYNDROME (ARDS)

This important syndrome is a high-permeability interstitial and alveolar edema associated with bilateral alveolar infiltrates, refractory hypoxemia, a rigid noncompliant lung and the absence of evidence of left ventricular failure. Most studies have required mechanical ventilation, a pulmonary capillary wedge pressure less than some defined value, a total static compliance of 50 ml/cm H_2O, and an arterial to alveolar partial pressure of oxygen ratio of 0.2 or less. Using criteria such as these, two recent studies[18,19] reported that 6.8% and 22.7% of those considered to be at risk developed the syndrome. The overall mortality for patients with ARDS was 64.8% and 68%, respectively. These mortality figures are similar to those reported in the many studies that appeared after the initial report of Ashbaugh et al.[7] (See Table 7–3)[20–30]. Etiology, diagnostic criteria, and treatment may affect the reported mortality.[31] Cotev et al.[17] described 57 patients treated with positive end-expiratory pressure delivered by conventional methods. All but two of the 28 nonseptic patients increased arterial oxygenation with positive end-expiratory pressure; the overall mortality was 18%. Only 20 of 29 septic patients responded with increased oxygenation and the increase was one-third that of the nonseptic patients; the overall mortality was 62%. Douglas and Downs[26] reported that 80% of 54 patients treated with intermittent mandatory ventilation were alive three months after leaving the hospital (see p. 240). Rinaldo[32] pointed out that the rigorous admission requirements developed by most investigators excluded many individuals with a less severe form of the syndrome, particularly those where pulmonary artery catheterization was not thought to be indicated. She reported an overall mortality of 30% in

TABLE 7–3.
Mortality in the Adult Respiratory Distress Syndrome

STUDY	YEAR	NUMBER	MORTALITY
Bartlett(20)	1975	45	53%
Kirby(21)	1975	28	39%
Klein(22)	1976	36	47%
Bone(23)	1976	30	77%
Lashminarayan(24)	1976	55	58%
Cotev(17)	1976	57	62% (septic)
			18% (others)
Lamay(25)	1976	45	67%
Douglas(26)	1977	54	20%
Zapol(27)	1977	30	80%
Yahav(28)	1978	15	29%
Gallagher(29)	1980	315	28%
Bell(30)	1983	141	74%

patients who would have been excluded. These patients included the entire trauma population and all patients under 30 years of age without multiple organ failure.

Table 7–4 presents the patients at risk, the percentage of the syndrome who died, and the mortality rate for each grouping reported by Fowler et al.[18] The median time for developing the syndrome was 22 hours; with aspiration or burns, it occurred much earlier. The close temporal relationship to the inciting event becomes an important differential point since pulmonary embolization usually occurs somewhat later in the hospital course.

Sepsis and multiple organ failure are interwoven with most reported incidence and mortality statistics. Fein et al.[33] showed that all of 21 patients with septic shock but only 12 of 95 with sepsis but without shock developed the syndrome. The study of Montgomery et al.[19] showed that sepsis was either a direct or contributing cause of death in three-quarters of those who died with respiratory failure. Other deaths were due to multiple organ failure or to severe central nervous system disease that developed prior to admission. Both the studies by Fowler et al.[18] and Fein et al.[33] demonstrated that the risk factors shown in Table 7–2 were cumulative; increased numbers of risk factors were associated with an increased risk of developing respiratory failure.

Pathology and Pathophysiology

Studies of respiratory failure demonstrated the importance of massive capillary leakage in the development of the syndrome. Granular leukocytes, red blood cells, macrophages, cell debris, and proteinaceous material filled the alveolar spaces while alveolar septa bulged with edema fluid and migrated cells.[25,34] A good correlation between morphologic changes and physiologic consequences has been demonstrated. Impairment of gas exchange in the early stages is caused mainly by the filling of alveoli with edema fluid and formed elements of the blood. A large veno-arterial shunt, hypoxemia, decreased pulmonary compliance, and a modest elevation of pulmonary vascular resistance are present.

TABLE 7–4.
Risk Factors for Developing the Adult Respiratory Distress Syndrome

	NUMBER AT RISK	INCIDENCE OF ARDS	MORTALITY FROM ARDS
Cardiopulmonary Bypass	237	1.7%	50.0%
Burn	87	2.3%	50.0%
Bacteremia	239	3.9%	77.8%
Hypertransfusion	197	4.6%	44.4%
Fracture	38	5.3%	0
Pneumonia in ICU	84	11.9%	60.0%
Disseminated Intravascular Coagulation	9	22.2%	50.0%
Pulmonary Aspiration	45	35.6%	93.8%
All Single Risk Patients	936	5.8%	66.7%
Multiple Risk Patients	57	24.6%	71.4%

Adapted from Fowler AA, Hamman RF, Good JT, et al: Adult respiratory distress syndrome: risk with common predispositions. *Ann Intern Med* 1983; 98:593–597.

It is in this stage that positive end-expiratory pressure seems most effective in increasing functional residual capacity and decreasing veno-arterial shunting. In later stages, the lungs become progressively less compliant as chronic inflammatory changes and fibrosis occur. Higher inflation pressures are required, pulmonary vascular resistance and alveolar dead space increase, and end-expiratory pressure becomes less effective in decreasing the veno-arterial shunt.

Elegant ultrastructural studies by Bachofen, Gehr, and Weibel[35] using the scanning electron microscope provide a startling image; lungs fixed between 60% and 100% of total lung capacity exhibit a remarkably smooth alveolar surface and resemble a group of concave mirrors fastened together. Pressure-volume curves observed when surfactant was destroyed by rinsing with detergent were markedly abnormal and resembled some of the problems seen in the acute respiratory distress syndrome. Higher pressures were needed for inflation at low lung volumes and a decrease in hysteresis led to the need for relatively high pressures to maintain lung inflation during deflation. In other words, there was a striking tendency for alveolar collapse during deflation. Even at high lung volumes there were areas of atelectasis; with deflation, thickened septa surrounded large airspaces suggesting multiple collapsed alveoli with tilted alveolar ducts. The collapsed units never involved entire segments or lobules but were scattered at random throughout the entire parenchyma.

The final common pathway linking together patients with the acute respiratory distress syndrome seems to be increased vascular permeability. The wet weight of the normal mammalian lung is about four times its dry weight after water has been removed; the wet/dry ratio rises remarkably whenever the lung's defenses are breached, and capillary fluid swirls through the interstitium, flooding the alveolar space and destroying the lung's ability to exchange gases. Starling, in 1896,[36] proposed that the exchange of fluid between capillary and tissue was related to (1) the hydrostatic pressure on each side of the capillary wall, (2) the osmotic pressure of protein in plasma and tissue fluids and (3) the permeability characteristic of the vascular membrane. Pappenheimer and Soto-Rivera[37] demonstrated that plasma proteins and their osmotic or oncotic pressure were the major forces preventing leakage into the perivascular tissues. Alterations of these Starling forces (hydrostatic pressure, plasma protein concentration and vascular permeability) play a major role in the pathogenesis of cardiogenic pulmonary edema, ascites, myxedema, development of a third space in seriously ill patients, and the adult respiratory distress syndrome. An important difference exists in the Starling forces acting across the pulmonary vascular bed compared to those in the periphery. Plasma oncotic pressure is about 25 mm Hg, while measurements of lung lymph have suggested the interstitial oncotic pressure to be close to 19 mm Hg. In consequence, the interstitial to capillary oncotic ratio is 0.8 and 0.5 for albumin and globulin in the lung respectively. The oncotic ratio for the periphery is much lower (0.23) explaining the clinical observation that fluid appears in the lung interstitium before the periphery.

The sheep model developed by Staub, Nagano, and Pearce[38] provided a method for estimating transvascular fluid exchange by measuring a major portion of the lymphatic drainage of the lung. These studies demonstrated that there was a continuous flow of lymph from the lung with baseline pressures and a linear increase in lymph flow with an elevation in pulmonary venous pressures. Lung water did not increase until pulmonary venous pressures were about 25 mm Hg because the lung lymphatics were able to remove water at lower transvascular filtration rates. The protein concentration of lung lymph was 60% that of plasma during basal flow; it fell to much lower levels when pulmonary vascular pressures were elevated, suggesting that edema fluid was actually a transudate. Note that the increased hydrostatic pressure washes out interstitial proteins, decreasing the interstitial oncotic pressure and reducing the transudation of fluid.

Brigham et al.[39] developed a permeability model for lung damage by infusing gram negative endotoxin into unanesthetized sheep. Pulmonary vasoconstriction, bronchoconstriction, a decline in cardiac output, and the development of a low protein content pulmonary edema occur within the first hour of endotoxin infusion. Several hours later, pulmonary vascular pressures fall and the identification of protein-rich pulmonary edema fluid signifies the development of increased vascular permeability. Serial biopsy studies show sequestration of neutrophils and lymphocytes within the lung parenchyma. Leukocytes then degranulate and pass between endothelial cells into the interstitium. Endothelial damage is observed within one hour of endotoxin administration. The model provides an opportunity for the evaluation of a variety of therapeutic interventions (see "Treatment" p. 224).

Vascular "permeability" reflects both permeability per vascular unit and the total surface area of vessels available for fluid exchange. A dilated vascular bed would increase fluid exchange and also magnify hypoxemia by enhancing the venoarterial shunt. Vasoconstriction, in contrast, would reduce fluid exchange and hypoxemia, but could increase right ventricular afterload. The release of vasodilator prostanoids such as PGI_2 (prostacyclin), perhaps released during endothelial injury, evokes generalized vasodilatation and could exaggerate the existing pulmonary capillary leak. Administration of a cyclooxygenase inhibitor, Ibuprofen, to animals with experimental permeability edema decreases the concentration of PGI_2, lung water, and the veno-arterial shunt.[40]

An understanding of the permeability/surface area relationship may explain certain relationships between abnormalities in gas exchange and lung water. Brigham, et al.[41] measured lung water using a multiple isotope-indicating dilution method and a "permeability/surface area" coefficient (P/S ratio) by measuring the exchange of the small molecule urea. Alveolar-arterial gas exchange could not be correlated with increases in extravascular lung water, but appeared related to the P/S ratio. Gas exchange and probability of survival were greater in patients with low P/S ratios, suggesting that vasoconstriction and derecruitment of exchanging vessels reduced the net capillary leak into the alveolar spaces.

Fluid must cross both endothelial and epithelial membranes to produce alveolar edema. The clearance of aerosolized technetium labeled diethylenetriamine pentasacetic acid increases with epithelial injury. An increased clearance is observed in patients with ARDS, but not in those with cardiogenic pulmonary edema.[42] Use of indicators that measure either epithelial or endothelial permeability indicates the initial locus of damage and may provide more precise evaluation of the locus of lung injury. Increased concentration of labeled albumin identifies patients with ARDS and signifies damage to both endothelial and epithelial cells.

Pathogenesis

A number of converging lines of evidence suggest that hypoxemia, sepsis, trauma, volume contraction, and hypotension can initiate an immunologic sequence that produces diffuse lung injury. Landis[43] found that the pulmonary capillary permeability for proteins was increased following three minutes of oxygen deprivation. McCabe[44] showed that complement levels were decreased in patients with bacteremic shock and postulated activation of the alternative pathway. A group of studies showed that complement activation during hemodialysis produced a hypoxemic syndrome, probably mediated by oxygen radicals, that damaged pulmonary endothelial cells.[45] Monocytes, granulocytes, and platelets have all been shown to participate in this process.

Bronchoalveolar lavage studies have confirmed pathologic findings and demonstrated a massive migration of granulocytes to the alveolar spaces. Only 3% of cells obtained from bronchoalveolar lavage fluid obtained from nonsmoking normal volunteers were granulocytes, while patients with the adult respiratory distress syndrome had an average of 85% neutrophils.[46] Fowler et al. found almost identical concentrations of protein and granulocytes in lavage fluid from patients at risk and those with established respiratory failure[47]; others have correlated the percentage of neutrophils in lavage fluid with the degree of alveolar-capillary gas exchange.

The lung is the major storage site for noncirculating or marginated granulocytes. Their migration to alveolar spaces after serious injury or illness but before the onset of clinical lung disease has focused attention on the appearance of chemotactic factors that might initiate the entire pathogenetic sequence. Gathering information suggests that the macrophage has many more purposes than the phagocytic function, which has been studied for many years.[48] It now appears that the alveolar macrophage, and perhaps other macrophages, are endocrine organs that prepare the entire organism for defensive action (Figure 7–6). A group of soluble macrophage products known as monokines function as modulators of the inflammatory response and immune, endocrine, and metabolic function. Macrophage products are clearly chemotactic[49–51] and appear to trigger the migration of granulocytes to the alveolar spaces. Other monocyte products attract and activate platelets, lymphocytes, and presumably other macrophages to the

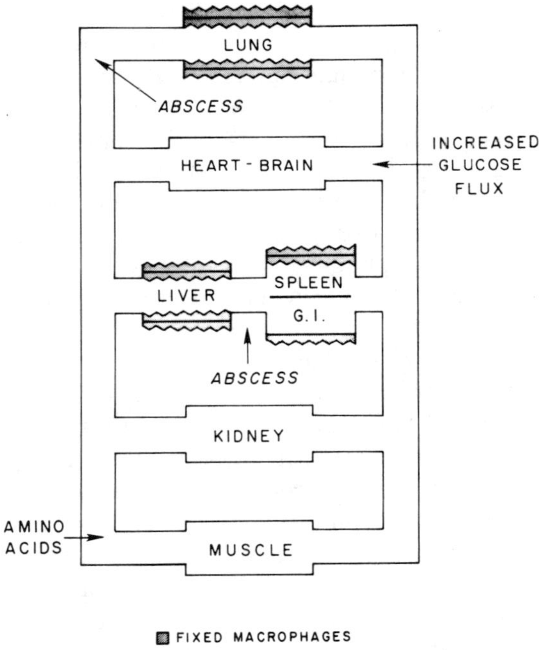

FIG 7–6.
The shaded areas in this diagram of the circulation represent the reticuloendothelial or macrophage system. Bacteria escaping from an abdominal abscess are phagocytosed by macrophages in the liver and spleen as well as those lining the peritoneum. Circulating bacteria are removed by macrophages located within the lungs. Also indicated is the macrophage-initiated increase in glucose flux to vital organs and release of amino acids from skeletal muscle. The amino acids are transported to the liver and used for the synthesis of acute phase reactants.

lung. The complement cascade, long implicated as part of the early warning system, collaborates with the monokines to attract and activate granulocytes to the alveolar spaces. The strategic position of the lung astride the returning venous blood and the presence of a large noncirculating pool of macrophages and granulocytes make diffuse lung damage a common early consequence of serious illness.

The pulmonary immune response is obviously a two-edged sword. Its importance to the defense of the lung is demonstrated by the observation that mortality is substantially higher in individuals who have less than 10% immature forms in their circulating blood.[52] On the other hand, noxious stimuli might change the nature of macrophage secretory products so that they become less effective in defensive functions. Perhaps the nature of the activating stimulus determines the character of the macrophage response. Jacobs, Kiel, and Balk[53] noted that macrophages obtained from animals with *E. coli* induced acute respiratory failure produce excessive amounts of hydrogen peroxide. These macrophages, however, also exhibited reduced phagocytosis of *E. coli* and *Staphylococcus aureus*, and were less able to kill these bacteria than unstimulated macrophages. Observations such as these may partially explain the pathogenesis of pneumonia in certain individuals, the common finding of pulmonary infection in association with acute respiratory failure, and the development of nosocomial infections in hospitalized patients.

ARDS is occasionally seen in patients with chemotherapy-induced leukopenia, suggesting either that a small number of granulocytes can initiate lung damage or that the noncirculating granulocyte pool is less sensitive to destruction by these agents. Ognibene et al. from Parrillo's laboratory[54] recently described 11 patients with severe neutropenia who developed classic ARDS. Lung biopsies revealed the typical histologic characteristics of the syndrome except for the leukocytic infiltration commonly observed. Rinaldo and Borovetz[55] observed that gas exchange worsened as granulocyte counts returned toward normal in granulocytopenic patients.

These observations emphasize that both activation and response in ARDS are diverse, and that the idea of complement activation followed by granulocytic chemorecruitment is only part of the story.[56] Macrophages, granulocytes, lymphocytes, and platelets contain most of the lipases, cyclooxgenases, lipooxygenases, and other necessary machinery to convert membrane phosopholipid into prostanoids and leukotrienes; thromboxane B_2, PGI_2, PGE_2, leukotriene B_4, and other mediators[57] have been found in lavage fluid. Interleukin-1 (IL-1) from macrophages produces fever, muscle proteolysis, enhanced liver synthesis of acute phase reactants, and recruits other elements of the immune system (see chapter 2). Macrophage-derived platelet activation factor and endothelial injury initiates the coagulation cascade, and infusion of thrombin has been shown to produce a model of ARDS.[58] Factor VIII, antithrombin, and fragments of the coagulation cascade also have been found in lavage fluid. While the macrophage-reticuloendothelial system, complement and coagulation cascades, and neuroadrenergic axis are probably all ultimately activated in the respiratory distress syndrome, it is likely that different insults enter the final pathway at different points. Trauma may initially activate the neuroadrenergic acid and coagulation cascade, while sepsis initially activates the macrophage and complement systems.

Many substances produced in the immune response directly affect cell function. Granulocytic enzymes such as lysozyme, elastase, and collagenase are cytotoxic; elastase and collagenase have been found in lavage fluid, and Weiland et al.[59] have shown this fluid to damage alveolar cells. The leukotrienes B, C and D all increase vascular permeability, and PGE_2 markedly potentiates the effects of the leukotrienes, presumably because of its vasodilator activity. PGE_2 has other diverse activities that are ultimately harmful. It plays a role in the activation of granulocytes, can enhance T cell activity, and amplifies the effects of peptide pyrogens.[60]

A lymphocyte product, interleukin-2 (see chapter 2), has received considerable recent attention because its use as an antitumor substance has produced a syndrome resembling sepsis. Administration of interleukin-2 for four days to four patients by Ognibene an colleagues at the National Institutes of Health[61] increased cardiac index by 1.88 L/min/M^2 and heart rate by 56 beats per minute. Mean arterial pressure decreased by 30 mm Hg and systemic vascular resistance by 480 dynes-sec-cm^5. All developed oliguria, plasma creatine increased by 120 mg/dl, and one patient developed ARDS. The C5a fragment of complement was increased, emphasizing the parallel nature of soluble monocyte factors and the complement cascade. All patients returned to normal after discontinuation of IL-2.

A great deal of current interest has centered on the production of toxic oxygen metabolites.[62] Each oxygen atom in the oxygen molecule contains but six electrons on its outer orbital ring and shares two electrons with its sister atom in order to complete its outer circle (Fig 1–12). The passage of electrons from a variety of substrates to these receptive atoms reduces oxygen and produces water (biological oxidation). Incomplete reduction of oxygen, in contrast, produces certain active substances. A gain of one electron to the oxygen molecule leads to the superoxide anion, while two electrons produce hydrogen peroxide. These irritant oxygen species are rapidly inactivated by superoxide dismutase and catalase, respectively. Since these reactive species appear rapidly inactivated, greater concern has been directed to the likelihood of the indirect peroxidation of lipids by superoxide anion. These peroxidation products and their free radicals are extremely cytotoxic and also increase the synthesis of prostanoids and leukotrienes (see chapter 2).

The early studies of Craddock et al.[63] have spawned a series of investigations focusing on the activation of macrophages, monocytes, granulocytes, and platelets. These must be viewed as related components of a complex defensive network that includes the nervous system and endocrine organs as well as the immune system itself. Different activators at different sites may produce different sequences, but ultimately converge to increase permeability and damage cells (see Figure 2-2).

Treatment

Experience based on many studies suggests that the key to prevention or early treatment of the adult respiratory distress syndrome is the maintenance of normal or even greater than normal oxygen delivery to all body tissues at the earliest possible moment after the recognition of serious injury or illness. Rapid correction of hypoxemia, acidosis, hypovolemia, infection, and inadequate blood flow appears to prevent amplification of the pulmonary macrophage-granulocyte response that explodes as the adult respiratory distress syndrome. It has been shown, for example, that early intubation and correction of fluid deficits in patients with multiple injuries prevent death from respiratory failure.[64] Assiduous attention to sources of nosocomial infection, such as endotracheal tubes and vascular catheters, is necessary to prevent hospital-acquired sepsis from initiating a late immunologic assault on the lung or other organs.

Considerable attention has recently focused on the use of pharmacologic agents that might interfere with the pathogenetic steps leading to increased pulmonary vascular permeability. Many proposed experimental interventions affect the synthesis of products of arachidonic metabolism, while others attempt to block the release of cytocidal products from granulocytes and other formed elements. Although promising, much of the work accomplished thus far must be considered experimental.

Glucocorticosteroids were introduced in 1948 for the treatment of rheumatoid arthritis and are known to have powerful effects on immune function. Their use in septic shock is controversial, although it is likely that the use of pharmacologic doses administered within several hours of an infectious insult may be efficacious. Brigham, Bowers, and McKeen[65], for example, showed that pretreatment with methylprednisolone prevented the high protein pulmonary edema that occurred following endotoxin administration in the sheep model. Corticosteroids inhibit phospholipase A_2, which releases arachidonic acid from membrane phospholipid sources. The specific action of cyclooxygenases and lipooxygenases produce the prostanoids and the leukotrienes (Fig 1-11). Corticosteroids appear to have more powerful anti-inflammatory effects than nonsteroidal anti-inflammatory agents. The latter agents inactivate cyclooxygenase, while corticosteroids appear to block the action of phospholipase A_2 affecting the synthesis of both prostanoids and leukotrienes. Recently it has been shown that both steroids and specific lipooxygenase inhibitors decrease the production of leukotriene B_4 which, in turn, inhibits T cell proliferation and the production by T cells of interleukin-2.[66]

The use of corticosteroids in patients with septic shock remains controversial because there have been no clinical studies clearly demonstrating improved survival with their use in patients with the adult respiratory distress syndrome. The Upjohn Pharmaceutical Company,[67] in an August 21, 1986 letter to the medical profession, presented preliminary results of a randomized, double-blinded study matching placebo against methylprednisolone, 30 mg/kg every six hours for a total of four doses. A higher mortality rate was observed in patients with an elevated plasma creatinine at entry or who developed a secondary infection after the institution of therapy. Since a complete statistical evaluation of the 382 patients has not been completed (it is known that certain problems in randomization may have complicated interpretation of results), the data must be regarded as preliminary. It is clear, however, that corticosteroids should be used with great care in seriously ill individuals.

Since the products of arachidonic metabolism are found in bronchoalveolar lavage fluid from patients with ARDS and in left atrial blood in animals treated with endotoxin, pharmacologic manipulation of leukotrienes and prostanoids might be useful therapeutically. While results from animal models never should be directly extrapolated to the human situation, a group of studies with the conscious sheep model provides important insights into the development of newer pharmacologic approaches. Shortly after infusion of endotoxin, the concentrations of metabolites of thromboxane A_2 and PGI_2 increase in blood and lung lymph; samples obtained from the left atrium appear to have greater concentrations of these substances than those from the pulmonary artery.[68] Cyclooxygenase inhibitors, thromboxane synthetase inhibitors, and agents decreasing the production of leukotriene D_4 but not leukocyte or platelet depletion markedly attenuate the early hypertensive response.[69] In contrast, neutrophil depletion and agents affecting leukotriene synthesis, but not cyclo-oxygenase inhibitors or platelet depletion, ameliorate the intensity of the later increased permeability phase.[70] Although thrombocytopenia does not accompany leukopenia in the sheep model, the data strongly suggest that the vasoconstrictor thromboxanes produce the initial vasoconstriction, while leukotrienes mediate the increase in permeability. Seilaff, et al.[71] have shown that ibuprofen given shortly after *Pseudomonas* infusion in pigs improves oxygenation and decreases veno-arterial shunting but does not decrease lung water. The addition of H_1 and H_2 blocking agents to ibuprofen, however, significantly decreased the capillary leak as measured by transvascular albumin flux.

Attention recently has been focused on the ability of activated granulocytes to release a group of oxygen radicals that include the superoxide ion (O_2^-), hydroxyl radicals (OH^-), and singlet oxygen. These free radicals are produced by the reduction of molecular oxygen and have been shown to produce endothelial cell damage in *in vitro* systems. N-acetylcystein is a free radical scavenger that has been shown to markedly decrease both the hypertensive and high permeability stages of endotoxin lung damage and to decrease the production of thromboxane and PGI_2.[72] The interwoven relationships among products of arachadonic metabolism, free radical generation, and alterations in immune cell function demonstrate the uncertainty of pharmacologic action in whole animal studies, however. Leukotrienes appear to enhance T cell production while monocyte derived PGE_2 can inhibit both T and B cell function.[73] Moreover, ibuprofen, a potent cyclooxygenase inhibitor, blocks the production of myeloperoxidase, lysozyme, superoxide ion, and both chemotactic and adherence factors by granulocytes.[74] A group of randomized clinical trials using some of these agents is currently underway. For most patients today, however, maintenance of adequate oxygenation and ventilation are the mainstay of therapy.

A confirmation of the importance of surfactant deficiency to the pathogenesis of the pediatric respiratory distress syndrome may have important implications for therapy of the adult syndrome. Hallman et al.[75] prepared surfactant from human amniotic fluid or bovine lungs and introduced the material through the endotracheal tube as a 3–5 ml bolus. The surfactants appeared to spread quickly throughout the lungs in very low birth weight infants with respiratory failure, improving oxygenation and pulmonary compliance and reducing the inspired oxygen requirements. In a subsequent study, workers from the same laboratory[76] demonstrated that prophylactic administration to similar size babies without respiratory distress prevented the respiratory distress syndrome or reduced its severity. Whether a similar approach in adults with AARDS will be effective remains to be determined.

Mechanical Ventilation

The evolving understanding of the use of mechanical ventilation has focused on several important considerations: (1) the circulatory effects of positive pressure ventilation, (2) the avoidance of lung collapse during expiration, and (3) the distribution of inspired air during inspiration.

Circulatory Consequences of Increased Intrapleural Pressure

Ventilator theorists of the early 1960s followed the doctrine enunciated by Cournand et al.[77] These studies showed that mean intrathoracic pressure was raised to a level capable of impeding venous return to the right ventricle when alveolar pressure was raised above atmospheric levels for more than 50% of the breathing cycle. Continuing investigation has emphasized the importance of rhythmic changes in intrapleural pressure to circulatory dynamics. These changes are consequent to shifts in the position of respiratory muscles and affect cardiac function by changing systemic venous flow, pulmonary vascular resistance, and the dimensions of the cardiac chambers. During spontaneous respiration, intrapleural pressure becomes progressively more negative, overcoming the retractive or collapsing tendency of the lung and producing airflow and alveolar expansion. The increasingly negative pressure increases the gradient between the sytemic venous reservoir and the right atrium, enhancing venous return. These upstream-downstream gradients that promote air and blood flow must be distinguished from the transmural pressure differences acting across vessel and chamber walls. The negative intrapleural pressure is transmitted to the right atrium, for example, so that it is lower than it would be if intrathoracic pressure were at atmospheric levels. A problem ensues since the usual hemodynamic measurements relate vascular pressure to atmospheric pressure rather than to intrapleural pressure. This convention leads to right atrial pressure falling during inspiration although the atrial pressure, relative to intrapleural pressure, is essentially unchanged. The major reason for considering these transmural pressure gradients is their effect on chamber or vessel size. A negative intrapleural pressure can be viewed as increasing atrial, ventricular, and vascular dimensions while positive intrathoracic pressure decreases them.

Guyton et al.[78] used a right heart bypass preparation to demonstrate that venous return and cardiac output could be manipulated simply by increasing or decreasing right atrial pressure (see Fig 4–12). Increasing right atrial pressure reduced the pressure gradient between the small veins and the right atrium so that flow diminished. Of great interest, increasing the rate of bypass pumping (the "heart rate") did not increase cardiac output, but merely caused the right atrium and the distal venous system to collapse. Pinsky[79] confirmed these observations in an intact canine preparation by using positive pressure ventilation to increase right atrial pressure and decrease venous return.

The driving pressure for venous return is the weighted average of pressure across the entire systemic vascular bed, which averages 12 mm Hg (mean systemic pressure). Versprille and Jansen[80] have shown that mean systemic pressure is equal to the pressure actually measured at the level of the small veins. Mean arterial pressure does not itself determine venous return because about 80% of the aortic pressure is lost by the time the blood reaches the small veins. Positive pressure ventilation would be disastrous to the heart if the peripheral circulation, independent of changes in cardiac output, did not increase venous return by redistributing systemic blood flow. This is accomplished by selective vasoconstriction in the splanchnic and renal vascular beds which reduces their blood volume and makes additional blood available to the right atrium. In addition, the velocity of blood flow is increased in the splanchnic and renal veins because their capacitance is decreased by venoconstriction. Volume deficient patients may be unable to maintain venous return by this mechanism unless volume is rapidly replaced to raise mean systemic pressure.

An elevated intrapleural pressure may aggravate the pulmonary hypertension and right ventricular dysfunction found in the adult respiratory distress syndrome. Positive pressure-associated increases in pulmonary vascular resistance add an additional afterload burden to the right ventricle and the effects of decreased venous return may be magnified in this situation. Left ventricular dysfunction may result from right ventricular dilatation and flattening of the ventricular septum; Prewitt and Wood[81] found that this mechanism accounted for about half of the reduction of cardiac output with high levels of positive end-expiratory pressure.

Left ventricular afterload may be increased by any substantial increase in lung volume, since the enhanced descent of the diaphragm increases intra-abdominal pressure and the resistance within the distal aorta. Increased lung volumes press on both ventricles and make ventricular filling more difficult. In addition, higher lung volumes increase pulmonary vascular capacity and may decrease left ventricular preload. There is also evidence that positive end-expiratory pressure depresses myocardial function by some neural or humoral mechanism.[81]

Kirby[82] has emphasized that while the effects of increased intrathoracic pressure are of concern, spontaneous breathing can also be harmful to individuals with severe ventricular failure. Deep inspirations with marked reductions in intrapleural pressure could increase lung water by increasing venous return to the heart; the deep descent of the diaphragm could increase left ventricular afterload.

The Prevention of Expiratory Collapse

Mead and Collier[83] found that lungs ventilated at constant volumes tended to develop regions of atelectasis. They observed that frequent deep inspirations or "sighs" reversed the tendency to atelectasis, and most ventilators designed in the 1960s incorporated automatic "sighing" devices because of those observations. The important text prepared by Bendixen and colleagues in 1965[84] advocated the use of high lung volumes and intermittent deeper inspirations to maintain oxygenation. Their work led to a substantial improvement in critical care practice, but unacceptable mortality in patients with acute respiratory failure remained. Several groups of investigators cautiously applied expiratory pressure during controlled mechanical ventilation. Ashbaugh et al.[7] systematically applied the technique to 14 patients with severe respiratory failure and observed improved oxygenation and a substantial decrease in overall mortality. Cardiac output did not fall, apparently because most of the positive airway pressure was spent in distending the rigid lung and was not transmitted to the pleural space. These authors proposed the principle that "absolute control of ventilation in these patients is mandatory."

Positive end-expiratory pressure works because it increases resting lung volume by increasing the transpulmonic pressure throughout expiration. Consider two alveolar units, one with normal surface properties and compliance, the other with reduced compliance and absent surfactant. When fully expanded, both are capable of oxygenating pulmonary capillary blood. As the individual expires, intrathoracic pressure becomes less negative, approaching -5 cm H_2O. At that point, the transpulmonic pressure difference is 5 cm H_2O, since airway pressure is zero. This distending pressure allows the normal unit to remain one-quarter inflated. Depending upon the pressure generated inwards by the diseased lung unit, it may completely collapse or may reduce itself to a lower than normal functional residual capacity. With end-expiratory pressure maintained at a greater than atmospheric level, transpulmonic pressure is increased and expiratory collapse is obviated. Figure 7–7 shows the dramatic effect of positive end-expiratory pressure on arterial oxygen tension and the alveolar-arterial oxygen gradient. Note that the arterial pulse pressure narrows in response to a decrease in venous return to the heart.

A number of studies have demonstrated that positive end-expiratory pressure improves gas exchange in seriously ill patients, and it is indicated in almost all patients receiving mechanical ventilation except those with chronic obstructive lung disease and hyperinflated lungs. Positive end-expiratory pressure reduced the alveolar-arterial oxygen difference and venoarterial shunt in a group of patients with extrathoracic trauma and relatively normal lungs.[85] Alveolar and arterial washout of argon revealed that positive end-expiratory pressure improved distribution of the inspired air and increased

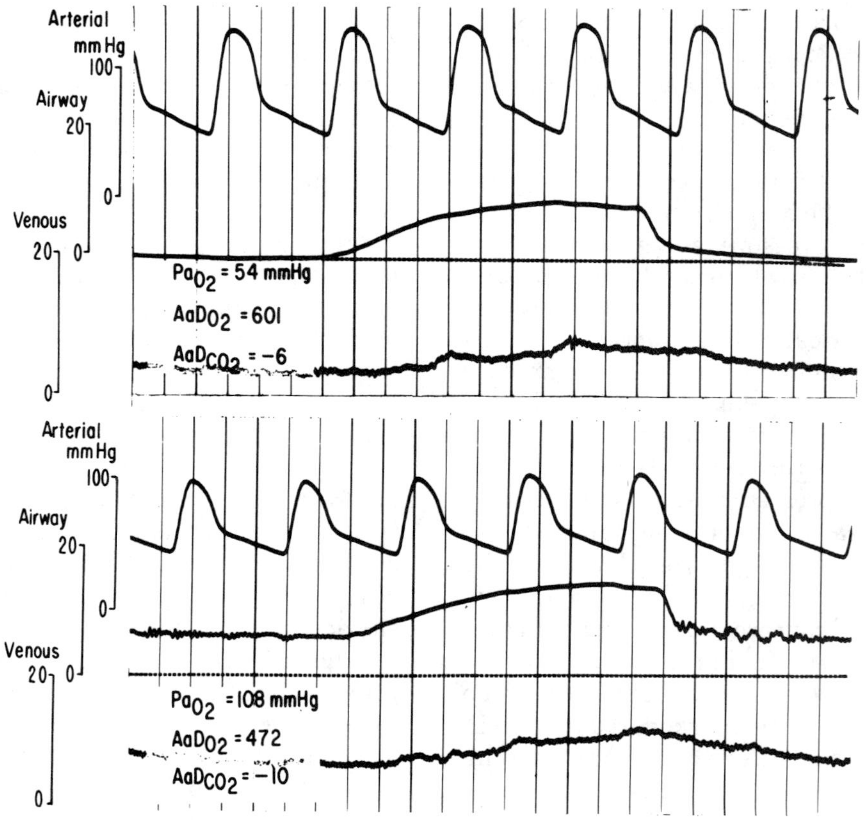

FIG 7–7.
Effect of continuous positive pressure breathing on arterial and venous pressure, airway pressure, and arterial gas tension. The level of airway pressure is higher and does not fall to atmospheric level with an increase in end tidal pressure. Continuous positive pressure ventilation in this patient markedly improved PaO_2, but decreased the arterial systolic and pulse pressure and increased the venous pressure. (From Ayres SM, et al: *Am J Cardiol* 1970; 26:588. Used by pemission.)

the functional residual capacity. The maintenance of lung expansion is not a function of positive end-expiratory pressure itself but rather a consequence of increasing transpulmonic or alveolar distending pressure throughout the breathing cycle. Continuous negative pressure applied to the thorax of newborn infants maintained an increased gradient between atmospheric pressure at the mouth and the negative extrathoracic pressure, later labeled "continuous distending pressure." The observation that the maintenance of increased transpulmonic pressure difference maintains alveolar inflation and appears to reverse progressive lung injury in the respiratory distress syndrome is important for the development of new techniques. One reason for the variable response of patients to high levels of PEEP is the existence of regional variations in lung mechanics. Oxygenation actually may deteriorate, for example, if PEEP is sufficiently high to impair blood flow in normal segments of the lung.

The Move Away from Controlled Ventilation

Experience over the past two decades has demonstrated that early intubation with positive pressure ventilation maintains alveolar integrity and provides the best chance for survival. The earlier emphasis on large tidal volumes with frequent sighs gave way to the realization that increasing functional residual capacity was more useful than increasing tidal volume. While most centers turned to positive end-expiratory pressure to improve oxygenation, and to reduced inspired oxygen concentrations in the adult respiratory distress syndrome, concern over the effects of increased intrathoracic pressure on cardiac output and blood pressure remained. The trade-off between respiratory and cardiovascular systems was starkly demonstrated by Lutch and Murray in 1972.[86] These investigators showed that positive end-expiratory pressure increased arterial oxygen tension but decreased cardiac output, venous oxygen tension, and overall oxygen delivery. In a study to determine the level of positive end-expiratory pressure that would improve oxygenation without affecting cardiac output, Suter, Fairley, and Isenberg in 1975[87] noted that when compliance increased to its maximum, cardiac output, oxygen transport, and venous oxygen tension were higher than they were initially. Increasing end-expiratory pressure from that point led to a decrease in compliance and a decrement in blood flow.

The theoretic basis for the optimization of lung-thorax compliance is best understood by plotting transpulmonic or distending pressure against lung volume. Figure 7–8 is based on the conceptual approach taken by Douglas and Downs.[88] The normal distending pressure when airway pressure is atmospheric is zero; the lung remains expanded at a functional residual volume related to the elastic properties of lung and thorax. Inspiration begins on a relatively steep segment of the pressure-volume curve so that a tidal volume is accomplished with minimal decrease in intrapleural pressure. Lung compliance is high, and the work of breathing is low. The increased stiffness of the lung in patients with the acute respiratory distress syndrome results in a rightward shift of that relationship. In consequence, functional residual capacity is reduced, and inspiration begins at a flatter segment of the curve; excessive distending pressures must be generated, and the work of breathing is increased. Note the contrasting effects of increasing end-expiratory distending pressure in different clinical situations. With the rightward shifted curve typical of the respiratory distress syndrome, increasing distending pressure moves the point at which inspiration is initiated to a steeper part

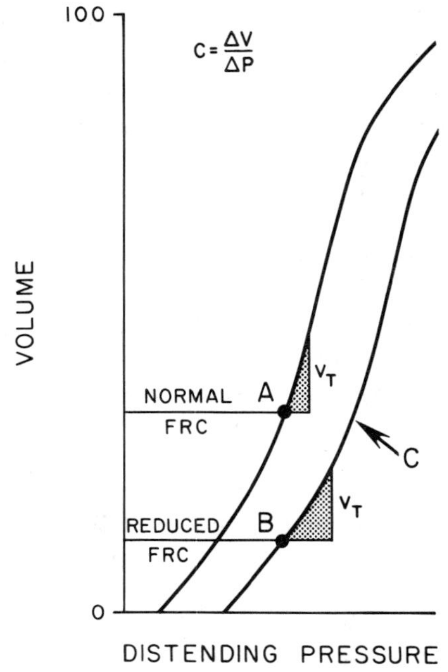

FIG 7–8.
The pressure-volume (P-V) curve of the lung and thorax. A tidal volume initiated at point A on the normal P-V curve requires much less pressure change than that initiated at a lower functional residual capacity (FRC), point C, on a rightward shifted curve due to decreased lung compliance V/P. Positive end expiratory pressure raises FRC to point C and reduces the pressure required for a tidal volume.

of the curve, improving lung compliance. In contrast, the same distending pressure in individuals with normally compliant lungs may move the point at which inspiration begins to the flatter top part of the curve and decreases lung compliance. The shapes and positions of pressure-volume curves vary widely among patients and change rapidly during hospitalization. Frequent titration of end-expiratory pressure to a level that allows tidal breathing with the lowest possible change in airway pressure is essential.

Early approaches to positive pressure ventilation had depended upon heavy sedation to permit total control of ventilation. Several observations caused many clinicians to question this approach: (1) controlled ventilation led to rapid deconditioning of systemic and ventilatory muscles, (2) the inspired air was not distributed as well with positive pressure ventilation, and (3) increased systemic venous pressure led to increased transvascular fluid filtration requiring the addition of replacement fluid such as albumin to augment alveolar ventilation. The technique of intermittent mandatory ventilation had been introduced to assist in the weaning of patients from mechanical ventilation but was soon used by Kirby[89] to exploit the advantages of spontaneous breathing with positive end-expiratory pressure (Table 7–5). The intermittent breaths delivered by the mechanical ventilator maintain minute ventilation. Arterial oxygen tension was much higher than that with controlled ventilation, presumably because spontaneous respiration was more effective in distributing the inspired air; cardiac output did not fall because mean intrathoracic pressure remained close to atmospheric most of the time. The advantages of intermittent mandatory ventilation with positive end-expiratory pressure are shown in Figures 7–9 and 7–10. Compared to data from a recently published series with controlled ventilation,[86] cardiac output is not depressed, and there is substantially better oxygenation because of better distribution of the inspired air with spontaneous breathing. IMV with either end-expiratory pressure or CPAP is particularly useful in patients who appear

TABLE 7–5.
Advantages of Spontaneous Breathing

Enhances Psychologic Well–Being
Maintains Respiratory Muscle Tone
Maintains Venous Return
Improves Distribution of Inspired Air

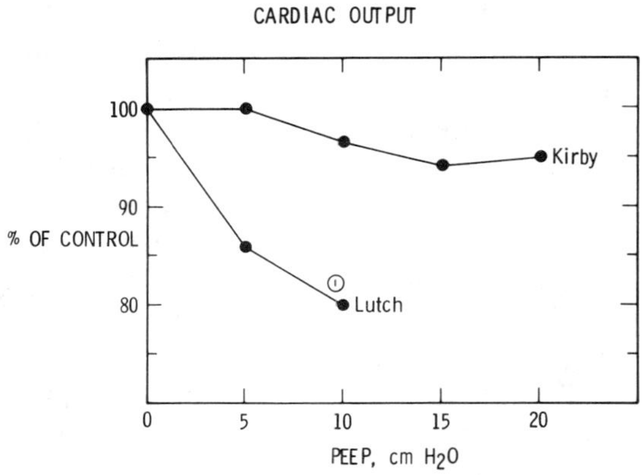

FIG 7–9.
Cardiac output and positive end-expiratory pressure in patients ventilated by intermittent mandatory ventilation compared to results with conventional controlled ventilation. See text for complete description.

to be ventilating adequately and who do not have excessive secretions. Kirby[82] has recently emphasized that patient selection is critical because some patients develop significant respiratory muscle fatigue and need continuous ventilatory support.

The Importance of Inspiratory Time, Flow and Pause

Not all patients can generate breaths of sufficient quality to allow use of intermittent mandatory ventilation, but the demonstrated value of spontaneous over controlled breathing has focused attention on the importance of the unassisted inspiratory process. When a normal animal lung is placed in a plethysmograph so that lung volume can be measured, lung volumes are observed to increase with constant or even decreasing airway pressure. This increased volume is due to the recruitment of additional alveolar units as they open in a sequence dependent upon their mechanical properties.[90] Differing resistances and compliances produce differing time constants in various lung regions. The inspired air is preferentially delivered to areas that fill and empty most easily. The problem of uneven distribution of inspired air is intensified by the spotty nature of lung damage in the adult respiratory distress syndrome. Conventional mechanical ventilation in the presence of marked variability in regional time constants increases the $\dot{V}/\dot{Q}$ mismatch and the degree of hypoxemia.

The mechanical properties of individual lung units affect overall lung function. The dynamic compliance of the total lung is not sensitive to inspiratory flow rate during spontaneous ventilation, but is strikingly dependent upon inspiratory flow rate during positive pressure ventilation.[91] The bolus of air applied to the airway simply cannot be distributed adequately to individual lung units. If patients cannot breathe spontaneously, mechanically derived inspiratory

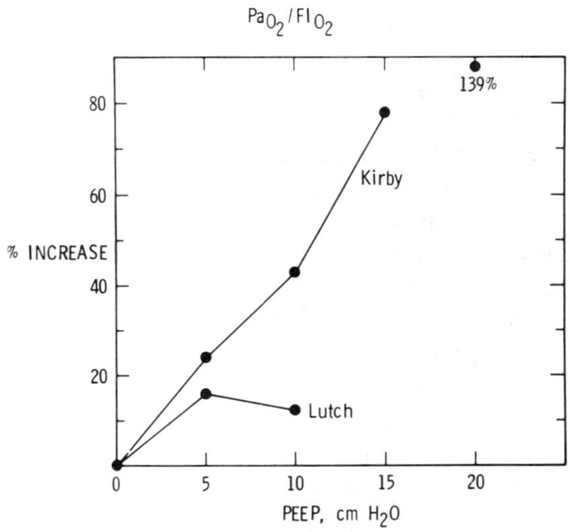

FIG 7–10.
Oxygenation, indicated by the ratio of arterial oxygen tension to inspired oxygen fraction and positive end-expiratory pressure compared to results with conventional ventilation. See text for complete description.

flow must be tailored to the individual needs of their abnormal lungs. An adequate tidal volume can be inhaled at a low flow rate only if the time of inspiration is prolonged or if the flow decreases during the inspiratory cycle.

Manginello et al., in 1978,[92] used a pressure limited ventilator with a prolonged inspiratory time and a reversed inspiratory/expiratory (I/E) ratio in a group of infants with hyaline membrane disease who could not be adequately oxygenated by conventional means. Peak pressures were about 50% lower with this technique, and improved oxygenation, enhanced survival, and less evidence of barotrauma were observed compared to those receiving conventional volume controlled ventilation.

Lachman et al.[93] used repeated bronchoalveolar lavage with normal saline to deplete surfactants in adult rabbits and beagles. An oxygen tension below 60 mm Hg during volume controlled breathing with 100% oxygen and an I/E ratio of 1:2 was reproducibly observed. They evaluated the importance of various breathing patterns in this model using a Servo ventilator 900 B (Siemens-Elema AB). Arterial oxygen tension and veno-arterial shunting improved remarkably as the inspiratory time was increased to 60% and 80% of total inspiration. Mean airway pressure increased, and cardiac output (and oxygen delivery) decreased as expected. A short inspiratory flow period with a prolonged pause produced the greatest improvement in oxygenation; higher frequency rates also had a better effect on oxygenation because the short inspirations kept airway pressures and alveolar units open. The investigators found that similar improvements in oxygenation could be achieved with either an I/E ratio of 4:1 and zero PEEP or an I/E ratio of 1:2 and 16 cm H_2O PEEP. The use of PEEP produced higher inflation pressures, a decrease in alveolar ventilation to 50% of control and major increases in carbon dioxide tension. They also observed substantial atelectasis, epithelial desquamation, and alveolar edema with an I/E ratio of 1:2. Animals ventilated with an I/E ratio of 4:1 showed well-expanded lungs with much less edema. This last observation is of particular importance since it suggests that high peak pressures delivered to open alveolar units may create shearing forces responsible for tissue damage.

Two patients treated with inverse ratio ventilation by Gurevitch et al.[94] confirm the value of this approach in certain situations. Each had deteriorated despite treatment with intermittent mandatory ventilation and positive end-expiratory pressure. They concluded that better oxygenation at lower airway pressures was due to "progressive alveolar recruitment with stabilization of surfactant-deficient regions."

High frequency ventilation (HFV) with cycling at rates in excess of 60 per second (1 Hz) includes high frequency positive pressure ventilation, high frequency jet ventilation, and high frequency oscillation. So many different approaches to HFV have been proposed that it is difficult to draw definitive conclusions. Frequent small tidal volumes lower peak airway pressures and improve convective gas exchange. These properties might be expected to lower complication rates, but patient outcomes did not vary appreciably when HFV was compared to conventional therapy in a randomized study of patients with acute respiratory failure.[95] Siegel et al.[96] have used advanced monitoring techniques to evaluate the effects of varying modes of ventilator support on lung mechanics, and have reported improved gas exchange at low inflation pressures in selected patients. They describe one patient treated at the Maryland Institute for Emergency Services where conventional volume controlled ventilation with optimized settings led to a 199 ml pleural air leak, a peak airway pressure of 83 cm H_2O, and marked arterial hypoxemia. They combined two ventilator techniques to obtain the advantage of rhythmic lung inflations with the lower peak pressure of HFV. Peak airway pressure was decreased to 65 H_2O and the veno-arterial shunt decreased from 57% to 31%. Their studies and others suggest the need for individualized approaches in the patient requiring high inflation pressures. HFV in particular may be indicated in patients with bronchopleural fistulae and in premature infants with hyaline membrane disease.

An additional approach to ventilatory support is extracorporeal membrane oxygenation (ECMO). ECMO does not appear to improve survival rates in the adult respiratory distress syndrome,[97] but may be useful in infants with respiratory distress[98] and following cardiac surgery.

Selection of Ventilators

Kirby,[82] in a detailed review of the design and application of positive pressure ventilators, suggested that they could be classified on the basis of (1) constant or variable inspiratory flow, (2) constant or nonconstant pressure generation, (3) presence of inflation hold, (4) method of shift from inspiration to expiration, (5) expiratory phase, and (6) shift from expiration to inspiration.

The shift from pressure cycling to volume cycling to signal the change from inspiration to expiration marked the beginning of modern ventilatory management. Pressure cycled ventilators are notoriously unreliable because air flows into the lung until a preselected pressure is achieved. At that point, the respirator cycles, flow ceases, and expiration occurs. The volume of air delivered depends upon the mechanical properties of airways, lungs, and thorax, as well as the preselected pressure and flow rates. For this reason it is sometimes called a pressure-constant, volume-variable ventilator. A leak in the apparatus may lead to a failure to cycle; a mucus plug obstructing a major bronchus may produce a rapid raise in airway pressure leading to a premature cut off of tidal volume. It is difficult to maintain a constant tidal volume with these ventilators because of frequent changes in resistance and compliance in the critically ill patient. If used, constant monitoring with expired air ventilometry and frequent arterial blood gas analysis is necessary.

The volume-cycled ventilator was designed because alveolar ventilation—not airway pressure—is the major determinant of arterial carbon dioxide tension. With this unit, air flows into the lung until a preselected volume is delivered. The pressure generated depends upon the mechanical properties of lung and airway, but volume depends upon the setting selected by the operator. Tidal volume does change as pressure is increased, however, because gas is compressed within the ventilator circuit. Two or three hundred ml of volume may be compressed and thus lost to the patient when lung compliance is extremely low.

A variety of techniques initiate inspiration. Controlled mechanical ventilation (CMV) is conceptually the simplest mode; preselected tidal volumes are delivered at the selected rate. This mode is usually undesirable in the awake patient, however, since it is not possible to breathe faster or slower than the set rate. The inability to match tidal volume to patient need limits the use of this technique.

Assist-control (A/C) ventilation is a refinement of CMV; the preselected tidal volume is delivered at the selected rate. Should the patient attempt to initiate a subsequent breath prior to the next scheduled breath, the ventilator senses the inspiratory effort and delivers an additional full tidal volume. The assist-control mode provides a minimum minute ventilation based on the rate selected, but much higher respiratory rates are attainable. The negative inspiratory pressure required to trigger the ventilator can be varied to control these extra breaths. Setting the trigger sensitivity at too high a level causes the expenditure of considerable effort to trigger a breath while setting it too low may predispose to hyperventilation and respiratory alkalosis. Some older ventilators have uncalibrated sensitivity controls and must be used with some care. A/C ventilation may be particularly suited to the needs of patients with marginal oxygen transport who cannot afford the energy required to breathe, or of patients with severe muscle fatigue who require a period of rest. This mode, coupled with progressively lengthened periods of ventilator withdrawal (T-tube trials), is considered by some physicians to be a superior method for weaning. Recent studies have suggested, however, that patients may perform substantial amounts of respiratory work during A/C ventilation because of delays between breath initiation and delivery.

Intermittent mandatory ventilation (IMV) delivers breaths at a selected frequency and, in addition, allows patients to breathe spontaneously from a continuous flow system by opening a one-way valve between ventilator breaths. Early modes of IMV were not synchronized; selected tidal volumes were delivered at random intervals in the patient's natural breathing cycle. IMV breaths delivered during spontaneous inspiration are added to the patient's own tidal volume, with unsynchronized techniques, and may cause peak pressure to rise to high values. Although many patients learn to breathe sychronously with this mode, others resist the ventilator and continuously exceed the high pressure limit causing ineffective ventilation. Synchronized IMV (SIMV) is similar to A/C ventilation in that additional breaths are triggered by patient effort; only the preset number of breaths are delivered, and the patient is permitted to breathe spontaneously between SIMV breaths by opening a demand valve.

Pressure support ventilation (PSV) has been introduced on the latest generation of ventilators.[99] PSV is a new mode of ventilation which has a significantly different method for triggering inspiration than that available with the original IPPB devices. Positive pressure breaths are triggered by patients in a method analagous to A/C ventilation but a preselected pressure rather than volume is delivered. Ventilators which provide this option also permit SIMV breaths to be interspersed between PSV breaths, permitting partial assistance with spontaneously initiated breaths. This technique appears particularly useful in discontinuation of mechanical ventilation in patients with marginal ventilatory function.

The Airway

The effectiveness of assisted or controlled ventilation depends upon the patency of the airway. Many individuals involved in critical care today may find it incredulous that the concept of translaryngeal intubation was not enthusiastically adopted by all when mechanical ventilation became available. In the earliest days of respiratory care, a tracheostomy was performed whenever a patient with pulmonary insufficiency or circulatory collapse could not be oxygenated by the usual techniques. The decision was frequently delayed until the situation became critical; a hasty tracheostomy performed at the bedside by a junior house officer frequently ended in disaster. The idea of immediate endotracheal intubation was not generally accepted for many years.

Until very recently, tracheostomies were performed in the operating room since it was believed that endotracheal tubes should not be left in place for more than several hours. Gradually endotracheal tubes were left in place for 24–48 hours and, at present, are commonly used for more than three weeks. Issues related to airway access are still controversial and have recently been reviewed by Berlauk.[100]

The artificial airway of choice is generally the largest endotracheal tube which readily passes through the glottis, reducing mechanical airway resistance to a minimum. This is an important consideration for subsequent weaning; although airflow resistance is equivalent for most tubes at low airflows, many patients generate high airflows during weaning, and the resistance presented by narrow tubes may become a limiting factor. It is sometimes appropriate to change a small caliber endotracheal tube to a large one to facilitate weaning. The tube should be of clear, plastic construction and should be pliable enough to conform with the airway but rigid enough to prevent kinking or flattening. The cuff should be firmly attached to the tube to prevent accidental dislodgement and should have a high compliance and high residual volume. Modern "floppy" cuff construction has greatly reduced the airway damage common with the older rigid low-compliance cuffs. Cuff pressure should be measured after inflation; a pressure higher than 30 mm Hg impedes blood flow within the adjacent trachea and predisposes to subsequent damage.

Nasotracheal intubation is sometimes preferred because it is somewhat more comfortable for the patient, although it can lead to nasal bleeding or to maxillary sinusitis. It is important to liberally anesthetize the nares with a topical agent and to dilate the nares with a gloved, lubricated 5th digit prior to inserting the tube. The posterior pharynx should be sprayed liberally with a topical anesthetic prior to oral or nasal intubation when time permits. A trained intensivist or other similarly prepared individual experienced in intubations in the awake patient should perform endotracheal intubation, since a prolonged and traumatic intubation attempt may be more harmful than not attempting it in the first place. Patients should receive positive pressure breaths by face mask between intubation attempts. Acute respiratory collapse should be anticipated and performed *before* the patient is comatose or moribund. Ideally, most patients should be conscious or semiconscious during the procedure and are tense, anxious, and afraid. During intubation, a nurse or physician should monitor vital signs, cardiac rhythm, and the duration of the intubation attempt. Every attempt should be made to make the patient as comfortable as possible by administering small doses of diazepam (valium) or morphine (as tolerated) and by encouraging the patient with calm, reassuring language. In the absence of such thoughtful precautions, tracheal intubation may be a brutal procedure.

Pain and discomfort are minimized by administering intravenous sedation several minutes before the procedure and by the use of local anesthesia. Cocaine (4%) may be sprayed on the nasal mucosa to produce anesthesia and shrink the mucosa. Lidocaine (1%) should be carefully sprayed into the posterior pharynx for oral endotracheal intubation. Lidocaine may be sprayed directly on to the vocal cords if larygnospasm is present.

The position of the tube is immediately checked by auscultation, and its position relative to the nares or mouth noted. A chest radiograph must be obtained as soon as possible to ensure that the tip of the tube is properly placed. A radiographic marker on the tip of the tube is mandatory. The cuff is then slowly inflated until resistance is met, using the minimum amount of air to prevent leaking during positive pressure ventilation. The tube is then secured by adhesive tape passed around the patient's neck. The manner of securing the tube is of major importance. Cloth ties generally slide down the patient's neck and permit spontaneous extubation. *It is essential that the tube be firmly anchored.* The distance of the proximal end of the tube from nares or lip must be observed regularly and recorded every two hours. All gases passing through the endotracheal tube must be warmed and humidified. Hypotension after intubation and initiation of positive pressure ventilation should be anticipated, particularly in dehydrated or septic patients, and treated with volume infusion.

A tracheostomy is performed initially only if nasal or oral obstruction is present. This may be a life-saving procedure when oral intubation is unsuccessful; however, the risks and benefits must be carefully considered. Literature and professional opinions regarding early or late tracheostomy (see beyond) are highly controversial. In general, tracheostomies are more comfortable for the patient and better protect the airway from aspiration of oral contents. However, tracheostomy should be performed only by experienced surgeons. A myriad of complications, such as puncture of the endotracheal tube cuff during local anesthesia, or hemorrhage from the thyroid gland may convert a routine procedure to an overt disaster.

Tracheostomies require approximately five days to "mature." Following this, tubes may be changed with increasing safety. Should a tracheostomy tube fall out prior to this time, oral intubation may be urgently indicated; tissue planes are rapidly lost despite attachment of sutures to the tracheal margins. *Failure to consider the oral approach to this situation has led to many deaths!*

The Design of Endotracheal Tubes

Both endotracheal and tracheostomy tubes produce airway damage. The tube itself, particularly if it is not secured firmly in place, directly traumatizes the posteromedial aspects of the true vocal cords and similar surfaces of the arytenoid cartilages. The cuff and even the tube distal to the cuff may injure the cricoid cartilage and the mucosa associated with the third through seventh tracheal rings. Laryngeal and tracheal damage also occurs with tracheostomy tubes; stricture formation at the site of the surgical stoma is commonplace. Tracheal stenosis produces respiratory symptoms in 11% of patients with tracheostomies;[101] patients managed with translaryngeal intubation experienced transient airway problems, but did not have persistent respiratory abnormalities.[102]

Major improvements in endotracheal tube design have reduced the severity of airway complications. The reusable red rubber tubes have been replaced by polyvinylchloride (PVC) or silicone rubber (Silastic). Both flexibility and resistance to collapse or kinking are essential and have been achieved by the addition of a variety of plasticizers and stabilizers. Modern high compliance, low pressure cuffs distribute the cuff to trachea pressure over a large area of mucosa so that blood flow continues even at pressures above 20–30 mm Hg. Berlauk[100] reviews literature that suggests that the minimal leak technique produces lower cuff pressures and may reduce mucosal damage. He states that the Lanz, Tek silicone disposable, and Argyle are cuffs which satisfy his requirements for an ideal cuff.

Complications of Mechanical Ventilation and Endotracheal Intubation

Two general categories of complications are observed: those due to inadequate understanding of ventilatory care, and those inherent in positive pressure ventilation and tracheal intubation. Zwillich et al.[103] identified mechanical problems in one-third of patients treated for acute respiratory failure. Failure of alarms to function and accidental disconnection of the respirator from the endotracheal tube are serious, but avoidable, hazards. A tension pneumothorax has been observed in up to 15% of patients treated in some units,[104] and can be recognized by sudden cyanosis with mediastinal shift and loss of breath sounds. Pleural air in the supine patient collects in the anterior costophrenic sulcus producing upper abdominal lucency,[105] but may be identified in upright or decubitus chest films. Immediate decompression with a large bore needle and insertion of a chest tube is indicated.

Stress ulceration with massive gastrointestinal hemorrhage may not be recognized for several hours after the development of circulatory collapse. Early diagnosis is facilitated by the measurement of venous pressure and frequent examination of the stool for occult blood. Stress ulceration can be minimized by titration of gastric juice with antacids to a pH of greater than 4.0. More et al.[106] found that neither cimetidine or ranitidine (both H_2 receptor antagonists) raised intragastric pH to adequate levels. Addition of the anticholinergic drug pirenzepine to ranitidine, however, did appear to control acidity.

Thrombosis *in situ* of the main pulmonary artery is most common in patients with severe chronic airway obstruction. It is characterized by signs of increasing right heart failure and should be treated with heparin and thrombolytic agents.

Complications are common with both tracheostomy and endotracheal intubation but those with tracheostomy are usually more serious. The mortality rate with emergency tracheostomy is as high as 15%,[107] and is 3% when performed electively.[108] Secondary bacterial invasion is eight times more common with tracheostomy compared to endotracheal intubation.[109] Tracheostomy is particularly dangerous in patients with burns, and may produce a 100% mortality in comparison with a 25% mortality in patients without tracheostomy.[110]

The endotracheal tube may be placed accidentally in the right main stem bronchus or the esophagus. Endotracheal tube obstruction may be caused by mucus within the tube or by kinking. Problems with the inflatable cuff are not uncommon. A leaking cuff may prevent adequate ventilation, while an overinflated cuff may occlude the tube. Cuff slippage may obstruct the tip of the tube.

Discontinuation of Mechanical Ventilation

Extubation and discontinuation of mechanical ventilation is frequently given the somewhat metaphorical name "weaning." Most approaches to discontinuation of support are based on evaluation of ventilatory reserve and overall physical status while the endotracheal tube is still in place. It is undesirable to allow the patient to develop respiratory muscle fatigue, since a period of rest then becomes necessary and the weaning process must be re-initiated again. If, on the other hand, the weaning process is more prolonged than necessary, increased deconditioning of respiratory muscles may occur. Three methods are presently used: attachment of a T-tube to the endotracheal tube for spontaneous breathing, assist control ventilatory mode, and intermittent mandatory ventilation (IMV). Our own preference is to begin T-tube trials for at least 30 minutes, three times daily, and reserve the use of IMV[111] or SIMV for patients who are too weak to tolerate this period of spontaneous breathing. Pressure support ventilation may be a valuable adjunct for patients who do not do well with either T-tube or IMV techniques. A moderately slow and fixed SIMV rate can be preset while spontaneous breaths are partially supported by PSV. The PSV can then be gradually eliminated.

It is often difficult to judge the moment at which fatigue is beginning during the weaning process. It is important to recognize that hypercarbia is a late finding, and that a normal carbon dioxide tension can exist with beginning patient decompensation. Tidal volumes decrease as the patient begins to tire. Minute ventilation must increase in order to compensate for decreased alveolar volumes so that decreasing tidal volumes at increased ventilatory rates are early evidence of fatigue. Tachycardia, diaphoresis, and a rising carbon dioxide tension soon develop.

Various criteria for extubation and discontinuation of mechanical ventilation have been proposed, and all require that the patient maintain reasonable levels of oxygen and carbon dioxide tension during unassisted breathing. Varying patient requirements make these criteria less useful than desirable, although measurement before and after weaning trials may indicate whether respiratory muscle fatigue has occurred. Bendixen et al.[112] suggested that the vital capacity should be in excess of 10 ml/kg, while Sahn and Lakshminarayan[113] suggested a peak negative pressure in excess of 20–30 cm H_2O and a maximum voluntary ventilation at least twice the minute ventilation. The importance of extrapulmonary factors is emphasized by Tahvanainen, Salmenpera, and Nikki,[114] who studied 47 patients who had been successfully weaned using the IMV method. Nine patients required re-intubation but this group could not be distinguished from those who did not require intubation on the basis of traditional weaning criteria or blood gases. Reduced urine volume, respiratory quotient, and positive blood cultures did discriminate between the two groups, emphasizing the importance of underlying patient condition. Indeed, indications for both intubation and extubation should be based in large part on the patient's overall status and some prediction about expected hospital course. Fluid retention during mechanical ventilation,[115] poor nutritional status,[116] and hypophosphatemia[117] may all reduce respiratory muscle power. Respiratory stimulants have been of questionable use in most weaning situation, but a recent report[118] suggests that the analeptic doxapram reversed ventilator dependence in a brain damaged patient.

Measurement of ventilatory reserve in intubated patients understates true reserve status because of the discomfort associated with breathing through an artificial airway. Vigorous therapy directed toward the underlying condition before and after intubation, maintenance of muscle function by encouraging spontaneous breathing with techniques such as IMV, and early attempts at extubation without slavish adherence to established criteria should reduce the number of ventilator dependent patients. The use of eclectic and creative attempts to extubate ventilator dependent patients referred from Veterans Administration Hospitals throughout the country has achieved a better than 75% success rate.[119]

Terminal Weaning

Grenvik[120] has written sensitively and eloquently about techniques for discontinuing ventilation in patients where decisions not to continue extraordinary forms of therapy have been made. Terminal weaning is accomplished rapidly and continues in spite of deterioration of monitored information. Blood gases are measured in order to predict the time of death, and morphine is added to prevent distressful respiratory efforts.

Continuous Positive Airway Pressure (CPAP)

While most attention in recent years has been placed on positive end-expiratory pressure during mechanical ventilation with inspiratory positive pressure, positive airway pressure can be used in spontaneously breathing patients. Bunnell[121] pointed out in 1912 that anesthetic gases could build up pressure in a face mask that was regulated by an exit valve "closed by a spring set at the desired pressure. . .the lungs will remain inflated to any desired degree." Gregory et al.[122] showed that a similar CPAP device applied to spontaneously breathing neonates with the acute respiratory distress syndrome remarkably decreased mortality. This demonstration that increased airway pressure could increase survivorship in respiratory failure remains one of the most important demonstrations to date of the value of the technique.

CPAP can be defined as positive pressure in the airway throughout the entire respiratory cycle. A typical CPAP circuit includes an oxygen blender with flow valve, an anesthesia bag for reservoir purposes, a humidifier, a unidirectional valve, a face mask and an exhalation pathway connected to a variable expiratory pressure valve. The gas flow must be adjusted to allow the bag to fill during the expiratory phase. The addition of an occasional ventilator breath into this circuit produces an IMV system. Lung expansion is maintained by the continuous positive airway pressure, and regularly spaced mechanical breaths maintain alveolar ventilation. CPAP can be administered by either face mask or endotracheal tube. It has been used with some success without intubation in certain clinical situations; intubation is indicated, however, whenever airway obstruction limits alveolar ventilation.

Treatment of the Adult Respiratory Distress Syndrome—Synthesis and Summary

The confusing and conflicting claims of the past 15 years form a coherent body of knowledge that can be used to develop workable approaches to individual patients. Clearly, maintenance of the functional residual capacity by positive end-expiratory pressure (PEEP) or continuous positive airway pressure (CPAP) is important. The level of intrapleural pressure throughout the ventilatory cycle determines the net effect on cardiac output, so that intermittent positive pressure falling to atmospheric at end-expiration may reduce cardiac output more than spontaneous inspirations with positive pressure at the end of expiration. Skillfully used increases in distending pressure preserve gas-exchanging capacity while incautious use of oxygen destroys the diffusing membrane. While earlier approaches maintained high-inspired oxygen concentrations while rapidly decreasing end-expiratory pressure, the reverse approach is much more rational. Inspired oxygen concentrations should be reduced below 50% as quickly as possible by maintaining an adequate functional residual capacity by positive end-expiratory pressure techniques. One must not focus exclusively on arterial oxyhemoglobin saturation in patients with respiratory failure, however; maintenance of all of the determinants of oxygen delivery must be constantly considered (see chapter 1). In addition, oxygen requirements vary widely and may be substantially greater than normal in many patients with acute respiratory failure. Shoemaker, Appel, and Kram,[123] for example, have shown that maintenance of cardiac index at 50% in excess of normal (4.5 L/min) and blood volumes 500 ml greater than normal, provided this can be done without producing wedge pressures that exceed 18–20 mm Hg, can improve survival in critically ill patients.

The group of 561 patients with severe acute respiratory failure treated by Douglas and Downs[26] in a military hospital provides an example of an integrated approach to patient care. Ten percent of the group required positive end-expiratory pressure in excess of 20 mm Hg in order to maintain adequate arterial oxygenation; 80% of this group was alive and asymptomatic three months after discharge from the hospital. Their nurse-technician ratio of 1.3:1 and an integral analytical laboratory allowed them to constantly adjust inspired oxygen concentrations, positive end-expiratory pressure, IMV rate, cardiac output, and blood volume to desired levels. They used respiratory support equipment that delivered an appropriate airway pressure pattern with little flow resistance, so the patient's work of breathing was minimized during spontaneous breathing, and exposure to high airway pressures was minimized during mechanical breaths. The incidence of pneumothorax was less than 1% in the entire group and 8% in those requiring more than 20 mm Hg positive end-expiratory pressure. Similar results were also reported by Kirby et al.[21]

A large experience using reversed I/E ratios has not been reported, but it is likely that similarly fine results could be achieved. Individualization of ventilatory management is essential. IMV with PEEP may be useful for many patients, but controlled pressure cycled ventilation with reverse I/E ratios, high frequency ventilation, independent lung ventilation, and extracorporeal membrane oxygenation may be necessary in specific situations.

RESPIRATORY FAILURE ASSOCIATED WITH CHRONIC AIRWAY OBSTRUCTION

Many names are applied to the syndrome (emphysema-bronchitis, chronic obstructive lung disease, chronic airway obstruction, or chronic airflow obstruction) which is characterized by airway obstruction and parenchymal destruction with hyperinflation. Both chronic lung disease and chronic coronary artery disease should be suspected in all critically ill patients. Either can lead to acute and chronic respiratory failure and also can complicate the clinical syndromes associated with trauma, sepsis, heart failure, and shock.

The first lesion in the development of chronic airflow obstruction is respiratory bronchiolitis.[124] In cigarette smokers this lesion is characterized by respiratory bronchioles filled with pigmented macrophages and nonalveolated bronchiolar walls infiltrated by mononuclear cells. Age increases the number of goblet and smooth muscle cells in bronchioles. Older patients also have increased mucous gland mass and evidence of centrilobular emphysema, suggesting at least three separate cigarette related lesions:[125] large airway disease, small airway disease, and respiratory bronchiolitis.

Terminal airway disease is associated with increased closing capacity. It is possible that inflammatory exudates inactivate bronchiolar surfactant and produce terminal airway collapse with air trapping and an increase in functional residual capacity. Supporting this belief is the observation that lungs with normal closing capacities developed airway closure when transpulmonary pressures fall to 0.97 cm H_2O.[126] Terminal airways close at an average value of 2.25 cm H_2O in patients with abnormal closing capacities and morphologic evidence of small airway disease.

Destruction of alveolar septa and dilatation of surviving alveoli and alveolar ducts produces the hyperinflated lung characteristic of emphysema. Decreased retractile force of the lung and airway collapse with increasing intrapleural pressure produce the characteristic physiologic abnormality of increasing airflow obstruction during expiration.

Regional distribution of respiratory bronchiolitis is accompanied by evidence of medial hypertrophy and intimal proliferation.[127] These lesions may account for the major changes in pulmonary blood flow and resistance seen in individuals with symptomatic chronic airflow obstruction. They also emphasize the importance of regional hypoxia in evoking regional vasoconstriction, and suggest that continued vascular contraction can lead to medial hypertrophy.

CHRONIC AIRWAY OBSTRUCTION

Perfusion and ventilation are decreased in parallel in many patients with chronic airways obstruction, so that arterial blood gases are close to normal. In other patients, significant abnormalities of ventilation/perfusion relationships are present, leading to a moderate reduction in arterial oxygen tension. These patients usually hyperventilate, however, so that carbon dioxide tensions are normal or even lower than normal. Hyperventilation accentuates the patient's dyspnea but tends to raise oxygen tension and saturation to satisfactory levels, giving rise to the descriptive term *pink puffer*. Marked reduction in ventilation relative to perfusion leads to hypoxemia, hypercapnia, and the syndrome of cor pulmonale—the *blue bloater*.

Factors which increase airway obstruction or decrease ventilatory drive lead to a reduction in alveolar ventilation and in ventilation/perfusion ratios. Bronchitis, bronchiolitis, and bronchopneumonia have long been incriminated as the major causes of acute hypoventilation in patients with chronic airways obstruction. Burk and George[128] studied 166 consecutive episodes of acute respiratory failure and incriminated infection in 91. These clinical observations are supported by the pathologic studies of Karpick, et al.[129] who observed alveolar inflammation in a high percentage of patients dying with acute respiratory failure. A peculiar lesion—goblet cell metaplasia producing bronchiolar obstruction (normally goblet or mucous cells are not found in bronchioles)—was also found in many of these patients.

A number of studies indicate that coexistent heart disease may lead to acute respiratory failure in patients with chronic airways obstruction. Burk and George[128] found congestive heart failure in 59 of the 166 episodes, and cardiac arrhythmias were noted in about one-third. Karpick et al.[129] found evidence of acute myocardial infarction in 25% of their patients dying from acute respiratory failure; in most this was not recognized during life.

Profound hypoxemia, marked elevation of carbon dioxide tension, pulmonary hypertension, right ventricular failure, polycythemia, and progressive obtundation constitute the syndrome of cor pulmonale. Figure 7–11 shows the presumed sequence of events. Characteristically, a respiratory infection decreases alveolar ventilation, raising carbon dioxide tension, and further reducing ventilation/perfusion ratios. Hypoxemia is intensified. Both hypoxemia and acidosis produce pulmonary arteriolar constriction. Polycythemia produced by chronic hypoxemia further increases pulmonary arterial pressure, and right ventricular failure develops. High cerebral carbon dioxide tensions increase the bicarbo-

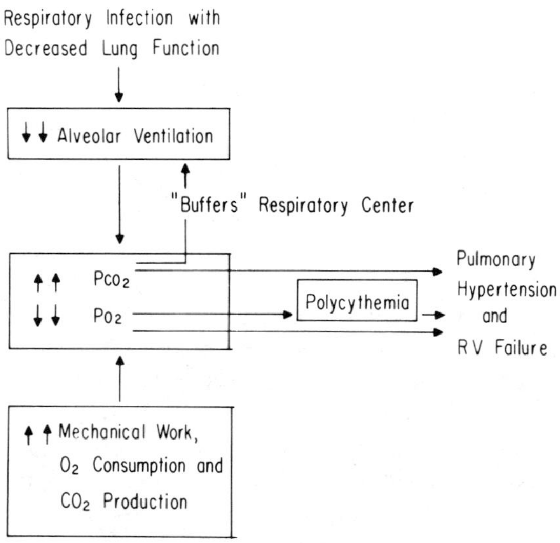

FIG 7–11.
Sequence of events leading to syndrome of respiratory acidosis and cor pulmonale in chronic obstructive lung disease. Increased mechanical work increases the carbon dioxide production of the body while decreased alveolar ventilation interferes with the clearance of carbon dioxide. While a respiratory infriction frequently initiates the sequence, decreased respiratory center activity due to bicarbonate buffering of medullary neurons and injudicious use of both sedation and oxygen lead to further retention of carbon dioxide. (From Ayres SM, Gregory, JJ: *Cardiology: A Clinicophysiologic Approach,* Appleton-Century-Crofts, 1971. Used by permission.)

nate concentration of the respiratory center, decreasing its sensitivity to carbon dioxide and further depressing alveolar ventilation. The increased work of breathing, produced by changes in airway resistance and decrease in pulmonary compliance, increases the carbon dioxide production and oxygen consumption of the respiratory muscles, aggravating hypoxemia and hypercapnia.

Respiratory Center Depression

Reversible respiratory center depression is characteristic of cor pulmonale and is commonly intensified by the injudicious use of oxygen or sedation. It is commonplace to observe patients with chronic airway obstruction and acute bronchial inflammation who deteriorate in the hospital following the overenthusiastic use of these agents. Respiratory center depression is probably due to increased brain bicarbonate concentration in response to chronic hypercapnia. The high levels of brain bicarbonate buffer the hydrogen ion response to increase in cerebral carbon dioxide tension. This increase in brain buffering capacity reduces the ventilatory response to rising carbon dioxide levels because the medullary pacemaker cells are responsive to changes in hydrogen ion concentration rather than to changes in carbon dioxide tension.

Figure 6–20 emphasizes that the medullary respiratory center may be stimulated by either the direct action of carbon dioxide on superficial chemoreceptor cells or by the effect of hypoxemia on the carotid and aortic bodies. When bicarbonate accumulation reduces the sensitivity of the medullary center to carbon dioxide, ventilation is stimulated primarily by the neural impulses reaching the brain stem from the carotid and aortic bodies. Unfortunately, the neural output of the carotid body is closely related to arterial oxygen tension (Fig 6-21). Elevating arterial oxygen tension to above 80 mm Hg by the administration of oxygen reduces the hypoxic drive mediated by the carotid body and leads to sudden hypoventilation. In a sense, raising arterial oxygen tension has "fooled" the respiratory center into assuming that alveolar gas exchange is adequate.

Figure 7–12 shows that this respiratory center depression is reversible. Arterial oxygen and carbon dioxide tensions before and after treatment are shown as coordinates on an oxygen carbon dioxide diagram. Prior to treatment, increasing arterial oxygen tension from 44 to 88

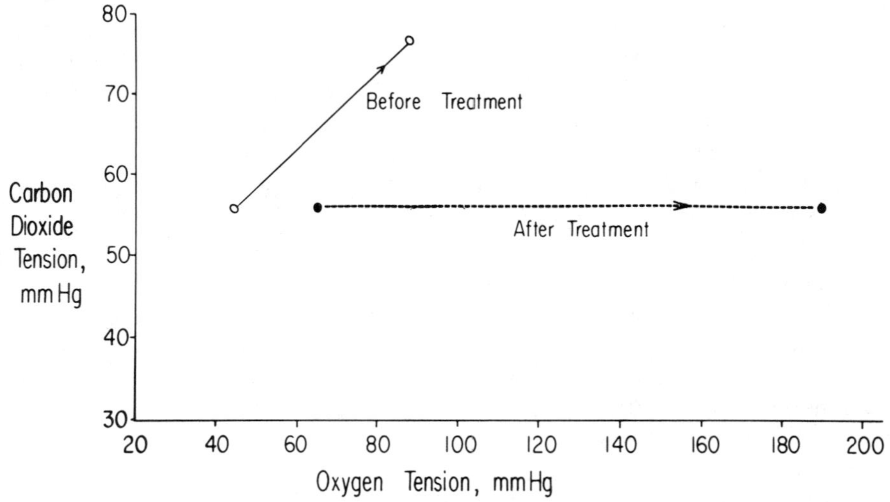

FIG 7–12.
Reversible depression of the respiratory center in a patient with chronic obstructive lung disease. Prior to treatment, a small increase in oxygen tension led to a decrease in alveolar ventilation and an increase in carbon dioxide tension. Following treatment, high oxygen tensions could be tolerated without changes in ventilation. See text for complete description.

mm Hg resulted in sudden hypoventilation; carbon dioxide tension rose from 56 to 77 mm Hg, and the patient became comatose. Following several days of vigorous treatment, which included administration of diuretics, acetazolamide, corticosteroids, and antibiotics, the response of the respiratory center to oxygen became normal. The dashed line in Figure 7–12 shows that in contrast to the situation prior to treatment, arterial carbon dioxide tension was unchanged as oxygen tension was raised from 65 to 190 mm Hg. Treatment had restored the sensitivity of the medullary respiratory center to carbon dioxide; removing the hypoxic drive by administering oxygen did not produce hypoventilation.

Treatment of Acute Respiratory Failure Associated with Chronic Airways Obstruction

Acute respiratory failure in patients with chronic airways obstruction usually is heralded by gradual deterioration in alveolar ventilation with increasing dyspnea, evidence of right heart failure, drowsiness, and stupor. Integrated respiratory therapeutic techniques that include low flow oxygen, humidification, use of nebulized bronchodilators, and physical therapeutic techniques designed to raise sputum frequently can lead to a return to baseline status. Intubation is rarely indicated and, if necessary, suggests an extremely poor prognosis.

The principles underlying the treatment of patients with respiratory failure in chronic obstructive lung disease were defined by E.J. Moran Campbell during the early 1960s.[130] Campbell pointed out that many patients in English hospitals (and presumably in the United States too!) exhibited much higher carbon dioxide tensions on their third or fourth hospital days compared to those on admission. Administration of high concentrations of oxygen and unwise sedation appeared to be responsible. Many of the patients were intubated and ventilated, but Campbell demonstrated that carefully controlled oxygen administration could raise oxygen tensions to adequate levels without decreasing ventilation. Oxygen therapy has become a cornerstone of treatment for all patients with respiratory failure, but the selection of the correct concentration of inspired oxygen remains a major challenge in patient care. Oxygen is obviously a life-giving substance, but it can easily produce lung tissue damage or hypoventilation. Its use is clearly supportive, not curative, and a variety of therapeutic techniques must be initiated in parallel with attempts to raise oxygen tension to levels between 55 and 60 mm Hg (see Table 7–6).

It was once believed that intermittent positive pressure ventilation was useful in the care of patients with chronic airways obstruction because it allowed the nebulization of bronchodilators, provided oxygen enrichment and humidification of the inspired air, and augmented alveolar ventilation. By 1974, the Second Edition of this text criticized those who viewed IPPB as a panacea or placebo and quoted Noehren[131] who asked the rhetorical question "is positive pressure breathing overrated?" A multi-institutional study sponsored by the National Institutes of Health was unable to demonstrate a difference in patients treated with either IPPB or a nebulizer-compressor and effectively answered Noehren's question in the affirmative.[6] The precise use of specific respiratory therapeutic techniques has replaced IPPB in the treatment of chronic airway obstruction.

Humidification

Particulate material including bacteria and viruses are cleared from the human tracheobronchial tree by a blanket of mucus overlying ciliated epithelial cells. Once particulate material reaches the level of the carina, afferent sensory impulses stimulate a cough, which forcibly ejects it from the airway. Ciliary action requires a moist mucous membrane. Normally, this is accomplished by nasal breathing so that the inspired air is humidified as it passes sequentially over the moist mucous mem-

Table 7–6
Treatment of Respiratory Failure in Patients with Chronic Obstructive Lung Disease

1. Administration of low concentrations of oxygen (24–35%) by nasal cannula at flow rate of 1–3 liters/minute or ventimask.

2. Vigorous treatment including:

Bronchodilators	Antibiotics
Physical Therapy	Steriods
Diuretics	Phlebotomy
Digitalis	Acetazolamide (Diamox)
Avoid Sedation	

3. Intubation and controlled ventillation probably indicated if:
   - PO_2 cannot be raised to above 60 mm Hg
   - pH remains below 7.25–7.35
   - PCO_2 rises at rapid rate
   - Clinical findings of somnolence, coma, hypertension, or cardiac arrhythmias.

branes of the nose, the convoluted choanae of the nasopharynx, and the oropharynx.

Humidity refers to the amount of water present as vapor. Since it is dispersed in molecular form, the water is invisible. Water dispersed in particulate form is visible and is termed fog, mist, or aerosol. Continuing the comparison with weather, condensation of water in respiratory therapy equipment is frequently called rainout.

The amount of water vapor carried in a gas increases as the gas is warmed, so that alveolar air contains more moisture than ambient air. Saturated alveolar air carries about twice as much water as saturated room air at 23° C. Since the relative humidity of room air is usually less than 50%, the mucous membranes of the airway must add considerably more water than in the example cited above.

Mouth breathing, hyperventilation, fever, and systemic dehydration all interfere with hydration of the mucosal carpet. If there is any reason to suspect abnormal airway function, the inspired breathing mixture should be humidified. The breathing moisture should always be humidified in patients with tracheostomies or endotracheal tubes because of nasopharyngeal bypass. Compressed gases are dry and cool as they flow from pressure tanks (adiabatic expansion of gases). Cold gas reduces the temperature of water in humidifying systems and thus reduces the amount of water added to the gas mixture. Subsequent rewarming in the lung markedly reduces the relative humidity of the gas delivered to the patient.

A bubble-jet humidifier is ordinarily used when oxygen is administered by either nasal cannula, partial rebreathing mask, or nonrebreathing mask. The unit is relatively inefficient, but lower concentrations of water vapor are adequate since the nasopharynx adds warmed water vapor when the nasal cannula is used; partial rebreathing of exhaled air with an appropriate mask, together with nose breathing, also adds additional water to the inspired mixture.

An aerosol generator must be used if additional water is required. Water and gas are heated to above body temperature by an immersion heater, increasing the amount of water vapor carried by the mixture. Additional water is added in the form of minute particles by directing the gas flow through a Venturi orifice. The high-velocity air flow physically strips off water particles which enter the gas mixture in aerosol form. A visible fog indicates the presence of suspended water particles. Another advantage of these units is that either oxygen or compressed air may be used. The mask is of special design and termed an aerosol mask. The connecting tubing is of much larger diameter than that used with nasal cannulas or partial rebreathing masks so that obstruction from condensation of aerosol particles may be prevented.

Ultrasonic nebulizers have been used with increasing enthusiasm during the past decade. The units produce particles of a uniform small size, but they are so effective that the patient may be overloaded with water. Even the heated nebulizer described above is capable of adding 200–400 ml of water to the body each day.[132] We prefer the heated Venturi-type aerosol generator (Puritan-type) to the ultrasonic generator because the high flow of cool water particles produced by the latter may irritate the lung and induce bronchospasm.[133]

It has been shown that humidification and aerosol equipment may harbor bacteria that are subsequently delivered to the airway, producing a necrotizing pneumonitis. Pierce et al.[134] demonstrated that 84% of samples from reservoir nebulizers were contaminated with gram-negative bacteria. Routine decontamination with 0.25% acetic acid dramatically reduces the frequency of such contamination. Similar bacterial contamination may involve all respiratory therapy equipment, making frequent change and sterilization of equipment an important aspect of patient care.

Bronchodilator and Aerosol Therapy

Nebulized bronchodilators are an important method for opening narrowed airways and improving alveolar ventilation. Airways of all sizes may be filled with purulent material or mucus. The degree of bronchoconstriction present varies from patient to patient, but clinical experience suggests that nebulized bronchodilators are useful in many patients. There is, in addition, evidence that they may improve mucociliary clearance.[135]

Isoproterenol, 1:200, is a potent bronchodilator and was used widely at one time. Although it was an excellent bronchodilator, its cardiac stimulatory effect and vasodilating effects limited its usefulness. Although all beta agonists with beta-2 activity may increase blood flow through poorly ventilated lung segments and produce transient decrements in arterial oxygen tensions, the magnitude of the changes seems less with the newer agents. In any case, modest increases in shunting can be overcome by oxygen administration.

Isoetharine (Bronkosol), metaproterenol (Alupent), terbutaline (Brethine or Bricanyl), and albuterol (Proventil or Ventolin) have generally replaced isoproterenol. These agents may be administered by a nebulizer-compressor or metered dose cannister. The activity of a group of bronchodilator drugs is shown in Figure 7–13.

Recent reports of sudden deaths in asthmatic patients using pressurized aerosols have prevented many clinicians form using nebulized isoproterenol as a bronchodilator. Although Speizer, Doll, and Heaf[136] suggested that a threefold increase in asthma mortality might be correlated with excessive use of aerosols containing isoproterenol, a significant cardiotoxic effect of either the catecholamine or the Freon propellant has not been demonstrated. A recent publication[137] listed the unsuccessful attempts to identify significantly harmful side effects of pharmacologic doses in man. While isoproterenol in ordinary doses is a safe and extremely effective bronchodilator, it should be administered with care in the critically ill patient. Adequate dilution with saline, correction of hypoxemia with oxygen, and continuous electrocardiographic monitoring should minimize the possibility of isoproterenol-induced cardiac arrhythmias.

The need to separate bronchodilatation from cardiac stimulation has led to the search for specific beta-2 adrenergic agonists. Both terbutaline and metaproterenol appear to have selective beta-2 activity in experimental models, but cardiac stimulation still occurs when used clinically. Both are available in oral form

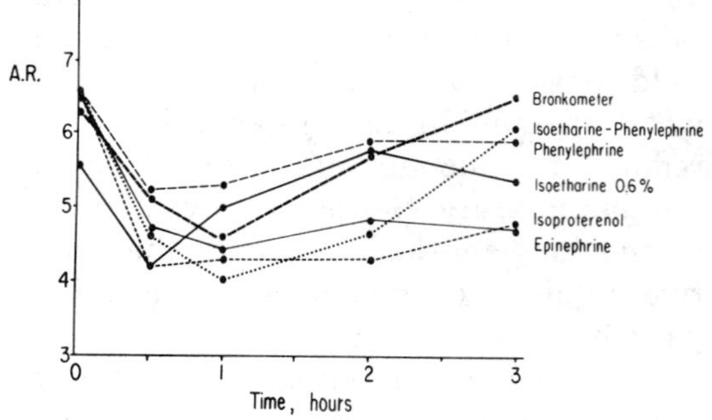

FIG 7–13.
Response of airway resistance (A.R.) to a group of sympathomimetic aerosols. Both isoproterenol and epinephrine produce sustained bronchodilatation.

and are useful for maintenance therapy. Albuterol is probably the only sympathomimetic bronchodilator available in the United States that appears to stimulate beta-2 adrenergic receptors selectively in a clinical setting. Albuterol is also an effective pulmonary vasodilator and has been used in patients with primary pulmonary hypertension. Agonist selectivity is always dose-related, however, and patients who receive sympathomimetic bronchodilators must be monitored carefully in order to avoid increasing heart rate, ventricular premature contractions, and other consequences of increased cardiac stimulation.

Glucocorticoids are bronchodilators with minimal cardiovascular side effects but important consequences for immune function. A recent controlled study[138] has shown their efficacy in the treatment of acute respiratory insufficiency associated with chronic obstructive lung disease. They are indicated for short-term use in this situation. Together with other techniques, they maximize alveolar ventilation while oxygenation is maintained by low-flow techniques. Although nebulized bronchodilators are useful in many clinical situations,[139] bronchospasm and bronchial obstruction may prevent delivery of nebulized medication in certain patients requiring mechanical ventilation. Radioactive material is poorly distributed throughout the tracheobronchial tree in patients on ventilators compared to normal controls. In addition, aerosolized metaproterenol did not produce physiologic changes, suggesting that the material did not reach the peripheral airways. The authors concluded that either improved methods for aerosolization must be developed, or increased dosages of medication must be used.

The use of agents promoting clearance of mucus has been advocated by many investigators. Propylene glycol, 2–5% in 0.5–1.0% saline is believed to be a better expectorant than water alone. Deoxyribonuclease (Dornavac), 50,000 units three time daily, is frequently recommended for purulent secretions. Acetylcysteine (Mucomyst or Respaire) attacks the polysaccharide bonds of mucin and is used in patients producing large volumes of mucus; 5–10 ml of the 20% solution is used. The agent occasionally produces bronchospasm and must be used with caution in patients with bronchial asthma.

Antibiotics have been nebulized for many years, but their efficacy remains in doubt. Toxic but nonabsorbable agents such as kanamycin (Kantrex), colistin (Coly-Mycin), or gentamicin (Garamycin) may be administered with little fear of systemic absorption. Nebulized antibiotics cannot penetrate poorly ventilated lung regions, but appear useful in treating extensive areas of tracheobronchitis. Prior treatment with a nebulized bronchodilator probably enhances distribution.

Veno-arterial shunting in pulmonary edema is caused largely by the stable foam which fills large areas of the tracheobronchial tree. Ethyl alcohol, 30–100%, is an antifoaming agent which may assist in the mobilization of high surface tension material from the periphery.

Antibiotic Therapy

Many clinical studies and at least two decades of experience have demonstrated that viral respiratory infections commonly initiate exacerbations of purulent bronchitis that reduce airway function and alveolar ventilation. Although bacterial infections usually are not the primary factor involved, prompt use of antibiotics has been shown to be useful and should be administered empirically and early in the patient's course. Either ampicillin or tetracycline are ordinarily administered; most physicians prefer ampicillin in patients without penicillin sensitivity. Antibiotics should be continued for five to seven days or until there is evidence of improved alveolar ventilation, decreased sputum production, less purulent sputum or decrease in systemic evidence of infection. Sputum examination and culture is necessary so that specific etiologic agents such as the *pneumococcus* or *H. influenzae* can be identified.

Oxygen Enrichment of Inspired Air

The decrease in oxygen delivery produced by arterial hypoxemia (Fig 1–9) could be easily corrected by raising arterial oxygen tension to normal. More complicated is the question of whether raising arterial oxygen tension above 80 mm Hg significantly enhances tissue oxygen delivery. Arterial blood at 80 mm Hg (hemoglobin, 15 g/100 ml) contains 19.5 ml of oxygen per 100 ml. Increasing the arterial oxygen tension to 400 mm Hg increases its oxygen content to 21.4 ml. The answer is related to the other variable of the oxygen delivery equation—the cardiac output. If cardiac output is normal, oxygen delivery is normal at an oxygen tension of 80 mm Hg, and further enhancement by raising arterial content is unnecessary and useless. In contrast, if cardiac output is depressed, raising arterial oxygen content may improve oxygen delivery enough to overcome tissue hypoxia.

The effect of raising arterial oxygen tension in a patient with both cardiac and pulmonary insufficiency is shown in Table 7–7. The patient had coronary artery disease with left ventricular failure, as evidenced by a left ventricular, end diastolic pressure of 38 mm Hg. He had experienced chronic pulmonary congestion interspersed with bouts of pulmonary edema and had a pulmonary arterial pressure of 88/36 mm Hg. (Normal left ventricular, end-diastolic pressure, 5–10 mm Hg; normal pulmonary arterial pressure 25/5 mm Hg.) His arterial oxygen tension was 51 mm Hg; his mixed venous oxygen tension was 30 mm Hg. Table 7–7 shows that as the inspired oxygen mixture was increased, arterial oxygen tension, cardiac output, and venous oxygen tension rose. The increase in venous oxygen tension, a reflection of tissue oxygenation, was due to both the improvement in cardiac output and the increase in arterial oxygen tension. Note that the optimal effect on cardiac output occurred between an arterial oxygen tension of 200 and 300 mm Hg.

The oxygen delivery may be calculated

Table 7–7
Effect of Oxygen Administration in a Patient with Combined Cardiopulmonary Failure

	INSPIRED OXYGEN TENSION (mm Hg)			
	150	219	304	766
Arterial oxygen tension (mm Hg)	51	63	125	214
Venous oxygen tension (mm Hg)	30	35	37	39
Arterial carbon dioxide tension (mm Hg)	41	49	50	46
Cardiac output (liters/minute)	1.66	1.94	2.30	2.26
Arterial oxygen content (ml/100 ml)	18.46	20.74	19.18	20.98
Total Oxygen Delivery (ml/minute)	306	402	441	475
Increase due to increased content (ml/minute)		36	12	42
Increase due to increased output (ml/minute)		58	123	127
Hemoglobin (gm/100 ml)	17.1	15.4	15.4	15.8

for each oxygen mixture using arterial oxygen content and cardiac output. Since both of these increased, oxygen delivery increased substantially with each increase in inspired oxygen concentration. It is also possible to calculate the fraction of oxygen delivery increase due to improved oxygenation or to improved blood flow. Table 7–5 shows that both factors contributed to the overall improvement in oxygen delivery, although the increase in output played a greater role. While cardiac output and arterial venous oxygen content differences were measured in this example, mixed venous oxygen tensions provided a simple indicator of the adequacy of tissue oxygenation and are recommended for general clinical use.

Cardiac output improved in this patient because increased coronary arterial oxygen content augmented myocardial oxygenation and contractility. The importance of maintaining myocardial oxygen delivery in patients with reduced coronary blood flow was emphasized in a recent study by Ganz and associates.[140] Myocardial oxygen delivery was low in a group of patients with coronary arterial disease and angina pectoris. Increasing arterial oxygen content by administering high concentrations of oxygen increased myocardial oxygen delivery, improved myocardial lactate metabolism, and raised the pacing threshold for the production of angina (Table 7–8).

Arterial oxygen tension should not exceed 80 mm Hg in patients with chronic obstructive lung disease because (1) cardiac output is usually normal in these patients; (2) higher arterial oxygen tensions may depress ventilation; and (3) higher tensions may injure the alveolar surface, producing atelectasis. In general, high oxygen tensions should be avoided in all patients unless absolutely essential for the maintenance of tissue viability.

Effects of Oxygen Administration

Addition of oxygen to the inspired air usually corrects hypoxemia produced by any of the factors discussed in Chapter 6. Such correction of hypoxemia, however, does not reverse underlying physiologic abnormalities; it is merely a supportive technique. High-oxygen mixtures, for example, may correct arterial hypox-

Table 7–8
Effect of Oxygen Breathing on Systemic and Myocardial Hemodynamics in Patients with and without Coronary Artery Disease

	CORONARY PATIENTS		NONCORONARY PATIENTS	
	CONTROL	OXYGEN	CONTROL	OXYGEN
Heart rate (beats/minute)	75	69	79	72
Blood pressure (mm/Hg)	93	99	106	107
Cardiac index (liters/minute/M^2)	2.9	2.6	3.6	3.2
Coronary blood flow (ml/100g/minute)	151	138	158	131
PO_2—coronary sinus (mm Hg)	19.2	24.0	18.8	22
PO_2—arterial (mm Hg)	75	403	77	425
Lactate extraction (%)	4	28	40	60

Adapted from Ganz W, Donoso R, Marcus H, Swan HJC: Coronary hemodynamics and myocardial oxygen metabolism during oxygen breathing in patients with and without coronary artery disease. *Circulation* 1972; 45:763.

All changes statistically significant except change in arterial blood pressure in noncoronary patients.

emia produced by atelectasis, but do not reexpand collapsed alveolar segments. Indeed, oxygen administration may actually increase the degree of atelectasis by injuring the surface-lining material of the lung.

The different effects of oxygen breathing in the presence of totally collapsed compared to poorly ventilated alveoli were demonstrated in Figure 6–15. While relatively low concentrations of oxygen restore arterial oxygen tension to normal in patients with unequal ventilation/perfusion distribution, high concentrations are frequently needed in overcoming the hypoxemia produced by venoarterial shunting.

Alveolar Hypoventilation

The effects of oxygen breathing in alveolar hypoventilation may be understood by considering the following calculations. Alveolar oxygen tension P_{AO_2} is readily calculated from the simplified form of the alveolar air equation:

$$P_{AO_2} = F_{IO_2}(713) - \frac{P_{CO_2}}{R}$$

Breathing room air inspired fraction of oxygen (F_{IO_2}) 0.21, respiratory quotient R 0.8—the alveolar oxygen tension would be 100 mm Hg when the arterial carbon dioxide tension was 40 mm Hg, but would fall to 50 mm Hg when arterial carbon dioxide tension rose to 80 mm Hg.

$$(0.21)(713) - \frac{40}{0.8} = 100 \text{ mm Hg}$$

$$(0.21)(713) - \frac{80}{0.8} = 50 \text{ mm Hg}$$

Since arterial oxygen tension is normally 5–15 mm Hg lower than alveolar oxygen tension unless distribution or shunting problems exist, it would fall from 90 to 40 mm Hg as the carbon dioxide tension rose from 40 to 80 mm Hg. This decrease in oxygen tension is due solely to the overall decrease in alveolar ventilation.

The effects of oxygen breathing may be readily estimated by changing the inspired oxygen fraction from 0.21 to 0.30 (30% oxygen).

$$(0.30)(713) - \frac{80}{0.8} = 114 \text{ mm Hg}$$

Low concentrations of oxygen are obviously effective in correcting the hypoxemia of pure hypoventilation.

Unequal Distribution of Ventilation/Perfusion

Although Figure 6–15 presented a theoretical description of oxygen enrichment in the presence of maldistribution of the inspired air, the actual result of such treatment may be seen in the treatment of patients with chronic airways obstruction. Mithoefer et al.[141] administered low concentrations of oxygen to 14 normal subjects and to 34 patients with chronic airways obstruction. They found that an inspired oxygen concentration of 40% increased arterial oxygen tension to acceptable levels in almost all patients, and, frequently, considerably lower concentrations were adequate to maintain oxygen tension above 60 mm Hg (Fig 7–14).

True Venoarterial Shunting

The fortunate effect of low concentrations of oxygen observed in chronic airways obstruction is not seen in patients with other forms of respiratory failure. There is a progressive fall of arterial oxygen tension with increasing venoarterial shunting in patients breathing 100% oxygen (Fig 7–1). Normal oxyhemoglobin saturation may be maintained in patients with venoarterial shunts up to 30% of the cardiac output if 100% oxygen is administered.

The response to 100% oxygen is a useful

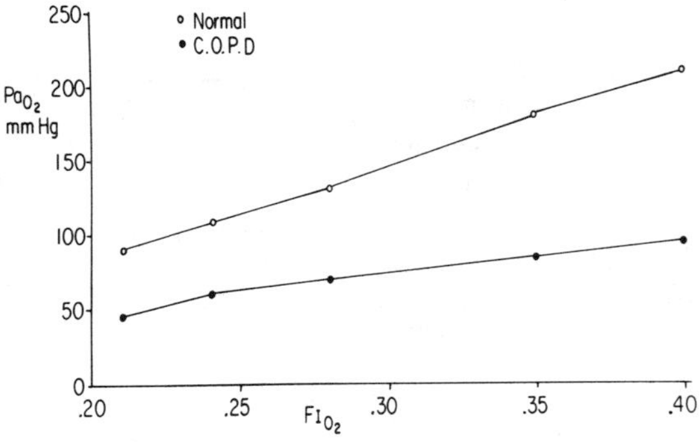

FIG 7–14.
Response of arterial oxygen tension (Pa_{O_2}) to increasing inspired oxygen tension (F_{LO_2}). (Adapted from Mithoefer JC, Keighley JF, Chir B, Karetzky MS: Response of the arterial P_{O_2} to oxygen administration in chronic pulmonary disease. *Ann Intern Med* 1971; 74:328.)

way of measuring the degree of venoarterial shunting, and also provides predictive information regarding the response of arterial oxygen tension to lower concentrations of inspired oxygen. Figure 7–15 shows the arterial oxygen tension breathing 100% oxygen in a group of patients with hypoxemia due to a variety of disease states. Note that patients with nonobstructive respiratory failure have large shunts and poor response to 100% oxygen compared to those with chronic airways obstruction.

Diffusion Block

Low concentrations of oxygen restore arterial oxygen tension to normal in patients with pure membrane diffusion blocks. Breathing 100% oxygen raises arterial oxygen tension to 650 mm Hg (Table 7–9). The explanation for this complete correction lies in the large alveolar-arterial oxygen gradient. Alveolar oxygen tension is 670 mm Hg, while blood entering the pulmonary capillary is at an oxygen tension of 40 mm Hg. The initial alveolar-capillary gradient of 630 mm Hg (670–40) produces such a large flow of oxygen across the alveolar membrane that even with a thickened membrane end-capillary oxygen tension equals alveolar oxygen tension.

Toxic Effects of Oxygen

Both too much and too little oxygen are harmful. Early clinical experiences demonstrated that patients with chronic airways obstruction frequently became pink, breathed more easily, and generally looked better when given oxygen. This period of apparent well-being was followed by either coma or death in many patients, suggesting that oxygen exerted a depressant effect on ventilation. The mechanism of oxygen-induced hypoventilation is discussed earlier. This phenomenon is widely known today, and ox-

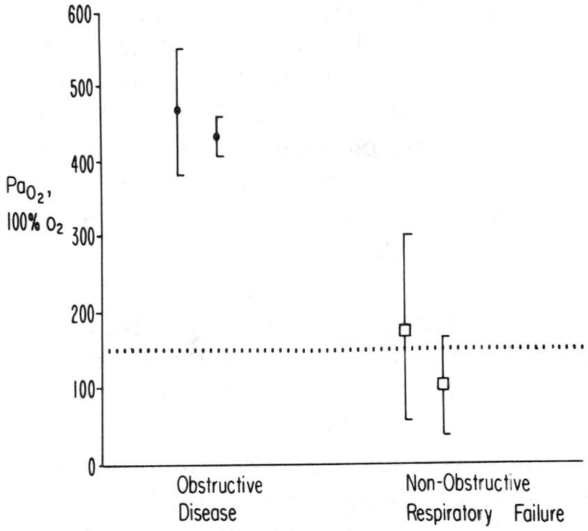

FIG 7–15.
Response to arterial oxygen tension (Pa_{O_2}) to breathing 100% oxygen. Patients with obstructive lung disease are compared to those with nonobstructive respiratory failure (acute respiratory distress syndrome). The presence of massive venoarterial shunting in nonobstructive respiratory failure limits increase in arterial oxygen tension. Many of the patients' levels fell below 150 m Hg, a level frequently selected as an indication for intubation and controlled ventilation.

Table 7–9
Effect of Oxygen Breathing on Oxygen Tensions

	PO_2 (mm Hg) ALVEOLAR	PO_2 (mm Hg) ARTERIAL	ALVEOLAR - ARTERIAL GRADIENT (mm Hg)	O_2 SATURATION
Diffusion block	670	650*	20	100
Unequal distribution	670	650*	20	100
Venoarterial shunt	670	200	470	100

* Arterial oxygen tension is slightly lower than alveolar tension because of the small physiologic shunt.

ygen is generally administered with great care to patients with chronic lung disease.

Recent experimental and clinical studies delineated another side effect of oxygen administration—oxygen damage to the lung. This problem is of great practical importance in the treatment of nonobstructive respiratory failure. Whenever massive shunting is present, high inspired oxygen concentrations are necessary to maintain adequate arterial oxygen tensions. Since high concentrations may further injure lung tissue and produce increased shunting, an important question is the relative safety of various oxygen concentrations and the relative hazards of high inspired oxygen tensions compared to low arterial oxygen tension.

A useful model is the study of Kapanci et al.[142] who administered 100% oxygen to a series of monkeys. Minimal changes were observed following 48 hours of continuous oxygen administration, but by 4 days, significant and serious morphologic changes were observed. Almost all of the type I membranous pneumocytes were destroyed, leading to a complete loss of the alveolar lining membrane. Many alveoli contained edema fluid with fibrin, desquamated cells, macrophages, and cellular debris. Capillary endothelial cells were swollen, and encroached upon the capillary lumen. By 7 days, a continuous layer of hypertrophied type II pneumocytes lined the alveolar septa. These type II pneumocytes were extremely abnormal in appearance and contained but few lamellar bodies—the storage sites for surfactant.

Direct extrapolation of these data to the clinical situation is hampered by the multiple factors which appear to modify oxygen toxicity. Sympathomimetic amines and corticosteroids appear to intensify the toxic effects of oxygen, while preexisting lung disease, venoarterial shunting, and alkalosis minimize oxygen toxicity. The variable human response to 100% oxygen is seen in two recent studies from the same institution. Singer et al.[143] administered 100% oxygen to 20 patients following open heart surgery for up to 7 days and could find no differences compared to a control group ventilated with low concentrations of oxygen. In contrast, Barber, Lee, and Hamilton[144] observed a steady decline in alveolar-capillary gas exchange in five patients with irreversible brain damage who were given 100% oxygen compared to a similar group ventilated with room air. Patients breathing room of air for 30 hours had an arterial oxygen tension of 400 mm Hg during a brief period of breathing 100% oxygen. Arterial PO_2 was reduced to an average of 120 mm Hg in patients breathing 100% oxygen for 30 hours.

While these conflicting human and animal studies complicate the development of rigid guidelines for oxygen administration, several important conclusions clearly emerge. High concentrations of oxygen administered for more than four days may produce alveolar damage in certain situations. Tissue hypoxia may develop if high concentrations of oxygen are not administered, however, leading to a classic therapeutic dilemma. Both oxygen toxicity and tissue hypoxia may generally be avoided if these guidelines for oxygen administration are followed.

1. Carefully adjust the inspired oxygen concentration to produce arterial oxygen tensions of 80–120 mm Hg in nonobstructive respiratory failure and 60–80 mm Hg in patients with chronic airways obstruction. Arterial oxygen tensions as low as 55 mm Hg may be tolerated in young individuals with normal cardiovascular systems.
2. Closely monitor inspired and arterial oxygen tensions.
3. Diminish atelectasis by using techniques such as high tidal volume ventilation, positive end-expiratory pressure, and physical therapeutic techniques in patients requiring high concentrations of oxygen. Be careful not to lower the P_{CO_2} precipitously with high tidal volume techniques.
4. Be sure all oxygen mixtures are well humidified.
5. Correct acidosis and avid alpha-adrenergic agents where possible.

Techniques of Oxygen Administration

Oxygen is a potent drug which must be dispensed with accuracy and caution. The precise inspired concentration is usually not known because the patient breathes a mixture of oxygen from an oxygen source and room air from the surrounding environment. If the patient hyperventilates, additional room air is added to the mixture, lowering the oxygen concentration. If hypoventilation occurs, the oxygen flow may be sufficient so that inspired concentrations approach high levels. The difference between average ventilation and instantaneous ventilation is important in understanding the dynamics of mixing. While the average ventilation may be 10 liters/minute, inspiration flows may reach 3–5 liters/second (180–300 liters/minute). The 5 liters/minute produced by a nasal cannula may be markedly diluted by a high inspiratory flow rate resulting in an oxygen concentration close to that of room air. The effect of a given method of oxygen administration on an individual patient can be evaluated only by serial measurement of arterial oxygen tension.

Equipment for Low Concentrations of Oxygen. The *nasal cannula* (or catheter) is a useful technique for delivering low concentrations of oxygen. Concentrations of 32–35% may be delivered with oxygen flow rates of 6 liters/minute; concentrations of 24–28% may be achieved with flow rates of 2–3 liters/minute. A major advantage of the oxygen cannula over masks of all types is that it remains in place during eating, talking, or coughing.

An alternative method for delivering low concentrations of oxygen is the *Venturi mask.*[145] This mask entrains fixed proportions of room air and thus delivers a constant concentration of oxygen. Available for delivery of 24, 28, 35, and 40% oxygen, these masks are extremely useful in the management of chronic airway obtructive disease. They suffer from the disadvantage that they must be removed for meals or other activities, so that they actually deliver intermittent rather than continuous oxygen.

Equipment for Intermediate Concentrations of Oxygen. The heated aerosol generator is used whenever higher concentrations of oxygen or high concentrations of moisture are necessary. Since hypoxemia is almost always due to atelectasis in the critically ill patient, high concentrations of moisture are almost always useful.

The oxygen concentration of the gas mixture leaving the generator must be carefully distinguished from the oxygen concentration available to the patient. The oxygen concentration leaving the generator is determined by setting the control at either 40, 70, or 100%. This setting adjusts a Venturi, which determines how much room air is entrained within the generator. Considerations discussed above emphasize that the concentration of oxygen presented to the patient is related to the total gas volume available. If the patient requires more gas volume than produced by the generator, room air is drawn into the face mask, diluting the final concentration.

The total flow of humidified gas leaving the aerosol generator is determined by the rate of oxygen flow and the concentration setting. Note that at the 100% setting, all of the total gas flow is supplied by the oxygen flow, while at the 40% setting, 75% of the total flow is entrained room air (Table 7–10).

In practice, the desired oxygen concentration is set on the generator, and the oxygen flow rate selected by estimating total ventilatory needs. The large-bore aerosol mask must be used to minimize the effects of condensation of water within the tubing.

Another method for delivering intermediate concentrations of oxygen is the *partial rebreathing mask*. The reservoir fills with oxygen during expiration so that high concentrations of oxygen are available for the subsequent inspiration. It is termed a partial rebreathing mask because the initial one-third of exhaled air (primarily dead space air high in oxygen concentration) together with its water vapor also enters the reservoir bag during each expiration and mixes with the incoming oxygen. This exhaled air is then rebreathed during the subsequent inspiration. Such a mask delivers 45–60% oxygen at oxygen flow rates of 6–10 liters/minute.

We prefer the heated aerosol generator to the partial rebreathing mask because it permits more precise adjustment of inspired oxygen concentration, and also allows large concentrations of water to be added to the inspired air.

Table 7–10
Gas Flow Rates with the Heated Aerosol Generator

OXYGEN CONCENTRATION (%)	TOTAL GAS FLOW AT THREE OXYGEN FLOW RATES (LITERS/MINUTE)		
	5	10	15
40	20	40	60
70	8	16	24
100	5	10	15

Equipment for High Concentrations of Oxygen. Oxygen concentrations of up to 100% may be administered by a nonrebreathing mask which contains one-way flutter valves. These masks are rarely used, since most patients requiring oxygen concentrations above 70% need intubation and artificial ventilation.

Postoperative Respiratory Failure

A major advance in postoperative management has been the recognition that many cardiopulmonary complications–including sudden, unexpected death–are related to atelectasis with venoarterial shunting. Adequate respiratory care may reverse these abnormalities; even more important, if used preoperatively it may prevent them.

Progressive atelectasis is known to occur in laboratory animals and in man unless periodic deep breaths or sighs reopen closed alveolar units. Bendixen, et al.[84] and others showed that venoarterial shunting developed during general anesthesia and could be partially corrected by deep-breathing techniques. Inability to reverse the venoarterial shunt completely suggested the presence of transient changes in the surface properties of the alveoli. Hypoxemia does not correlate with temperature elevation, pulse rate, respiratory rate, or chest x-ray, and frequent measurements of arterial oxygen tension are necessary to evaluate the status of lung expansion.

The major pathophysiologic event leading to postoperative complications appears to be a decrease in pulmonary compliance and an increase in minute ventilation (Fig 7–16). These two factors produce a marked increase in respiratory work which is considerably greater in surgical procedures lasting more than 4 hours, compared to shorter procedures.

The importance of an orderly preoperative pulmonary program is emphasized in the study by Stein and Cassara.[146] They measured pulmonary function in patients undergoing general surgery and identified a group of high-risk patients with low forced expiratory volumes. Half of these patients were given an intensive period of respiratory care, while no special treatment was given to the remainder. Postoperative pulmonary complications were seen in 15 of the 25 untreated high-risk patients but only in 5 of the 23 specially treated high-risk patients.

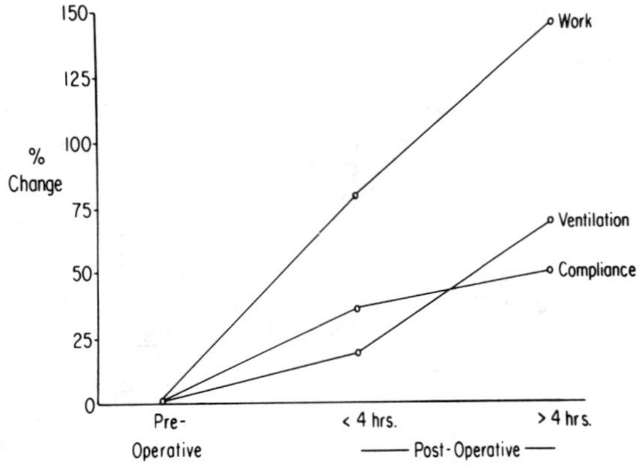

FIG 7–16.
Postoperative lung rigidity produces a decrease in pulmonary compliance and an increase in minute ventilation leading to an increase in pulmonary work. If the patient is unable to maintain the required increase in pulmonary work, progressive atelectasis with venoarterial shunting and hypoxemia may develop. (Adapted from Neely, Robinson, Hardy, Bobo: *Ann Thorac Surg* 1971; 11:565.)

Respiratory Failure in Left Ventricular Failure

Acute respiratory failure in myocardial infarction, coronary shock, and pulmonary edema all appear related to acute elevations of left atrial pressure. Arterial hypoxemia is common in acute myocardial infarction; Figure 7–17 shows that the alveolar-arterial oxygen difference is closely related to the level of pulmonary arterial pressure. Reversible atelectasis presumably associated with inactivity is also a factor, since periodic deep breathing decreases venoarterial shunting in these patients (Fig 7–18).

Pulmonary edema represents sudden respiratory failure that may be quickly fatal unless properly treated. High pulmonary capillary pressure floods alveoli with fluid that washes out surface-lining material, forming a high-surface-tension material readily forming bubbles. This material produces atelectasis and, in addition, obstructs all levels of bronchi and bronchioles, leading to massive venoarterial shunting with hypoxemia. While hyperventilation occurs commonly, Aberman and Fulop[147] found carbon dioxide tensions above 45 mm Hg in 11 of 50 patients with acute pulmonary edema. Hypercapnia may reflect severe airway obstruction, but also could indicate coexistent chronic bronchitis.

Routine treatment of pulmonary edema includes the use of oxygen, aminophylline when wheezing due to cardio-

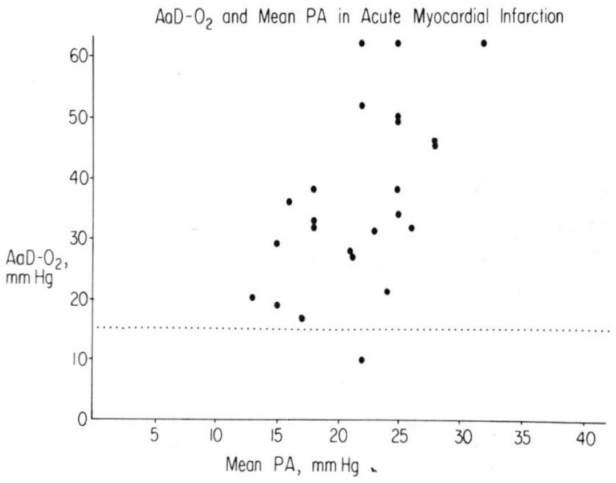

FIG 7–17.
Increase in alveolar-arterial oxygen difference with increasing mean pulmonary arterial pressure. Dotted line represents upper limits of normal for the alveolar-arterial oxygen difference.

genic bronchoconstriction is present, and intravenous morphine. Morphine is especially useful because its venodilator action pools blood within the venous reservoir. Furosemide is not only an effective diuretic, but is also a venodilator; it decreases pulmonary capillary wedge pressure even before an increase in urine output is observed. Insertion of a pulmonary artery catheter is useful for several reasons. It confirms the diagnosis of cardiogenic pulmonary edema and allows monitoring of oxygen delivery as left ventricular preload is reduced by diuretic agents. Some patients may require additional vasodilator agents or the use of inotropes. An occasional patient with cardiogenic pulmonary edema will exhibit normal or reduced pulmonary capillary wedge pressures because of volume depletion or markedly reduced ventricular compliance. Integration of hemodynamic data with clinical observations should confirm that the patient has cardiogenic pulmonary edema.

Endotracheal intubation should be avoided when possible in patients who are otherwise stable, since pulmonary edema often resolves rapidly following diuretic therapy. On the other hand, oxygen delivery may not be sufficient for the increased oxygen consumption of the vigorously contracting respiratory muscles, and a period of assisted or controlled ventilation may be necessary to prevent major deficits in peripheral oxygenation. The decision to intubate is made primarily on clinical grounds; intubation is probably indicated if it appears unlikely that the edema will clear rapidly or if the patient appears unable to tolerate either the increased work of breathing or hypoxia (see Fig 7–19).

Asthma: The Problem of Bronchospasm

Spasmodic bronchospasm is common in patients with chronic bronchitis and emphysema, as well as those with classic allergic asthma. Acute respiratory fail-

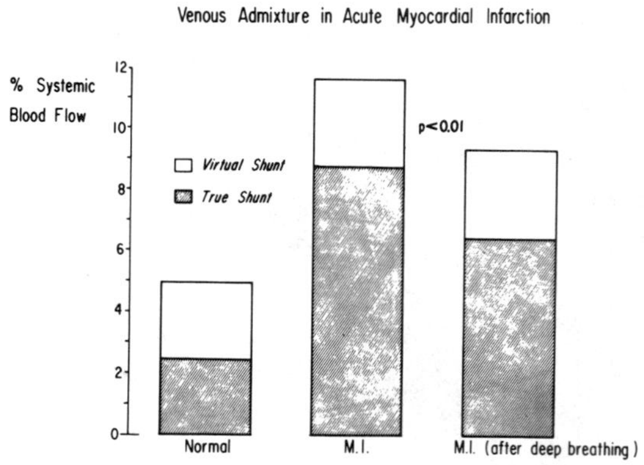

FIG 7–18.
Venous admixture expressed as a percentage of systemic blood flow in acute myocardial infarction. The true shunt represents blood flow completely bypassing alveolar tissue. The virtual shunt is an index of ventilation/perfusion inequality and reflects perfusion of poorly ventilated areas. Note the marked increase in true venoarterial shunting in acute myocardial infarction. Following several deep breaths, the true shunt decreases by about one-third. The importance of reversible atelectasis in acute myocardial infarction is described in detail in the text.

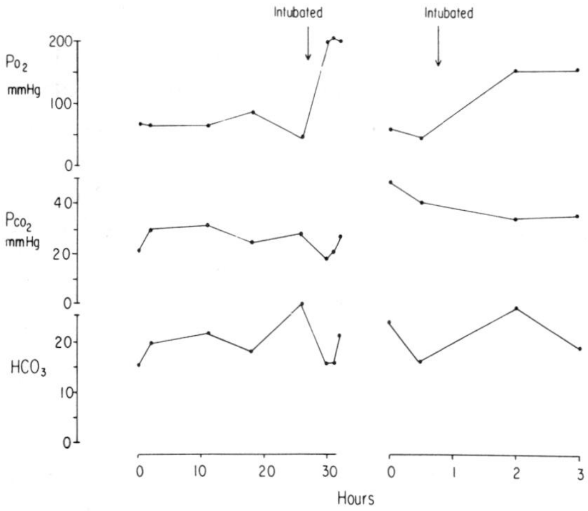

FIG 7–19.
Both buffer base deficits and arterial hypoxemia, the two common metabolic abnormalities seen in acute pulmonary edema, may be readily corrected. The arterial oxygen tension (Po_2) was measured during the breathing of 100% oxygen. This should approach 650 mm Hg if shunting is not present. Profound shunting was demonstrated in both patients by the failure of arterial oxygen tension to rise above 60 mm Hg during 100% oxygen. Endotracheal intubation and ventilation with a volume cycled ventilator produced a prompt decrease in shunting and a striking rise in arterial oxygen tension. Carbon dioxide tension was low in one patient and elevated in the other. Both patients had buffer base deficits, evidenced by the low plasma bicarbonate, which responded to the administration of sodium bicarbonate.

ure (status asthmaticus) may occur with great rapidity in these patients but be unrecognized until cardiac or respiratory arrest occurs.[5] Asthma is probably best defined as an increase in airway responsiveness to a variety of stimuli; enhanced responsiveness may be identified by measuring pulmonary function before and after administration of parasympathetic agents such as methacholine or carbachol. The diagnosis in critically ill patients must be inferred from historical information and physical examination. Before diagnosing asthma, the following other causes of wheezing must be ruled out: chronic airways obstruction, foreign body, bronchogenic carcinoma, bronchial adenoma, endobronchial granuloma, allergic bronchopulmonary aspergillosis, tracheal stenosis, pulmonary embolism, upper airway obstruction, left ventricular failure, polyarteritis nodosa, Wegener's granulomatosis, and the carcinoid syndrome. Recording of flow-volume curves provides important clues to the diagnosis of airway obstruction. Expiratory flow is much lower than inspiratory flow in lower airway obstruction; in contrast, inspiratory flow is attenuated in upper airway obstruction. A syndrome of laryngeal dysfunction associated with an inspiratory plateau can be treated by speech therapy.

Diffuse airway obstruction with thick mucus plugs is the causal factor in most asthmatics who develop acute respiratory failure. Poor response to sympathomimeteic agents does not necessarily mean that smooth muscle is unresponsive (so called epinephrine-fastness) but usually suggests that factors other than bronchospasm are responsible for the airway obstruction. Mucus plugging and incipient respiratory failure may be recognized by the presence of severe dyspnea together with a decrease or disappearance in breath sounds. Since wheezing decreases as alveolar ventilation and air flow through the bronchial tree decrease, agitation and unusual behavior may be attributed to emotional instability rather than to alterations in alveolar-capillary gas exchange. Only analysis of arterial blood or measurement of the first second forced expiratory vital capacity ($FEV_{1.0}$) will separate the critically ill asthmatic from the asthmatic with severe wheezing but relatively normal gas exchange. The initiated might even mistake a severely obstructed asthmatic without wheezing for an individual with acute anxiety; refusal to hospitalize or the administration of barbiturates in that situation might well lead to the patient's death.

An important study by McFadden and Lyons[148] demonstrated the behavior of oxygen and carbon dioxide tensions in asthma. These authors used the $FEV_{1.0}$ as an index of airway obstruction and found strikingly different relationships between severity of obstruction and oxygen or carbon dioxide tensions. Arterial oxygen tension decreased linearly with decreases in $FEV_{1.0}$ (Fig 7–20). Carbon dioxide decreased with decreasing $FEV_{1.0}$ because of hyperventilation, then became normal and rose sharply when $FEV_{1.0}$ fell below 25% of predicted. Inspection of the data shown in Figure 7–20 reveals that a normal carbon dioxide tension could occur at either point A, representing minimal airway obstruction, or point B, representing severe airway obstruction. A low oxygen tension with a normal carbon dioxide tension suggests severe obstruction; a normal oxygen tension in the same individual suggests minimal obstruction.

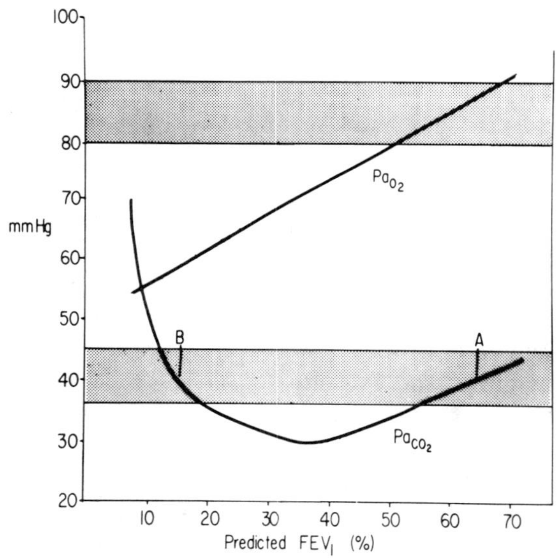

FIG 7–20.
Arterial blood gases in asthma. Note different behavior of arterial oxygen and carbon dioxide tension as airway obstruction, indicated by the $FEV_{1.0}$ expressed as a percentage of normal, decreases. While oxygen tension decreases linearly with increasing obstruction, arterial carbon dioxide tension decreases with mild obstruction and becomes normal with moderate degrees of obstruction. It suddenly rises as airway obstruction becomes severe. Note that it would be impossible from the carbon dioxide data alone to predict the amount of airway obstruction at points A or points B. Correlation of carbon dioxide and oxygen tensions help define the current status of the patient. (Adapted from McFadden ER Jr, Lyons HA: Arterial blood gas tensions in asthma. *N Engl J Med* 1968; 278:1027.)

The initial treatment in patients with normal mental status and reduced carbon dioxide tensions should be either adrenergic agonists (subcutaneous epinephrine or terbutaline) or aminophylline, the soluble salt of theophylline. It is important to achieve theophylline levels of 10–20 μg/ml; lower levels are generally ineffective, and higher levels may produce insomnia, anorexia, nausea, vomiting, sinus tachycardia, cardiac arrhythmias, or seizures. The knowledge of prior plasma levels and doses previously administered is helpful in understanding atypical responses. Cigarette smokers and individuals receiving barbiturates have increased clearances of theophylline; reduced clearances are seen in patients with impaired liver, kidney, or cardiac function, in alcoholics, and in patients receiving erythromycin.

A recent study involving the house staff from the Peter Bent Brigham Hospital[149] demonstrated that subcutaneously administered epinephrine increased $FEV_{1.0}$ an average of 0.76 liter, nebulized isoproterenol 0.79 liter, and aminophylline 0.23 liter when given as initial therapy to patients arriving at an emergency room. Side effects for all agents and differences between the two beta agonists were not observed. These data suggest that short-acting sympathomimetic agents produce better and more rapid improvement in acutely ill asthmatics than intravenous theophylline, and also emphasize the importance of $FEV_{1.0}$ to monitor therapy. If objective improvement cannot be demonstrated, both sympathomimetic drugs and theophylline should be used; but hospitalization should be considered, since the combination substantially increases the likelihood of cardiovascular side effects.

While there is no clear-cut evidence that administration by intermittent positive pressure breathing is more effective than by metered inhalation, the delivery with large tidal volumes and slow flow rates and concurrent nebulization of water may be valuable. In theory, the use of specific beta-2 agonists may be useful because of the reduction of cardiovascular side effects and because of an extended length of action. The longer action derives from the resistance of these compounds to activation by the enzyme catecholamine transferase.

Corticosteroids are very useful in the treatment of acute exacerbations and of status asthmaticus. Initial doses of 40–60 mg or more of prednisone may be required; rapid reduction in dose is usually possible and should be based on clinical status and sequential spirometry. Three relatively new agents have been effective in long-term management. Cromolyn prevents mast cell mediator release and is indicated in patients with allergic asthma. Nebulized beclamethasone apparently alters immune responses directly and allows for major reductions in oral corticosteroid dosage. Parasympathetic agents like atropine may be useful in individuals where evidence for vagal-induced larger airways obstruction is present.

The sharp increase in carbon dioxide tension as airway obstruction increases makes it important to consider intubation whenever hypercapnia or normocapnia with hypoxemia is present in the asthmatic. It is a mistake to attempt conservative treatment in the agitated, severely obstructed asthmatic with evidence of hypoxemia and normal or slightly elevated carbon dioxide tensions. The cautious approach advised for the treatment of chronic airway obstruction is dangerous in the patient with asthma and developing respiratory failure. Vigorous therapy, including hydration, high doses of corticosteroids, endotracheal intubation, and controlled ventilation is almost always lifesaving if instituted early. Most deaths from asthma result from ignorance of the severe prognosis associated with even mild abnormalities of oxygen and carbon dioxide exchange in these patients.

Acute Pulmonary Embolism

Acute pulmonary embolization (APE) may produce sudden cardiorespiratory collapse, but the diagnosis may be difficult; 50–60% of patients with evidence of APE were not diagnosed during life.[150] The incidence of APE at autopsy is 15–30%, depending upon the patient population, and about 40% of individuals diagnosed as APE had other conditions such as bronchopneumonia, congestive heart failure, or viral pneumonia. APE is usually multiple, more common in the lower than in the upper lung fields, and more than 80% arise from the leg veins so that impedence plethysmography of the lower extremity provides a method for suspecting its presence. Infarction complicates embolization in 25% of instances, but rises to 90% in cardiac patients.

Two-thirds of deaths from acute pulmonary emboli occur within 30 minutes of the embolism, and they are presently the third leading cause of sudden death in the United States. These massive emboli may not be associated with evidence of deep vein thrombosis, so that the correct diagnosis may not be immediately apparent. Acute cardiovascular effects are secondary to sudden elevations of pulmonary arterial pressure due to humorally mediated pulmonary arteriolar constriction and to obliteration of vascular bed by clot. While pulmonary hypertension is usually associated with obliteration of more than 60% of the pulmonary vascular bed, humoral mechanisms in the early minutes of embolization can produce acute vasoconstriction and sudden death with lesser degrees of anatomic obliteration. Occlusion of a major pulmonary artery or segmental artery suggests serious obstruction. Estimation of the degree of vascular occlusion by ventilation/perfusion scanning and measurement of right-sided cardiac pressures are useful in determining the severity of an embolic episode. Obviously, the physician responsible for the care of a patient with suspected acute pulmonary embolism must *personally* view the $\dot{V}/\dot{Q}$ scan as soon as it is obtained!

A national cooperative study conducted between 1968 and 1970[150] randomized 160 patients to either heparin or urokinase. Mortality was 9% and 7%, respectively, in the two groups, but a number of measurements demonstrated more rapid resolution with urokinase. When both treatment groups were combined, perfusion defects resolved in 55% at 14 days; 78% at 6 and 12 months; and, at 12 months, 16% had residual defects greater than 10% of total perfusion. Since all diagnoses were confirmed by angiocardiography, the following frequency of clinical manifestations appear reliable.

Fifty percent had normal values for LDH, SGOT and bilirubin. LDH was elevated in 40% , bilirubin in 12%, and SGOT in 27%. Wacker's triad (elevated LDH and bilirubin with normal SGOT) was found in 4%; 54.2% had fibrinogen levels above 450 mg/dl; 22.7% had plasminogen levels below 1.75 units/ml. Right ventricular pressures averaged 44/9 mm Hg; right atrial pressure was six. Twenty-four hours later, right ventricular pressures in patients given urokinase had fallen to an average of 33.7/6.5; there was no change in diastolic pressure in the heparin group, but the right ventricular systolic pressure fell to 41 mm Hg. Arterial oxygen tension was below 80 mm Hg in 90% and below 70 mm Hg in 75% of patients.

Heparin should be administered as *soon* as possible by either continuous or intermittent methods. It is good practice to begin heparin if APE is suspected *before* moving the patient to a radiographic diagnostic area. Most believe the best technique is a loading dose of 75 IU per pound followed by 10 IU/pound/hour by a constant infusion pump into a plastic catheter placed above the antecubital fossa. Subsequent dosage should be adjusted to maintain the partial thromboplastin time (PTT) at 1.5–2.5 times normal or the Lee-White clotting time (CT) to 2.0–2.5 times normal. If this is not possible, intermittent administration with 10,000 units every four hours for the first day, with subsequent dosages based on measurement of PTT or CT one hour before the next dose is scheduled. Bleeding may be controlled by the slow intravenous administration of protamine diluted in physiologic saline. One approach is to administer an amount equal to half of the last dose of heparin but not in excess of 100 mg; each 100 units represents one mg. Increasing heparin requirements suggests active thrombosis.

Heparin therapy should be continued for 7–10 days. Warfarin should be initiated several days before discontinuation of heparin and continued for at least six weeks. The duration of warfarin therapy is controversial; some authorities recommend continuation for three to six months depending on the clinical situation. An uncommon complication of heparin therapy is thrombocytopenia.

The national urokinase study described above defined massive APE as one with obstructions or significant filling defects in two or more lobar pulmonary arteries or an equivalent amount of emboli in other vessels; submassive APE was an obstruction or filling defect in at least one segmental pulmonary artery. A 12-hour urokinase infusion in addition to heparin therapy is probably indicated with massive APE, particularly if the patient is in shock. The expense of urokinase and the improvement in streptokinase formulation has led many to substitute the latter for the former. The efficacy of the newly synthesized tissue plasminogen activator in acute pulmonary embolism remains to be determined.

Insertion of a vena caval umbrella or filter (probably more desirable than other vena caval interruption techniques) is indicated if anticoagulants are contraindicated or if another massive APE occurs while the patient is on anticoagulant therapy. It is not indicated with a minor recurrence, since this may be related to the initial embolus.

REFERENCES

1. McCann WS, Lovejoy FW Jr, Yu PNG: The failing lung. *NY State J Med* 1952; 52:1983.

2. Noehren TH: Relief of carbon dioxide narcosis by simple intermittent positive pressure breathing therapy. *Dis Chest* 1955; 28:515.

3. Miller FL, Zerbi-Ortiz A, Elkins JT Jr: Use of the tank respirator in overwhelming bacterial pneumonia. *N Engl J Med* 1960; 262:1264.

4. Anthonisen NR, Smith HJ: Respiratory acidosis as a consequence of pulmonary edema. *Ann Intern Med* 1965; 62:991.

5. Gregory JJ, Ayres SM, Giannelli S Jr, et al: Treatment of acute respiratory acidosis complicating status asthmaticus. *J Thorac Cardiovasc Surg* 1968; 55:426.

6. The IPPB trial group. Intermittent positive pressure breathing therapy of chronic obstructive pulmonary disease. *Ann Intern Med* 1983; 99:612–620.

7. Ashbaugh DG, Petty TL, Bigelow DB, et al: Continuous positive pressure breathing (CPPB) in adult repiratory distress syndrome. *J Thorac Cardiovasc Surg* 1969; 57:31.

8. Extracorporeal Support for Respiratory Insufficiency: A collaborative study in response to RFP-NHLI-73-20. US Department of Health, Education, and Welfare Public Health Service, National Institutes of Health, National Heart, Lung, and Blood Institute Division of Lung Diseases, 1979.

9. Ayres SM, Grace WJ: Inappropriate ventilation and hypoxemia as causes of cardiac arrhythmias: The control of arrhythmias without antiarrhythmic drugs. *Am J Med* 1969; 46:495.

10. Richardson DW, Kontos HA, Raper AJ, et al: Modification by beta-adrenergic blockade of the circulatory responses to acute hypoxia in man. *J Clin Invest* 1967; 46:77.

11. Filley GF: *Pulmonary Insufficiency and Respiratory Failure.* Philadelphia, Lea & Febiger, 1967.

12. Otis AB: Some physiological responses to chronic hypoxia, in *Oxygen in the Animal Organism.* New York, Pergamon Press, 1964.

13. Benesch R, Benesch RE: The effect of organic phosphates from the human erythrocyte on the allosteric properties of hemoglobin. *Biochem Biophys Res Commun* 1967; 26:162.

14. Hurtado A: Adaptation to the environment, in Dill, DB (ed): *Handbook of Physiology.* Section 4. Washington, DC, American Physiological Society, 1964, chap 54, p 851.

15. Lenfant C. , Torrance J. , English E, et al: Effect of altitude on oxygen binding by hemoglobin and on organic phosphate level. *J Clin Invest* 1968; 47:2652.

16. Brackett NC Jr, Cohen JJ, Schwartz WB: Carbon dioxide titration curve of normal man: Effect of increasing degrees of acute hypercapnia on acid-base equilibrium. *N Engl J Med* 1965; 272:6.

17. Cotev S, Perel A, Katzenelson R, et al: The effect of PEEP on oxygenating capacity in acute respiratory failure with sepsis. *Crit Care Med* 1976; 4:186–192.

18. Fowler AA, Hamman RF, Good JT, et al: Adult respiratory distress syndrome: Risk with common predispositions. *Ann Intern Med* 1983; 98:593–597.

19. Montgomery AB, Stager MA, Carrico CJ, et al: Causes of mortality in patients with the adult repiratory distress syndrome. *Am Rev Resp Dis* 1985; 132:485–489.

20. Bartlett RH, Gazzaniga AB, Wilson AF,

et al: Mortality prediction in adult respiratory insufficiency. *Chest* 1975; 67:680–684.

21. Kirby RR, Downs JB, Civetta JM, et al: High level positive end-expiratory pressure (PEEP) in acute respiratory insufficiency. *Chest* 1975; 67:156–163.

22. Klein JJ, van Haeringen JR, Sluiter JF, et al: Pulmonary function after recovery from the adult respiratory distress syndrome. *Chest* 1976; 69:350–355.

23. Bone RG: Treatment of adult respiratory distress syndrome with diuretics, dialysis, and positive end-expiratory pressure. *Crit Care Med* 1978; 6:136.

24. Lakshminarayan S, Stanford RE, Petty TL: Prognosis after recovery from adult respiratory distress syndrome. *Am Rev Resp Dis* 1976; 113:7–16.

25. Lamy M, Fallat RJ, Koeniger E, et al: Pathologic features and mechanisms of hypoxemia in the adult respiratory distress syndrome. *Am Rev Resp Dis* 1976; 114:267–284.

26. Douglas ME, Downs JB: Pulmonary function following severe acute respiratory failure and high levels of positive end-expiratory pressure. *Chest* 1977; 71:18–23.

27. Zapol WM, Snider MT: Pulmonary hypertension in severe acute respiratory failure. *N Engl J Med* 1977; 296:476–480.

28. Yahav J, Lieberman P, Molho M: Pulmonary function following the adult respiratory distress syndrome. *Chest* 1978; 74:247–250.

29. Gallagher TJ, Civetta JM: Goal-directed therapy of acute respiratory failure. *Anesth Analg* 1980; 59:831–834.

30. Bell RC, Coalson JJ, Smith JD, et al: Multiple organ system failure and infection in adult respiratory distress syndrome. *Ann Intern Med* 1983; 99:293–298.

31. Downs JB: Intensive care and the adult respiratory distress syndrome, in Parillo JE, Ayres SM (eds): *Major Issues in Critical Care Medicine*. Baltimore, Williams & Wilkins, 1984.

32. Rinaldo JE: Letter to the editor, *Am Rev Resp Dis* 1986; 133:343.

33. Fein AM, Lippmann M, Holtzman H, et al: The risk factors, incidence, and prognosis of adult respiratory distress syndrome after septicemia. *Chest* 1983; 83:40–42.

34. Bachofen M, Weibel ER: Alterations of gas exchange apparatus in adult respiratory insufficiency associated with septicemia. *Am Rev Resp Dis* 1977; 116:589.

35. Bachofen H, Gehr P, Weibel ER: Alterations of mechanical properties and morphology in excised rabbit lungs rinsed with detergent. *J Appl Physiol* 1979; 47:1002.

36. Starling EH: On the absorption of fluids from the connective tissue spaces. *J Physiol* 1896; 19:312.

37. Pappenheimer JR, Soto-Rivera A: Effective osmotic pressure of the plasma proteins and other quantities associated with the capillary circulation in the hind limbs of cats and dogs. *Am J Physiol* 1948; 152:471.

38. Staub NC, Nagano H, Pearce ML: Pulmonary edema in dogs, especially the sequence of fluid accumulation in the lungs. *J Appl Physiol* 1967; 22:227.

39. Brigham KL, Woolverton WC, Blake LH, et al: Increased sheep lung vascular permeability caused by pseudomonas bacteria. *J Clin Invest* 1974; 54:792.

40. Sprague RS, Stephenson AH, Dahms TE, et al: Effect of cyclooxygenase inhibition on etchlorvynol-induced acute lung injury in dogs. *J Appl Physiol* 1986; 61:1058–1064.

41. Brigham KL, Kairman K, Harris TR, et al: Correlation of oxygenation with vascular permeability-surface area but not with lung water in humans with acute respiratory failure and pulmonary edema. *J Clin Invest* 1983; 72:339–349.

42. Cooper JA, Feustel PJ, Line BR, et al: Pulmonary epithelial clearance of ^{99m}Tc-DTPA after thrombin-induced pulmonary microembolism. *Amer Rev Resp Dis* 1986, 134:734.

43. Landis EM: The capillary pressure in frog mesentery as determined by microinjection. *Am J Physiol* 1926; 75:548.

44. McCabe WR: Serum complement levels in bacteremia due to gram-negative organisms. *N Engl J Med* 1973; 288:21.

45. Sacks T, Moldow CF, Craddock PR, et al: Oxygen radicals mediate endothelial cell damage by complement-stimulated granulocytes. *J Clin Invest* 1978; 61:1161.

46. Fowler AA, Walchak S, Giclas PC, et al: Characterization of antiprotease activity in the adult respiratory distress syndrome. *Chest* 1982; 81: 50S–51S.

47. Fowler AA, Fisher BJ, Webster RO, et al: Lavage fluid from patients at risk for ARDS promotes neutrophil adherence. *Am Rev Resp Dis* 1985; 131S:137.

48. Filkins JP: Monokines and the metabolic pathophysiology of septic shock. *Fed Proc* 1985; 44:25.

49. Parsons PE, Fowler AA, Hyers TM, et al: Chemotactic activity in bronchoalveolar lavage fluid from patients with adult respiratory distress syndrome. *Am Rev Resp Dis* 1985; 132:490–493.

50. Hunninghake GW, Gadek JE, Fales HM, et al: Human alveolar macrophage-derived chemotactic factor for neutrophils. *J Clin Invest* 1980; 66:473–483.

51. Merril WW, Naegel GP, Matthay RA, et al: Alveolar macrophage-derived chemotactic factor. *J Clin Invest* 1980; 65:268–276.

52. Fowler AA, Hamman RF, Zerbe GO, et al: Adult respiratory distress syndrome: prognosis after onset. *Am Rev Resp Dis* 1985; 132:472–478.

53. Jacobs RF, Kiel DP, Balk RA: Alveolar macrophage function in a canine model of endotoxin-induced lung injury. *Am Rev Resp Dis* 1986; 134:745–751.

54. Ognibene FP, Martin SE, Parker MM, et al: Adult respiratory distress syndrome in patients with severe neutropenia. *N Engl J Med* 1986; 315:547–551.

55. Rinaldo JE, Borovetz H: Deterioration of oxygenation and abnormal lung microvascular permeability during resolution of leukopenia in patients with diffuse lung injury. *Am Rev Resp Dis* 1985; 131:579–583.

56. Rinaldo JE, Rogers RM: Editorial adult respiratory distress syndrome. *N Engl J Med* 1986; 315:578.

57. Fowler AA, Hyers TM, Stephenson AH, et al: The appearance of neutrophils and metabolites of arachidonic acid in bronchial fluid of patients at risk for ARDS. *Am Rev Resp Dis* 1985; 131S:135.

58. Johnson A, Tahamont MV, Malik AB: Thrombin-induced lung vascular injury: Roles of fibrinogen and fibrinolysis. *Am Rev Resp Dis* 1983; 128:38–44.

59. Weiland JE, Davis WB, Holter, JF, et al: Lung neutrophils in the adult respiratory distress syndrome. *Am Rev Resp Dis* 1986; 133:218.

60. Ford-Hutchinson, AW: Leukotrienes: Their formation and role as inflammatory mediators. *Fed Proc* 1985; 44:25.

61. Ognibene FP, Rosenberg SA, Skibber J, et al: Interleukin-2 hemodynamics mimic septic shock. *Clin Res* 1986; 34:413A.

62. Martin WJ: II. Neutrophils kill pulmonary endothelial cells by a hydrogen-peroxide dependent pathway. *Am Rev Resp Dis* 1984; 130:209–213.

63. Craddock PR, Fehr J, Brigham KL, et al: Complement and leukocyte mediated pulmonary dysfunction in hemodialysis. *New Engl J Med* 1977; 296:769.

64. McAslan TC, Cowley RA: The preventive use of peep in major trauma, in *The American Surgeon*. Philadelphia, JB Lippincott, 1979.

65. Brigham K, Bowers R, McKeen C: Methyl-prednisolone prevention of increased lung vascular permeability following endotoxemia in sheep. *J Clin Invest* 1981; 67:1103.

66. Goodwin JS, Atluru D, Sierakowski S, et al: Mechanism of action of glucocorticosteroids: Inhibition of T cell proliferation and interleukin-2 production by hydrocortisone is reversed by leukotriene B_4. *J Clin Invest* 1986; 77:1244.

67. Parrillo JE: Corticosteroid therapy of septic shock: Preliminary evaluation of a multicenter trial. Update in *Crit Care Med* 1986; vol 1.

68. Kubo K, Kobayashi T: Effects of OKY-046, a selective thromboxine synthetase inhibitor, on endotoxin-induced lung injury in unanesthetized sheep. *Am Rev Resp Dis* 1985; 132:494–499.

69. Ogletree ML, Brigham KL: Effects of

cyclooxygenase inhibitors on pulmonary vascular responses to endotoxin in unanesthetized sheep. *Prostaglandins Leukotrienes Med* 1982; 8:489–502.

70. Tate RM, Repine JE: Neutrophils and the adult respiratory distress syndrome. *Am Rev Resp Dis* 1983; 128:552.

71. Seilaff TD, Sugerman HJ, Tatum JL, et al: Successful treatment of ARDS by histomine and prostaglandin blockade in a porcine pseudomonas model. *Surgery* (in press).

72. Bernard GR, Lucht WD, Niedermeyer ME, et al: Effect of N-acetylcysteine on the pulmonary response to endotoxin in the awake sheep and upon in vitro granulocyte function. *J Clin Invest* 1984; 73:1772.

73. Jelinek DF, Thompson PA, Lipsky PE: Regulation of human B cell activation by prostaglandin E_2. Suppression of the generation of immunoglobulin-secreting cells. *J Clin Invest* 1985, 75: 1339.

74. Webster RO, Nielson V: Unpublished data.

75. Hallman M, Merritt TA, Jarvenpaa A-L, et al: Exogenous human surfactant for treatment of severe respiratory distress syndrome: A randomized prospective clinical trial. *J Pediatr* 1985; 106:963–969.

76. Merritt TA, Hallman M, Bloom BT, et al: Prophylactic treatment of very premature infants with human surfactant. *New Engl J Med* 1986; 315:785–790.

77. Cournand A, Motley HL, Werko L, et al: Physiological studies of the effects of intermittent positive pressure breathing in cardiac output in man. *Am J Physiol* 1948; 152:162.

78. Guyton AC, Lindsey AW, Abernathy B, et al: Venous return at various right atrial pressures and the normal venous return curve. *Am J Physiol* 1957; 189:609–615.

79. Pinsky MR: Instantaneous venous return curves in an intact canine preparation. *J Appl Physiol* 1984; 56:765–771.

80. Versprille A, Jansen JRC: Mean systemic filling pressure as a characteristic pressure for venous return. *Pjlugers Archiv* 1985; 405: 226–233.

81. Prewitt RM, Wood LH: Effects of positive end-expiratory pressure on ventricular function in dogs. *Am J Physiol* 1972; 236:H534–544.

82. Kirby RR: Positive airway pressure: System design and clinical applications, in Shoemaker WC (ed): *Critical Care: State of the Art.* Fullerton, CA, Society of Critical Care Medicine, 1985.

83. Mead J, Collier C: Relation of volume history of lungs to respiratory mechanics in anesthetized dogs. *J Appl Physiol* 1959; 14:669.

84. Bendixen HH, Egbert LD, Hedley-Whyte J, et al: *Respiratory Care.* St Louis, MO, CV Mosby, 1965.

85. Dammann JF, McAslan TC: PEEP: Its use in young patients with apparently normal lungs. *Crit Care Med* 1979; 7:14.

86. Lutch JS, Murray JF: Continuous positive pressure ventilation: Effects on systemic oxygen transport and tissue oxygenation. *Ann Intern Med* 1972; 76:193.

87. Suter PM, Fairley B, Isenberg MD: Optimum end-expiratory airway pressure in patients with acute pulmonary failure. *N Engl J Med* 1975; 292:284.

88. Douglas ME, Downs JB: Respiratory therapy for ventilatory failure, in Shoemaker WC, Thompson WL, Holbrook PR (eds): *Textbook of Critical Care.* Philadelphia, WB Saunders, 1984.

89. Kirby RR: Intermittent mandatory ventilation. *Refresher Courses in Anesthesiology* 1979; 7:169.

90. Giannelli S, Ayres, SM, Buehler ME with the technical assistance of Armstrong DR, Stuart ME: Effects of pulmonary blood flow upon lung mechanics. *J Clin Invest* 1967; 46:1625–1642.

91. Ayres SM, Kozam RL, Lukas DS: The effects of intermittent positive pressure breathing on intrathoracic pressure, pulmonary mechanics and the work of breathing. *Am Rev Resp Dis* 1963; 87:370–379.

92. Manginello FP, Grassi AE, Schechner S, et al: Evaluation of methods of assisted ventilation in hyaline membrane disease. *Arch Dis Child* 1978; 53:878–881.

93. Lachmann B, Jonson B, Lindroth M, et al: Modes of artificial ventilation in severe respiratory distress syndrome: Lung functions and morphology in rabbits after washout of alveolar surfactant. *Crit Care Med* 1982; 10:724–32.

94. Gurevitch MJ, Van Dyne J, Young ES, et al: Improved oxygenation and lower peak airway pressure in severe adult respiratory distress syndrome. *Chest* 1986; 89:211.

95. Carlon GC, Howland WS, Ray C: High frequency ventilation: A prospective, randomized evaluation. *Chest* 1983; 84:551.

96. Siegel JH, Stoklosa JC, Borg U, et al: Quantification of asymmetric lung pathophysiology as a guide to the use of simultaneous independent lung ventilation in posttraumatic and septic adult respiratory distress syndrome. *Ann Surg* 1985; 202:425.

97. Kirby RR: Membrane oxygenators: What role (if any) in acute ventilatory insufficiency? *Crit Care Med* 1978; 6:19.

98. Bartlett RH, Jeffries MR, Haiduc N, et al: Extracorporeal membrane oxygenation (ECMO) cardiopulmonary support in infancy. *Trans Am Soc Artif Intern Organs* 1976; 22:80.

99. MacIntyre NR: Respiratory function during pressure support ventilation. *Chest* 1986; 89:677–683.

100. Berlauk JF: Prolonged endotracheal intubation vs. tracheostomy. *Crit Care Med* 1986; 14:742.

101. Hedenstierna G, Friman L, Schildt B: Stenosis following tracheostomy. *Anaesthesia* 1976; 31:479.

102. Stauffer JL, Olson DE, Petty TL: Complications and consequences of endotracheal intubation and tracheostomy. A prospective study of 150 critically ill adult patients. *Am J Med* 1981; 70:65.

103. Zwillich CW, Pierson DJ, Creagh CD, et al: Complications of assisted ventilation. *Am J Med* 1974; 57:161.

104. Cullen DJ, Caldera DL: The incidence of ventilator-induced pulmonary barotrauma in critically ill patients. *Anesthesiology* 1979; 50:185.

105. Chiles C, Ravin CE: Radiographic recognition of pneumothorax in the intensive care unit. *Crit Care Med* 1986; 14:677.

106. More DG, Raper RF, Watson CJ, et al: Combination therapy with ranitidine and pierenzepine for control of intragastric pH in the critically ill. *Crit Care Med* 1985; 13:651–655.

107. el-Kilany SM: Complications of tracheostomy. *Ear Nose Throat J* 1980; 59:123.

108. McGovern FH, Fitz-Hugh GS, Edgemon LS: The hazards of endotracheal intubation. *Ann Otol* 1971; 80:556.

109. Bernard GR, Lucht WD, Niedermeyer ME, et al: Effect of N-acetylcysteine on the pulmonary response to endotoxin in the awake sheep and upon in vitro granulocyte function. *J Clin Invest* 1984; 73: 1972.

110. Eckhauser FE, Billote J, Burke JF, et al: Tracheostomy complicating massive burn injury. A plea for conservatism. *Am J Surg* 1974; 127:418.

111. Downs JB, Klein EF, Desautels D, et al: Intermittent mandatory ventilation: A new approach to weaning patients from mechanical ventilators. *Chest* 1973; 64:331.

112. Bendixen HH, Egbert LD, Hedley-Whyte J, et al: Management of patients undergoing prolonged artificial ventilation, in *Respiratory Care*. St Louis, CV Mosby, 1965, p 149.

113. Sahn SA, Lakshminarayan S: Bedside criteria for discontinuation of mechanical ventilation. *Chest* 1973; 63:1002.

114. Tahvanainen J, Salmenpera M, Nikki P: Extubation criteria after weaning from intermittent mandatory ventilation and continuous positive airway pressure, in Parillo JE, Ayres SM (eds): *Major Issues in Critical Care Medicine*. Baltimore, Williams & Wilkins, 1983.

115. Sladen A, Laver MB, Pontoppidan H: Pulmonary complications and water retention in prolonged mechanical ventilation. *N Engl J Med* 1968; 279:448.

116. Larca L, Greenbaum DM: Effectiveness of intensive nutritional regimes in patients who fail to wean from mechanical ventilation. *Crit Care Med* 1982; 10:297.

117. Varsano S, Shapiro M, Taragan R, et al: Hypophosphatemia as a reversible cause of refractory ventilatory failure, in Parillo JE, Ayres SM (eds): *Major Issues in Critical Care Medicine*. Baltimore, Williams & Wilkins, 1983.

118. Gilbert J, Rice WH, Johnston J: Possible doxapram reversal of ventilator dependence in a brain-damaged patient. *Crit Care Med* 1985; 13:605.

119. Goldberg NS, Danon J, Sharp JT: Treatment of acute respiratory failure in the patient with chronic obstructive lung disease. *Chicago Medicine*. 1973; 76:357–360.

120. Grenvik A: "Terminal weaning", discontinuance of life-support therapy in the terminally ill patient. *Crit Care Med* 1985; 11:394.

121. Bunnell S: The use of nitrous oxide and oxygen to maintain anesthesia and positive pressure for thoracic surgery. *JAMA* 1912; 58:835–838.

122. Gregory GA, Kitterman JA, Phibbs RH, et al: Treatment of the idiopathic respiratory distress syndrome with continuous positive airway pressure. *N Engl J Med* 1971; 284:1333–1340.

123. Shoemaker WC, Appel PL Kram, HB: Comparison of two monitoring methods (central venous pressure versus pulmonary artery catheter) and two protocols as therapeutic goals (normal values versus values of survivors) in a prospective randomized clinical trial of critically ill surgical patients. *Crit Care Med* 1985; 13:304 (abst).

124. Niewoehner DE, Kleinerman J, Rice DB: Pathologic changes in the peripheral airways of young cigarette smokers. *N Engl J Med* 1974; 291:755.

125. Thurlbeck WM: Smoking, airflow limitation, and the pulmonary circulation. *Am Rev Resp Dis* 1980; 122:183.

126. Petty TL, Silvers GW, Stanford RE, et al: Small airway pathology is related to increased closing capacity and abnormal slope of phase III in excised human lungs. *Am Rev Resp Dis* 1980; 121:449.

127. Hale KA, Niewoehner DE, Cosio MG: Morphologic changes in the muscular pulmonary arteries: Relationship to cigarette smoking, airway disease, and emphysema. *Am Rev Resp Dis* 1980; 122:273.

128. Burk RH, George RB: Causes of acute respiratory failure in chronic airway obstruction: Relationship to immediate and long-term prognosis. Abstract of paper presented at annual meeting of the American Thoracic Society, May 21–24, 1972.

129. Karpick RJ, Pratt PC, Asmundsson T, Kilburn KH: Pathological findings in respiratory failure: Goblet cell metaplasia, alveolar damage, and myocardial infarction. *Ann Intern Med* 1970; 72:189.

130. Campbell EJM: The management of acute respiratory failure in chronic bronchitis and emphysema. *Am Rev Resp Dis* 1967; 95:626.

131. Noehren TH: Is positive pressure breathing overrated? *Chest* 1970; 57:507.

132. Herzog P, Norlander OP, Engström CG: Ultrasonic generation of aerosol for the humidification of inspired gas during volume-controlled ventilation. *Acta Anaesthiol Scand* 1964; 8:79.

133. Mitchell RI: Retention of aerosol particles in the respiratory tract: A review. *Am Rev Resp Dis* 1960; 82:627.

134. Pierce AK, Sanford JP, Thomas GD, et al: Long-term evaluation of decontamination of inhalation-therapy equipment and the occurrence of necrotizing pneumonia. *N Engl J Med* 1970; 282:528.

135. Mussberg B, Strandberg K, Philipson K, et al: Tracheobronchial clearance and beta-adrenoceptor stimulation in patients with chronic bronchitis. *Scand J Respir Dis* 1976; 57;281.

136. Speizer FE, Doll R, Heaf P: Observations on recent increase in mortality from asthma. *Br Med J* 1968; 1:335.

137. Resistance to β-adrenoceptor stimulants, editorial. *Br Med J* 1972;

138. Albert RK, Martin TR, Lewis RW: Controlled clinical trial of methylprednisolone in patients with chronic bronchitis and acute respiratory insufficiency. *Ann Intern Med* 1980; 92:753.

139. Miller WF: Fundamental principles of aerosol therapy. *Resp Care* 1972; 17:295.

140. Ganz W, Donoso R, Marcus H, et al: Coronary hemodynamics and myocardial oxygen metabolism during oxygen breathing in patients with and without coronary artery disease. *Circulation* 1972; 45:763.

141. Mithoefer JC, Keighley JF, Chir B, et al: Response of the arterial PO_2 to oxygen administration in chronic pulmonary disease. *Ann Intern Med* 1971; 74:328.

142. Kapanci Y, Weibel ER, Kaplan HP, et al: Pathogenesis and reversibility of the pulmonary lesions of oxygen toxicity in monkeys: II: Ultrastructural and morphometric studies. *Lab Invest* 1969; 20:101.

143. Singer MM, Wright F, Stanley LK, et al: Oxygen toxicity in man: A prospective study in patients after open-heart surgery. *N Engl J Med* 1970; 283:1473.

144. Barber RE, Lee J, Hamilton WK: Oxygen toxicity in man: A prospective study in patients with irreversible brain damage. *N Engl J Med* 1970; 283:1478.

145. Campbell EJM: Methods of oxygen administration in respiratory failure. *Ann NY Acad Sci* 1965; 121:861.

146. Stein M, Cassara EL: Preoperative pulmonary evaluation and therapy for surgery patients. *JAMA* 1970; 211:787.

147. Aberman A, Fulop M: The metabolic and respiratroy acidosis of acute pulmonary edema. *Ann Intern Med* 1972; 76:173.

148. McFadden ER Jr, Lyons HA: Arterial blood gas tensions in asthma. *N Engl J Med* 1968; 278:1027.

149. Rossing TH, Fanta CH, Goldstein DH, et al: Emergency therapy of asthma: Comparison of the acute effects of parental and inhaled sympathomimetic and infused aminophylline[1–3]. *Am Rev Resp Dis* 1980; 122:365.

150. National Cooperative Urokinase-Pulmonary Embolism Trial. *Circulation* 1973; 47 (suppl II):1.

8 THE KIDNEY AND BODY FLUIDS

The mammalian kidney evolved to conserve salt and water and to maintain a blood pressure sufficient to perfuse the multiple organ systems characteristic of mammalian development. This is accomplished by diverting a major proportion of the cardiac output through approximately one million nephrons. Most of these nephrons are located in the outer two-thirds of the renal cortex and have relatively short loops of Henle that enter only the outer part of the renal medulla. About 15% of nephrons are called juxtamedullary nephrons because they extend through the medulla to the papillary region of the kidney (inner medulla). The ascending limb of the loop of Henle has a short segment that is near to the glomerulus and contains the macula densa. Adjacent to the macula densa are the juxtaglomerular cells of the afferent arteriole, and the two comprise the juxtaglomerular apparatus, which plays a major role in the control of renin secretion. Eighty percent of the total blood flow perfuses the outer cortex, 15% the inner cortex and outer medulla, and 3% the inner medulla.

Glomerular capillary pressure in the normal kidney is kept within close limits by the tone of the afferent and efferent arterioles. If blood pressure rises, an increase in afferent resistance keeps glomerular pressure within normal limits. A fall in arterial blood pressure leads to afferent arteriolar dilatation and maintains perfusion pressure. These autoregulatory changes may be overcome by the general increase in sympathetic tone that occurs in critical illness. Sympathetic stimulation increases afferent arteriolar resistance and reduces glomerular blood flow. An increase in efferent resistance raises glomerular pressure and maintains filtration pressure initially, but total flow is markedly decreased. Blood flow is also redistributed from the outer cortex to the juxtamedullary glomeruli, which have long loops of Henle and appear to reabsorb sodium more efficiently than those in the outer cortex.

A group of recently identified humoral agents also affect renal blood flow and its distribution. Reduction in circulating blood volume, blood pressure, sodium concentration of renal arterial blood, or beta-adrenergic activation stimulates the secretion of renin from the juxtaglomerular apparatus. Renin is a proteolytic enzyme that transforms a plasma precursor to angiotensin I. Angiontensin II, produced from angiotensin I by a converting enzyme contained in pulmonary vascular endothelial cells, is the most potent vasoconstrictor known and also stimulates the adrenal cortex to secrete aldosterone. McGiff and Wong[1] have emphasized that the presence of cyclooxygenase in a variety of renal tissues provides an opportunity for compartmentalization of renal prostaglandin production. Increased concentrations of prostaglandin E_2, produced by medullary interstitial cells, have been found following hemorrhage, administration of a loop diuretic, or with surgical stress. Its concentration parallels that of renin and appears to partially counteract the vasoconstriction of sympathetic neural activity and angiontensin II release. Its production by the inner medulla leads to redistribution of cortical perfusion to the inner medulla, further favoring the activity of the juxtamedullary nephrons. The use of a cyclooxygenase inhibitor such as indomethacin in patients with impaired renal function can block PGE_2 synthesis and further decrease renal blood and function. PGI_2 (prostacyclin) is produced by the vascular bed and also increases renal blood flow. In addition, PGI_2 appears to stimulate the production of renin. The renal production of the vasoconstrictor prostanoid thromboxane A_2 is increased in severe stress and acts to decrease renal blood flow. Still another humoral agent, atrial natriuretic factor or atrin, increases blood flow in response to volume overload. It increases glomerular filtration by dilating the afferent glomerular arteriole and constricting the efferent arteriole so that higher glomerular pressures are available for filtration.[2]

BODY FLUIDS

Water is the most abundant material in the human body, and regulation of its volume and composition is a primary function of the kidney. Water comprises 70–80% of muscle, skin, and the parenchymal organs, and 10% of adipose tissue. The amount of adipose tissue present determines the percentage of water in the whole body and accounts for the observation that water may constitue but 45% of total body weight in obese individuals and up to 75% of body weight in lean individuals.

Body Fluid Compartments

It is convenient to consider the body as an aqueous solution of electrolytes divided into compartments: the intravascular space,[3,4] the interstitial space, and the intracellular space. As much as 30–40% of body weight is occupied by intracellular water. Extracellular fluid includes blood plasma (4.5% of body weight), interstitial fluid (16%), and lymph (2%).

Electrolyte Concentrations

Electrolyte concentrations are conventionally described in milliequivalents (mEq) per unit volume rather than in absolute weight. In this system of notation, quantities are expressed in terms of equivalent ionic activity, so that 1 mEq of a positive ion (cation) balances one of a negative ion (anion). In the reaction of hydrochloric acid and sodium hydroxide

$$Na^+ + OH^- + H^+ + Cl^- \rightarrow Na^+ + Cl^- + HOH$$

equivalent weights of each reactant react with each other.

The equivalent weight of a substance equals the molecular weight* of that substance in grams, divided by its valence. The gram molecular weight of sodium therefore is 22.99 and its valence is one; the equivalent weight of sodium is 22.99g. This is too large a value for convenient biologic usage, and electrolyte concentrations are expressed as milliequivalents (1/1,000 of an equivalent) per liter of fluid. The serum sodium concentration,

*Molecular weights have been designated for different compounds based on an arbitrary molecular weight of 16.000 assigned to oxygen.

$[Na^+]$,* is about 136 mEq/liter or 0.136 equivalents per liter. In another example, for calcium, with a valence of two and a molecular weight of 40.09, the equivalent weight is 40.09/2 or 20.05.

Table 8–1 lists the electrolyte composition of extracellular and intracellular compartments in muscle.[5,6] There are several striking differences: sodium is the major extracellular cation and potassium the major intracellular cation. Chloride is the principal extracellular anion, while phosphate is the major intracellular anion. Undoubtedly cells with different functions have different compositions. Tissue analysis is difficult, and it is impossible to state with certainty the fraction of total tissue water and electrolytes that are intracellular. Muscle, the largest single tissue mass, has been carefully investigated, and the values listed in Table 8–1 are probably quite accurate. These differences in ion concentration across cellular membranes are not due to ionic membrane impermeability. Inorganic ions diffuse freely across cell membranes, and concentration differences must be maintained by active ion transport against concentration gradients. Potassium and sodium gradients are maintained by an "ionic pump" powered by cellular energy. More sodium is actively "pumped" out than passively "leaks" in. The relationship of ion influx to ion efflux determines the gradient between intracellular and interstitial concentrations. Specialized functions—such as gastric hydrochloric acid production, pacemaking activity of cardiac cells, and muscular contraction—depend upon ionic gradients.

In most ion pumps, the outward pumping of sodium is linked with the inward pumping of potassium. Figure 8–1, from Glynn[7] illustrates the functioning of such a pump. The dashed arrows show the expected direction of ion flow if such flow followed a simple concentration gradient. Potassium would flow from the interior outward; sodium from the exterior inward. The energy-dependent ion pump opposes this tendency by pumping sodium out of and potassium into the cell.

Hypoxia, cold temperature, and certain metabolic inhibitors inactivate the potas-

*Concentration is conventionally indicated by enclosing the symbol for the substance in brackets—e.g., $[K^+]$ = 5.0 mEq/liter.

TABLE 8–1.
Electrolyte Composition of Muscle

	EXTRACELLULAR FLUID (mEq/liter)	INTRACELLULAR FLUID (mEq/liter)
Cations		
Na^+	142	10
K^+	4	160
Ca^{++}	5	–
Mg^{++}	3	35
Anions		
Cl^-	103	2
HCO_3^-	27	8
$PO_4^{\equiv}$	2	140
SO_4^-	1	–
Organic acid	5	–
Protein	16	55

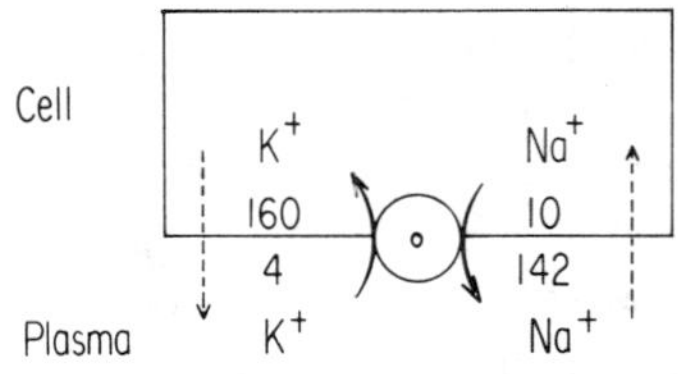

FIG 8–1.
The sodium potassium pump maintains an intracellular concentration of potassium of 160 mEq/liter compared to a plasma concentration of 4 mEq/liter. The sodium potassium pump requires adenosine triphosphate (ATP) as an energy source. The enzyme ATPase releases high energy phosphates and activates the pump. The ATPase dependency of the sodium-potassium pump is probably of great clinical significance. Recent studies have shown, for example, that digitalis partially inhibits ATPase, decreasing the activity of the pump and allowing sodium to leak into myocardial cells. (Adapted from Glynn IM: Sodium and potassium movements in human red cells. *J Physiol* 1956; 134:278.)

sium-sodium pump, decreasing ionic gradients and impairing cellular function. Pitts[8] pointed out that the most familiar example of this is the loss of potassium and gain in sodium observed when banked blood is stored in the cold. Rewarming restores the ion pump, and potassium reenters the red blood cells.

The myocardial ion pump plays a major role in intiating the contractile process. Depolarization appears to inhibit ion pumping and allows sodium to enter myocardial cells where it alters the distribution of calcium, making it available for the contractile process. The pump is reactivated during repolarization, restoring intracellular sodium and potassium concentrations. (See pp. 104 and 150).

Osmotic Pressure

The various compartments are in osmotic equilibrium despite the differences in ionic composition. This is a useful concept for guiding therapy because alterations in plasma osmolarity mirror parallel changes in intracellular osmolarity. Osmotic equilibrium is related to the diffusion of water molecules. Figure 8–2 shows water molecules on either side of a membrane which allows them to diffuse back and forth freely. If molecules of another substance—such as glucose that cannot pass the membrane—are dissolved in one compartment, water concentration decreases in that compartment. This produces a net passage of water molecules into the compartment containing the dissolved substance. The water molecules diffuse out of the compartment of higher water concentration faster than water molecules leave the compartment containing the solute. The process is similar to the diffusion of gas molecules described in Chapter 6. Theoretically, this difference in diffusion rates would occur indefinitely because there would always be a diffusion gradient favoring passage of water molecules into the compartment containing the solute. However, in enclosed compartments, the hydrostatic pressure rises because of the influx of water molecules. Equilibrium is established when this increased hydrostatic pressure causes the same net number of water molecules to return per unit time as enter the solute compartment, due to the osmotic diffusion effect. The hydrostatic pressure at equilibrium is called the osmotic pressure of the solution containing the solute that cannot penetrate the membrane.

Osmotic pressure is measured in osmols. A gram molecular weight of a substance that does not dissociate, such as glucose, is called 1 osmol. The dissolution of 1 mole in 22.4 liters of water creates an osmotic pressure of 760 mm Hg. If, instead, 1 mole, is dissolved in 1 liter, the osmotic pressure is 22.4 times greater. As with milliequivalent weights, milliosmols are more convenient units than osmols. The milliosmol (mosmol) is 1/1,000 of an osmol.

In electrolyte solutions, osmotic pressure is approximately proportional to

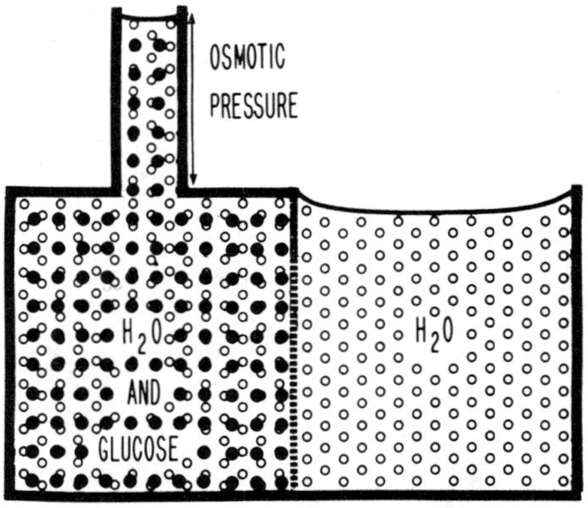

FIG 8–2.
Water molecules (open circles) freely diffuse across a semipermeable membrane separating the two compartments. The membrane is not permeable to glucose (closed circles) which is dissolved in the left compartment. The concentration of water molecules is greater on the right, and there is a net diffusion of water across the membrane into the left compartment until equilibrium is established. Hydrostatic pressure rises in the left compartment because of the influx of water molecules and causes the column of water above the compartment to rise. The difference in hydrostatic pressure between the two compartments at equilibrium is the osmotic pressure of the solution containing the glucose.

the ionic concentration. NaCl forms two osmotically active particles, Na^+ and Cl^-, giving an osmotic effect of almost 2 osmols for each mole of NaCl per liter of water. (The osmotic effect of these two ionic particles varies slightly with their concentration, and only if the 1 mole of NaCl were dissolved in an infinite volume of water would a 2-osmolar effect be produced. At the concentration of solutes in body fluids, 1 mole of dissolved NaCl in a liter of water exerts an osmotic effect of 1.85 osmol.)

A given weight of dissolved protein exerts an osmotic pressure that is inversely proportional to its molecular weight. There are more molecules in a gram of albumin than in a gram of globulin, so that a gram of the former is osmotically more active than a gram of the latter (dissolved in the same volume of water). The total osmotic pressure developed when plasma is separated from pure water by a membrane permeable only to water molecules is very large—5,100 mm Hg.

The osmotic effect of a solution is referred to as a colligative property, because it depends upon the number of particles in solution rather than the chemical characteristics of the particles. Another colligative effect of solutions is depression of the freezing point. A solution containing 1 osmol/liter of water freezes at −1.86° C. Because freezing point depression is proportional to osmotic activity, the osmolality of body solutions is usually determined by the easily performed measurement of freezing point depression.

Biologic osmotic activity depends upon the amount of solute per unit volume of water, not upon the amount of solute per unit volume of solution. An *osmolal solution* contains 1 osmol/kg of *water.* An *osmolar solution* contains 1 osmol/liter of *solution.* Usually the difference between plasma osmolality and osmolarity is not great. In lipemic serum, however, the water content of plasma can be markedly diminished. Thus, the freezing point depression is greater than one would expect from the total plasma electrolyte concentration, which would be low, because appreciable plasma volume is taken up by fat.

Electrolytes and water molecules pass freely across capillary walls, while plasma proteins cannot penetrate the small pores of the capillary membrane of most vascular beds and are confined to the vascular space. This has two effects: (1) the osmotic pressure of the plasma is greater than that of interstitial fluid. This osmotic pressure difference is only about 25 mm Hg, but it is approximately the same as the blood pressure in the capillary. (2) The negative charge of plasma proteins produces slight differences in electrolyte composition between plasma and interstitial fluid because of the Gibbs-Donnan principle.

The total milliequivalents of anions and cations must balance in each compartment to preserve electrical neutrality. The plasma must therefore contain more diffusible cations than the interstitial fluid in order to balance the negatively charged plasma proteins. The interstitial fluid contains more anions than does plasma.

RENAL REGULATION OF BODY COMPOSITION

On the average, about 25% of the total cardiac output perfuses the kidney each minute, giving that organ an opportunity to monitor and adjust the composition of the circulating blood. This is accomplished by first filtering a volume of plasma (glomerular ultrafiltration), reabsorbing more than 90% of this volume, secreting certain other components, and finally excreting in the urine a small fraction of the glomerular filtrate. Changes in urinary flow result from changes in water reabsorption, not from changes in glomerular filtration or renal blood flow. These changes in reabsorption maintain body water constant in spite of varying water intake. For example, the changes observed in a dehydrated individual compared to a well-hydrated individual who had just ingested an extra liter of water are seen in Table 8–2.

Decreased glomerular filtration rates are found in renal disease and in states associated with decreased renal blood flow. The plasma concentrations of urea, creatinine, phosphate, sulfate, and uric acid all increase and may be used as indicators of abnormal filtration rates. Blood urea concentrations are frequently used to estimate the glomerular filtration rate, but the broad range of normal renders the determination relatively insensitive. A 50% decrease in glomerular filtration rate would increase the urea concentration twofold, but the level might still be within normal limits. In addition, increases in urea concentration may also be due to increased protein intake or breakdown with normal glomerular filtration. Plasma creatinine concentrations are believed by many investigators to be a better indicator of decreased glomerular filtration.

Renal Reabsoroption and Excretion of Ions

The ultimate fate of the glomerular filtrate (which resembles plasma in electrolyte concentration and osmolarity) depends upon the balance of reabsorption and secretion as the filtrate moves successively through the proximal tube, loop of Henle, distal tubule, and collecting ducts. Proximal tubular reabsorption is isosmotic—water and solute are removed in equal proportion so that proximal tubular fluid has the same osmotic pressure as plasma. Both sodium and potassium reabsorption are thought to be active

TABLE 8–2.
Body Fluids After Ingestion of 1 Liter of Water in a Dehydrated and a Well-Hydrated Individual

	VOLUME (ml/minute)	
PARAMETER	DEHYDRATED INDIVIDUAL	WELL-HYDRATED INDIVIDUAL
Renal plasma flow	700	700
Plasma filtered	125	125
Water filtered	116	116
Water reabsorbed	115.5	100
Urine excreted	0.5	16

metabolic processes requiring the expenditure of cellular energy, while water and chloride reabsorption appear to be passive, occurring down an electrochemical gradient.

The familiar sodium-potassium ion pump described above operates between tubular cell and interstitial fluid to keep intracellular potassium concentration high and sodium concentration low (Fig 8–3). The low cellular sodium favors diffusion of sodium from tubular lumen to cell. Influx of potassium from the glomerular filtrate requires an active potassium pump which is efficient enough to result in almost complete removal of potassium from proximal luminal fluid. Chloride diffuses passively from cell to interstitial fluid. There is some evidence that active transport of neutral sodium chloride from lumen to cell is also present. The dashed lines in Figure 8–3 refer to ion transport down electrochemical gradients; the solid lines indicate active transport.

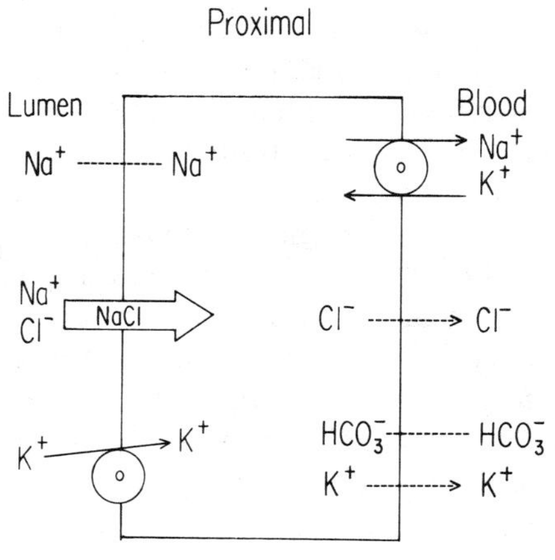

FIG 8–3.
A proximal tubular cell interposed between the tubular lumen and the renal capillary blood. Upper right, the sodium potassium pump described in Figure 8–1. More than 80% of the glomerular filtrate is reabsorbed by the proximal tubule. See text for complete description of proximal tubular fluxes. (Adapted from Pitts RF: *Physiology of the Kidney and Body Fluids*, ed 2. Chicago, Year Book Medical, 1968, p 102.)

The proximal tubule reabsorbs more than 80% of the glomerular filtrate; the remaining tubular fluid is variably reabsorbed by the distal tubule depending upon body requirements. The distal tubules possess the sodium-potassium ion pump of the proximal tubule as well as a potassium pump for further reabsorption of tubular potassium (Fig 8–4). Potassium may be secreted into tubular fluid down an electrochemical gradient. Aldosterone appears to modulate distal tubular activity by enhancing sodium and decreasing potassium reabsorption.

Regulation of Osmolarity

Osmolarity is maintained at about 283 mosmol/liter by the appropriate secretion of antidiuretic hormone (ADH). If osmolarity falls because of ingestion of hypotonic fluids, there is a prompt outpouring of dilute urine. If osmolarity rises because of dehydration, then concentrated urine is elaborated and water is conserved. This regulation is effected by osmoceptors, which are in the area of distribution of the internal carotid arteries in the supraoptic nuclei. The receptors are vesicles which probably swell when the surroundings become hypotonic and shrink when the surrounding interstitial fluid is hypertonic. With shrinkage, nerve endings in the receptors are stimulated, and their impulses release ADH from the hypophysis. Experimentally, a change of 2% in the osmotic pressure of carotid blood is sufficient to cause elaboration of ADH.

As indicated above, proximal tubular fluid is isotonic with respect to plasma. It leaves the loop of Henle somewhat hypotonic, indicating that more salt than water has been reabsorbed by that structure. Clearly, concentration of the urine must occur in either distal tubule or collecting ducts.

Current understanding of the nature of renal concentration of tubular fluid is

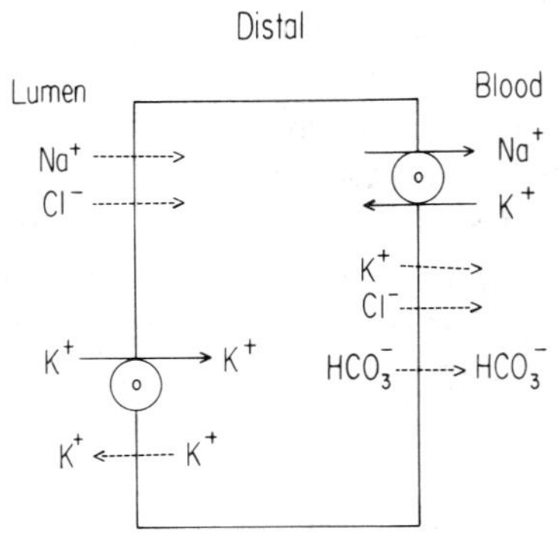

FIG 8–4.
The distal tubular cell, like the proximal tubular cell, contains a sodium-potassium pump between cell and capillary blood and a potassium pump between tubular lumen and cell. Potassium may be secreted into the tubular fluid down an electrochemical gradient. (Adapted from Pitts RF: *Physiology of the Kidney and Body Fluids*, ed 2. Chicago, Year Book Medical, 1968, p 102.)

based on the early experimental evidence of Wirz and associates suggesting the existence of a countercurrent multiplier system.[10] While it has been known for many years that the loop of Henle was necessary for the production of concentrated urine, recent studies indicate the actual function of that segment of the convoluted tubules. Tubular fluid entering the descending limb becomes progressively concentrated as it flows toward the renal papilla owing to reabsorption of water and active secretion of sodium. The ascending limb is impermeable to water but not to sodium, which is actively pumped from ascending limb fluid. So much sodium is removed from this fluid that it is actually hypotonic by the time it reaches the distal tubule. This extrusion of sodium by the loop of Henle results in the production of very hypertonic interstitial fluid in the renal papillae; the highest osmolarity is at the tips of the papillae.

The tubular fluid next enters the distal convoluted tubules and the collecting tubules, which pass back through the hypertonic papillae. The distal convoluted and the collecting tubules have a variable permeability to water, which is controlled by ADH. When ADH is secreted, the tubules become more permeable to water molecules, and water leaves the tubules owing to the increased osmotic pressure of the papillae. This water first enters the interstitial fluid of the papillae and then the capillaries in this tissue, and is returned to the general body water pool. In the absence of ADH, the tubules are relatively impermeable to water molecules and less water passes into the papillae, despite the osmotic gradient. Thus, an increased volume of dilute urine is produced.

The production of hypertonic interstitial fluid in the renal papillae is the key process in the ability of the kidneys to vary urine concentration.

Regulation of Vascular Volume

The control of total body water—in contrast to the regulation of electrolyte concentration and osmolarity—is a more complex, integrated mechanism involving a number of volume-sensitive receptors and a group of effectors that include vasopressin (ADH), aldosterone, and the recently discovered "third factor" or atrial natriuretic factor. Although historically the sensing of hyperosmolarity by the superoptic nuclei of the hypothalamus was first observed to elicit vasopressin release, the ability to measure vasopressin in body fluids has led to a more complete understanding of its role in volume regulation. Acute blood loss, hypoxia, hypercapnia, and factors associated with the syndrome of inappropriate secretion of ADH as well as hypertonicity of body fluids lead to increased concentrations in blood, cerebral spinal fluid, and urine.[11] Changes in blood volume appear to stimulate both low pressure mechanoreceptors in the central veins and atria and high pressure mechanoreceptors in the arterial circulation. Considerable difference of opinion exists regarding the importance of atrial receptors in mediating volume change in man,[12] although the stretching of left atrial stretch receptors by negative pressure breathing and the antidiuresis observed with positive pressure breathing suggests their importance.

Fluid volume may also be adjusted by regulating body sodium stores; sodium retention produces parallel fluid retention by stimulating vasopressin release in order to maintain isotonicity. Salt excretion is a function of the amount of sodium reaching the glomerulus (the "filtered load") and the amount reabsorbed by the renal tubule. Sodium reabsorption in the distal tubule is under the direct control of aldosterone, which stimulates a potassium-sodium exchange system, increasing plasma sodium and decreasing plasma potassium. A number of stimuli cause the zona glomerulosa of the adrenal gland to secrete aldosterone: increased plasma potassium concentration, decreased blood pressure in certain branches of the internal carotid artery, ACTH secretion, and renin production stimulated by decreased blood flow to the juxtaglomerular apparatus of the kidney.

The recent identification of the atrial natriuretic factor, a polypeptide perhaps best termed "atrin," allows a better understanding of mammalian volume control. Atrin is found within specific granules in mammalian atria. The material is released by experimental procedures that increase atrial pressure and has been shown to bind to receptors in the renal glomeruli and medullary vessels as well other vessels, including mesenteric artery. Atrin produces a striking salt and water diuresis. Atrin inhibits aldosterone synthesis, the rate of renin release, and renal vasoconstriction.[13]

The three volume control factors, vasopressin, aldosterone, and atrin, act in an integrated or amplifying manner. Increased sympathetic activity directly increases vasopressin and renin secretion. Renin, atrin, and vasopressin all lead to the increased release of aldosterone. Significant interspecies differences in volume control exist, and it is likely that the human responses vary greatly with the nature and intensity of the environmental stress. Increases in all three factors and renin have been observed in the critically ill patient, suggesting an all out effort to retain salt and water!

ACUTE RENAL FAILURE

Renal failure represents the acute deterioration of renal function from a previously defined baseline over a period of several weeks, and it may be superimposed on preexisting chronic renal failure. Many factors, some reversible and some irreversible, can lead to a rise in plasma creatinine levels or to a fall in urine output. A fall in renal blood flow produces some evidence of renal dysfunction in many critically ill patients; ischemic renal cell damage leads to irreversible renal disease (postischemic acute tubular necrosis or vasomotor nephropathy), nephrotoxins such as the aminoglycosides are commonly used in critical care units, and a variety of other forms of renal dysfunction may be encountered. An elevated creatinine, just like a reduced arterial oxygen tension, frequently suggests a poor prognosis, even if the cause is not well understood. Knaus et al.,[14] in their study of prognosis in multiple organ failure, arbitrarily diagnosed renal failure when the urine output was lower than 479 ml in 24 hours or the creatine was above 3.5 mg/dl, and found it to influence survival regardless of the cause. The clinician responsible for a single patient must make a precise diagnosis and may well use different criteria for the presence of renal failure, but their studies emphasize the importance of almost any evidence of renal failure to outcome.

Creatinine is formed by the degradation of muscle phosphocreatine at a relatively constant rate. Plasma creatinine concentrations are a much better measurement of renal function than urea nitrogen. The renal clearance of creatinine is closer to that of inulin than any other endogenous substance; about half of the filtered urea diffuses back into the blood from renal tubules, making urea clearance dependent on urine flow and a less reliable indicator of glomerular filtration. Creatinine clearance may be measured by obtaining a 24-hour urine sample and a single sample of blood during this period. Normal values for men are 97–140 ml/minute and for women, 85–125 ml/minute. A 2-hour creatinine clearance has recently been shown to be as accurate as the 24- hour clearance.

Urea is a simple compound containing two amino groups joined to a keto group. It may be measured as urea itself or, more commonly, as the nitrogen of urea (BUN). The molecular weight of urea is 60, and the plasma urea is actually 2.14 times the BUN concentration. Ammonia from the deamination of amino acids and the intestinal metabolism of urea itself by urease is synthesized into urea by the liver. In critical illness, when amino acids are used by the Krebs cycle for energy, ammonia nitrogen is converted to urea by the liver. The urea load is related to total caloric and protein intake, the ratio of essential and nonessential amino acids, nitrogen balance, the synthetic capacity of the liver, activity of bacterial urease in the gut, and renal function.

Two important forms of acute renal failure are commonly found (and confused with one another) in the critically ill patient. Hemodynamic instability causes marked variation in glomerular filtration rate (GFR) and plasma creatinine concentrations. Irreversible renal disease after battle wounds was first recognized during World War II and has been called acute tubular necrosis, postischemic acute tubular necrosis, vasomotor nephropathy, or simply acute renal failure.[15] The term acute tubular necrosis (ATN) will be used in this text to describe parenchymal renal failure in critically ill patients.

Renal Failure Due to Hemodynamic Instability

Extrarenal abnormalities are common causes of acute renal failure. The term prerenal is used because a decrease in glomerular filtration rate is due to the reduction in renal blood flow associated with a reduction in cardiac output or to increased sympathetic neural activity rather than to intrinsic renal or postrenal disease.

Hypotension of any cause, including sepsis, ventricular failure, or hypovolemia, can markedly reduce the GFR by exceeding the ability of the kidney to autoregulate its glomerular circulation. The afferent arteriole becomes maximally dilated when the mean renal perfusion pressure falls below 80 mm Hg and is no longer able to maintain glomerular hydrostatic pressure. Further decreases in arterial perfusion pressure lead to decreases in GFR. Since changes in stroke output, heart rate, vascular volume, sympathetic tone, the presence of intimal hyperplasia due to long standing hypertension, and other factors affect afferent arteriolar pressure, the changes in creatinine concentration and urine output may occur earlier than in vasomotor nephropathy. Characteristically urine output is fixed, and plasma creatinine rises at the rate of 1–4 mg/dl per day in ATN (vasomotor nephropathy); wide swings in creatinine, in contrast, are seen in the renal failure associated with hemodynamic instability.

Renal failure due to hemodynamic instability should be strongly suspected in individuals with obvious evidence of blood or fluid loss, fever, or recent weight loss. It is common in the elderly who are unable to compensate for even minor reductions in blood volume. Clinical recognition is difficult because changes in skin turgor or mucous membrane hydration are unreliable at best. Most elderly individuals appear to have poor skin turgor even when they are well hydrated. A fall of 15–20 mm Hg systolic and 5–10 mm Hg diastolic pressures upon standing indicate reduced venous return to the heart and are good signs of hypovolemia. Orthostatic hypotension, however, is neither specific nor sensitive for hypovolemia, and measurement of atrial filling pressures are indicated in most critically ill patients to assess volume status. Hypernatremia and the excretion of a concentrated urine provide good supportive evidence of dehydration.

Subacute or even chronic renal failure is seen in a variety of edematous states such as congestive heart failure, hepatic cirrhosis, and the nephrotic syndrome. Renal blood flow is reduced by low cardiac output in congestive heart failure, and increased portal pressures initiate the problem in cirrhosis. Hypoalbuminemia and permeability changes in the nephrotic syndrome produce hypovolemia and decrease renal blood flow. In each of these situations, renal salt and water retention is the response to a decrease in renal blood flow. Initially, the attempt to increase blood volume appears useful; water retention and increased venous tone increase preload and stroke output. These responses set up the classic critical care dilemma; use of diuretic may improve pulmonary gas exchange but at the same time decrease cardiac output and vital organ blood flow.

The hepatorenal syndrome represents reversible prerenal failure and is a good example of potential reversibility in a clinical situation where improvement in renal blood flow is difficult. Increased portal pressure, abnormal hepato-cellular function with hypoalbuminemia, and markedly elevated plasma aldosterone concentrations are found in most individuals with the hepatorenal syndrome, but the role of each factor in contributing to renal failure is not well understood. Patients are oliguric and excrete a concentrated urine that is low in sodium. Hyponatremia, when present, is probably dilutional. Reinfusion of ascitic fluid improves renal function by increasing circulating volume.[16] The reversibility of the organ dysfunction, but not the overall patient problem, is demonstrated by the normal function of kidneys transplanted from patients with the hepatorenal syndrome to a recipient with normal liver function.

Postischemic Acute Tubular Necrosis

Tubular necrosis may result from a variety of causes. In critically injured or ill patients, it commonly follows renal hypoperfusion and is termed postischemic. Acute tubular necrosis occurs early in the course of critical illness and was a major cause of mortality in many combat situations. The importance of early recognition and treatment is strikingly demonstrated in combat mortality statistics. The delay between injury and treatment in World War II was 79 hours, and the incidence of acute renal failure was 12%. In Korea, the delay in treatment and incidence were reduced to four hours and 0.2%, respectively. It did develop, however, in 35% of severely wounded individuals surviving more than three days. Acute renal failure occurred in only 0.08% of severely injured soldiers in Viet Nam, in large part because of early fluid replacement and an air evacuation system that reduced delays to 35–40 minutes.[17]

Postischemic ATN may present as either oliguric (less than 400 cc of urine per day) or nonoliguric renal failure. Nonoliguric renal failure is much more common than in the past, and has a substantially better prognosis than that of oliguric renal failure. The increased use of nephrotoxic antibiotics has been suggested as one reason for the recent prevalence of this form of renal failure. In both forms, pathologic examination reveals tubular necrosis and dissolution of the basement membranes. The abnormalities are usually patchy and can involve any portion of the nephron. Both granular and pigmented casts frequently can be seen blocking the tubules. The precise pathophysiologic sequence is unclear, and three main abnormalities have been suggested as responsible for the acute renal failure seen in acute tubular necrosis: tubular obstruction, cessation of glomerular filtration, and the back leak of ultrafiltrate.

Both granular and pigmented casts are seen blocking the tubules and, in fact, in a variety of experimental models early increases in intratubular pressure are noted. These changes are observed for relatively short periods of time, and GFR remains depressed even when intratubular pressures fall to normal. Tubular obstruction may be an important initiating factor in acute renal failure, and the resultant decrease in GFR may operate to perpetuate it.

The marked reduction in GFR seen in acute tubular necrosis is probably multifactoral. Reductions in renal blood flow, glomerular hydrostatic pressure, glomerular capillary permeability, and glomerular surface area can all contribute to decreasing GFR. Although it is easy to understand the reduction in renal blood flow seen in hypotension, it is not so easy to see why the GFR remains depressed long after the systemic blood pressure returns to normal. Presumably, production of renal or extrarenal humoral agents maintains afferent arteriole constriction and also redistributes blood flow from cortex to medulla. Increasing glomerular capillary permeability also could reduce GFR, but the biochemical mediators responsible for altering permeability properties are not well understood. Back leaking of filtrate through damaged tubular epithelium appears likely, but its precise contribution to the reduction in GFR is not known.

Regardless of the precise pathogenic pathways, it seems clear that tubular necrosis is mediated by decreased blood flow and oxygen delivery to the kidneys. Evidence of hemodynamic instability and actual renal cell necrosis are overlapping phenomena. The longer the kidney is deprived of adequate oxygen delivery, the more likely the progression to irreversible renal failure. The clinician must prevent where possible the development of irreversibility while carefully watching for signs of its appearance.

The careful recording of plasma creatinine concentration is essential for diagnosis. A substantial elevation of creatinine on admission suggests preexisting renal disease, while the fixed glomerular filtration rate of acute tubular necrosis produces a steady increase of 1–3 mg/dl per day. The daily urine output is relatively constant and below 400 ml/day unless superimposed hypotension leads to further reductions in glomerular filtration. Renal tubular dysfunction is expressed by the excretion of a dilute urine with a specific gravity of 1.010 and an osmolarity approaching that of the plasma. In addition, 30–90 mEq/l of sodium are excreted in the urine and a nonhyperglycemic glycosuria is found.

A variety of laboratory analyses have been suggested to differentiate acute tubular necrosis from vasomotor instability due to renal hyperfusion. Since glomerular filtration is markedly reduced in acute tubular necrosis, a urine/plasma creatinine ratio below 15 favors ATN, as does a urinary sodium greater than 10 mEq/l. A urine osmolarity close to plasma osmolarity (or a urine/serum osmolarity ratio of less than 1.5) favors ATN because it reflects an inability to concentrate urine. A BUN/creatinine ratio less than 10 favors ATN because creatinine clearance is markedly limited. Two of these physiologic abnormalities can be expressed by a ratio that attempts to measure the fractional excretion of sodium.[18] The urine/plasma sodium ratio estimating the clearance of sodium is divided by the urine/plasma creatinine ratio, which estimates the clearance of creatinine. A ratio above 1–3% has been suggested as evidence for ATN. The presence of casts and cellular debris suggests ATN, but red blood cells, leukocyte casts, or eosinophilia suggest another parenchymal abnormality. While these tests are useful guidelines, they should not be considered *absolute* evidence of acute tubular necrosis. Oken[19] has emphasized that preexisting mild renal disease or asymptomatic nephrosclerosis in the elderly may blunt the renal concentrating ability, and might mimic the chemical findings of tubular necrosis.

Electrolyte disturbances that include hyperkalemia, metabolic acidosis, hypocalcemia, and hyperphosphatemia are common in acute renal failure and often require prompt correction. Rarely, hypercalcemia may be seen during the diuretic phase because of mobilization of previously sequestered calcium. It is most common in renal failure associated with rhabdomyolysis. Infection is common in patients with renal failure because of reticuloendothelial and granulocytic depression. Pulmonary and urinary tract infections are common and should be suspected if renal function suddenly deteriorates even in the absence of fever and leukocytosis.

The renal failure phase of acute tubular necrosis can last from one to four weeks; occasional patients have had renal failure for up to six months. In general, nonoliguric renal failure resolves more quickly than oliguric renal failure. The gradual increase in GFR and decline in plasma creatinine heralds the diuretic phase of renal failure. GFR frequently improves before the restoration of tubular function, so that large amounts of salt and water may be excreted. Urine flow may be several times normal and may produce volume depletion which produces an exacerbation of renal failure. A fluid challenge leads to a fall in creatinine in this situation.

Nephrotoxic Acute Tubular Necrosis

Many drugs required for the treatment of critically ill patients are excreted primarily by the kidney, and some of these are nephrotoxic. Modest degrees of renal failure, in consequence, could lead to dangerous accumulations of nephrotoxic drugs within the kidney and amplify the initial renal insufficiency. Some drugs are relatively safe in the presence of normal renal function, while others are excreted primarily by the liver and do not present a problem even with markedly reduced renal function. A knowledge of the pharmacokinetics of therapeutic agents in patients with renal failure is essential.[20]

Aminoglycosides are probably the most common cause of nephrotoxic ATN.[21] The agent appears to be concentrated in the cortex, where significant concentrations can be detected as long as a month after the last dose. Although the exact mechanism of the acute tubular necrosis induced by Gentamicin is not known, the possibility of nephrotoxicity appears to be enhanced by dehydration, preexisting renal disease (diabetes, for example), inadvertent excessive dosing, and administration with cephalosporins such as cephalothin (an increased incidence of nephrotoxicity has been observed when cephalosporins are administered with aminoglycosides). Great care should be taken in calculating aminoglycoside maintenance dosage schedules, and the computer kinetic dosing protocols available in many hospitals may minimize the toxic effects of the agents.

Filtered myoglobin and hemoglobin can cause acute tubular necrosis and acute renal failure. Rhabdomyolysis due to heat stroke, trauma, seizures, hypokalemia, and other causes, and intravascular hemolysis can all lead to precipitation of pigments with the renal tubules.[22] Renal failure is particularly likely to occur in the volume-depleted patient and can be suspected by the finding of free hemoglobin or myoglobin in serum or urine or by finding pigmented casts in the urinary sediment. When volume depletion and/or hypotension are present along with the heme pigments, renal failure can be potentiated.

The diagnosis of heme pigment-induced ATN can be suspected by history and confirmed by laboratory data, including the presence of pigmented casts in the urine sediment and positive urine dipstick for blood when no red cells are seen on the microscopic. Serum-free hemoglobin and/or serum and urine myoglobin levels may be diagnostic in the presence of ARF. Some investigators advocate alkalinization of the urine since a urine pH less than 5.6 promotes production of the potentially toxic ferrihemate.

Renal failure may also follow the intravenous or intra-arterial injection of radiocontrast media. It is frequently seen following intravenous pyelography, but may be observed after any type of contrast study. The exact mechanism is unknown, but probably is related to a direct toxic effect on the renal tubule, increases in uric acid secretion, and a decrease in renal blood flow. Patients with diabetes and multiple myeloma are more likely than others to develop renal failure following injection of contrast media. Many clinicians administer mannitol, 12 grams, within an hour of contrast exposure as a prophylactic measure in patients at increased risk of renal failure.

Patients in renal failure are predisposed to infection.[23] Although the mechanism is not well understood, uremia (BUN greater than 80 mg per dl) depresses several components of the host's immune system including white cell function and the ability of the reticuloendothelial system to phagocytize foreign bodies. Two common sites of infection are the lungs and the urinary tract. A high degree of suspicion for infection should be maintained even in the absence of the usual signs, such as fever and elevated white count, when any patient with ARF suddenly decompensates without apparent reason.

Other Forms of Renal Failure

While hemodynamic instability, acute tubular necrosis, and nephrotoxicity are common causes of renal failure in the critically ill patient, acute interstitial nephritis and atheromatous embolic disease are also occasionally responsible. A variety of drugs including the beta lactam antibiotics[24] produce renal failure in certain hypersensitive patients. Fever, hematuria, rash, arthralgias, and eosinophilia or eosinophiuria may suggest the diagnosis. Atheroembolic disease may be suspected if evidence of peripheral embolization is found. Oken[19] has called attention to ischemic gangrene of toes and fingers, livedo reticularis (a bluish cutaneous mottling of skin at areas of small vessel occlusion), petechiae, ischemic ulcers, and retinal arterial embolization as evidence of peripheral embolization. The fever and eosinophilia of atheroembolism may suggest allergic vasculitis, and a muscle biopsy may sometimes be necessary to establish the diagnosis.

Treatment of Renal Failure

Correction of water and electrolyte abnormalities require frequent monitoring of electrolytes. Concentrations of electrolytes change rapidly, especially in hypercatabolic patients, and several determinations may be necessary within each 24-hour period. Hyperkalemia can frequently be controlled by potassium restriction with the addition of cation exchange resins if necessary. Resins such as Keyexalate exchange sodium for potassium and may lead to water retention. Doses of drugs excreted by the kidneys must be modified, and serum levels regularly monitored where possible. Daily fluid balance must be estimated by measuring all fluid intake and output. Insensible losses are usually between 500 and 1,000 cc per day, but may be much less in patients receiving humidified oxygen and/or on ventilators. Nutritional support is essential, but may complicate the control of urea concentration and fluid balance. Hyperphosphatemia, hypocalcemia, hypercalcemia, and hypermagnesemia must be identified and aggressively corrected.

Decreases in cardiac output or arterial blood pressure lead quickly to renal vasoconstriction and marked decreases in renal blood flow. Hemodynamic monitoring is indicated in most critically ill patients whenever hypovolemia or hypotension is present or likely; recovery of renal function requires immediate restoration of renal blood flow because early determination of cardiac output is necessary whenever post-ischemic renal injury is suspected. Renal hemodynamics cannot be directly measured, but maintenance of adequate systemic hemodynamics can lead to direct improvement of renal blood flow.

Persistent and uncorrectable hyperkalemia, acidosis, or fluid overload require either peritoneal or hemodialysis.[25] Although classic teaching warns against basing dialysis decisions on the level of BUN or creatinine, urea concentrations greater than 80–100 usually are accompanied by platelet dysfunction and white blood cell defects, which translate clinically into infections and bleeding disorders. Hemorrhagic diatheses in these patients appear related to reduced concentrations of factor VIII and Von Willebrand activity. Administration of cryoprecipitate may be necessary (see chapter 12). Other complications of uremia such as pericarditis and colitis are also seen. Since any of these complications will have serious consequences in critically ill patients, dialysis is generally indicated when the BUN rises to this range. Hemodialysis has a greater capacity to clear solutes and is the method of choice in hypercatabolic states. However, peritoneal dialysis can be useful in hypotensive patients and usually does not produce the hemodynamic instability frequently seen with hemodialysis.

Slow Continuous Ultrafiltration (SCUF)

SCUF[26] has been used successfully in the oliguric and anuric ICU patient and in cardiac surgical patients. Ultrafiltration is a technique by which an ultrafiltrate of plasma is formed by the passage of circulating blood across a semipermeable membrane. The technique resembles glomerular filtration in that water and solutes are filtered from the circulating plasma by a pressure gradient. Continuous ultrafiltration requires lower perfusion pressures than the older hemofiltration methods and produces ultrafiltration rates of up to 20 ml/min. Either arterial or venous catheters, or a Scribner shunt, allow arterial pressure to maintain blood flow rates of 30–120 ml/min without a mechanical pump if mean arterial pressure is at least 60 mm Hg. Veno-venous ultrafiltration using a roller pump may be necessary in hypotensive patients. Systemic anticoagulation is not always necessary; one technique involves administering heparin into the proximal line so that the filter is directly anticoagulated. The ultrafiltrate generally consists of water, electrolytes and small to medium sized molecules less than 50,000 daltons. Electrolytes and other molecules are removed in the same concentration as they are found in plasma. The technique has been used in a variety of settings including the management of fluid overload in acute renal failure. It also has been used in patients who require nutritional support where impaired renal function may preclude the administration of large volumes of fluid. SCUF may be preferable to dialysis when volume overload is the predominant problem and uremia and hyperkalemia are not present. SCUF is advantageous because large volumes of fluid may be removed without producing hypotension if the ultrafiltration rate approximates the rate at which fluid enters the vascular compartment from the interstitial space. The technique is ideal for patients requiring large volumes of fluid for the administration of antibiotics or nutritional support. Lesser volumes of fluid are frequently removed with hemodialysis because of the short time of dialysis and the inability of the patient to rapidly mobilize interstitial fluid. Many drugs are also removed in the ultrafiltrate, and clearance calculations may be made from blood and ultrafiltrate concentrations. Infused fluids should continue to approximate the concentrations of electrolytes desired in the plasma. The rapid appearance of severe hyponatremia or hypomagnesemia may occur if infused electrolyte concentrations are not accurately calculated.

DISTURBANCES OF SALT, WATER, AND ELECTROLYTE BALANCE

Hypo-osmolar States

Hyponatremia

Hyponatremia is one of the most frequent electrolyte disorders encountered in a general hospital population.[27] It may be dilutional, depletional, or due to the presence of increased insoluble large molecules such as proteins or lipids which displace water (pseudohyponatremia). The distinction is of great importance: use of 5% NaCl solution in a patient with congestive heart failure and dilutional hyponatremia might normalize sodium concentration but produce acute pulmonary edema by increasing total body sodium and water. As a general rule, depletional hyponatremia does not occur in a patient with edema; dilutional hyponatremia is common in the critically ill patient.

Dilutional or hypo-osmolar hyponatremia occurs when sodium loss exceeds water loss or when free water excretion is impaired. Dilutional hyponatremia in the critically ill patient may be due to decreases in the effective circulating volume, the use of diuretics, acute renal failure, adrenal insufficiency, and the syndrome of inappropriate ADH secretion (SIADH). The decrease in free water excretion may be either appropriate or inappropriate. Hemorrhage, gastrointestinal losses, salt wasting nephropathies, positive pressure ventilation, burns, abdominal surgery, heart failure, and cirrhosis all decrease the effective circulating plasma volume or stimulate ADH release by other mechanisms even though total plasma volume may be close to normal. This decrease in effective circulating volume stimulates thirst and ADH release in an attempt to restore vascular volume to normal. The combination of the falling GRF produced by the decreased renal blood flow and the increase in proximal sodium and water absorption reduces the delivery of water to the ascending limb of Henle and, in consequence, free water clearance is reduced.

Water retention in response to injury is an important evolutionary advance. Prior to the availability of infusional therapy, stress-related increases in water retention maintained reasonable homeostasis even though oral intake was impossible because of unconsciousness, ileus, or immobility. These ancient stimuli of pain, stress, and sepsis continue to cause fluid retention even though fluids are infused. Fluid retention evolved as a very appropriate response, but may appear "inappropriate" to the modern intensivist. Critically ill patients often remain hyponatremic and retain fluid inappropriately even though intravascular volume and oxygen transport are normal. Some patients, particularly the elderly, develop pulmonary edema and anasarca even though all measured variables indicate good perfusion of all vascular beds including the kidney. Such patients usually respond to small doses of diuretics.

Diuretics, particularly the loop diuretics, cause secondary hyponatremia because of their volume and potassium depleting effects, particularly when replacement fluids contain little sodium. The patient who receives 5% dextrose and water with large doses of diuretics is destined to become hyponatremic. Even those individuals who are volume overloaded should receive replacement fluids with sodium concentrations, but not volume, approximating that of the urine when pharmacologic diuresis is undertaken. Potassium depletion produces hyponatremia because intracellular potassium is exchanged for plasma sodium. Adrenal insufficiency may cause hyponatremia because the ADH action on the water permeability of the collecting ducts is dependent on cortisol. Without cortisol, water excretion is impaired and hypo-osmolality results.

Increased ADH secretion not attributable to stimuli like hyperosmolarity or hypovolemia is considered "inappropriate." It is frequently difficult to diagnose the classic SIADH syndrome in the critically ill patient because of the necessity to demonstrate normal cardiac, renal, and adrenal function, as well as normal plasma volume and osmolarity. A variety of neurologic and pulmonary abnormalities, a variety of drugs, and ectopic production of ADH can all cause inappropriate ADH release. The coexistence of inappropriate and appropriate ADH release probably occurs but would be difficult to diagnose in critically ill patients.

Some substances like glucose or mannitol are distributed throughout the extracellular water but poorly penetrate cell membranes. In consequence, hyperglycemia produces an osmotic gradient that favors the movement of water from cells to the extracellular space and decreases the plasma sodium concentration. This has been called pseudohyponatremia with hyperosmolarity and is a form of dilutional hyponatremia. Urea, on the other hand, penetrates cell membranes freely and so is osmotically inactive.

Under normal circumstances, the concentration of osmoles in plasma can be reported as either osmolarity (milliosmoles per liter) or osmolality (milliosmoles per kg of plasma). Plasma proteins and lipids occupy about 70 ml of each liter of plasma but exist as a separate phase. The fraction of plasma occupied by this nonaqueous phase rises dramatically in patients with hyperlipidemia or hyperproteinemia. The plasma sodium concentration measured per liter of plasma will be much lower than if it were measured per liter of water. Osmolarity measured in an osmometer will be normal. As a general rule, the plasma sodium falls 2 mEq/L for every 100 mg/dl of glucose above normal.

The measurement of urine sodium excretion and the estimation of the extracellular fluid volume facilitates the differential diagnosis of hyponatremia (Table 8–3). Central venous pressure is used to estimate blood volume in this analysis, but should be supported by clinical evaluation of the state of hydration. Either renal or extrarenal sodium loss produces volume contraction, but the urine sodium is low with extrarenal loss as the kidney reabsorbs the ion in an attempt to replace body stores. Disorders of the heart, liver, or kidney are associated with decreased effective circulation and hypervolemia, as decreased GFR and increased secretion of ADH and other humoral agents lead to sodium retention. Edema is frequently present as a sign of increased interstitial water. Inappropriate secretion of ADH is frequently confused with true volume depletion, but the lack of evidence of hypovolemia and an increased urinary sodium excretion provides useful differential information. Increased sodium excretion in SIADH reflects an appropriate cardiorenal response to hypervolemia and implies the presence of relatively normal kidneys. Bartter's syndrome is a rare disease associated with increased renin secretion, perhaps due to enhanced prostaglandin production by the kidney. Increased aldosterone production produces hypokalemia but an associated tubular defect leads to increased sodium excretion.[30]

Treatment should be directed to the underlying cause. Volume depletion should be treated with the appropriate fluids, diuretics should be discontinued, and cortisol replaced as necessary. Fluid restriction (1,200–1,500 cc per day) and replacement of sodium and potassium deficits will usually correct hyponatremia in the syndrome of inappropriate secretion of ADH. Patients requiring large volumes of fluid to deliver therapeutic substances usually require diuretics to maintain fluid balance. Ten grams of NaCl added to an enteral solution yields a final concentration similar to that of normal saline. It may seem paradoxical to administer

TABLE 8–3.
Differential Diagnosis of Hyponatremia

URINARY SODIUM	HYPERVOLEMIA/ NORMOVOLEMIA	HYPOVOLEMIA
20 mEq/L	SIADH	Addisons Renal salt loss Bartter's syndrome
10 mEq/L	Heart Liver Kidney	Extrarenal salt loss

sodium to volume overloaded patients, but it is necessary as long as diuretic therapy produces massive sodium losses (see discussion above).

A major problem in designing therapy is the rate of sodium replacement. Arieff[31] recently described 15 previously healthy women who developed hyponatremia, convulsions, respiratory arrest, and permanent brain damage after elective surgery (average serum sodium, 108 mEq/L). Narins,[32] in editorial comment, questioned whether the neurological consequences were the result of too little or too much treatment? He concluded that most experts believe that an increase of 2 mEq/L per hour in sodium concentration represents a reasonable replacement rate in symptomatic patients with hyponatremia. The editorial writer queried a group of nephrologists, who generally suggested the combined use of 3% saline and a diuretic to reduce volume and raise serum sodium levels.

If hypo-osmolality and fluid overload is secondary to acute renal failure, diuretics are occasionally useful. Furosemide generally produces a hypo-osmotic urine in the fact of a hypo-osmotic serum. If ineffective, ultrafiltration can be considered while replacing the volume deficit with the appropriate fluids. While formulas for calculating volume deficits are useful guidelines (see hypernatremia), monitoring of plasma osmolarity and sodium concentration is essential.

Hyperosmolar States

Increased serum osmolarity in critically ill patients leads to lethargy, confusion, and coma by promoting dehydration of vital tissues. The usual equilibrium between body compartments is disturbed when a substance that is not readily distributed within total body water is introduced into the extracellular spaces. A hyperosmolar fluid leads to intracellular dehydration as water follows an osmotic gradient and flows into the extracellular spaces. In an analagous manner, failure of bicarbonate to cross the blood-brain barrier leads to a disequilibrium in cerebral acid/base balance.

Hypernatremia

Water depletion in excess of sodium results in hypernatremia (increased serum sodium concentration). The usual causes include insufficient water intake or excessive loss due to diarrhea, polyuria (as in renal disease or diabetic ketoacidosis), and the lack of, or unresponsiveness to, ADH (diabetes insipidus). The prolonged use of diuretics may also cause this type of dehydration. Clinically, the patient's skin is dry and flushed, the mucous membranes are dry, and skin turgor is normal. Laboratory findings are compatible with dehydration. BUN, hematocrit, serum sodium, and serum osmolality are elevated. Urine volume is decreased with a high specific gravity and osmolality. Treatment includes replacement of the water deficit either orally or parenterally, but care should be taken to correct hypernatremia slowly. Too rapid correction of the sodium excess may result in cerebral edema and death.

Water deficits can be estimated from formulas based on the assumption that total body sodium and red blood cells are unchanged and that their increased plasma concentration represents the effects of dehydration. Isotonic water deficits, previously unrecognized anemia, or active bleeding could lead to significant errors, however, and it is usually advisable not to attempt to replace the entire calculated deficit.

$$\text{Water deficit} = 0.6 \times \text{body weight} \times \left(\frac{\text{plasma sodium}}{140}\right) - 1$$

$$\text{Extracellular fluid deficit} = 0.2 \times \text{body weight} \times \left(\frac{\text{Hct}}{\text{normal Hct}}\right) - 1$$

Some degree of diabetes insipidus is not infrequently seen in patients with basilar skull fractures, pituitary tumors both before and after surgery, increased intracranial pressure, and after infections of the brain or meninges. Nephrogenic diabetes insipidus can be produced by hyperkalemia, hypercalcemia, postobstructive neuropathy, and drugs such as amphotericin B, lithium carbonate, and demeclocycline. Thirst, polydipsia, polyuria, and hypernatremia suggest the syndrome. A low urine specific gravity and osmolarity confirm the diagnosis. Water replacement with 5% dextrose in water is usually effective, since much more water than electrolyte is lost. Aqueous vasopressin, administered either intramuscularly or intravenously may be necessary in some patients to control hypernatremia and dehydration.[33]

Hyperglycemia

A classic example of the hyperosmolar syndrome is the hyperosmolar nonketotic coma occasionally seen in diabetics.[34] Serum osmolarity averaged 373 mosm/liter in one report; in this group of patients, serum glucose averaged 979 mg/dl, while bicarbonate was almost normal. These patients usually are dehydrated because of the osmotic diuresis; continued glycogenolysis and gluconeogenesis in the presence of decreased glomerular filtration lead to extremely high plasma glucose concentrations. Very often administration of normal saline or lactated Ringer's alone reduces serum glucose rapidly by dilution and by permitting glucosuria. Insulin eventually is necessary, but must be administered with care since such patients are frequently inordinately sensitive to insulin administration.

Mannitol

Mannitol is now used in a variety of critical situations, including cerebral edema and in the prevention and treatment of acute renal failure. It may also be used in some centers as a volume expander. Hyperosmolar states secondary to mannitol may be seen, particularly in renal failure where mannitol cannot be excreted in the urine. In this case, mannitol is retained in the extracellular fluid, and subsequently will increase the osmolality by acting as an osmotic agent and lowering the plasma sodium concentration in a manner similar to that of high glucose concentrations.

Disturbances of Potassium Balance

Hyperkalemia

Increased plasma potassium is caused by renal failure, which decreases the excretion of potassium, or by increased potassium stores, caused by either excessive intake or protein breakdown. Systemic acidosis in the presence of diminished urinary output may also produce hyperkalemia.

The electrocardiographic changes of hyperkalemia are first evident at a serum potassium concentration of 6.0 mEq/liter; this constitutes a medical emergency. Prompt institution of therapy with sodium bicarbonate, calcium gluconate, or glucose and insulin is warranted. Prolonged control of hyperkalemia can be maintained with a sodium-exchange resin (Kayexalate), although repeated dialysis may also be required.

Hypokalemia

Hypokalemia is extremely common in the critically ill patient and may precipitate serious ventricular arrhythmias. Unfortunately, the magnitude of potassium depletion cannot be estimated accurately from serum potassium measurements, since most of the total body potassium is intracellular. A deficit of 100 produces but a 1 mEq/liter lowering of serum potassium. Since hypokalemia leads to metabolic alkalosis (see section on bicarbonate reabsorption by kidney), an elevated bicarbonate concentration is frequently an indication of total body potassium depletion, even if serum potassium is close to normal.

Probably the most common cause of hypokalemia in cardiac patients is the chronic use of diuretics. Potassium loss may also occur from the gastrointestinal tract and is seen in patients with renal tubular dysfunction or primary aldosteronism. Chronic alkalosis also causes hypokalemia since the distal tubule attempts to conserve hydrogen ion by excreting potassium.

Although conventional teaching suggests that potassium should not be replaced at rates exceeding 20–40 mEq/liter of intravenous fluids, more rapid replacement rates may be used in critically ill patients with severe hypokalemia.[35] Higher concentrations of potassium may be safely infused as long as uniformity of infusion is guaranteed by use of a constant infusion pump, phlebitis is excluded by use of the cava vein, and hyperkalemia is avoided by continuous electrocardiographic and serum electrolyte monitoring.

Treatment of Volume and Electrolyte Disturbances

The correction of volume, acid-base, and electrolyte abnormalities is a daily activity for the ICU physician. This area is more of an "art" and less of a "science" than some other fields of knowledge, and considerable differences in philosophy and practice are evident in various geographic locations.

Correction of Volume Deficits

The majority of critically ill patients require volume expansion during at least one phase of their ICU stay. Hemorrhage leads to loss of intravascular volume directly. Postoperative and traumatized patients develop increased exudation or transudation of fluid in the injured area, due presumably to an impaired capillary-endothelial barrier, and "leak" fluid slowly from the intravascular space. Patients who have suffered a severe insult such as prolonged septic or hemorrhagic shock may have generalized capillary-endothelial damage; the consequent diffuse capillary leak adds further to the intravascular volume deficit and to gross anasarca after volume resuscitation. Septic shock is characterized by "vasomotor paralysis," rendering a previously adequate intravascular volume inadequate due to the consequent increased capacitance of the circuit. Patients on positive-pressure ventilation often develop higher than normal mean venous pressure, and therefore frequently require volume resuscitation in order to raise mean systemic pressure. A number of options for volume resuscitation of these various states are available, leading to considerable controversy. The ultimate goal of volume resuscitation, by whatever means, is preservation of oxygen transport to all tissues (see chapter 1).

Dextrose solutions provide free water because glucose is rapidly metabolized to carbon dioxide and water or stored as glycogen or triglyceride. Electrolyte-free dextrose solutions, of course, distribute to the entirety of the total body water and should never be used alone for intravascular volume resuscitation. Of a liter of free water administered to a patient, only approximately 80 cc remains in the intravascular space. Crystalloid solutions capitalize on the cellular membrane; sodium enters the intracellular space only in small quantities, and is extruded by the sodium-potassium ATPase pump. The quantity of crystalloid solution which remains in the extracellular space, therefore, is proportional to its sodium content. Since the intravascular space is about one-fifth of the extracellular space, about 200 cc of a liter of normal saline remains in the intravascular space of a normal patient; presumably less remains in an edematous patient. Only slightly more than half as much of a half-normal saline solution remains in the intravascular space. Half-normal saline is suited to the patient who, in addition to intravascular volume depletion, suffers from free water depletion. Half-normal saline is rarely indicated for resuscitation. Administration of large volumes of normal saline may lead to mild hypernatremia since the sodium concentration of this solution is 154 mEq/liter. In addition, hyperchloremia acidosis may result due to acutely rapid dilution of available bicarbonate in an expanded cellular space. Ringer's lactate contains lactate as a sodium salt (not as lactic acid); lactate is converted to bicarbonate in the liver. Due to its lower sodium content, Ringer's lactate produces slightly less volume expansion.

Colloid resuscitation capitalizes on the integrity of the capillary-endothelial membrane. Normal capillary oncotic pressure is 28 mm, and interstitial oncotic pressure is 5. Albumin, dextran, and hetastarch are retained largely in the intravascular space. Five percent albumin increases intravascular volume in a quantity nearly equal to that administered when the capillary-endothelial barrier is intact. Twenty-five percent albumin draws fluid from the interstitium, if the capillary-endothelial barrier is intact; this effect may not become fully manifest for several hours. Fresh frozen plasma (FFP) is a valuable resource which may contain infectious agents; FFP should not be used as a volume expander unless the patient suffers in addition from a coagulopathy. Packed red blood cells are, of course, the best volume expander; this therapy, in addition to increasing intravascular volume, increases oxygen carrying capacity of the blood.

The heat of the colloid/crystalloid controversy has frequently obscured the need to design individually the replacement fluids for specific clinical situations. Demling, Monohan, and Belzer[36] have attempted to sort out the indications for various replacement fluids. Isotonic crystalloid can restore plasma volume if enough is given, but will produce edema if more than 50% of the blood volume is replaced by crystalloid. Hypertonic saline solutions containing 240–30 mEq/L appear to produce less edema because the extracellular hyperosmolarity recruits fluid from the intracellular space. Monafo and Ayvazian[37] have demonstrated that urine output increased but, cardiac output decreased in burn patients treated with hypertonic saline, compared to Ringer's solution. Protein solutions remain in the vascular space for varying time periods as long as permeability is normal and can increase plasma volume without increasing body water to the level observed with crystalloid solution. Many critically ill patients, particularly those with sepsis, burns, and the respiratory distress syndrome, develop a progressively worsening capillary leak. In this situation, colloid solutions may leak rapidly into the interstitial space where they could exert an oncotic pressure, favoring additional fluid transfer from the vascular space. There is little evidence supporting the concern that this increase in interstitial protein concentration will increase interstitial lung water, and the replacement fluid which best maintains cardiac output and tissue perfusion should be selected. Hauser et al.[38] compared the effects of colloids and crystalloids in a group of seriously ill patients with the respiratory distress syndrome. Plasma volume, oxygen consumption, and cardiac output were increased to a much greater degree with colloid compared to crystalloid, and the improvement persisted for at least one hour.

Much more important than the type of fluid used is the rate at which it is given. It is certainly reasonable to administer crystalloid solutions at least until colloid or blood infusion is located and has begun infusing. Patients who are most profoundly hypotensive should be infused with fluid through multiple large-bore I.V.s. In this situation, colloid solution should be utilized until blood pressure begins to respond. The maintenance of adequate arterial filling pressures as well as arterial pressures is an important goal for fluid therapy. The perfect replacement colloid is not yet available. Newer synthetic colloids such as hetastarch may be useful in many situations.[38,39]

Estimation of a total electrolyte deficit requires knowledge of the plasma concentration, body weight, and distribution space of that electrolyte expressed as a percentage of total body weight. Such estimates are usually extremely inaccurate and good clinical practice usually suggests administration of half of the calculated deficit followed by repeat measurement.

Rapid restoration of plasma bicarbonate is frequently desirable although sudden return of pH to normal may lead to potassium depletion[40] or to increased cerebral acidosis.[41] While extracellular fluid constitutes 20% of total body weight, recent studies have suggested that the bicarbonate space is actually increased in patients with acidosis.[42] The use of a 30% estimate of bicarbonate space, aiming for 20–22 mEq/liter of plasma bicarbonate rather than complete normality, and initial administration of half of the calculated dose is a reasonable clinical approach.

For example, calculate the bicarbonate deficit in a 70-kg patient with a plasma bicarbonate of 15 mEq/liter. Bicarbonate space is probably 30% of 70 kg or 21 liters. Bicarbonate deficit is 22 minus 15 or 7 mEq/liter (aiming for 22 mEq/liter after replacement). Total calculated deficit is 7 mEq/liter times 21 liters or 147 mEq. Good clinical practice would suggest administration of 50–70 mEq of bicarbonate solution. Since bicarbonate may be rapidly consumed during periods of acidosis, bicarbonate concentration following administration of bicarbonate could be unchanged or actually lower than before replacement.

The calculation of sodium deficit in a patient with depletional hyponatremia further illustrates the problems associated with calculation of total body deficits. This example also demonstrates how infused solutions may shift water from one body compartment to another. Prior to infusion of sodium, tissue and extracellular osmolarity are identical. Infusion of sodium chloride raises the plasma osmolarity; since water moves from regions of lower osmolarity to high osmolarity, pure water flows from the intracellular space to the extracellular space. This water does not contain sodium and thus dilutes the infused sodium. Calculations of this type have shown that the calculation of the total sodium deficit in such a patient requires the assumption that the sodium space is actually total body water.[43] In practice, as indicated above, good clinical practice would be the administration of half the calculated dose—the sodium space might be estimated at 30% of body weight.

The Use of Diuretics in the Critically Ill Patient

A group of pharmacologic agents produces a salt and water diuresis by selectively inhibiting reabsorption of these substances at some point in the renal tubule.

The glomeruli and tubules work together to maintain blood volume (glomerulotubular balance), and so an agent which decreases absorption high in the tubule may be ineffective because of a distal compensatory increase in absorption of salt and water. The loop diuretics, furosemide and ethacrynic acid, act in the thick segment of the medullary ascending limb of Henle. Interference with the concentration and dilution function of this segment leads to the excretion of large volumes of isotonic urine. These agents also increase renal blood flow, particularly to the outer cortex, and increase vascular capacitance. The relationship between the vascular and tubular actions is not known, but the former may account for the rapid improvement in pulmonary edema observed with furosemide.[44] Potassium secretion is linked to sodium reabsorption in the distal tubule. Diuretics that deliver a large volume of urine to the distal tubule increase potassium secretion and produce hypokalemia. Potassium-sparing diuretics like triamterene inhibit both sodium reabsorption and potassium secretion in the distal tubule.

Thiazide Derivatives

This large group of compounds has gained wide popularity both as oral diuretic agents and as mild antihypertensives. They are weak carbonic anhydrase inhibitors, but their primary diuretic action is probably in the distal tubule, where they inhibit sodium and chloride reabsorption.[45] Their administration results in mild hypochloremic alkalosis and may be attended by significant urinary potassium loss. Therefore serum potassium should be checked intermittently, particularly if potassium levels may be achieved by potassium-rich diets or by addition of 30–60 mEq of elixir of KCl per day. Enteric-coated preparations combining KCl with a diuretic should be avoided because of the danger of small intestinal ulceration attending their use. Uncommon side effects of thiazide therapy include agranulocytosis and thrombocytopenia, cholestatic jaundice, pancreatitis, and glomeruloephritis. More common are hyperglycemia, hyperuricemia, and azotemia. Elevations in urea nitrogen and uric acid frequently follow pronounced diuresis and may be due to contraction of the intravascular volume and decreased glomerular flow. These metabolic changes are seldom troublesome and usually reverse by decreasing or withdrawing the diuretic agent.

Spironolactone and Triamterene

Both these agents are useful in combined diuretic therapy because of their ability to conserve potassium. Spironolactone does so by competitive inhibition of aldosterone, while triamterene causes potassium retention and sodium loss independently of aldosterone levels.[46] Despite the emphasis above on aldosterone activity in the pathogenesis of sodium and water retention, the aldosterone antagonists currently available are not usually effective as single diuretics in the management of congestive heart failure.

Ethacrynic Acid and Furosemide

These recently developed, extremely potent diuretics have assisted immeasurably in the control of fluid retention seen in refractory heart failure.[47] Ethacrynic acid is a ketone derivative of aryloxyacetic acid, completely unrelated to the thiazide drugs, while furosemide differs by the replacement of the thiadiazine ring with a furfuryl group on the amino nitrogen of anthranilic acid. They differ from thiazide drugs by inhibiting sodium reabsorption in the loop of Henle, as well as in the proximal and possibly distal tubules. Because of their potency and rapid onset of action intravenously (almost immediate), these agents are being used extensively in acute pulmonary edema—50 mg ethacrynic acid diluted in 50 ml dextrose and water or 40 mg furosemide can be given intravenously over a 5 minute period and repeated in 2–4 hours if necessary. Sudden and transient loss of hearing has been reported during or following intravenous injection of ethacrynic acid. Hyponatremia, hypokalemia, hypochloremia, alkalosis, azotemia, and severe dehydration may accompany massive diuresis associated with the oral or intravenous administration of either drug. This may usually be avoided by careful monitoring of serum electrolytes, urea nitrogen, and clinical status, and discontinuing therapy at an appropriate time. Potassium chloride supplement, 100–120 mEq per day, should be initiated at the onset of therapy. Another approach is to combine therapy, using a potassium sparing drug to avoid potassium depletion. As with the thiazides, elevations in blood glucose and uric acid may be observed during therapy.

Acidifying Agents

Most of the diuretic agents described above, particularly when used in maximal doses, result in hypochloremic alkalosis, which tends to limit the effectiveness of the diuretic agent. While the more potent agents (ethacrynic acid and furosemide) tend to produce continued diuresis despite this development, it is useful to be aware of methods to correct this disturbance in blood chemistry. By restoring pH and chloride level toward normal, more effective diuresis may again be accomplished. Acetazolamide, a carbonic anhydrate inhibitor, causes impaired secretion of hydrogen ion, increased excretion of sodium bicarbonate, and conserves chloride ion, tending to produce a hyperchloremic acidosis. Other agents, such as ammonium chloride and arginine and lysine hydrochloride, by supplying chloride with a metabolizable radical, produce a similar effect.

REGULATION OF HYDROGEN ION CONCENTRATION

The metabolic processes detailed in Chapter 1 yield energy by splitting off hydrogen from substrate. Some hydrogen atoms lose electrons, forming hydrogen ions, while other hydrogen ions accept these electrons and become negatively charged hydride ions, which are then transferred to the coenzyme nicotinamide adenine dinucleotide (NAD). These electrons are transferred to the cytochrome system (respiratory enzyme chain) and ultimately form high energy phosphates; the hydrogen ions combine with oxygen, producing harmless water. Additional hydrogen ions are produced by the hydration of carbon dioxide, which is also split off from substrate during oxidation, and from the oxidation of certain other substrates which yield other acids.

These three sources of hydrogen ions are summarized in Figure 8–5 and emphasize the hydrogen disposal problems facing the organism. Hydrogen ions from most oxidative metabolism are bound by oxygen and excreted as water; carbonic acid forms carbon dioxide, which is removed by the lungs; hydrogen ions produced by the so-called fixed acids are removed by the kidneys. The practical implication here for the care of the critically ill patient is that disturbances of pulmonary, circulatory, and renal function may interfere with one or more of these mechanisms for hydrogen ion disposal.

Nature of Acids, Bases, and Buffers

Chemical elements exist as atoms, which are themselves composed of a central

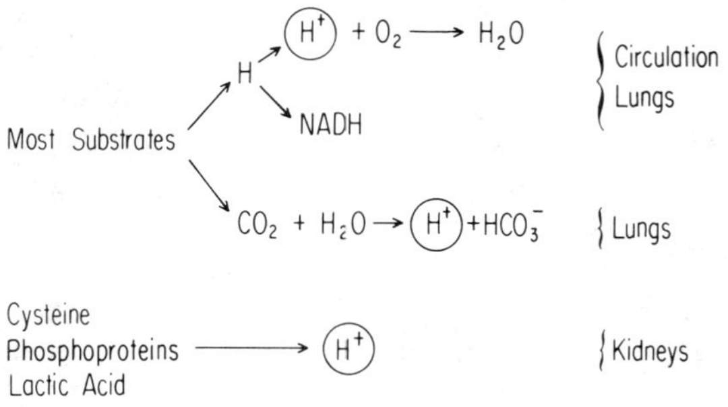

FIG 8–5.
Sources of hydrogen ions. See text for complete description.

nucleus containing positively charged protons (as well as neutrons) surrounded by rings of negatively charged electrons. The positive charges in the nucleus balance the negative charges of the orbital electrons so that the atom is electrically neutral. Much of modern chemical theory is based on the behavior of these orbital electrons. Either gain or loss of orbital electrons unbalances the charge of the nucleus; the charged particles produced are termed ions. Loss of an electron produces a positively charged cation, while gain of an electron produces a negatively charged anion.

Acids ionize into hydrogen ions and a variety of anions—the conjugate bases of the various acids. Hydrogen atoms contain but one proton and one orbital electron; loss of the orbital electron leaves the central proton unprotected and produces the positively charged hydrogen ion. The chemist Bronsted revolutionized thinking in this area when he proposed that acids should be viewed as proton donors since a hydrogen ion is actually a single proton.

A number of somewhat confusing aspects of acid-base behavior are simplified by accepting the concept that acids are proton (or hydrogen ion) donors while bases are proton (or hydrogen ion) acceptors. A strong acid is one which almost completely dissociates into hydrogen ions and conjugate base, making a large supply of hydrogen ions available for subsequent reaction. The conjugate base of such a strong acid must be quite weak since it "allows" hydrogen ions to escape. A weak acid holds on to its hydrogen ions and in consequence has a strong conjugate base. The strength of a base and its ability to bind hydrogen ions is a central theme in physiologic homeostasis.

For example, consider the following two acids:

$$HCl \rightleftharpoons H^+ + Cl^-$$
$$H_2CO_3 \rightleftharpoons H^+ + HCO_3^-$$

Hydrochloric acid (HCl) is a strong acid which readily dissociates, indicating that its conjugate base is weak. Carbonic acid (H_2CO_3) is a weak acid, indicating that bicarbonate ion is a strong base anxious to bind hydrogen ions. If these two acids are mixed, hydrogen ions from the hydrochloric acid are bound by bicarbonate ion, and chlorine gas is liberated.

The binding of hydrogen ion by a base is termed buffering. The hydrogen ion concentration of biologic systems is maintained by a group of buffers which minimize the effect of added acid or base and are then regenerated by pulmonary and renal mechanisms. While bicarbonate, phosphate, protein, and hemoglobin all function as buffer systems, bicarbonate is perhaps the most important because carbonic acid formed by the reaction is rapidly excreted by the lungs. For this reason, the buffering ability of the carbonic acid-bicarbonate system in vivo is far greater than its efficiency in a closed in vitro situation.

The law of mass action explains the buffering action of a system containing a weak acid and its salt. In an ordinary chemical reaction, the concentrations of the constituents in a reaction at equilibrium

$$A + B \rightleftharpoons C + D$$

are related by the equation

$$\frac{[C][D]}{[A][B]} = K$$

The right hand reactants are placed in the numerator by convention. K is the equilibrium constant. (If more than one molecule of substance A reacts with substance B, the molar concentration of A is raised to the power numerically equal to the number of molecules of substance A present.)

Both hydrochloric and carbonic acids follow the laws of mass action and dissociate into hydrogen ions and their respective anions. The equilibrium constant for hydrochloric acid is close to 1.0, so that a mole of hydrochloric acid produces a mole of hydrogen ions and a mole of chloride ions. In contrast, carbonic acid is a weaker acid because it only slightly dissociates into hydrogen ions.

$$H_2CO_3 \rightleftharpoons H^+ + HCO_3^-$$

$$\frac{[H^+][HCO_3^-]}{[H_2CO_3]} = K$$

Henderson demonstrated that hydrogen ion concentration could be determined by a rearrangement of the mass action equation.

$$[H^+] = K\frac{[H_2CO_3]}{[HCO_3^-]}$$

The hydrogen ion concentration in biologic fluids is extremely small (4.47–3.55 $\times 10^{-8}$). Sorenson found this notation cumbersome and introduced the concept of pH, the negative logarithm of the hydrogen ion concentration. A 0.01 molar solution of hydrochloric acid contains 0.01 or 1×10^{-2} moles of hydrogen ion. The logarithm of 0.01 is -2; the negative logarithm of 0.01 is 2, so the pH of this solution is 2.

Hasselbalch applied the Sorenson notation system to the original Henderson equation by expressing K and the ratio $[H_2CO_3]/[HCO_3^-]$ as their negative logarithms:

$$\text{pH} = \text{p}K + \log\frac{HCO_3^-}{H_2CO_3}$$

Note that in the Henderson-Hasselbalch equation the negative logarithmic transformation inverts the ratio and places bicarbonate ion in the numerator. The pK for carbonic acid is 6.1.

The addition of sodium bicarbonate to a solution of carbonic acid drives the dissociation reaction to the left according to the law of mass action.

$$H_2CO_3 \rightleftharpoons H^+ + HCO_3^-$$

This type reaction is referred to as the common ion effect. The bicarbonate ion is common to the salt and the carbonic acid. The anions of weak acids—such as carbonic, lactic, or phosphoric acid—act as biologic buffers and protect the internal environment from wide variations in hydrogen ion concentration. If hydrochloric acid is added to a solution containing carbonic acid, the following reaction is driven toward the right.

$$H^+ + Cl^- + Na^+ + HCO_3^- \rightleftharpoons H_2CO_3 + Na^+ + Cl^-$$

Carbonic acid is poorly ionized, so that the added hydrogen ions may be said to be buffered by the bicarbonate. Most of the strong hydrochloric acid is in effect converted to the weaker carbonic acid. The relationships between pH, bicarbonate, and carbonic acid (P_{CO_2}) are shown in Figure 8–6.

Proteins also serve as buffers by virtue of various reactive groups on the protein molecules. An amino group accepts a hydrogen ion and reduces the concentration of hydrogen ion in solution.

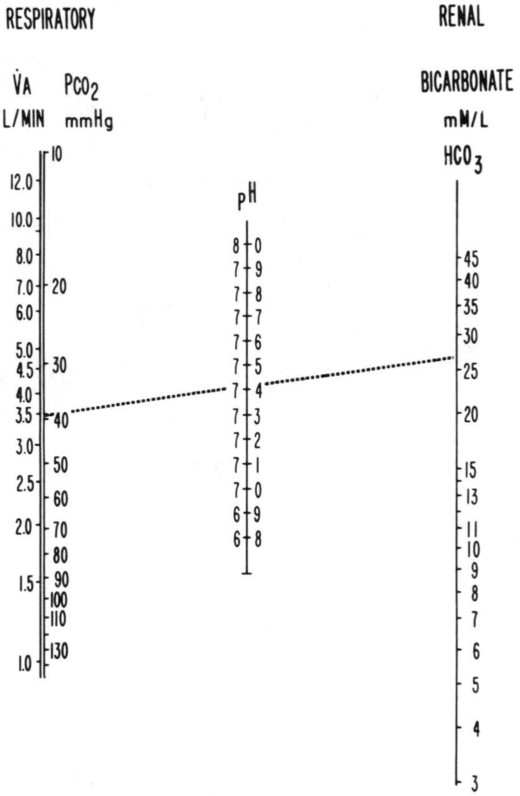

FIG 8–6.
Blood pH is determined by carbon dioxide tension P_{CO_2} and bicarbonate concentration. The former is directly related to alveolar ventilation, whereas the latter is determined by the rate of tubular reabsorption of bicarbonate. The straight line intersecting any two of the variables fixes the third variable. The calculations of alveolar ventilation were made assuming a carbon dioxide production of 180 ml per minute.

$$\text{Protein-NH}_2 + H^+ = \text{protein-NH}_3^+$$

Protein and electrolyte buffers are present in the plasma, as well as in the interstitial and intracellular spaces. Experimentally infused hydrochloric acid is primarily buffered intracellularly.

A very important aspect of buffering action is that all buffers must be in equilibrium for any given hydrogen ion concentration.

$$[H^+] = K_1\frac{[H_2CO_3]}{[HCO_3^-]} = K_2\frac{[H_2PO_4^-]}{[HPO_4^=]} = K_3\frac{[\text{H lactate}]}{[\text{lactate}^-]} = K_4\frac{[HPr]}{[Pr^-]}$$

In addition to these buffer pairs, all the others also conform to this relationship. The ratio of each buffer constituent *must change to satisfy the above relationship with a change in hydrogen ion concentration.* Conversely, if one ratio is changed by addition of salt, hydrogen ion concentration changes due to the common ion effect and all the other buffer ratios must change.

At pH 7.4 the ratio of carbonic acid to bicarbonate concentration is 1:20. This ratio is carefully maintained in the body by the interrelated activities of the lungs and the kidneys. The respiratory control of the carbonic acid level was described in Chapter 6.

Carbonic acid dissociates to water and carbon dioxide, and the level of carbon dioxide directly affects the carbonic acid concentration. If carbon dioxide is "blown off," carbonic acid concentration falls, the ratio $[H_2CO_3]/[HCO_3^-]$ falls, and the hydrogen ion concentration also falls. The ratio of all the other buffer pairs also changes. For example, the reaction

$$H_2PO_4^- \rightleftharpoons HPO_4^= + H^+$$

would proceed toward the right and hydrogen ions would be liberated, tending to lessen the effect of hyperventilation.

Bicarbonate ion concentration is regulated by the kidney at a level between 24 and 26 mEq/liter, and thus the lungs and kidneys combine to maintain the $[H_2CO_3]/[HCO_3^-]$ ratio at 1:20, fixing the pH at about 7.4.

Carbon Dioxide Transport and Bicarbonate Ion

The buffer pair H_2CO_3/HCO_3^- described above reveals that blood carbon dioxide may exist in one of two forms. Total plasma carbon dioxide content is 26–28 mEq/liter; less than 5% of this is dissolved carbon dioxide, the remainder being bicarbonate ion. The volume of dissolved carbon dioxide is determined by the carbon dioxide tension, which is in turn determined by the rate of alveolar ventilation (Fig 8–6; see also Fig 6–14). The solubility constant for carbon dioxide is 0.03 mEq/mm Hg so that the amount dissolved equals the arterial carbon dioxide tension (P_{CO_2}) times the solubility constant.

$$\text{Dissolved } CO_2 = 0.03 \times P_{CO_2}$$
$$1.2 \text{ mEq/liter} = 0.03 \times 40 \text{ mm Hg}$$

Bicarbonate ion is produced by an important two-step chemical reaction.

$$CO_2 + H_2O \overset{CA}{\rightleftharpoons} H_2CO_3 \rightleftharpoons H^+ + HCO_3^-$$

The right-hand reaction, the dissociation of carbonic acid into hydrogen and bicarbonate ions, is an inherently rapid reaction. The left-hand reaction, the hydration of carbon dioxide to form carbonic acid, is relatively slow. Meldrum and Roughton[48] identified a zinc-containing enzyme, carbonic anhydrase (CA), which is found in erythrocytes, kidney tissue, and gastric mucosa and which catalyzes the hydration of carbon dioxide. The presence of this enzyme permits efficient transportation of carbon dioxide from cell to alveolar air.

The exchange of hydrogen ions between bicarbonate and hemoglobin buffer systems demonstrates many aspects of physiologic buffer action and is responsible for the transportation of carbon dioxide with little change in hydrogen ion concentration. Figure 8–7 shows these reactions within an erythrocyte traversing a systemic capillary (**A**) and within another erythrocyte traversing a pulmonary capillary (**B**).

Carbon dioxide diffuses from tissue into the erythrocyte (Figure 8–7A) where, under the influence of carbonic anhydrase, it hydrolyzes into carbonic acid, which then dissociates into hydrogen and bicarbonate ions. The next reaction

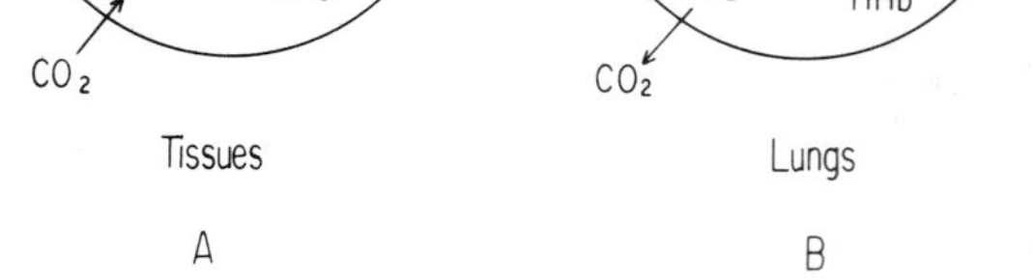

FIG 8–7.
The transport of carbon dioxide from tissue to erythrocyte and thence to the lungs. The enzyme carbonic anhydrase (CA) catalyzes the formation of bicarbonate in the erythrocyte at the tissue level and then catalyzes the release of carbon dioxide from bicarbonate in the lungs. Hydrogen ions produced by the hydrolysis of carbon dioxide are buffered by hemoglobin. In the lung, oxygenation of hemoglobin changes its buffer capacity and releases hydrogen ions for the subsequent release of carbon dioxide. **A.** Tissue-erythrocyte reactions. **B.** Erythrocyte-lung reaction. See text for complete description.

is dependent upon the fact that reduced hemoglobin is a stronger base than oxyhemoglobin, and is able to bind hydrogen ions like any base. Reduced hemoglobin binds hydrogen ion produced from carbonic acid, pulling the reaction to the right by the law of mass action and generating bicarbonate ion, which diffuses from erythrocyte to plasma. The hydrogen exchange between these two systems may be expressed as:

$$H_2CO_3 \rightarrow H^+ + HCO_3^-$$
$$\downarrow$$
$$HHb \leftarrow H^+ + Hb^-$$

Chloride diffuses into the erythrocyte in exchange for the bicarbonate ion, which has diffused out—the chloride shift.

The reverse action occurs within pulmonary capillaries (Figure 8–7B). Oxyhemoglobin is a weaker base, so that hydrogen ions are released in the erythrocyte and react with bicarbonate ion to form carbonic acid. Carbonic anhydrase catalyzes the dehydration of carbonic acid to carbon dioxide, which diffuses through the erythrocyte and alveolar-capillary membranes into the lung. The efficiency of this system is such that 200 ml of carbon dioxide is transported each minute with a pH drop of only 0.04 units.

Bicarbonate and Total Body Buffering

Bicarbonate plays a major role in the defense of hydrogen ion because it is readily available for hydrogen ion binding and because it forms carbonic acid, which is readily excreted as carbon dioxide. It is a valuable indicator of total body buffer stores. It is not, however, the major buffer system of the body. Figure 8–8 shows the buffering of exogenous hydrogen ions. Swan and Pitts[49] administered hydrochloric acid to nephrectomized dogs and observed that 57% of the hydrogen ions were bound by intracellular buffers, the remainder by extracellular buffers. Hydrogen ions are bound by plasma bicarbonate, releasing carbon dioxide for pulmonary excretion but depleting bicarbonate reserves. Additional hydrogen ion is buffered by interstitial bicarbonate ion. Cellular buffers— hemoglobin in erythrocytes and phosphate and protein buffers in other cells—further engage hydrogen ions. The efficiency of this buffering may be seen by comparing the effect of infusing 156 ml of 1.0*N* HCl into a 19.7-kg dog (containing 11.4 liters of water) to that of pouring the same amount of acid into a beaker containing 11.4 liters of water. The pH of the beaker drops from 7.44 to 1.84; plasma pH in the dog drops from 7.44 to 7.14. Moreover, the pH in the beaker remains acidic while the dog gradually excretes hydrogen ion over the next several days and replenishes his stores of bicarbonate. Other experiments by Swan

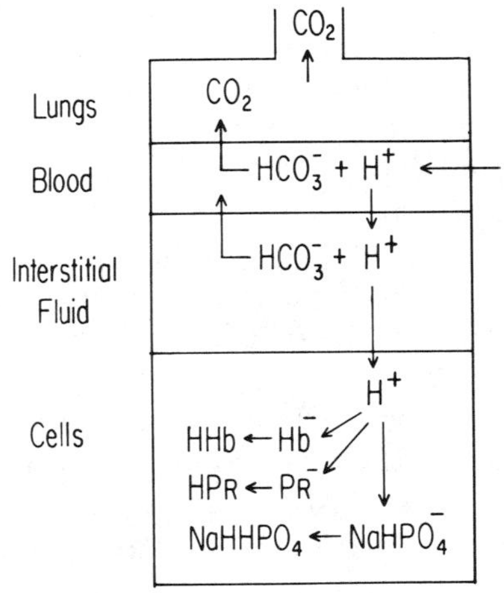

FIG 8–8.
Buffering of exogenous hydrogen ions (see text for complete description). Note that 57% of the hydrogen ions were bound by intracellular buffers. (Adapted from Swan RC, Pitts RF: Neutralization of infused acid by nephrectomized dogs. *J Clin Invest* 1955; 34:205.)

and Pitts[49] showed that intracellular reactions accounted for 32% of buffering in metabolic alkalosis, 97% in respiratory acidosis, and 99% in respiratory alkalosis.

Renal Excretion of Hydrogen Ions

The kidney regulates hydrogen ion concentration by maintaining the plasma bicarbonate concentration between 24 and 26 mEq/liter. Pitts[9] emphasized that *the tubular secretion of hydrogen ions in exchange for sodium ions* is the basic mechanism underlying acidification of the urine and maintenance of plasma bicarbonate concentration within a narrow range. This tubular secretion of hydrogen ions is responsible for the reabsorption of bicarbonate, the generation of titratable acidity, and the excretion of ammonium salts.

In normal man, bicarbonate reabsorption dominates the ion exchange process; 30–50 mEq of acid is excreted each day by ammonium salt generation and 10–30 mEq by the excretion of titratable acidity—compared to approximately 13,000 mEq excreted by the lung as carbon dioxide. This is possible because the aerobic metabolism of most food material results in the production of carbon dioxide and water. The metabolism of cystine-containing protein leads to the production of sulfate, and that of phosphoprotien to the production of phosphate, which must be disposed of in other ways. The anaerobic mechanisms presented in Chapter 1 lead to the production of lactate and hydrogen ions, which must be excreted by the kidney unless the subsequent availability of oxygen permits the complete oxidation of lactate to water and carbon dioxide. This shift in the renal pattern of hydrogen ion-sodium ion exchange is seen in the patient with diabetic ketoacidosis who may excrete 300–500 mEq daily as ammonium salts and 75–250 mEq daily as titratable acidity.

Bicarbonate Reabsorption by the Kidney

The key chemical reaction in the acidification of urine is the production of hydrogen ions within renal tubular cells from carbon dioxide and water. Carbon dioxide is produced by tubular cells and also transported to them from other cells. This important overall reaction is closely dependent upon the enzyme carbonic anhydrase found in high concentrations in renal tubular cells.

$$CO_2 + H_2O \rightarrow HCO_3^- + H^+$$

The hydrogen ions so produced are exchanged for sodium ions (and excreted into the tubular lumen) and bicarbonate ions (which diffuse into peritubular blood). Sodium is actively pumped as described above so that the net result is the reabsorption of sodium bicarbonate and the excretion of hydrogen ion.

The tubular excretion schemes presented in Figures 8–3 and 8–4 must be expanded to include a hydrogen ion pump, which actively secretes hydrogen ion into tubular urine against a concentration gradient. Figure 8–9 shows such a pump and demonstrates how the active extrusion of hydrogen ion is balanced by the influx of sodium ion into the tubular cell and its subsequent active extrusion into peritubular blood. The secreted hydrogen ions combine with filtered bicarbonate within the tubular urine to form carbonic acid, which rapidly dissociates to form carbon dioxide and water. The molecular carbon dioxide freely diffuses back into tubular cells where it recombines with water to form carbonic acid and ultimately makes more hydrogen and bicarbonate ions available.

The rate of bicarbonate reabsorption is controlled by five major factors:

1. *Arterial carbon dioxide tension:* The Henderson-Hasselbalch ratio described earlier is kept constant

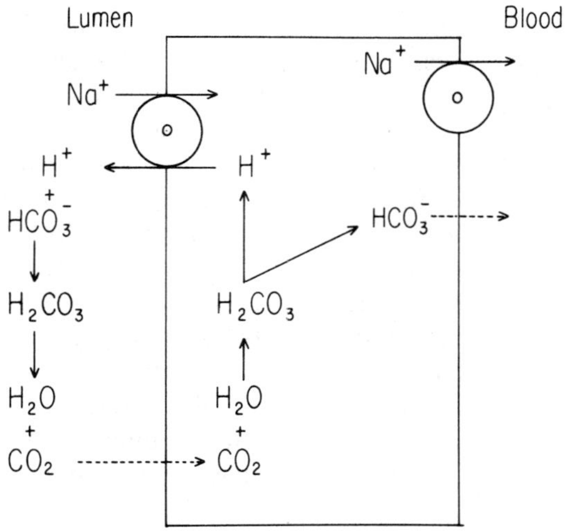

FIG 8–9.
The hydrogen ion pump actively secretes hydrogen ions into tubular urine against a concentration gradient. The net effect of hydrogen ion excretion is carbon dioxide reabsorption and intracellular bicarbonate production. (Adapted from Pitts RF: *Physiology of the Kidney and Body Fluids*, ed 2. Chicago, Year Book Medical, 1968, p 31.)

by increased reabsorption of bicarbonate in the presence of increased arterial carbon dioxide tensions. The actions portrayed in Figure 8–9 explain this phenomenon; increased arterial and cellular carbon dioxide levels make more hydrogen ions available for tubular secretion and bicarbonate reabsorption. The converse occurs with reduced carbon dioxide tensions, where a decrease in the supply of available hydrogen ions reduces bicarbonate reabsorption.

2. *Plasma chloride level:* Renal mechanisms appear to adjust chloride and bicarbonate reabsorption reciprocally, maintaining the sum of these anions at a relatively constant level. Recent evidence suggests that the plasma chloride level and filtered chloride load play a role in regulating bicarbonate reabsorption. If tubular fluid is deficient in chloride, the anions required to balance sodium reabsorption must come from bicarbonate reabsorption. Bicarbonate reabsorption, in turn, increases the availability of intracellular hydrogen ions and further augments bicarbonate reabsorption. Potassium ions are also lost from tubular cells, but the resultant hypochloremic alkalosis may be corrected by chloride replacement alone.[50] *In other words, chloride reabsorption prevents or "holds back" the excretion of potassium and hydrogen.* If sufficient chloride is not present in tubular fluid, sodium reabsorption must be accompanied by both potassium and hydrogen in order to maintain electroneutrality.
3. *Plasma potassium level:* A number of clinical and experimental observations suggest that potassium and hydrogen ions have a reciprocal relationship across cellular membranes. Infused potassium rapidly enters the intracellular space, combining with cellular anions (collectively termed buffer or buf$^-$) and displacing hydrogen ions, which diffuse out into the extracellular space (Fig 8–10A). Infused potassium thus produces a hyperkalemic acidosis. The reverse occurs when plasma potassium is low. Cellular potassium diffuses out of the cell, making intracellular anions available for hydrogen ions, which diffuse in to replace potassium. The result is hypokalemic alkalosis (Fig 8–10B). Primary alterations in hydrogen ion concentration produce the same reciprocal change in potassium. If there is an increased produc-

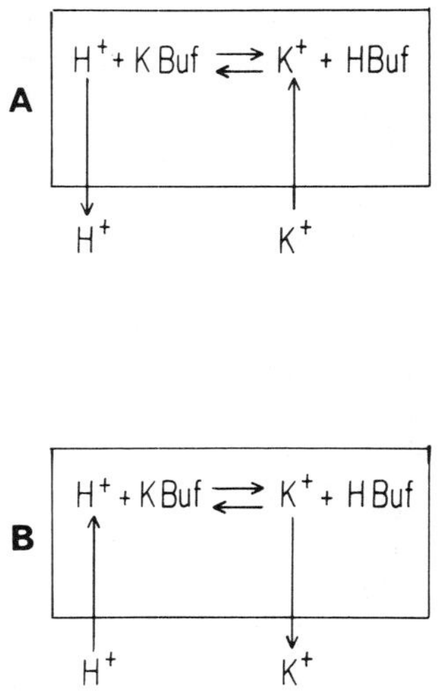

FIG 8–10.
Reciprocal relationship of potassium and hydrogen ions across cellular membranes. **A.** Hydrogen ions diffuse out into the extracellular space when extracellular potassium is elevated, producing acidosis. **B.** Alkalosis is produced when cellular potassium is reduced.

tion of intracellular hydrogen ions, they compete for potassium, which then diffuses into the extracellular fluid. In the reverse situation, potassium leaves extracellular fluid and diffuses into cells when the intracellular hydrogen ion concentration is low. *Acidosis leads to hyperkalemia; alkalosis leads to hypokalemia. Hyperkalemia leads to acidosis; hypokalemia leads to alkalosis.* The reciprocal relationships between hydrogen and potassium ions explains the changes in bicarbonate reabsorption seen with changing potassium levels. Kennedy and Berliner,[51] emphasized the importance of this concept and suggested that potassium and hydrogen compete for a common secretory mechanism. Recent work of Rector, Bloomer, and Seldin[52] suggests that this may not be the case since hydrogen ion secretion occurs along the entire renal tubule while potassium secretion is limited to the distal nephron. When renal tubular potassium concentration is reduced, hydrogen ions diffuse in from peritubular blood (as in Figure 8–11) for all cells. These hydrogen ions are secreted into tubular urine and combine with bicarbonate ion to form carbonic acid, which then dehydrates to carbon dioxide and water. The carbon dioxide diffuses back into renal tubular cells and ultimately forms bicarbonate, which raises extracellular bicarbonate concentration. The resultant hypokalemic alkalosis is characterized by extracellular alkalosis, intracellular acidosis, and excretion of acidic urine.

4. *Aldosterone secretion:* Increased mineralocoticoid secretion decreases plasma potassium and increases bicarbonate reabsorption. While the precise mechanism is not clear,

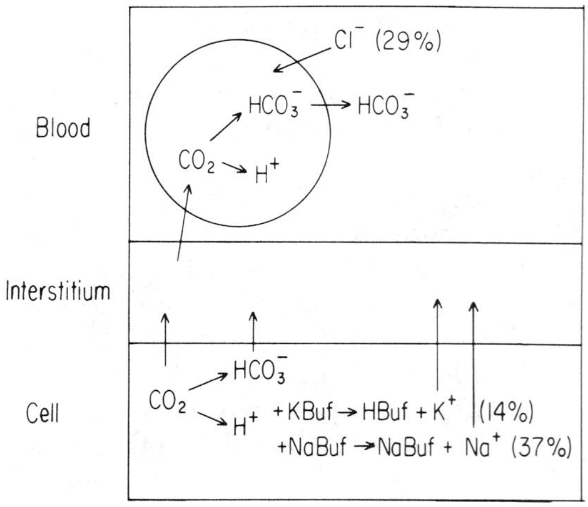

FIG 8–11.
Body buffering in respiratory acidosis. Carbon dioxide produced by the tissues is buffered by hemoglobin (29% of total buffering) and intracellular proteins buffers (51%).

these agents appear to increase sodium retention at the expense of potassium excretion.

5. *Hydration:* Dehydration appears to enhance bicarbonate reabsorption. One recent study related alveolar hypoventilation associated with metabolic alkalosis to systemic dehydration.

Preservation of Bicarbonate Stores by Secretion of Ammonia Salts and Titratable Acidity

Bicarbonate reabsorption is the dominant mechanism for stabilization of plasma bicarbonate levels in normal man. When bicarbonate is depleted, hydrogen ions are buffered by phosphate; dibasic phosphate (Na_2HPO_4) is the major filtered buffer. The key process described above—by which carbon dioxide and water produce intracellular hydrogen ions and bicarbonate ions— works with phosphate buffer to restore bicarbonate stores and excrete hydrogen ion. Hydrogen ions are excreted into the tubular lumen, combining with dibasic phosphate to form monobasic phosphate.

$$Na_2HPO_4 + H^+ \rightarrow NaH_2PO_4 + Na^+$$

The hydrogen ion is excreted as monobasic phosphate; sodium diffuses into the tubular cell (note the common feature of sodium-hydrogen exchange) and is then actively pumped into extracellular fluid where it combines with bicarbonate ion (the other ion resulting from the combination of carbon dioxide and water described above).

When phosphate buffer is depleted, the accumulation of intracellular hydrogen ions blocks the hydrogen ion-sodium ion exchange mechanism. Ammonia is formed from glutamine and diffuses into the acidic tubular urine where it binds hydrogen ions to form ammonium ion. The bound hydrogen ion is then excreted as ammonium chloride, releasing a sodium ion which is reabsorbed.

Note that the following common events occur in all three mechanisms for excreting hydrogen ion: (1) Hydrogen ions and bicarbonate ions are produced from carbon dioxide and water. (2) Hydrogen ions exchange for sodium ions. (3) Hydrogen ions are excreted in tubular urine. (4) Sodium is reabsorbed in combination with bicarbonate.

ACIDOSIS AND ALKALOSIS

The important distinction between hypoxia and hypoxemia was pointed out in Chapter 1. A similar distinction should be made between acidosis and acidemia, and between alkalosis and alkalemia. Analysis of a sample of plasma may show evidence of acidemia or alkalemia which suggests the presence of abnormal cellular hydrogen ion concentration—acidosis or alkalosis. The critically ill patient presented in Table 1–3 demonstrates that this is more than an academic distinction. A low erythrocyte pH suggests the possibility of increased cellular hydrogen ion concentration (acidosis), while marked hyperventilation produces arterial alkalemia.

Respiratory Acidosis

A decrease in alveolar ventilation decreases the clearance of carbon dioxide, raising arterial, venous, and tissue carbon dioxide tensions (see Fig 1–14). In contrast to the response to addition of fixed acid (Fig 8–8), 97% of the buffering of hydrogen ion produced from carbonic acid requires the participation of intracellular mechanisms. Figure 8–11 shows three compartments representing intracellular, interstitial, and plasma fluid. The plasma compartment is disproportionately large in order that events occurring within the red blood cell may be shown. Carbon dioxide is produced in the tissues and diffuses to interstitial and plasma compartments. Unable to be excreted by the lungs, it enters the red blood cell in large quantities where, under the influence of carbonic anhydrase, hydrogen and bicarbonate ions were formed. This process is described in greater detail in Figure 8–7. Studies of Giebisch et al.[54] show that hemoglobin binding of hydrogen ion with subsequent exchange of chloride for bicarbonate ion accounts for 29% of total buffering. Additional hydrogen ions produced in tissue or extracellular fluid diffuse back into cells and are exchanged for sodium and potassium. The intracellular buffers, collectively labeled buf (mainly protein and phosphate buffers), bind hydrogen ion and release cation into the extracellular fluid. Sodium exchange accounts for 37% of the buffering, potassium exchange for 14%. The end effect of these three intracellular mechanisms is to increase plasma bicarbonate concentration.

The normal relationship*

$$pH = 7.40 \propto \frac{HCO_3^- = 26 \text{ mEq/liter}}{P_{CO_2} = 40 \text{ mm Hg}}$$

has shifted to

$$pH = 7.24 \propto \frac{HCO_3^- = 29 \text{ mEq/liter}}{P_{CO_2} = 70 \text{ mm Hg}}$$

This immediate increase in bicarbonate attempts to restore the bicarbonate-carbonic acid ratio to 20:1. While not completely successful, it represents a first line of defense. Had the bicarbonate remained at 26 mEq/liter, the pH would have fallen to 7.19 instead of 7.24.

This initial response is inadequate as a defensive maneuver; and within several hours the renal absorption of bicarbonate increases plasma bicarbonate concentration, buffering more carbonic acid, and increasing pH.

$$pH = 7.32 \propto \frac{HCO_3 = 38 \text{ mEq/liter}}{P_{CO_2} = 70 \text{ mm Hg}}$$

This is generally termed a compensated respiratory acidosis, although it obviously does not represent complete compensation. High bicarbonate levels with normal and even alkalemic pH values are commonly observed in patients with carbon dioxide retention and suggest an associated increase in bicarbonate stores, perhaps due to potassium deficiency.

The study of Giebisch, Berger, and Pitts[54] shows the effect of experimental acute hypercapnia in a nephrectomized dog (Table 8–4). Removal of the kidneys eliminates the possibility of increased bicarbonate reabsorption and also prevents potassium excretion.

Respiratory Alkalosis

Hyperventilation leads to a decrease in arterial carbon dioxide tension and an increase in pH. Total body buffering follows the same pathways shown in Figure 8–11 but in reverse direction. Plasma bicarbonate decreases somewhat so that:

$$pH = 7.62 \propto \frac{HCO_3^- = 20 \text{ mEq/liter}}{P_{CO_2} = 20 \text{ mm Hg}}$$

Later, renal excretion of bicarbonate leads to partial compensation:

*p*K*, logarithm, and solubility coefficient have been omitted from this and following equations in the interest of clarity. For this reason, the equality sign has been replaced with proportionality sign.

TABLE 8–4.
Values Obtained from Nephrectomized Dogs Under Various Experimental Conditions

CONDITION	P_{CO_2}	pH	HCO_3^-	Na^+	K^+	Cl^-	LACTATE
Acute respiratory acidosis [29]							
Control	33	7.30	17.2	154	3.8	115	3.1
Experimental	146	6.87	28.0	160	4.7	113	1.4
Acute respiratory alkalosis [29]							
Control	30	7.42	21	155	3.9	116	1.0
Experimental	7	7.57	7.5	151	3.9	124	5.9
Acute metabolic acidosis [24]							
Control	38	7.40	25	156	4.0	119	–
Experimental	24	7.11	7	145	10.3	134	–

$$\text{pH} = 7.52 \propto \frac{HCO_3^- = 16\ \text{mEq/liter}}{P_{CO_2} = 20\ \text{mm Hg}}$$

Also seen in Table 8–4 are values from the study of Giebisch et al.[54] for experimentally produced acute respiratory alkalosis. Note that lactate ion migrates into the extracellular space. This increase in lactate should not be considered evidence of anaerobic metabolism.

Metabolic Acidosis

Hydrogen ions liberated from fixed acids are bound by tissue and extracellular buffers (Fig 8–8). Plasma bicarbonate concentrations and pH decrease. Common causes include increased production of fixed acids (diabetes, uremia, lactic acidosis in shock) or loss of bicarbonate (diarrhea, fistulas, renal tubular acidosis).

$$\text{pH} = 7.08 \propto \frac{HCO_3^- = 10\ \text{mEq/liter}}{P_{CO_2} = 35\ \text{mm Hg}}$$

In primary metabolic abnormalities, respiratory attempts at compensation may occur almost immediately. Increased hydrogen ion concentration stimulates peripheral and central chemoreceptors. augmenting ventilation and decreasing carbon dioxide tension. This response has been well known for many years and is termed Kussmaul breathing. The net result is to lower carbon dioxide tension and attempt to restore the balance of the carbonic acid- bicarbonate buffer pair.

$$\text{pH} = 7.30 \propto \frac{HCO_3^- = 10\ \text{mEq/liter}}{P_{CO_2} = 20\ \text{mm Hg}}$$

Swan and Pitts[49] produced acute metabolic acidosis by the acute addition of hydrogen ions in a series of animal experiments. (Table 8–4).

Metabolic Alkalosis

Excessive intake of bicarbonate, loss of fixed acid in vomiting, and potassium depletion lead to increased plasma bicarbonate.

$$\text{pH} = 7.60 \propto \frac{HCO_3^- = 38\ \text{mEq/liter}}{P_{CO_2} = 40\ \text{mm Hg}}$$

Respiratory compensation is variable, but is apparently more common in dehydrated patients. A recent study showed significant hypoventilation with hypercapnia and hypoxemia, which responded to correction of the bicarbonate excess.[53]

$$pH = 7.55 \propto \frac{HCO_3^- = 34 \text{ mEq/liter}}{Pco_2 = 45 \text{ mm Hg}}$$

Mixed Abnormalities

The combination of a metabolic deficit together with primary hypoventilation may produce a combined acidosis (or alkalosis) that is difficult to analyze. It is sometimes not easy to determine whether a given bicarbonate concentration is appropriate for the observed carbon dioxide tension—or conversely, if the carbon dioxide tension is appropriate for the bicarbonate concentration. In the following example, the bicarbonate concentration observed in a patient with a sudden increase in carbon dioxide tension was such that the pH fell to 7.15.

$$pH = 7.15 \propto \frac{HCO_3^- = 21 \text{ mEq/liter}}{Pco_2 = 60 \text{ mm Hg}}$$

Why is the bicarbonate lower than normal? Is this an appropriate response in acute respiratory acidosis? The decrease in bicarbonate clearly indicates an associated metabolic defect and suggests the coexistence of circulatory insufficiency. The problem is even more complicated when a low carbon dioxide concentration coexists with a low bicarbonate concentration.

$$pH = 7.40 \propto \frac{HCO_3^- = 15 \text{ mEq/liter}}{Pco_2 = 25 \text{ mm Hg}}$$

What is the explanation for this almost perfect compensation? Has the bicarbonate been reduced in response to the hyperventilation and a reduction in carbon dioxide tension? Has the carbon dioxide tension been reduced in response to a metabolic deficit in bicarbonate? This particular constellation is frequently seen in critically ill patients in whom hyperventilation coexists with circulatory insufficiency and a metabolic deficit. "Perfect" physiologic compensation is rare. A normal pH associated with abnormalities of both Pco_2 and bicarbonate generally indicates combined respiratory and metabolic abnormalities.

The following is an obvious example of what might be called double acidosis, since it followed combined circulatory and respiratory arrest. The former led to an increase in lactic acid and a decrease in bicarbonate, while the latter led to an increase in carbon dioxide tension.

Before cardiac arrest

$$pH = 7.40 \propto \frac{HCO_3^- = 26 \text{ mEq/liter}}{Pco_2 = 40 \text{ mm Hg}}$$

After arrest

$$pH = 6.92 \propto \frac{HCO_3^- = 14 \text{ mEq/liter}}{Pco_2 = 70 \text{ mm Hg}}$$

This situation is obviously life-threatening. Its lethal nature is intensified by its rapid onset, allowing little time for the development of adaptive mechanisms. The acidotic myocardium cannot be defibrillated; sympathomimetic amines are ineffective, and little hope for salvage is present, unless the severe abnormalities are corrected by the immediate administration of bicarbonate solution and the initiation of assisted ventilation.

Carbon Dioxide Titration Curve

Participation of the entire body in buffering hydrogen ions complicates the interpretation of blood bicarbonate and pH data. While the bicarbonate concentration is frequently used as an indicator of metabolic or nonrespiratory abnoralities, considerations presented above emphasize that it may also be changed by changes in carbon dioxide tension alone. Determining the carbon dioxide combining power, standard bicarbonate level, and buffer base value are all attempts to measure the metabolic component independent of the respiratory abnormality. Filley[55] lucidly reviewed the theory behind these various approaches and showed that differences between base excess and bicarbonate concentrations in a given patient are relatively small and clinically insignificant.

A recent approach has been the construction of a carbon dioxide titration curve in both experimental animals and man. A series of important investigations from Schwartz's[56,57] laboratory showed the effect of graded increases in carbon dioxide tension on bicarbonate concentration and pH. Arterial pH falls rapidly when carbon dioxide is increased, but the fall in pH is much less when animals become chronically adapted to high carbon dioxide tensions (Fig 8–12). The explanation is seen in Figure 8–13, which shows differing bicarbonate responses in acute and chronic hypercapnia. These differences are what might be expected from the concepts presented in previous pages, but Figure 8–12 and 8–13 provide quantitative predictions of these relationships.

These titration curves were recently performed in anesthetized man by the same group of investigators. Bicarbonate concentrations and pH values were obtained over a range of carbon dioxide tensions from 15 to 78 mm Hg. Mean values and confidence limits could be established from these data. Figure 8–14 is a bicarbonate-carbon dioxide curve constructed from the data of Schwartz and bicarbonate-carbon dioxide curve constructed from the data of Schwartz and associates.[56,57] Bicarbonate and carbon dioxide tension are preferred as the coordinates for a study of hydrogen ion relationships because they represent the numerator (bicarbonate) and denominator (car-

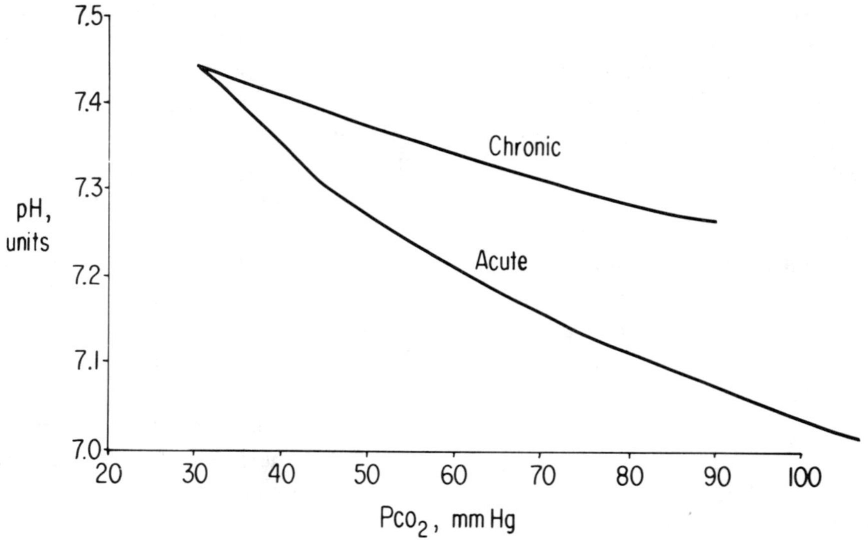

FIG 8–12.
Response of pH to acute and chronic elevation of carbon dioxide tension. (Adapted from Brackett NC Jr, Cohen JJ, Schwartz WB: Carbon dioxide titration curve of normal man. *N Engl J Med* 1965; 272:6.)

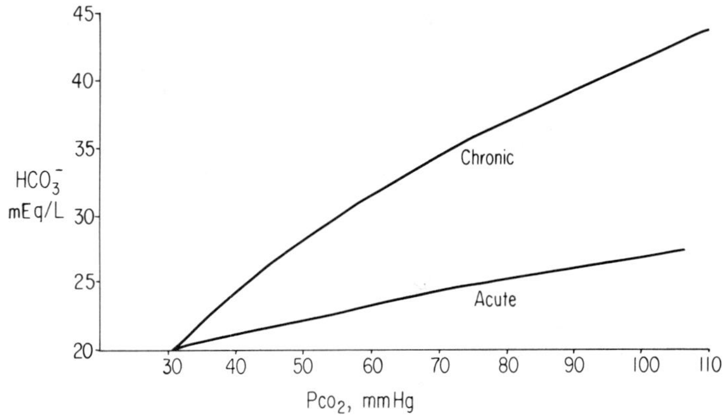

FIG 8–13.
The difference in the acute and chronic pH responses to hypercapnia is due to differing rates of bicarbonate generation.

bon dioxide tension) of the Henderson-Hasselbalch buffer pair. Since all points with the same ratio have the same pH, lines radiating from the origin represent isopleths of pH, as any point on a line has the same slope. The confidence limits for hypocapnia and hypercapnia are shown by the hatched area. Bicarbonate-carbon dioxide tension points lying below the area represent a decreased bicarbonate, while those above the area represent an increased bicarbonate for a particular carbon dioxide tension.

Also included is an upper limb indicating confidence limits for patients with chronic hypercapnia. While these points are extrapolated from animal studies, recently performed studies in humans suggest that they are valid. It is suggested that the bicarbonate-Pco_2 diagram be used for evaluating complicated (and simple) problems in acid-base regulation. Points may be plotted and the patient's progress followed as a series of points connected by appropriate arrows.

DISTURBANCES OF CALCIUM AND MAGNESIUM HOMEOSTASIS

Hypocalcemia

Serum calcium may be bound to albumin (40%), complexed with the bicarbonate, phosphate, and citrate (10%) and ionized (50%). The ionized fraction is physiologically active and not closely correlated to measurements of total calcium. Total hypocalcemia is extremely common in critically ill patients, in part because of alterations in plasma proteins, but abnormally low concentrations of ionized calcium are unusual. As a general rule, total serum calcium changes 0.8 mg/dl for every 1 gm/dl change in serum albumin. Alkalosis increases calcium binding to protein and decreases ionized calcium so that hyperventilation may produce clinical evidence of hypocalcemia.

Hypocalcemia may be suspected by the presence of weakness, fatigue, muscular irritability, Chvostek and Trousseau's signs, apnea, and laryngeal spasm. Cardiac arrhythmias, ventrical dysfunction, insensitivity to beta-adrenergic agonists, and prolongation of QT and ST segments may be found.

Depression of parathyroid function is the most common cause of hypocalcemia. Severe hypomagnesemia suppresses parathyroid function and leads to hypocalcemia. Hyperphosphatemia leads to calcium precipitation and decreased renal vitamin D synthesis, producing hypocalcemia. Hypocalcemia in the critical care setting is best treated by the I.V. administration of 10 ml of 10% calcium gluconate over ten

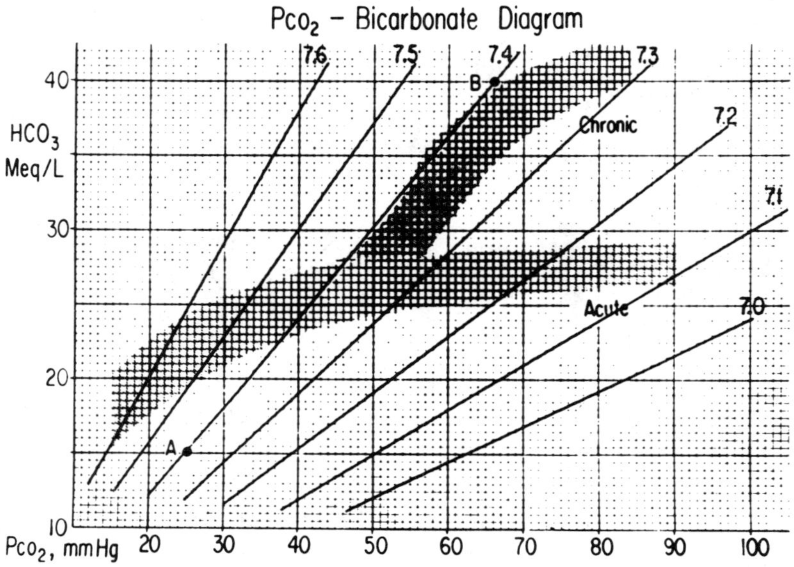

FIG 8–14.
Bicarbonate-carbon dioxide diagram. Bicarbonate and carbon dioxide tension are chosen as the ordinate and abscissa because they are the primary determinants of hydrogen ion concentration. Since pH is related to the logarithm of the bicarbonate–P_{CO_2} slope, linear isopleths radiate out from the origin of the graph. The line marked 7.4, for example, includes all of the possible bicarbonate-P_{CO_2} values with a slope of about 20. The hatched areas show the physiologic regions for acute and chronic change in carbon dioxide tension. Any point falling within either hatched area reveals an appropriate bicarbonate response for a particular carbon dioxide tension. (Data from Brackett NC Jr, Cohen JJ, Schwartz WB: Carbon dioxide titration curve in normal man. *N Engl J Med* 1965; 272:6. and Arbus GS, Herbert LA, Levesque PR, Etsten BE, Schwartz WB: Characterization and clinical application of the "significance band" for acute respiratory alkalosis. *N Engl J Med* 1969; 280:117.)

minutes. This approach has been called the rule of 10s by Chernow and Zaloga.[58]

Hypomagnesemia

Parathormone also regulates the renal reabsorption of magnesium, and important intracellular cation necessary for many enzymatic processes. Hypomagnesemia is relatively common in critically ill patients because of dietary deficiencies, increased losses from the gastrointesintal tract, and failure of renal reabsorption. Diuretics, aminoglycosides, digoxin, cis-platinum, and ethyl alcohol inhibit renal reabsorption of magnesium and lead to hypomagnesemia. This normal serum magnesium is between 1.7 and 2.4 mg/dl, and clinical manifestations are found when the level falls below 1.5 mg/dl. Neuromuscular irritability is similar to that found with hypocalcemia; convulsions may occur with severe hypomagnesemia. Cardiac arrhythmias, flattened T waves, prolonged QT and PR intervals and ST depression are also observed. Decreased intracellular magnesium inhibits the sodium-potassium ATPase, which produces electrophysiologic abnormalities similar to those seen with hypokalemia.

Hypomagnesemia is treated with 10% and 50% solutions of magnesium sulfate. 600 mg may be given initially, followed by an additional 900 mg over the next 24 hours.

Hypercalcemia

Hypercalcemia is found with malignant disease, hyperparathyroidism, and immobilization. Hypercalcemia is particular common in cancers of the breast, lung, kidney, head and neck, and hematopoetic system. Tumor secretion of parathormone and direct involvement of bone are both responsible for hypercalcemia with these tumors, although the aberrent production of PTH seems the more common. Hypercalcemia produces malaise, thirst, weight loss, dehydration, and weakness.

The initial treatment of hypercalcemia is sodium diuresis. Two to three liters of normal saline are infused over the first 3–6 hours; furosemide 10–40 mg I.V. every two hours is added to increase the calcium diuresis. Calcitonin inhibits osteoclastic bone resorption, and Mithramycin inhibits osteoclastic activity and vitamin D metabolism. It is indicated in most patients with hypercalcemia associated with malignant disease.

Hypermagnesemia

Hypermagnesemia is rare and usually due to the use of magnesium-containing medications. It is treated by eliminating the offending medications and may be transiently antagonized by the administration of intravenous calcium.

REFERENCES

1. McGiff JC, Wong P Y-K: Compartmentalization of prostaglandins and prostacyclin within the kidney: Implications of renal failure. *Fed Proc* 1979; 38:89–93.

2. Ballermann BJ, Brenner BM: Biologically active atrial peptides. *J Clin Invest* 1985; 76:2041–2048.

3. Gregersen MI, Rawson RA: Blood volume. *Physiol Rev* 1959; 39:307.

4. Sjostrand T: Volume and distribution of blood and their significance in regulating the circulation. *Physiol Rev* 1953; 33:202.

5. Korge P, Viru A: Water and electrolyte metabolism in skeletal muscle. *J Appl Physiol* 1971; 31:1.

6. Korge P, Viru A: Water and electrolyte metabolism in myocardium of exercising rats. *J Appl Physiol* 1971; 31:5.

7. Glynn IM: Sodium and potassium movements in human red cells. *J Physiol* 1956; 134:278.

8. Pitts RF: *Physiology of the Kidney and Body Fluids*, ed 2, Chicago, Year Book Medical, 1968, p 31.

9. Pitts RF: *Physiology of the Kidney and Body Fluids*, ed 2, Chicago, Year Book Medical, 1968, p 102.

10. Ullrich KJ, Kramer K, Boylan JW: Present knowledge of the counter-current system in the mammalian kidney. *Prog Cardiovasc Dis* 1961; 3:395.

11. Wang BC, Share L, Goetz KL: Factors influencing the secretion of vasopressin into cerebrospinal fluid. *Fed Proc* 1985; 44:72–77.

12. Menninger RP: Current concepts of volume receptor regulation of vasopressin release. *Fed Proc* 1985; 44:55–58.

13. Huang CL, Lewicki J, Johnson LK, et al: Renal mechanism of action of rat atrial natriuretic factor. *J Clin Invest* 1985; 75:769–773.

14. Knaus WA, Draper EA, Wagner DP, et al: Prognosis in acute organ-system failure. *Ann Surg* 1985; 202:685.

15. Oken DE: Nosologic considerations in the nomenclature of acute renal failure. *Nephron* 1971; 8:505–510.

16. Clermont FJ, Vlahcenic ZR, Chalmers TC, et al: Intravenous therapy of massive ascites in patients with cirrhosis: II. Long-term effects on survival and frequency of renal failure. *Gastroenterology* 1967; 53:220–228.

17. Fischer RP: High mortality of post-traumatic renal insufficiency in Vietnam: A review of 96 cases. *The American Surgeon*, 1974.

18. Miller TR, Anderson RJ, Linas SL, et al: Urinary diagnostic indices in acute renal failure. *Ann Intern Med* 1978; 89:47–50.

19. Oken DE: Hemodynamic basis for human

acute renal failure. *Am J Med* 1984; 76:702–710.

20. Bennett WM, Muther RS, Parker RA, et al: Drug therapy in renal failure: dosing guidelines for adults. *Ann Intern Med* 1980; 93:62–89.

21. Schentag JJ, Cumbo TJ, Jusko WJ, et al: Gentamicin tissue accumulation and nephrotoxic reactions. *JAMA* 1978; 240:2067–2069.

22. Rubin E, Kantz AM, Lieber CS, et al: Muscle damage produced by chronic alcohol consumption. *Am J Pathol* 1976; 83:499–515.

23. Tourane JL, Touraire F, Revillard JP, et al: T-lymphocytes and serum inhibitors of cell-mediated immunity in renal insufficiency. *Nephron* 1975; 14:195.

24. Linton AL, Clark WF, Driedger AA, et al: Acute interstitial nephritis due to drugs. *Ann Intern Med* 1980; 93:735–741.

25. Conger J: A controlled evaluation of prophylactic dialysis in post-traumatic acute renal failure. *J Trauma* 1975; 15:1056–1063.

26. Quellhorst E, Doht B, Schuenermann B: Hemofiltration: Treatment of renal failure by hemofiltration and substitution. *J Dial* 1977; 1:529.

27. Anderson RJ, Chung H-M, Kluge R, et al: Hyponatremia: A prospective analysis of its epidemiology and the pathogenetic role of vasopressin. *Ann Intern Med* 1985; 102:164–168.

28. Fichman MP, Vorkerr H, Kleeman CR, et al: Diuretic-induced hyponatremia. *Ann Intern Med* 1971; 75:853.

29. Bartter FC, Schwartz WB: The syndrome of inappropriate secretion of antidiuretic hormone. *Am J Med* 1967; 42:790.

30. Landis E, Pappenheimer JR: Exchange of substances through the capillary walls, in Hamilton WF, Dow P (eds), *Handbook of Physiology*, Sec 2, Circulation, vol II. Washington DC, American Physiological Society, 1963.

31. Arieff AI: Hyponatremia, convulsions, respiratory arrest, and permanent brain damage after elective surgery in healthy women. *N Engl J Med* 1986; 314:1529–1535.

32. Narins RG: Therapy of hyponatremia: Does haste make waste? Editorial. *N Engl J Med* 1986; 314:1573–1575.

33. Balestrieri FJ, Chernow B, Rainey TG: Post-craniotomy diabetes insipidus: Who's at risk? *Crit Care Med* 1982; 10:108.

34. Gerich JE, Martin MM, Recant L: Clinical and metabolic characteristics of hyperosmolar nonketotic coma. *Diabetes* 1971; 20:4.

35. Beigelman PM: Potassium in severe diabetic ketoacidosis. *Am J Med* 1973; 54:419–420.

36. Demling RH, Monohan M, Belzer FO: Effect of plasma oncotic pressure on the pulmonary microcirculation after hemorrhagic shock. *Surgery* 1979; 86:323–332.

37. Monafo W, Ayvazian V: Hypertonic sodium solutions in the treatment of burn shock. *Am J Surg* 1973; 126:778–783.

38. Hauser CJ, Shoemaker C, Turpin I, et al: Hemodynamic and oxygen transport responses to body water shifts produced by colloids and crystalloids in critically ill patients. *Surg Gynecol Obstet* 1980; 150:811.

39. Lazrove S, Waxman K, Shippy C: Hemodynamic blood volume and oxygen transport responses to albumin and hydroxyethyl starch infusions in critically ill postoperative patients. *Crit Care Med* 1980; 8:302–306.

40. Soler NG, Bennett MA, Dixon K, et al: Potassium balance during treatment of diabetic ketoacidosis with special reference to the use of bicarbonate. *Lancet* 1972; 30:665.

41. Posner JB, Plum F: Spinal-fluid pH and neurologic symptoms in systemic acidosis. *N Engl J Med* 1967; 277:605.

42. Russell CD, Illickal MM, Maloney JV, et al: Acute response to acid-base stress in the dog. *Am J Physiol* 1972; 223:3:689–694.

43. Goldberger E: *A Primer of Water, Electrolyte and Acid-base Syndromes*, ed 4, Philadelphia, Lea & Febiger, 1970.

44. Dikshit K, Vyden JK, Forrester JS, et al: Renal and extrarenal hemodynamic effects of furosemide in congestive heart failure after acute myocardial infarction. *N Engl J Med* 1973; 288:1087.

45. Laragh JH: The mode of action and

use of chlorothiazide and related compounds. *Circulation* 1962; 26:121.

46. Crosley AP Jr, Ronquillo LM, Strickland WH, et al: Tramterene, a new natriuretic agent—Preliminary observations in man. *Ann Intern Med* 1962; 56:251.

47. Cannon PJ, Heinemann HO, Stason WB, Laragh JH: Ethacrynic acid: Effectiveness and mode of diuretic action in man. *Circulation* 1965; 31:5.

48. Meldrum NU, Roughton FJW: Carbonic anhydrase, its preparation and properties. *J Physiol* 1933; 80:113.

49. Swan RC, Pitts RF: Neutralization of infused acid by nephrectomized dogs. *J Clin Invest* 1955; 34:205.

50. Kassirer JP, Schwartz WB: Correction of metabolic alkalosis in man without repair of potassium deficiency: A reevaluation of the role of potassium. *Am J Med* 1966; 40:19.

51. Berliner RW, Kennedy TJ Jr, Orloff J: Factors affecting transport of potassium and hydrogen ions by renal tubules. *Arch Int Pharmacodyn Ther* 1954; 97:299.

52. Rector FC Jr, Bloomer HA, Seldin DW: Effects of potassium deficiency on the reabsorption of bicarbonate in the proximal tubule of the rat. *J Clin Invest* 1964; 43:1976.

53. Tuller MA, Mehdi F: Compensatory hypoventilation and hypercapnia in primary metabolic alkalosis. *Am J Med* 1971; 50:281.

54. Giebisch G, Berger L, Pitts RF: The extrarenal response to acute acid-base disturbances of respiratory origin. *J Clin Invest* 1955; 34:231.

55. Filley G: *Acid-Base and Blood Gas Regulation*. Philadelphia, Lea & Febiger, 1971.

56. Brackett NC Jr, Cohen JJ, Schwartz WB: Carbon dioxide titration curve of normal man. *N Engl J Med* 1965; 272:6.

57. Arbus GS, Herbert LA, Levesque PR, Etsten BE, Schwartz WB: Characterization and clinical application of the "significance band" for acute respiratory alkalosis. *N Engl J Med* 1969; 280:117.

9 THE CENTRAL NERVOUS SYSTEM IN THE CRITICALLY ILL

The brain and the heart share a group of common attributes. Each is exquisitely sensitive to oxygen deprivation and can adjust its own blood flow to metabolic need (autoregulation). Each holds a privileged position in the oxygen economy of the body as blood flow is shunted from less critical organs to heart and brain during periods of oxygen or perfusion deficits. The blood flow and metabolism of each organ may be measured by sampling its venous effluent, and the arterial circulation of each organ is commonly imperiled by atheromatous obstruction. The adult brain comprises 2% of total body weight but consumes 20% of total body oxygen and 25% of total body glucose uptake (the heart requires even more oxygen;[1] it consumes 12% of total body oxygen requirement, even though it weighs but 0.4% of total body weight).

The high levels of brain oxygen consumption are necessary to maintain electrical potentials across neuronal membranes. The neuron is the functional unit of the nervous system and consists of a cell body (perikaryon), afferent processes termed dendrites, and a single efferent axon extending from the cell body to other neurons or to effector organs. Three types of non-neuronal or glial cells are found in the central nervous system. *Oliogodendrocytes* form the myelin sheaths of white matter while *microglia* are phagocytic cells. *Astrocytes* appear to regulate the extracellular concentration of potassium and neurotransmitters by storing and releasing these substances. Multiple reciprocal connections between neurons are made possible by the afferent and efferent neuronal processes. Neurons within the cerebral cortex are arranged in columnar packages, which extend through the cortex and communicate with adjacent columns forming neuronal units or modules. These units receive afferent impulses from other cortical and subcortical structures.[2] In the normal brain, cortical functions appear to be regionalized so that damage to one region may affect specific cognitive functions. Increasing loss of neural tissue, however, appears to have a general effect on decreasing mental function.

STRUCTURAL ARRANGEMENTS WITHIN THE BRAIN

The gray matter of the cerebral hemispheres is a convoluted surface containing layers of cells. The *neocortex* occupies 90% of the cerebral hemispheric surface and has six layers of neurons. The paleocortex (olfactory cortex) and archicortex (hippocampus and dentate gyrus) contain three cellular layers, while the cingulate gyrus and part of the parahippocampal gyrus contain from three to six layers.

Pyramidal neurons are the major efferent cells of the cortex and project to the brainstem and spinal cord. Stellate cells serve as connecting links among other cortical neurons, and fusiform cells project mainly to the thalamus. The olfactory (I) and optic (II) nerves connect to the cerebral cortex; the olfactory fibers of the retinal cross (decussate) in the optic chiasm and reach the optic cortex as the optic tracts.

The *thalamus* lies deep in the brain just beyond the midbrain. It receives sensory afferents from peripheral sensory nerves and, after synaptic interruption, projects to the cerebral cortex. The *hypothalamus* lies ventral to the thalamus and is responsible for integrating the homeostatic responses of the entire body. Hypothalamic neurons initiate the secretion of a group of hormones, provide central direction to the autonomic nervous system, and serve as the seat of emotions.

The midbrain is a short segment containing the cerebral aqueduct, which connects the third and fourth ventricles. The pons is a much larger segment, lying caudal to the midbrain. Together, the midbrain and pons give rise to the oculomotor (III), trochlear (IV), trigeminal (V), abducens (VI), and facial (VII) nerves.

The medulla is continuous with the spinal cord. The caudal part of the medulla contains the reticular formation and extends through the medulla, pons and midbrain. The auditory (VIII), glossopharyngeal nerve (IX), vagus nerve (X), spinal accessory nerve (XI), and hypoglossal nerve (XII) arise from the medulla. Nuclei in this system are responsible for the control of blood pressure and respiration. Part of the formation serves as a reticular activating system which regulates the level of brain activity and determines sleep and wakefulness.

There are three covering membranes or meninges. The pia mater is attached to brain tissue. The arachnoid covering lies outside of the pia mater, and the subarachnoid space lies between the two. The dura mater is a tough layer that lines the cranial cavity and vertebral canal. The ventricles are spaces within the brain. They are filled with cerebrospinal fluid which is formed by special capillary tissues called the choroid plexus and the brain itself. About 100–150 ml of cerebrospinal fluid fill the four ventricles and surround the brain and spinal cord. Constant secretion and reabsorption result in replacement of the total volume several times each day. Intraventricular pressure is maintained by a series of outflow resistances which impede flow of cerebrospinal fluid into the subarachnoid spaces. The cerebral aqueduct between the third and fourth ventricles constitutes the smallest canal; fluid leaves the fourth ventricle by three small openings, the two foramina of Luschka and the foramen of Magendie.

NEUROTRANSMITTER CONTROL OF SYNAPTIC TRANSMISSION

Nerve impulse conduction occurs when an action potential leads to a flow of current along neural tissue. During the resting state, the inside of the cell is strongly negative with respect to the extracellular fluids because of an energy-requiring pumping mechanism that maintains a high intracellular potassium concentration. In a manner analagous to nerve conduction in cardiac tissues, an action potential is generated when sodium rushes into the neuron and reverses polarity for a short period of time. Electrical currents can form synaptic connection in areas of low resistance, but many mammalian synapses are mediated by chemical transmitters.

The discovery of high concentrations of norepinephrine in the dog hypothalamus by Vogt in 1954[3] signalled a new era in the understanding of brain function; the brain was no longer to be considered a black box but could be viewed as a central endocrine organ that modified the function of all body tissues. Dopamine had been thought to be important only as a precursor of norepinephrine, for example, until Carlsson's discovery[4] that large amounts could be found in the brain. Histochemical fluorescence staining methods have permitted the localization of neurotransmitters. High concentrations are found in the hypothalamus and maps of the distribution of noradrenergic, dopaminergic, and serotonergic fibers[5] have been prepared, and the extent of their connections carefully analyzed. In the years following these seminal discoveries, more than 20 neurotransmitter molecules have been identified. Most fall into four groupings: acetylcholine, monoamines, peptides, and amino acids. Their importance for critical care medicine seems obvious; pharmacologic agents which modify neurotransmitter action may modify many organ responses.

A neurotransmitter may be defined as a substance that is (1) synthesized in a presynaptic neuron, (2) bound to a postsynaptic receptor (3) alters membrane potential of the postsynaptic neuron, and (4) is removed from the synaptic site by dilution or chemical destruction. Multiple receptors for single transmitters are common (alpha- and beta-adrenergic, for example) and can be identified by radioactive ligand binding.

Norepinephrine and *epinephrine* selectively inhibit a variety of cortical and subcortical functions. *Serotonin* appears to play a role in sleep, pain transmission, and behavioral patterns. *Dopamine* binds to a number of pre- and postsynaptic receptors; the role of these receptors in vascular regulation and the effects of blocking agents are discussed in chapter 4. Dopamine-containing neurons inhibit the release of prolactin and melanocyte-stimulating hormone from the pituitary. Multiple CNS dopamine receptors (DA) exist and explain the activity of a variety of pharmacologic agents.[6] One receptor type is coupled to adenyate cyclase and is competitively antagonized by the phenothiazines. Halolperidol (Haldol), a butyrophenone, blocks another receptor type that apparently is not linked to adenylate cyclase. The importance of dopaminergic neurons in motor control demonstrates the possibilities of neurotransmitter manipulation. Degeneration of the dopamine-synthesizing neurons of the substantia nigra leads to Parkinson's Disease. A similar syndrome can be produced in animals by chemically ablating DA cells with 6-hydroxydopamine with subsequent increase in the number of DA receptors and increased responsiveness to DA agonists. Up-regulation of receptors following denervation, as has been noted previously, represents an adaptive response. A similar supersensitivity of DA receptors appears to be responsible for the tardive dyskinesia that is associated with antipsychotic medication.[7] Lithium appears to stabilize DA receptors and may be useful in the treatment of tardive dyskinesias as well as other affective disorders. The increase in DA receptors found in schizophrenic brains is a tantalizing reminder of the pervasive importance of this neurotransmitter.[8]

Peptide neurotransmitters mediate many body functions. The general stress response discussed widely in this text appears mediated by corticotrophin releasing factor (CRF), which leads to the simultaneous release of ACTH and beta endorphins. Recent information indicates that the endorphins are important humoral mediators between the brain and the immune system; lymphocytes have surface receptors for endorphins, and receptor occupancy influences antibody production, lymphocyte proliferation, and natural killer cytotoxicity.[9]

Many peptide neurotransmitters are found in the gastrointestinal tract as well as in the brain. *Substance P* is found in dorsal root ganglia and is probably a neurotransmitter for certain somatic afferent nerves.[10] Peptide neurotransmitters frequently have multiple functions. Thyroid releasing hormone (TRH), for example, suppresses appetite and stimulates gastric function as well as leading to the release of thyroid stimulating hormone (TSH). Cholecystokinin (CCK) influences gastrointestinal function and stimulates a central receptor that is dependent on an intact vagus and appears to regulate satiety.[11]

Acetylcholine is the neurotransmitter of the peripheral nervous system and plays a major role in autonomic neural transmission (see chapter 4). Cholinergic neurons within the central nervous system are limited to areas where they give rise to linkages that communicate with cortical and subcortical areas of the brain. Alterations in acetylcholine terminals in the cerebral cortex may play an important role in the development of Alzheimer's disease.

A group of amino acid transmitters produced by enzymatic steps related to carbohydrate metabolism have profound effects on neural activity. Gamma-aminobutyric acid (GABA) has an inhibitory effect on transmission, while glutamate and aspartate have excitatory effects. GABA appears to interfere with the balance of dopamine and acetylcholine in the striatum and produce choreiform movement. Loss of GABA-producing neurons has been observed in Huntington's Chorea.

CEREBRAL METABOLISM AND BLOOD FLOW

The Regulation of Cerebral Blood Flow

Cerebral blood flow (CBF) is governed by the factors expressed in the Pouiseille relationship (chapter 4). Like pulmonary blood flow, cerebral blood flow is sensitive to the extramural pressure surrounding its conduits. The brain, however, is encased in bone so that its total intracranial volume is fixed at 1,800 to 2,000 ml in the adult. The rigid cranium provides the brain with important protection against external injury, but also imposes constraining pressure-volume relationships so that effective compliance drops dramatically as cranial volume increases (see Figure 9–1). The intracranial contents may be conveniently divided into neural, vascular, and cerebrospinal fluid compartments. An increase in the volume of either compartment must lead to an increase in ICP unless one of the compartments shrinks; one response to increased brain volume is a shift of cerebrospinal fluid through the foramen magnum and into the spinal subarachnoid space. Cerebral venous pressure is close

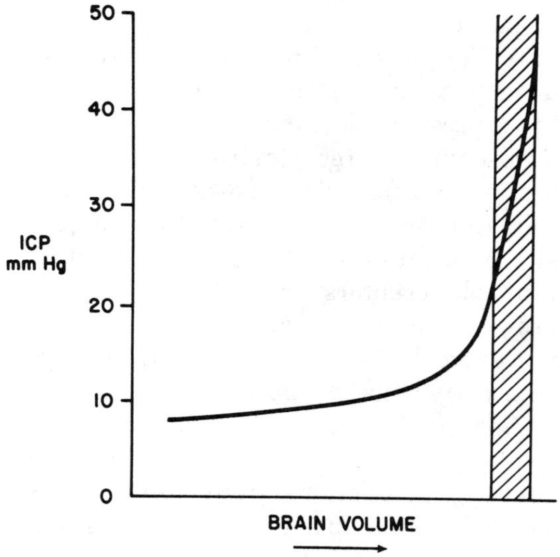

FIG 9–1.
The rigid cranium produces a rapid rise in intracranial pressure (ICP) as the brain swells following illness or injury. Treatment directed towards lowering ICP should be instituted when pressure rises to 20–25 mm Hg because that pressure zone is on the steep segment of the intra-cranial pressure-volume curve (hatched area). Note that a modest reduction in brain volume can dramatically reduce ICP.

to ICP, so the mean perfusion pressure of the brain is generally calculated as the difference between mean arterial pressure (MAP) and ICP. This gradient is termed the cerebral perfusion pressure (CPP) and can be calculated whenever ICP measurements are available. The following equation describes that relationship and becomes important in critically ill patients with elevations of ICP.

$$CBF = \frac{MAP - ICP}{CVR}$$

where CVR = cerebral vascular resistance.

Cortical blood flow is several times greater than flow through white matter because of increased neuronal activity,[12] emphasizing the importance of metabolic activity in its regulation. The major end product of oxygen consumption, carbon dioxide, is a potent vasodilator, acting through a change in hydrogen ion concentration in the extracellular fluid.[13] Increased mental activity results in increased oxygen consumption, carbon dioxide production, and regional blood flow. Figure 4–16 shows that cerebral blood flow decreases as carbon dioxide tension is decreased. Controlled hyperventilation is used to decrease ICP, but levels below 20–25 mm Hg are usually avoided.[14]

Cerebral blood flow is also sensitive to changes in oxygen tension. It increases dramatically when arterial P_{O_2} approaches 50 mm Hg. At lower levels, flow may increase to levels that are three to five times greater than normal.[15] Hypoxic hyperventilation produces hypocapnia, so that the response of cerebral blood flow to reduced oxygen tensions may be partially blunted by hypocapnic vasoconstriction. This latter phenomena was first observed in hyperventilating pilots flying at high altitudes; addition of carbon dioxide markedly improved their mental acuity.

Important autoregulatory responses maintain cerebral blood flow in spite of wide swings in arterial perfusion pressure. Vasodilatation occurs whether CPP falls as a result of a fall in mean arterial pressure or a rise in intracranial pressure. Conversely, vasoconstriction protects the brain from increased blood flow up to a CPP of about 160 mm Hg. Both the lower and upper thresholds for autoregulation are shifted upwards in chronic hypertension or with increased sympathetic activity. These threshold shifts become particular important when individuals with chronic hypertension become critically ill. (see chapter 5).

Kontos et al.[16] examined the control of cerebral blood flow with a technique that permitted direct observation of blood vessels in the pia mater. They observed that reduction in oxygen tension at sites remote from the vessel wall led to vasodilation even though oxygen tension in at the vessel wall was maintained at normal tensions by exposure to oxygenated cerebrospinal fluid. Subsequent studies showed that enzymatic destruction of adenosine ablated the vasodilator response. Hypoxic vasodilatation is thus mediated by the release of adenosine, which then binds to adenosine receptors on the vascular wall. Similar studies by the same group[17] showed that the autoregulatory vasodilation observed with hypotension was also due to adenosine release mediated through regional hypoxia, although intrinsic myogenic responses could also be identified.

The Response of the Brain to Hypoxia

Experimental increases in altitude or decreases in oxygen concentration produce reproducible physiologic responses to hypoxia. Dark adaptation and visual acuity decrease with alveolar oxygen tensions close to 65 mm Hg. Memory and the ability to perform complicated tasks become abnormal with oxygen tensions close to 50 mm Hg. Unconsciousness develops when oxygen tension is reduced to 20–30 mm Hg. These findings were obtained in healthy young individuals, usually pilots, with presumably normal cerebral vascular beds. More serious functional changes at higher levels of oxygenation could be expected with individuals with impaired cerebral circulations.

Studies in the normal rat demonstrate that brain lactate content and lactate/pyruvate ratios rise as the arterial oxygen tension falls below 50 mm Hg. At about 35 mm Hg, phosphocreatine concentration is reduced, but ATP, ADP, and AMP remain normal until oxygen tension levels of 20 mm Hg are reached.[18] If hypotension is combined with hypoxia, however, high energy phosphates are depleted at higher oxygen tensions.

The importance of perfusion pressure to brain integrity during hypoxia can be shown by experiments occluding one carotid artery prior to inducing hypoxia.[19] In this model, one half of the brain is hypoxic, the other is hypoperfused with hypoxemic blood. High energy phosphates are markedly reduced in the ischemic and hypoxemic hemisphere but relatively normal in the normally perfused hypoxic hemisphere. Lactate concentrations are extremely high and are closely correlated to decreases in high energy phosphates. The extremely high lactate concentrations obtained from poorly perfused and hypoxic brain tissue are almost ten times higher than those seen with complete ischemia, suggesting that continued availability of glucose and glycogen was necessary to produce severe lactic acidosis. Partial ischemia in fasted animals does not produce the degree of lactic acidosis found in well-nourished animals because of glycogen and glucose depletion.

A graded relationship between brain function and oxygen deficits exists. At moderately reduced oxygen tensions, hypoxia appears to interfere with neurotransmitter synthesis and blocks or disorganizes synaptic connections. With increasing cellular hypoxia, reduced energy availability produced membrane depolarization with accumulation of potassium in extracellular fluid. Two separate mechanisms may then lead to irreversible cell damage. Siesjo and Wieloch[20] have suggested that a pathologic calcium "cascade" is produced as membrane alterations lead to increased cytosolic calcium concentrations. Calcium triggers enzymatic breakdown of cell membrane lipids and promotes increased amounts of neurotransmitters. Intracellular swelling occurs as sodium, chloride, and water enter cells which have lost their normal volume-regulating ability. In addition to the calcium cascade, free radicals are produced and destroy lipid and protein structures (see chapters 1, 2).

CEREBRAL EDEMA AND THE BLOOD-BRAIN BARRIER

Intercellular channels or gap junctions permit communication between cells and appear to play a significant role in determining capillary permeability. These 10 angstrom diameter channels are controlled by intracellular Ca^{++}. Toxic inhibition of the sodium-calcium pump, or decreased ATP generation, leads to increased intracellular calcium closing the communicating channels.[21] In contrast to most capillary beds, tight junctions exist between cerebral capillary cells, and their exchange channels are much less active, creating a blood-brain barrier that restricts the entry of proteins, ions, water soluble nonelectrolytes, and water into brain tissue. Cerebral edema is considered "vasogenic" if the blood-brain barrier is violated and "cytotoxic" if the barrier remains intact. The two forms of edema are not mutually exclusive. Brain injury produces vasogenic edema as the blood-brain barrier is broken; secondary ischemia may then lead to cytotoxic edema.

The increased volume of the edematous brain leads to an elevation of intracranial pressure, and more than 75% of patients with post-traumatic coma have an elevated ICP.[22] There is increasing evidence that cerebral edema may be due to altered cell regulatory function, and that control of edema may reduce the mortality of severe head trauma.[23]

Most animal cells have homeostatic mechanisms that return disordered cell volume to normal; the swollen cell shrinks and the shrunken cell expands. Isolated cells increase their volume when exposed to hypotonic solutions but reduce their volume to almost normal levels within 5–10 minutes. A calcium-activated calmodulin mechanism opens potassium and chloride channels, which reduce volume by ejecting those ions and water. Altered neurotransmitter release in early trauma may interfere with volume correcting responses and lead to sustained cell swelling. Edema formation in patients with abnormal cerebral capillary permeability is sensitive to changes in hydrostatic pressures. Transient hypertension due to increased sympathetic neural activity or loss of local autoregulation may lead to increased cerebral edema. Failure of volume homeostasis sets the stage for prolonged edema.

Cerebral edema does not directly impair neuronal function but leads to increased ICP, which compresses the capillary bed and decreases cerebral perfusion pressure leading to global ischemia. Edema is further increased by a syndrome of vasoparalysis, described by Langfitt.[24] Normal autoregulation cannot occur because of vasoparalysis, and even mild hypertension leads to substantial increases in cerebral blood flow and volume.

Global ischemia is found with cardiac arrest, shock, sepsis, and after blunt trauma to the head. A syndrome characterized by coma can be produced by a variety of etiologic processes and careful differential diagnosis is necessary (see Table 9–1).

CEREBRAL ISCHEMIC SYNDROMES

Abnormalities in the determinants of oxygen delivery discussed in Chapter 1 lead to cerebral hypoxia or ischemia. It is important to remember that cellular oxygen deficits may be recognized by decreases in venous oxygen saturation and are termed either hypoxia or anoxia. Anoxic anoxia is the result of decreased arterial oxyhemoglobin saturation, anemic anoxia the result of decreased oxygen carrying capacity, and ischemic anoxia the result of reductions in blood flow insufficient to meet metabolic needs. Rarely is direct tissue damage or histotoxic anoxia present (the best example is cyanide poisoning). Almost always, decreased oxygen delivery is due to cardiopulmonary problems related to a variety of etiologic situations. Cardiac arrest in an individual with subclinical cerebral vascular disease, for example, can produce global hypoxia. Cardiac ejection with extremely low stroke outputs of incompletely saturated arterial blood produces diffuse ischemia as blood pressure falls below the thresholds for autoregulation. Atheromatous segments of cerebral vessels fail to autoregulate under any circumstance and are particularly sensitive to decreases in arterial pressure. *Hypotension is the major cause of focal or diffuse ischemia in the critically ill patient; it is also the most readily preventable cause.*

TABLE 9–1.
Causes of Coma

(1)	DEFICIENCY OF OXYGEN, SUBSTRATE OR COFACTORS
	Hypoxia
	Ischemia
	Hypoglycemia
	Deficiency of Thiamin, niacin, pyridoxine, cyanocobalmin, folic acid
(2)	DISEASES OF OTHER ORGANS
	Liver, kidney, lung, pancreas
	Pituitary, thyroid, parathyroid, adrenal or pancreas
	Cancer, porphyria, sepsis
(3)	SUBSTANCE INGESTION
(4)	ELECTOLYTE ABNORMALITIES
	Hypo and hypernatremia
	Acidosis
	Alkalosis
	Hypo and hypermagnesemia
	Hypo and hypercalcemia
	Hypophosphatemia
(5)	DISORDERED TEMPERATURE REGULATION
(6)	INFECTIONS OF THE CENTRAL NERVOUS SYSTEM
(7)	PRIMARY NEURONAL DISEASES
(8)	ACUTE DELIRIUM STATES

Adapted from Plum F, Posner JB: *The Diagnosis of Stupor and Coma, 3rd ed.* Philadelphia, FA Davis Co, 1982.

Complete cessation of the circulation leads to unconsciousness in 6–8 seconds.[25] Unconsciousness, convulsions, pupillary dilatation, and bilateral extensor plantar responses occur within several seconds. Complete recovery after one to two minutes of anoxia occurs in individuals with normal cerebral vascular beds, but significant disability occurs after much shorter periods of circulatory interruption in individuals with cerebral vascular disease. Total ischemic anoxia for more than four minutes produces cell death, beginning with the cerebral cortex (particularly the hippocampus) and the cerebellum. Severe anoxia lasting more than 10 minutes begins to damage large segments of brain tissue.[26] Siesjo's studies,[27] mentioned earlier, emphasize that careful maintenance of perfusion pressure can prevent hypoxic damage even with extremely low arterial oxygen tensions. The importance of maintaining blood pressure in patients with the adult respiratory distress syndrome is obvious!

Cerebral ischemia may be caused by vascular obstruction, embolism, or hemorhage into the brain or the subarachnoid space. Restriction of blood flow to part of the brain produces focal manifestations usually called strokes, while global ischemia leads to rapid loss of consciousness. Transient ischemic attacks are analagous to angina pectoris; transient ischemia produces regional abnormalities that disappear completely in a short period of time but suggest the presence of severe cerebral vascular disease. Critical illness in a patient with a history of transient ischemic attacks challenges the physician to maintain cerebral blood flow at all costs to prevent structural brain damage. There is a spectrum of cellular damage ranging from reversible ischemia to irreversible infarction.

ALTERATIONS IN CONSCIOUSNESS

This text emphasizes the prevention, consequences, and treatment of individual or multiple organ failure; alterations in mental status suggest brain *dysfunction*, while stupor or coma mean *brain failure*. The parallels to failure of other organs are obvious; the early signs of brain dysfunction may be subtle but should be recognized by all members of the critical care team.

Content and *arousal* are the primary components of consciousness. The ability to maintain arousal lies in the reticular activating system of the brainstem, and disorders involving that region may produce coma. Coma represents complete brain failure, and is defined by Plum and Posner[28] as the "total absence of awareness of self and environment even when the patient is externally stimulated. Between the extreme states of consciousness and coma stand a variety of altered states of consciousness . . . to which have been applied a bewildering number of terms." The authors go on to emphasize that isolated impairments of function such as aphasia or memory loss usually are not considered as altered states of consciousness. The degree of brain failure is related to the amount of brain damage; the nature is frequently related to the chronicity of the insult. Acute or subacute processes produce stupor or coma while more slowly developing processes may manifest as dementia. Brain reserve is extensive so that states of altered consciousness imply either extensive bilateral disease or involvement of the brainstem reticular activating system (the arousal mechanism), or both.

The importance of structural damage to the reticular activating system (RAS) in producing coma was based on morphologic and clinical studies. Hayes et al. recently have challenged this view by demonstrating that coma may occur without obvious damage to the RAS.[29] These investigators demonstrated that concussive injury produced a reversible, flaccid comatose state not associated with observable damage to the RAS. The concussive injury appeared to increase glucose utilization and produce increased cholinergic neural activity in the dorsolateral pontine tegmentum. These effects could be blocked by atropine and simulated by the injection of carbochal, a cholinergic agonist. Studies in the 1940s had shown the appearance of increased quantities of acetylcholine in cerebral spinal fluid and Hayes et al.[29] have suggested that pharmacologic blockade of muscarinic cholinergic systems can reduce neurological deficits in experimental situations. The idea of functional rather than structural alterations as important causes for coma presents exciting therapeutic possibilities.

A group of clinical syndromes describes increasing brain damage. *Obtundation* indicates mild to moderate impairment of consciousness. There is decreased awareness of the external environment, drowsiness, and increased duration of sleep. *Stupor*, on the other hand, indicates a state of unresponsiveness; arousal is possible only with vigorous stimulation, and those in this state are unresponsive as soon as the stimuli are withdrawn. The patient with *coma* is unarousable and demonstrates no response to the external environment. The eyes are closed. Motor abnormalities may or may not be present. Sleeplike coma rarely lasts more than 2–4 weeks. After that period, patients exhibit an unresponsive state that resembles wakefulness even though there is no evidence of cognitive activity or environmental awareness. These comalike states have been called vegetative states, akinetic mutism, coma vigil, or the apallic syndrome.

The confusional states may be associated with altered consciousness. *Delerium* is frequently due to toxic and metabolic causes. Patients are disoriented, afraid, misinterpret environmental stimuli, and may have visual or auditory hallucinations. Delerium is common in the critical care setting where depressed brain function and a frightening environment cause continuous confusion and fear, particularly at night. *Dementia* refers to a chronic abnormality in thinking and usually is not associated with alterations in consciousness.

CARE OF THE BRAIN-DAMAGED PATIENT

Monitoring Brain Function

Close clinical evaluation identifies early evidence of brain dysfunction. More advanced brain damage leads to an elevation of intracranial pressure (ICP). Figure 9–1 shows the familiar rectangular hyperbola which describes so many biologic processes (see chapter 1). The pressure-volume characteristics of the brain are determined by the rigid encasing cranium; increased volume produces little change in pressure until a critical point is reached; at that point, relatively small increases in brain volume lead to rapidly rising pressure, ICP is a useful surrogate for evaluating brain function in the edematous syndromes that follow trauma and ischemic brain damage.

For many years, ICP was measured by lumbar puncture. This technique may cause brain herniation through the foramen magnum if mass lesions are present, and is not able to accurately mirror ICP when obstructions exist between the spinal and brain subarachnoid spaces. Normal ICP averages 10 mm Hg, and pressures between 20 and 25 mm Hg indicate a brain volume on the steep portion of the pressure-volume curve.[30]

Two techniques are commonly used to measure ICP. An intraventricular catheter may be inserted at the mid-pupillary line of the coronal suture. These catheters reliably measure ICP but penetrate the brain and may lead to infection. The Richmond group[31] developed a subarachnoid screw which obviates brain penetration. Both the dura and arachnoid membranes are opened and the device inserted in the subarachnoid space. Infection rates of 2–3% have been reported, and cerebrospinal fluid cannot be removed through the screw. Newer implantable devices are presently under evaluation.

Imposed on the pressure forms related to cardiac events, intracerebral pressure tracings show several slower wave-forms. Type A waves begin abruptly, rise to 50–100 mm Hg and then fall rapidly after five to 20 minutes. These occur in seriously ill patients, may be related to loss of autoregulation with increased blood flow, and suggest increasing deterioration. B waves are short-duration increases of up to 20–50 mm Hg. These may be due to changes in breathing patterns. Type C waves are due to changes in blood pressure.

Protecting the Brain from Progressive Damage

The parallels between the brain and the heart discussed at the beginning of this chapter extend to the issues of treatment. With both situations, there is good evidence that a zone of potentially viable but critically ischemic tissues exists adjacent to a central nonviable core. These potentially salvageable regions in the heart were termed "jeopardized" by Braunwald's group[32] and an "ischemic penumbra" in the brain by Siesjo's group.[33] Blood flow in the ischemic penumbra is reduced from 60 ml/100 gm to 12–15 ml/100 gm. Salvage strategies for both organs include techniques that increase blood flow, decrease metabolic need, interfere with cellular autolysis, or alter neurotransmitter release.

Maintenance of arterial blood pressure is probably the single most important approach to protecting brain tissue. Fluid replacement should be used initially, followed by inotropes or vasopressor agents. Cerebral vascular autoregulation is markedly decreased following brain damage so that both hypotension and hypertension are undesirable. Even a moderate amount of hypotension may decrease blood flow and damage critically ischemic segments. Hypertension commonly occurs in the early recovery phases following resuscitation for cardiac arrest. It could lead to increased cerebral edema, but usually is transient and does not require treatment.

Mechanical hyperventilation produces cerebral vasoconstriction and decreases both brain water and blood flow. The decrease in ICP may actually increase cerebral blood flow by increasing the mean arterial pressure-ICP gradient. Tidal volumes of 10–15 ml/kg are usually selected to reduce P_{CO_2} to 27–30 mm Hg. Bicarbonate concentrations gradually decline (the half-life is about four hours) leading to a reduction in pH and a gradual reduction in vasoconstriction.

Osmotic and loop diuretics are commonly used to reduce brain edema. Mannitol, 0.25–1.0 gm/kg of a 20% solution every four hours, will produce an osmotic gradient between capillary and brain tissue as long as the blood-brain barrier is intact. Mannitol accumulates in brain tissue even with a normal blood-brain barrier and constitutes an osmotic force increasing brain water. Abrupt discontinuation of mannitol infusions reduces blood osmolarity and can reverse the osmotic gradient in a way that favors the accumulation of brain edema fluid. Furosemide also reduces ICP and can be used in combination with mannitol. A volume-contraction derived reduction in cardiac output must be carefully avoided. Loop diuretics also decrease the production of cerebrospinal fluid.[34]

Reductions in brain metabolic requirements may be accomplished by hypothermia and the use of anesthetics. The barbiturates were one of the first agents to be carefully evaluated and have been shown to reduce cerebral metabolism, edema formation, intracranial pressure, seizure activity, and brain damage.[35] A recent multiinstitutional study[35] is of considerable interest even though it failed to demonstrate a clear advantage of thiopental loading.

Twelve hospitals in nine countries were coordinated by the Resuscitation Research Center team at the University of Pittsburgh.[35] A total of 262 patients with "cardiac arrest or severe global ischemic-anoxic cerebral insults without actual cardiac arrest who had no purposeful motor response to pain after the restoration of adequate spontaneous circulation and oxygenation" were randomized into control and treatment groups. The control group received standard therapy (see Table 9–2) and the treatment group received thiopental 30 mg/kg intravenously as early as possible after restoration of circulation. Most of the deaths occurred within the first month, and 77% of the thiopental group and 80% of the standard therapy group were dead in one year. At one year, 18% of the thiopental group and 15% of the control group had returned to their prearrest level of mental function. None of these differences were statistically significant. Systolic blood pressure fell to below 70 mm Hg in 60% of

TABLE 9–2.
General Brain-Oriented Intensive Care

(1) Maintain blood pressure between 90–100 mm Hg by fluids and vasopressors as needed.
(2) Mechanical ventilation
(3) Maintain arterial P_{CO_2} between 25–35 mm Hg and arterial P_{O_2} above 100 mm Hg
(4) Maintain arterial pH between 7.3–7.5
(5) Immobilization and sedation
(6) Anticonvulsants (diazepam or phenytoin) as needed
(7) Normalization of electrolytes
(8) Glucose 5–10% in 0.25–0.5% NaCl; 30 ml/kg/24 hr.
(9) 50 kcal/kd/24 hours of carbohydrate, amino acids and vitamins beginning 48 hours after restoration of spontaneous circulation
(10) Short term use of steroids for increased ICP; dexa-methasone 0.2 mg/kg i.v. and 0.04 mg/kd/6 hr or methylprednisolone, 1mg/kg/i.v. and 0.2 mh/kg/6 hr preferably for not more than four days
(11) Osmotic diuresis with mannitol as needed
(12) Normothermia

Adapted from Brain Resuscitation Clinical Trial I Study Group[35]: Randomized Clinical Study of thiopental loading in comatose survivors of cardiac arrest. *N Engl J Med* 1986, 314:397.

the thiopental group compared to 29% of the standard group. Mortality was 78% in hypotensive patients who received thiopental and 92% in those who received standard treatment. Yatsu,[36] in editorial review, suggested that "the concept of brain resuscitation cannot be simply jettisoned as fundamentally flawed. . . . the use of barbiturate coma on the pretense of preserving brain function after cardiac arrest or stroke has no clinical basis and should be abandoned."

Prevention of autolysis or mediated injury has been attempted; corticosteroids, calcium channel blockers, free radical scavengers, and cholinergic blockage all have been proposed to reduce brain damage after ischemic or traumatic injury. Corticosteroids reduce ICP in patients with brain tumors[37] but have not been shown to be effective following head trauma.[38] Calcium channel blockers may prevent activation of calcium-mediated cascades, which may mediate cell damage. They increase ICP, however, and should not be used when ICP is elevated.[39] A number of agents including vitamins C and E, superoxide dysmutase, dimethylsulfoxide, n-acetyl cysteine, and glutathione inactivate free radicals. Barbiturates, mannitol, calcium entry blockers, and corticosteroids also inactivate free radicals, which might account for part of their observed activity in improving brain function. The development of free radical scavenging agents shows great promise and could come to dominate the field of brain protection.

Correcting disturbed neurotransmitter release has been exploited in treating the ischemic myocardium and also may be useful in preventing brain injury. Studies reviewed earlier suggest that injury to certain brainstem regions leads to a release of acetylcholine, which disturbs the function of the reticular activating system. Pharmacologic inhibition of acetylcholine release has been shown to improve brain function both clinically and in experimental studies.[29]

BRAIN DEATH

Modern resuscitative and supportive techniques are able to maintain cardiopulmonary function for sustained periods of time so that traditional definitions for death such as cessation of heart beat are obsolete. Intensive care units could become filled rapidly with patients who were essentially dead and would die if ventilatory support was terminated. Transplantation of organs added another urgency to the development of new criteria for death. A major diagnostic concern for clinicians requiring expert consultation is distinguishing coma from brain death or other irreversible syndromes.

Brain death is a term for irreversible brain damage that is so severe that cardiopulmonary function cannot be maintained without mechanical means. Plum and Posner[28] have suggested that brain death can only be diagnosed if the cause of brain damage is irreversible and if the "vital structures necessary to maintain consciousness and independent vegetative survival are damaged beyond all possible repair." A variety of criteria beginning with those of Mollaret and Goulon[40] have attempted to define the presence of brain death.

Two general criteria must be met. Brain death cannot be diagnosed unless the possibility of coma due to reversible metabolic processes or drug poisoning has been ruled out. Detailed metabolic and toxicologic examination by experienced physicians is mandatory; one study showed that physicians frequently overlooked the possibility of narcotic overdosage as a cause of coma.[41] In addition, any evidence of brain function should be absent for at least 12 hours.

The Clinical Recognition of Brain Death

Diagnosis of brain death is based on the evaluation of cortical and brainstem function. Teasdale and Jennett,[42] Plum and Posner[28] and Grenvik[43] all have presented detailed approaches to the diagnosis of brain death. The level of consciousness first must be evaluated by examining eye opening, verbal responses, and responses to noxious stimulation of the face and extremities. The ease of arousal provides an important guide to the level of consciousness. Complete lack of electrical activity in an electroencephalogram obtained with full electronic gain confirms the clinical observation of absent cortical activity.

The Vegetative or Brain Stem Functions

Circulation

The complex spinal and supraspinal neural connections to the circulatory centers located in the reticular formation of the pontomedullary region have been discussed in chapter 4. Hypotension, hypertension, bradycardia, or tachycardia may result from destruction of stimulatory or inhibitory structures. The central role of the brainstem in controlling the circulation is graphically demonstrated by the severe ischemic and dysrhythmic changes observed in subarachnoid hemorrhage. Electrocardiographic changes include large upright T waves with long QT intervals and the appearance of Q waves with ST segment depression. These changes may resemble acute myocardial infarction and lead to significant misdiagnosis. Early ischemic changes probably are due to massive autonomic discharges secondary to brainstem compression by rising intracranial pressure.[44] A variety of arrhythmias and conduction disturbances occur somewhat later, probably due to sustained vagal and sympathetic neural activity.

Respiration

The respiratory centers are also located in the brainstem reticular system; changes in respiratory pattern provide evidence of serious injury to that region. Cheyne-Stokes respiration consists of alternating phases of hyperpnea and apnea with smooth increments and decrements in respiratory rates up to and following a peak. Bilateral disturbance of cortical or subcortical structures, a prolonged circulation time, and hypoxemia are associated with its development.

Tachypnea is common in critically ill patients but probably results from peripheral neural stimulation. Hypoventilation suggests toxic suppression of the respiratory centers, and sustained apnea, of course, is an important sign for brain death. Other abnormal breathing patterns may indicate brainstem damage.

Pupillary Reactions

The pupillary pathways are resistant to metabolic injury. An absent light reflex strongly suggests that loss of consciousness is due to structural causes. Both parasympathetic and sympathetic pathways are involved in pupillary control, and centers controlling pupillary size are located close to those areas regulating consciousness.

Ocular Motion

The neural structure regulating eye movements also lie close to the brainstem reticular activating centers. Changes in eye motions may indicate structural abnormalities; asymmetrical abnormalities in eye motion strongly suggest structural rather than metabolic abnormalities.

The Importance of Brainstem Abnormalities in Evaluating Brain Function

Evidence of absent brainstem function is of great value in confirming the diagnosis of brain death because many processes can produce temporary absence of cortical activity. Flaccidity and areflexia indicate severe brainstem damage but can be found in severe drug overdosage. Extensor responses indicate lesions in the upper pons and midbrain (decerebrate behavior) and also are present in reversible metabolic states.

Evidence of apnea is critical. The lack of spontaneous breathing after temporary discontinuation of mechanical ventilation with an elevation of P_{CO_2} to more than 60 mm Hg, fall in pH to below 7.3, and P_{O_2} below to 50 mm Hg constitute a positive *apnea test*. The threshold for apneic stimulation of respiration is close to a P_{CO_2} of 60 mm Hg, and the period of apnea necessary to reach this level varies widely. Caronna[45] and Grenvik[43] recommend obtaining arterial blood gases and then administering 100% oxygen at a rate of 6 L/min via endotracheal tube after disconnection of ventilator. The reservoir bag can be observed for respiratory activity and repeat arterial sampling should be made at ten minutes. Evidence of respiratory activity is an indication for reinstitution of mechanical ventilation. This procedure prevents cardiac arrest and is useful if organ removal for transplantation is contemplated.

The absence of *brainstem* reflexes provides important evidence for brain death. Plum and Posner[28] provide a detailed discussion of the pathologic basis for abnormal brainstem function. The pupils must be fixed to light stimulation. Bilateral dilated and fixed pupils are seen after cardiac arrest and become small and reactive if cardiopulmonary resuscitation is successful. Pupils may remain small in some individuals with severe brain hypoxia and many drugs may alter pupillary size. Atropine and scopolamine produce dilated pupils, while opiates and metabolic encephalopathies result in small pupils. Glutethimide (Doriden) intoxication is an example of a reversible situation presenting with moderately dilated and fixed pupils.

Corneal, oculovestibular, and oculocephalic responses must be absent. The *corneal reflex* is elicited by tactile stimulation of the cornea. The *oculovestibular reflex* is evaluated by irrigating each auditory canal with 50 ml of ice water for 30–45 seconds and observing whether any movement of eyes toward the stimulated tympanum is observed. The *oculocephalic reflex* is elicited by performing lateral rotation, extension, and flexion of the neck. These maneuvers should not be performed until the possibility of cervical spinal injury has been ruled out. Positive responses to lateral movement are contraversive conjugate eye deviation; both eyes deviate to the side opposite the direction of rotation. A positive response to neck flexion is upward movement of the eyes and downward movement with extension. The doll's head phenomenon is eye opening with flexion.

The concept of brain death is generally accepted in the United States and was endorsed by the President's Commission Report entitled "Deciding to Forego Life-Sustaining Treatment."[46] Since Mollaret and Goulon,[40] a number of brain death criteria have been published including Harvard, Minnesota, Swedish, British, U.S. Collaborative, New York Hospital, and Presbyterian Hospital–University of Pittsburgh. The Pittsburg criteria were developed in collaboration with an outstanding critical care group and are extremely useful for general hospital use. These criteria stipulate that there be a flat electroencephalogram recorded at high gain and that two clinical examinations be performed at least two hours apart. The clinical requirements are:

1. Coma of established cause with absence of hypothermia below 34°C or evidence of toxic drug ingestion
2. No spontaneous movements or evidence of decerebrate behavior
3. Absent cranial nerve responses
   - Fixed pupils with absent light reflex
   - Absent corneal reflexes
   - No response to painful stimuli with supraorbital pressure
   - Absent responses to upper and lower airway stimulation during suctioning
   - Absent ocular response to head turning
   - Absent ocular response to irrigation with 50 ml of ice water
   - Apnea test with recording of P_{CO_2} and P_{O_2} at beginning and end of test
   - Failure to increase heart rate by more than five beats per minute with atropine

Plum and Posner[28] compiled ten published series including 877 patients and demonstrated that not a single individual with established criteria for brain death survived. Most died (cessation of heartbeat) within several days or a week, most in spite of resuscitative efforts. Some electroencephalographic activity was still present in 37 of the 449 instances where the test had been performed. Others also have noted brain death in the presence of some electrical activity. Jennett, Gleave, and Wilson[47] reversed the study and evaluated 1,003 patients in three neurosurgical units who survived coma lasting at least six hours. No patient met the clinical criteria for even a brief period.

PERMANENTLY LOST CONSCIOUSNESS

Jennett and Plum,[48] described a group of patients who survived for prolonged periods after severe brain trauma with coma. They appeared to awaken after several weeks of coma but exhibited no evidence of cognitive function. Plum and Posner[28] suggest that "an operational definition is that the eyes open spontaneously in response to verbal stimuli. Sleep-wake cycles exist. The patients spontaneously maintain normal levels of blood pressure and respiratory control. They show no discrete localizing motor responses and neither offer comprehensible words nor obey any verbal commands. They called this syndrome the *persistent or chronic vegetative state*; the public has come to know it as the Karen Quinlan syndrome.

A number of neuropathologic studies have described the elements of the syndrome.[49] Most of the patients had severe anoxic insults and were initially in coma. They survived for as long as 17 years because of exceptional care and had normal brainstem activity but no recognizable evidence of cognitive function. Pathologic studies usually showed severe cortical laminar necrosis, although occasionally relatively mild abnormalities were observed.[50] Persistent vegetation with a mildly abnormal brain at postmortem examination is a startling observation and suggests depletion of important functional substances. Brainstem damage was usually minimal. The contrast between brain death and the persistent vegetative state is perhaps best described by Korein's term *cerebral death*.[51] Cerebral death differs from brain death since the midbrain, pons, brainstem, and cerebellum are capable of maintaining some function.

The persistent vegetative state must be distinguished carefully from the *locked-in or deefferented syndrome*. In these patients, an extensive pontine lesion destroys the brainstem efferent motor tracts but spares the reticular activating system. These patients have paralysis of all four extremities and the lower cranial nerves and appear unconscious because they cannot communicate. Often their only means of communication is by vertical eye movements, and some patients have been able to communicate by eye signals.[52]

ETHICAL AND LEGAL CONSIDERATIONS IN THE CARE OF BRAIN-DAMAGED PATIENTS

Physicians and other care-givers always must maintain a presumption in favor of life. Those who enter the medical, nursing, and other related health care professions pledge to themselves and to others that they will do all in their power to preserve and support human life. But, as the pages above have shown, life may appear to be at an end even though mechanical support permits blood to course through an otherwise lifeless person. Failure to understand that death must be properly identified as much as any other human health problem can produce devastating consequences for patients, families, hospital staff, and the public at large.

William Harvey[53] discovered the circulation of the blood in the latter half of the seventeenth century and also decided that the heart was the seat of human life.

> Since death is a corruption which takes place through deficiency of heat, and since all living things are warm, all dying things cold, there must be a particular seat and fountain, a kind of home and hearth, where the cherisher of nature, the original of the native fire, is stored and preserved; from which heat and life are dispensed to all parts as from a fountain head; from which sustenance may be derived; and upon which concoction and nutrition, and all vegetative energy may depend. Now, that the heart is this place, that the heart is the principle of life, and that all passes in the manner just mentioned, I trust no one will deny.[53]

At almost the same time in history, Sir Francis Bacon[54] chided Seneca and his stoic philosophy for his complicated approach to death:

> Just as I choose a ship to sail in or a house to live in, so I choose a death for my passage from life . . . Nowhere should we indulge the soul more than in dying . . . A man's life should satisfy other people as well, his death only himself, and whatever sort he likes best.[54]

Bacon went on to add that "it is as natural to die as to be born; and to a little infant, perhaps, the one is as painful as the other."[54] He was echoing the moving and significant words of the author of Ecclesiastes: "For every life there is a season, and a time for every purpose under heaven: a time to be born, and a time to die; a time to plant, and a time to pluck up that which is planted."[55]

Definitions of death changed little in the subsequent 400 years and tended to follow William Harvey's conclusions as embodied in English common law: death is "the cessation of life" indicated primarily by "a total stoppage of the circulation of the blood."[56] The development of mechanical ventilation, ventricular assist devices, cardiopulmonary resuscitation, and other life-sustaining techniques challenged Harvey's views. Intensive care units became filled with ventilator-dependent patients who had little hope for survival. Physicians and hospitals made operational decisions that varied widely, but little general attention was paid to the problem until April 15, 1975. On that day, the Karen Quinlan tragedy began to unfold.

The Supreme Court of New Jersey ordered that Karen Quinlan be disconnected from mechanical ventilation and based its judgment on the right of an incompetent patient's guardian, in consultation with a hospital "ethics committee," to make informed decisions. The court held that "we consider that a practice of applying to a court to confirm such decisions would generally be inappropriate, not only because that would be a gratuitous encroachment upon the medical profession's field of competence, but because it would be impossibly cumbersome." Two other courts followed the view of the New Jersey Court, but the Supreme Judicial Court of Massachusetts, in contrast, rejected that position. That court, in a case labeled "Saikewicz," stated that it took "a dim view of any attempt to shift the ultimate decision-making responsibility away from the duly established courts of proper jurisdiction to any committee, panel, or group, ad hoc or permanent."

On March 21, 1983, the President's Commission for the Study of Ethical Problems in Medicine and Biomedical and Behavioral Research[46] sent a most significant document to the President of the United States, the President of the Senate, and the Speaker of the House of Representatives:

> We are pleased to transmit our report on *Deciding to Forego Life-Sustaining Treatment*. This subject was not part of our original legislative mandate but was added as a natural outgrowth of our studies on informed consent, the "definition' of death, and access to health care and because it seemed to us to involve some of the most important and troubling ethical and legal questions in modern medicine.

The letter went on to say:

> We have concluded that the cases that involve true ethical difficulties are many fewer than commonly believed and that the perception of difficulty occurs primarily because of misunderstandings about the dictates of law and ethics. Neither criminal nor civil law precludes health practitioners or their patients and relatives from reaching ethically and medically appropriate decisions about when to engage in or to

> forego efforts to sustain the lives of dying patients.

The President's Commission presented over 500 tightly reasoned pages to the United States government. The report generally supported the Quinlan decision rather than the Saikewicz decision and provided a basis for ethical decision making in the critical care unit. It should be available to all involved in those decisions. The first chapter of the report contains a summary and is briefly reviewed here.

The report emphasizes that "primary responsibility for ensuring that morally justified processes of decision making are followed lies with physicians." Institutions also have similar responsibilities and should develop policies regarding these important decisions. There is, however, "no substitute for the dedication, compassion, and professional judgment of physicians." According to the report:

> The voluntary choice of a competent and informed patient should determine whether or not life-sustaining therapy will be undertaken . . . Health care institutions and professionals should try to enhance patients' abilities to make decisions on their own behalf and to promote understanding of the available treatment options. . . . Health care professionals serve patients best by maintaining a presumption in favor of sustaining life, while recognizing that competent patients are entitled to choose to forego any treatments, including those that sustain life.

The report went on to emphasize that health care professionals do not have to take actions that violate their own professional judgment of conscience, but they may not abandon patients. Institutions may limit the availability of certain scarce resources in order to make them available where they will be most useful.

There is a more difficult problem with patients who are *incompetent* to make appropriate decisions. A surrogate, usually a family member, should be named to make decisions for incompetent patients. As the report states:

> The decisions of surrogates should, when possible, attempt to replicate the ones that the patient would make if capable of doing so. When lack of evidence about the patient's wishes precludes this, decisions by surrogates should seek to protect the patient's best interests. Because such decisions are not instances of self-choice by the patient, the range of acceptable decisions by surrogates is sometimes not as broad as it would be for patients making decisions themselves.

Families, health care institutions, and professionals should work together to make decisions for incompetent patients. The medical staff, administrators, and trustees should develop arrangements for consultation and review, including the formation of "ethics committees."

Legislatures and courts should develop methods for allowing individuals to designate in advance that others may make health care decisions on their behalf. According the The President's Commission:

> Durable powers of attorney are preferable to 'living wills' since they are more generally applicable and provide a better vehicle for patients to exercise self-determination, though experience with both is limited.
>
> Recourse to courts should be reserved for the occasions when adjudication is clearly required by state law or when concerned patients have disagreements that they cannot resolve over matters of substantial import. Courts and legislatures should be cautious about requiring judicial review of routine health care decisions for patients with inadequate decision making capacity.

Ethical problems surrounding patients

with the chronic vegetative state are particularly difficult. Robert Veatch, a noted bioethicist, has supported the idea that whole brain death is an incomplete and inappropriate concept: "Death is the irreversible loss of what is essentially significant to the nature of man, including the capacity to integrate bodily function, for rationality, to experience, and for social interaction.[57] A statement of the American Medical Association, reprinted in appendix C of the President's Report, endorses Veatch's position by stating that "where a terminally ill patient's coma is beyond doubt irreversible and there are adequate safeguards to confirm the accuracy of the diagnosis, all means of life support may be discontinued."

The President's Commission[46] also considered the institution of cardiopulmonary resuscitation and the writing of orders prohibiting its use. The Presbyterian-University of Pittsburgh Hospital has provided an unusually complete set of guidelines for foregoing life-sustaining treatment.[58] Drawing heavily on the President's Commission,[46] they provide important guidance for the documentation of decisions and entry of orders. They emphasize that whenever a decision to withhold lifesupporting techniques has been made, a specific order must be written. The order must be accompanied by a detailed entry in the progress notes describing the patient's condition and the details of the decision. The guidelines suggest three categories of acceptable orders: (1) "all but cardiac resuscitation," (2) "limited therapy," and (3) "comfort measures only."

Decisions in the critical care unit must be made on medical grounds. Frequently these decisions involve ethical and legal implications. It is frequently important to obtain consultative advice, and it is essential to seek consensus among the professional staff, patient, and family members.

REFERENCES

1. Sokoloff L: Circulation and energy metabolism of the brain, in Siegel CJ, Albers RW, Katzman R, Agranoff BW (eds): *Basic Neurochemistry*, ed 2, Boston, Little, Brown, 1976, p 388.

2. Hubel DH, Wiesel TN: Sequence regularity and geometry of orientation columns in the monkey striate cortex. *J Comp Neurol* 1974; 158:267–294.

3. Vogt, M: The concentration of sympathin in different parts of the central nervous system under normal conditions and after administration of drugs. *J Physiol* 1954; 123:451–481.

4. Carlsson A: The occurrence, distribution and physiological role of catecholamines in the nervous system. *Pharmacol Rev* 1959; 11:490–493.

5. Ungerstedt W: Stereotaxic mapping of monoamine pathways in the rat brain. *Acta Physiol Scand Suppl* 1971; 367:1–48.

6. Synder SH, Bruns RF, Daly JW: Multiple neurotransmitter receptors in the brain: amines, adenosin and cholyecystokinin, *FASEB* 1981; 40:142.

7. Klawans HL, Weiner WJ, Nausieda PA: The effect of lithium on an animal model of tardive dyskinesia. *Prog Neuro-Psychopharm* 1977; 1:53–60.

8. Lee T, Seeman P: Elevation of brain dopamine-stimulated cyclic AMP formation. *Naunyn Schmiedebergs Arch Pharmacol* 1978; 304:141–145.

9. Wybran J: Enkelphalins and endorphins as modifiers of the immune system: Present and future. *FASEB* 1985; 92.

10. Buck SH, Walsh JH, Yamamura HI: Burks TF: Neuropeptides in sensory neurons. *Life Sci* 1982; 30:1857–1866.

11. Smith GP, Gibbs J: Gut peptides and postprandial satiety. *FASEB* 1984; 43:2889.

12. Sokoloff L, Fitzgerald GG, Kaufman EE: Cerebral nutrition and energy metabolism, in Wurtwan RJ, Wurtman JJ (eds): *Nutrition and the Brain*, vol 1. New York: Raven Press, 1977, p 87.

13. Kontos HA, Raper AJ, Patterson JL: Analysis of vasoactivity of local pH, PCO_2 and bicarbonate on pial vessels. *Stroke* 1977a; 8:358.

14. Tyson GW, Jane JA: Pathophysiology of head injury, in Cowley RA, Trump BF (eds), *Pathophysiology of Shock, Anoxia and Ischemia*, Baltimore, MD, Williams & Wilkins, 1982.

15. Borgström L, Jóhannsson H, Siesjö BK: The relationship between arterial PO_2 and cerebral blood flow in hypoxic hypoxia. *Acta Physiol Scand* 1975; 93:423–432.

16. Kontos HA, Wei EP, Raper AJ, et al: Role of tissue hypoxia in local regulation of cerebral microcirculation. *Am J Physiol* 1978; 234:H582–H591.

17. Kontos HA, Wei EP, Navari RM, et al: Responses of cerebral arteries and aterioles to acute hypotension and hypertension. *Am J Physiol* 1978; 234:H371–H383.

18. Siesjö BK, Nilsson L: The influence of arterial hypoxemia upon labile phosphates and upon extracellular and intracellular lactate and pyruvate concentration in the rat brain. *Scand J Clin Lab Invest* 1971; 27:83–96.

19. Salford LG, Siesjö BK: The influence of arterial hypoxia and unilateral carotid artery occlusion upon regional blood flow and metabolism in the rat brain. *Acta Physiol Scand* 1974; 92:130–141.

20. Siesjö BK, Wieloch T: Cerebral metabolism in ischemia: Neurochemical basis for therapy. *Br J Anaesth* 1985; 57:47–62.

21. DeMello WC: Modulation of junctional permeability. *FASEB* 1984; 2692.

22. Miller JD, Becker DP, Ward JD, et al: Significance of intracranial hypertension in severe head injury. *J Neurosurg* 1977; 47:501.

23. Becker DP, Miller JD, Ward JD, et al: The outcome from severe head injury with early diagnosis and intensive management. *J Neurosurg* 1977; 47:491.

24. Langfitt TW: Intracranial volume-pressure relationship, in Lundberg N, Ponten U, Brock M (eds): *Intracranial Pressure II*. New York, Springer-Verlag, 1975, p 69.

25. Rossen R, Kabat H, Anderson JP: Acute arrest of cerebral circulation in man. *Arch Neurol Psychiatr* 1943; 50:510–528.

26. Levy DE, Brierley JB, Silverman DG, et al: Brief hypoxia-ischemia initially damages cerebral neurons. *Arch Neurol* 1975; 32:450–456.

27. Siesjö BK: Cerebral circulation and metabolism. Review article. *J Neurosurg* 1984; 60:883–908.

28. Plum F, Posner JB: *The Diagnosis of Stupor and Coma, ed* 3. Philadelphia, FA Davis Co, 1982.

29. Hayes RL, Pechura CM, Katayama Y, et al: Activation of pontine cholinergic sites implicated in unconsciousness following cerebral concussion in the cat. *Science* 1984; 223:301–303.

30. Miller JD, Sullivan HG: Severe intracranial hypertension. *Int Anesthesiol Clin* 1979; 17(2,3):19.

31. Vries JK, Becker DP, Young HF: A subarachnoid screw for monitoring intracranial pressure. *J Neurosurg* 1973; 39:416.

32. Sobel BE, Shell WE: Jeopardized, blighted, and necrotic myocardium. *Circulation* 1973; 47:215.

33. Siesjö BK: The biology of cerebral ischemia. Part 1: Pathology and pathophysiology. *Neuro & Neurosurg* 1985a; 6(15): 1–8 and Part 2: Neurochemical Pathology. *Neuro Neurosurg* 1985a; 6(16):1–8.

34. Tornheim PP, McTaurin RL, Sawava R: Effect of furosemide on experimental traumatic cerebral edema. *Neurosurg* 1979; 4:48.

35. Brain Resuscitation Clinical Trial I Study Group: Randomized clinical study of thiopental loading in comatose survivors of cardiac arrest. *N Engl J Med* 1986; 314:397.

36. Yatsu FM: Cardiopulmonary-cerebral resuscitation, *N Engl J Med* 1986; 314:440–441.

37. Galich JH, French L: Use of dexamethasone in treatment of cerebral edema resulting from brain tumors in brain surgery. *Amer Pract Dig* 1961; 12:169–174.

38. Molofsky WJ: Steroids and head trauma. *Neurosurg* 1984; 15:424–426.

39. Bedford RF, Dacey R, Winn HR, et al: Adverse impact of calcium entry blocker (verapamil) on intracranial pressure in patients with tumors. *J Neurosurg* 1983; 59:800–809.

40. Mollaret P, Goulon M: Le coma dépassé. *Rev Neurol* 1959; 101:3–15.

41. Walker AE: Cerebral death, in Tower DB (ed): *The Nervous System*, vol 2. *The Clinical Neurosciences*. New York, Raven Press, 1975, pp 75–87.

42. Teasdale G, Jennett B: Assessment of coma and impaired consciousness: a practical scale. *Lancet* 1974; 2:81–84.

43. Grenvik A: Brain death and permanently lost consciousness, in Shoemaker WC, Thompson WL, Holbrook PR (eds): *Textbook of Critical Care*. Philadelphia, WB Saunders Co, 1984.

44. Hammer WJ, Luessenhop AJ, Weintraub AM: Observations on the electrocardiographic changes associated with subarachnoid hemorrhage with special reference to their genesis. *Am J Med* 1975; 59:427–433.

45. Caronna JJ: The neurological intensive care unit, in Parrillo JE, Ayres SM (eds): *Major Issues in Critical Care Medicine*. Baltimore, Williams & Wilkins, 1984.

46. President's Commission for the Study of Ethical Problems in Medicine and Biomedical and Behavioral Research. *Deciding to Forego Life-Sustaining Treatment*.

47. Jennett B, Gleave J, Wilson P: Brain death in three neurosurgical units. *Br Med J* 1981; 282:533–539.

48. Jennett WB, Plum F: The persistent vegetative state: a syndrome in search of a name. *Lancet* 1972; 1:734–737.

49. Brierley JB, Adams JH, Graham DI, et al: Neocortical death after cardiac arrest. *Lancet* 1971; 2:560–565.

50. Dougherty JH Jr, Rawlinson D, Levy DE, et al: Hypoxic-ischemic brain injury and the vegetative state. Clinical and neuro-pathologic correlation. *Neurology* 1979; 29:591.

51. Korein J: The problem of brain death: Development and history. *Ann NY Acad Sci* 1978; 315:19.

52. Feldman MH: Physiological observations in a chronic case of locked-in syndrome. *Neurology* 1971; 21:459–478.

53. Harvey W: Circulation of the blood, 1628, in Eliot CW (ed): *The Harvard Classics*. New York, 1909, vol 38, p 129.

54. Bacon F: Of death, 1625, in Eliot CW (ed): *The Harvard Classics*. New York, 1909, vol 3, p 9.

55. Ecclesiastes III, 1.

56. Black's Law Dictionary 488 (4th ed. 1968). In its latest edition, Black's (5th ed. 1979) now includes an entry under "brain death" at p 170.

57. Veatch RM: Choosing not to prolong dying, in Beachamp TL, Walters L (eds): *Contemporary Issues in Bioethics*. Wadsworth Belmont, 1978, pp 301–306.

58. Benesch K, Abramson NS, Grenvik A, et al: *Medicolegal Aspects of Critical Care*. Rockville, MD, Aspen Publication, 1986, appendix A.

10 NUTRITIONAL SUPPORT OF CRITICALLY ILL PATIENTS

Recognition that many critical disease states are associated with accelerated malnutrition began with the pioneering work of Cuthbertson in the early 1930s.[1] Little could be done to correct this metabolic abnormality until the 1960s when beagle puppies were successfully raised to adulthood using intravenous mixtures of essential nutrients. Since a growing body of evidence suggested that malnutrition led to impaired host defenses, it seemed reasonable to believe that appropriate nutritional support could improve survival from critical illness by replacing catabolic losses. Currently, hyperalimentation, either enteral or intravenous, is widely used in many intensive care units. Few studies are available, however, to substantiate the belief that nutritional support of seriously ill individuals can improve morbidity or mortality rates.

PROTEIN CATABOLISM IN HEALTH AND CRITICAL ILLNESS

The urinary loss of nitrogen has been intensively studied since it largely reflects conversion of endogenous protein to urea in the fasting state. Excess urinary nitrogen loss implies loss of structural and enzymatic protein. The loss of one gram of urinary nitrogen is considered equal to the catabolism of 30 grams of fat-free tissue.[2]

A healthy 70 kg man loses approximately 12 grams of nitrogen per day during the first several days of an acute fast. Within a week, however, nitrogen loss falls to 8 grams per day and within several weeks to 3 grams per day.[3] Adaptive mechanisms limiting nitrogen loss include increased hepatic synthesis of amino acid activating enzymes and decreased total body protein turnover. In addition, preferential utilization of ketone bodies by the central nervous system leads to decreased glucose utilization.

Critically ill patients with high rates of catabolism, however, generally continue to lose large quantities of nitrogen for the duration of their illness, although losses are somewhat variable. The key factor appears to be the nonsuppressibility of nitrogen loss by glucose in this patient group. One hundred grams of glucose per day reduces fasting nitrogen loss to 5–6 grams per day in normal individuals[4] but has little effect on stressed patients.[5] In general, younger patients lose more nitrogen than older patients, and well-nourished patients lose more nitrogen than malnourished patients. Since mechanisms which normally limit nitrogen loss for normal individuals do not become operative in stressed patients, the continuous accelerated "leak" of nitrogen may profoundly impact body protein within a very short period of time. Nitrogen leak in patients with prolonged illness such as multiple trauma, unremitting sepsis, or severe burns may independently affect survival as vital host defenses become compromised (Table 10–1).

TABLE 10–1.
Approximate Fasting Nitrogen Loss for 70 kg Individuals, gm N/24 Hours.

Normal, acute	10–15
Normal, adapted (4–6 weeks)	3–5
Elective surgery	14–18
Multiple trauma	20–25
Gunshot injuries	20–25
Sepsis	20–30
Burns (extensive)	20–40

Pathogenesis of Nitrogen Loss

Current understanding of *normal* starvation, while somewhat teleological in orientation, suggests that glucose deficits are the initial stimulus for nitrogen loss. Following an acute fast in a normal individual, leakage of amino acids from muscle tissue is preceded by a period of hypoglycemia as glycogen stores become depleted. Hypoglycemia in turn inhibits pancreatic secretion of insulin. Low circulating insulin levels enhance amino acid release from the muscle protein pool. At the same time, elevated glucagon levels stimulate gluconeogenesis from these and other precursors to provide substrate for obligate glucose consumers—CNS, formed elements, and renal medulla.[6]

The pathogenesis of accelerated protein catabolism appears to be strikingly different during *critical disease states*. Early observations and recent reviews suggest that increased nitrogen excretion in that setting reflects the need for increased glucose and amino acids because of an increased metabolic rate. Either decreased nutrient availability or enhanced metabolic need could, according to this theory, account for proteolysis. Recent studies, however, do not support the idea that the appearance of excess nitrogen in the urine is due to a relative deficiency of metabolic substrate. Hyperglycemia with high insulin levels is commonly observed during the catabolic stages of critical illness; the periods of hypoglycemia and decreased insulin levels observed during unstressed starvation are not observed. In addition, although fasting glucose consumption is higher than normal, the rate of glucose synthesis exceeds the rate of glucose oxidation. This phenomenon is accounted for only partially by anaerobic glucose consumption with resynthesis of glucose from lactate in the liver. Finally, correlation between metabolic rate and nitrogen excretion is poor both within the various "ebb and flow" stages of a single illness and among various critical disease categories. In fact, nitrogen loss is frequently higher during the most critical periods when metabolic rate is abnormally low. Thus, it appears that the increased rate of conversion of amino acids to urea is not stimulated primarily by an enhanced requirement for glucose fuel.

Nitrogen lost in the urine is derived mainly from skeletal muscle, since excretion rates of 3-methylhistidine are very high. This amino acid is synthesized during muscle protein formation and cannot be reutilized after muscle protein is broken down. While other tissues may contain 3-MEH, muscle which comprises 40% of the fat free body mass is the obvious primary source of catabolized amino acids. This point is important to remember when one considers the relationship of urinary nitrogen loss to clinical morbidity (see below).

During the mid-1970s a number of investigators provided evidence to support an "energy deficit" hypothesis in an attempt to elucidate the pathogenesis of accelerated nitrogen loss. Substrate flow studies across the uninjured legs of critically ill patients failed to demonstrate significant utilization of glucose or fat by these extremities.[7] This was attributed to insulin resistance, carnitine deficiency, and/or lipoprotein lipase deficiency. Since it was known that skeletal muscle can oxidize branched-chain amino acids (BCAA) but not other amino acids, it was hypothesized that muscle, in a desperation measure to maintain its fuel supply, was forced to cannibalize its own BCAA. The residual nonbranched-chain amino acids could not be used for protein synthesis in the absence of BCAA, could not be retained in the muscle pool, and would be excreted into venous blood and cleared by the liver. It was, in fact, demonstrated that the amino acid mixture released from skeletal muscle was deficient in BCAA relative to the BCAA content of muscle. The problems with this theory, however, are several. First, the BCAA-deficient pattern of release by skeletal muscle during critical illness is identical to that of normal starvation, a state for which no "energy deficit" is apparent.[8] Second, approximately half of the BCAA mobilized from muscle protein is not oxidized, but rather is released to the circulation.[8] Third, infusion of BCAA mixtures into normal, starving, or critically ill patients, while increasing muscle oxidation of the exogenous BCAA, has failed to stop the outpouring of amino acids from limbs of these patients.[9,10]

More recent evidence suggests that net amino acid release from skeletal muscle serves an adaptive function by providing building materials for the vast array of proteins that must be rapidly synthesized in order to survive many critical illnesses—mucus, fibroblasts, leukocytes, complement components, clotting factors, immunoglobins, and other "acute phase reactants". Viewed in this manner, the magnitude of amino acid release from skeletal muscle is less surprising. In fact, total body synthetic rate consistently has been found to be elevated during critical illness, although the location of increased synthesis is not clear. Most interestingly, interleukin-1 or a related substance, "proteolysis-inducing factor," appears simultaneously to induce lysosomal muscle autolysis and hepatic protein synthesis.[11] Thus, a peripheral to visceral translocation of amino acids for stress protein synthesis may largely account for the amino acid mobilization observed. The relationship which this phenomenon may have to urinary nitrogen loss is not clear. However, it is interesting to speculate that the amino acid mixture released from skeletal muscle, being relatively deficient in essential amino acids necessary for protein synthesis, may be only partially utilized for stress protein synthesis. The remaining amino acids would then be cleared by the liver and other tissues and converted to urea. Alternatively, elevated glucagon levels may direct a substantial proportion of the mobilized amino acids towards glucogenesis.[12]

Hormonal mediation of amino acid mobilization remains to be clarified. Endogenously synthesized steroids alone do not appear important at physiological concentrations. Glucagon, cortisol, and epinephrine were recently infused into normal volunteers at rates to simulate levels characteristic of critical illness; although none of these hormones alone had a significant effect, infusion of all three together produces small but statistically significant increases in nitrogen excretion. However, nitrogen losses may have been reduced by the 30 kcal/kg, 1 gram/kg protein diet consumed by these individuals.[13] Relative insulin insufficiency may permit amino acid leakage from muscle since infusion of insulin into highly catabolic (but not mildly catabolic) patients markedly reduces nitrogen loss.[14–16] Although insulin levels are generally higher than normal, hyperglycemia generally prevails, indicating a relative deficiency. Interleukin-1, as discussed, may play a central role. Glucagon secretion appears to be stimulated by high amino acid levels and favor conversion of these and other substrates to glucose.

Effect of Nitrogen Loss on Host Defense

Muscle catabolism releases amino acids into the circulation, and these are utilized by the liver for the synthesis of acute-phase proteins. The loss of protein may lead to both cardiac and diaphragmatic muscle dysfunction. Cardiac muscle clearly atrophies during the course of unstressed states such as anorexia nervosa and during hospitalization for acute illness; the decrease in cardiac mass, however, is proportionately less than the decrease in body weight.[17] Although cardiac function appears adequate under normal circumstances, ventricular dysfunction may prevent stroke output from increasing to the high levels required in sepsis and other forms of critically illness. The adequacy of the atrophied myocardium during states of increased oxygen consumption has not been studied.

Diaphragmatic muscle also becomes atrophied during states of chronic malnutrition, producing a significant effect on maximal attainable inspiratory and expiratory muscle strength.[18,19] Changes in both the mass and length of the diaphragm have been documented in autopsy studies.[17] The rate of diminution of diaphragmatic mass is approximately the same as the rate of loss of body mass. Again, this may be of little consequence for patients without pulmonary or cardiac disease, but may predispose to respiratory arrest or hinder weaning of ventilator-dependent patients.

Immune function deteriorates markedly during unstressed starvation.[20] Accelerated catabolism may play an important pathogenetic role in the development of the serious impairment of cell-mediated immunity and neutrophil bacteriocidal activity seen in critical illness. Nutritional deficiencies might be expected to interfere with the synthesis of granulocytes, complement, immunoglobulins, fibronectin, and other components of the immune response, but other facts also appear important.

The ability of the protein-depleted critically ill patient to synthesize adequate quantities of other acute phase reactants is not well understood. Diminished levels of interleukin-1 have been found in a depleted critically ill population, suggesting a possible impaired ability to mobilize amino acids.[21] Many groups of intensivists believe that the nutritional support early in the course of a prolonged critical illness prevents deterioration of host defenses. Aggressive nutritional support is considered by most burn surgeons, for example, as a cornerstone of burn therapy. Other groups are not convinced that the vigorous application of nutritional support improves outcome.

CLINICAL STUDIES

Obviously, nutritional support is necessary in situations of severe nutritional deprivation. Healthy young men who starve themselves as a form of political protest live for an average of 60 days.[22] Clearly, malnutrition becomes an independent factor limiting survival for everyone. It is not clear, however, when malnutrition limits survival in critical illness and whether patients recover from critical illness before malnutrition becomes a limiting problem.

A group of studies suggest that nutritional support with amino acid solutions may favorably affect outcome. Two prospective randomized studies of 53[23] and 120[24] patients and one retrospective nonrandomized study of 40 critically ill patients[25] with acute renal failure found statistically significant differences in survival when nutritional solutions containing essential amino acids were provided. Twenty patients with isolated acute head injuries who were randomly assigned to receive early TPN similarly manifested a statistically significant survival advantage compared to 18 controls who did not.[26] Two retrospective studies of 23[27] and 48[28] ventilator-dependent patients demonstrated a markedly improved likelihood of successful weaning for patients who received nutritional support compared to those who did not. While these studies are by no means conclusive, they do suggest that nutritional support may be important in *some* critically ill patients.

Nutritional Assessment

It is difficult to measure the nutritional status of individual patients because unambiguous indicators that correlate with the adequacy of host defenses are not available. Two techniques—*in vivo* neutron activation analysis and isotope dilution technique—appear to be accurate in determining total body nitrogen or total body cell mass, respectively. These techniques may not describe the status of specific organ systems or the adequacy of host defenses because various key protein systems may not all deteriorate at the same time.

Serum proteins, while easily obtained from patients' records, may be misleading since metabolism of these substances is markedly altered during critical illness. While it is generally assumed that serum protein levels correlate with the nutritional integrity of the liver, recent studies of hepatic-derived protein levels during critical illness found that while albumin levels fell, levels of acute-phase reactants rose, suggesting a "reprioritization" of hepatic protein synthesis.[29] *Levels* of a substance, of course, are the resultant of both synthesis and metabolism and cannot be used to estimate the rate of synthesis. The catabolism of albumin for example, increases markedly during critical illness so that a depressed level may not necessarily imply decreased synthesis.[30,31] In addition, fluid loading and assumption of the recumbent position have been shown to cause levels to fall.[32,33] The kinetics of other serum proteins commonly measured as nutritional parameters during critical illness has not been adequately studied. Although the shifts in serum proteins with critical illness are uncertain indicators of nutritional status, they are of some value. An increase in serum proteins usually reflects improved nutritional status, while a decline could be due to a severely catabolic state, extracellular volume expansion, or a true decline in nutritional status.

Lymphocyte counts are a very imprecise measure of nutritional status, since the overlap between "normal" levels and "malnourished" levels is considerable.[34,35] Furthermore, a "normal" count may be "abnormal" for an illness requiring increased numbers of lymphocytes for host protection. Skin testing is of little value since powerful non-nutritional forces produce anergy in the majority of these patients.

Maximal expiratory pressure was recently found to correlate with body cell mass in ventilator-dependent patients. The correlation was highly significant ($p \ll 0.01$) although the correlation coefficient was only 0.27, suggesting poor predictive value. Obviously a large number of other factors such as degree of diaphragmatic muscle fatigue, chest wall tenderness, or serum phosphorus may also affect maximal expiratory pressure.[36]

Triceps skinfold thickness is of dubious

value since fat stores serve no vital function other than as a fuel reservoir. Serial determinations may identify a patient who is in negative fuel balance; however, measurements may be influenced by skin edema, a common finding in this population.[37] Creatinine/height index assumes a given muscle mass based on a constant rate of release of creatinine from skeletal muscle. This method overestimates muscle mass in highly catabolic patients since muscular release of creatinine is abnormally high.[38] The relation between noncardiac, nonrespiratory muscle function and vulnerability to medical stress is tantalizing, but remains to be demonstrated.

NUTRITIONAL SUPPORT IN CRITICAL ILLNESS

When to Begin Nutritional Support

It is obvious that malnutrition, even by itself, will ultimately produce death and that nutritional support can save lives. The problem in caring for critical care patients is *timing*. For each individual with sustained inability to eat, there must be a point where risk/benefit considerations for nutritional support shift from unfavorable to favorable. Unfortunately, it is not possible to identify that time in individuals or groups of patients with reasonable certainty. Several factors may be helpful, however, in estimating when to begin nutritional support.

The *degree of nutritional depletion* is obviously important. Provision of intravenous nutrition to *well-nourished* surgical patients in the postoperative period following elective procedures generally has not been found to influence morbidity or mortality. Since these individuals generally lose 50–75 grams of nitrogen over a three to five day period of reduced nutritional intake, that degree of negative nitrogen balance might be considered a baseline phenomena that does not effect morbidity or mortality.

Malnourished patients, on the other hand, clearly experience higher morbidity and mortality with elective surgery. It is not clear whether preoperative nutritional support can improve survival in this group of individuals; most studies failing to identify improvement with nutritional support have been in patients with malignant disease. Most studies indicate that nutritional reconstitution of these patients is not possible; only adipose tissue may increase. The host defenses of critically ill patients, on the other hand, are severely challenged; nutritional support of these individuals may, by preserving the structural integrity of body protein, improve the likelihood of survival.

In addition, it may be advisable to consider early nutritional intervention for the well-nourished new arrival to the ICU, based on the measured or estimated *nitrogen excretion rate* and the estimated duration of highly catabolic illness. Achievement of a positive nitrogen balance is frequently difficult in individuals who are severely protein catabolic (nitrogen loss greater than 20 grams per day), so it may make sense to begin nutritional support early, before a significant degree of malnutrition is reached. Early nitrogen loss must be identified, just as the intensivist attempts to identify early hypoxemia or early hypovolemia.

Certain risks are associated with nutritional support. Adequate nutritional support to the critically ill patient with oliguric renal failure leads to more frequent dialysis or ultrafiltration because of the volume of fluid which must be administered. Carbohydrate in particular increases carbon dioxide production, which may increase arterial and venous carbon dioxide tension if alveolar ventilation is not increased. Additional transvenous catheters may increase the likelihood of catheter infection, although an improvement in immune status might balance any additional risk. Clearly, decisions for nutritional intervention must be made on an individual basis.

Derivation of Nutritional Formula

Intermediary metabolism during critical illness deviates widely from normal and complicates the provision of adequate fuel and amino acid replacement. A growing number of formulations, championed by individual groups, has complicated the matter even more an emphasized the need for a general understanding of nutritional requirements in these patients.

Caloric Requirements

It has been known for some time that an elevated metabolic rate may accompany most critical illnesses,[39] although several recent reports have failed to document this finding.[40] Most investigators have clearly demonstrated that oxygen consumption varies widely in different stages of most critical illness. During the "ebb" phase, oxygen consumption may be lower than normal while the reverse is true during the "flow" phase. This phenomenon is most likely due to variations in blood flow and distribution. Since oxygen and substrate delivery and metabolic rate (oxygen consumption) are the determinants of oxidative phosphorylation, the concept of the ebb and flow of the peripheral circulation may be important. In addition, the blood flow and metabolic status of individual organ systems vary widely during critical illness (Table 10–2); it is clear that the individual contributions of various organs and metabolic functions may vary independently of each other, and thereby also account for the variability of metabolic rate reported by various groups. For example, respiratory muscle oxygen consumption may account for as much as 25% of total body oxygen consumption during severe respiratory distress;[41] institution of mechanical ventilation reduces metabolic rate appropriately.[42] Similarly, cardiac muscle work increases dramatically during high flow sepsis. Other factors which increase metabolic rate include increased thermogenesis during temperature elevations, increased protein synthetic rate, increased sodium potassium ATPase activity, and increased catecholamine levels. Provision of excessive quantities of nutrients may raise oxygen consumption because of the energy required to incorporate unused fuel into storage forms.[43]

Relationship Between Caloric Intake and Nitrogen Balance

Replacement of 100% of caloric expenditure appears desirable since, at any given nitrogen intake, nitrogen retention increases linearly with caloric intake. The degree to which nitrogen balance improves beyond the point where caloric intake is equal to caloric expenditure is controversial, but it is generally unwise

TABLE 10–2.
Factors Which May Influence "Metabolic Rate" in Critically Ill Patients.

Work of breathing
Myocardial stroke work
Elevated catecholamine levels
Adequacy of regional vascular perfusion
Protein synthetic rate
Altered thermoregulation
Increased sodium potassium ATPase activity
Increased hepatic metabolic rate
Free radical formation
Skeletal muscular work (agitation, seizures, etc.)
Infusion of nutrients at excessive rates

to overfeed critically ill patients with calories. Increases in oxygen consumption and CO_2 production will result, and the degree of improvement in nitrogen balance is small. Glucose leads to improved nitrogen balance by decreasing the catabolic rate and by stimulating insulin secretion. Insulin is an anabolic hormone which enhances muscle and hepatic protein synthesis. Fat by itself does not have a nitrogen conserving effect, at least when viewed from the perspective of total body nitrogen balance.[44] The effect of lipid-glucose regimens on nitrogen is discussed below.

Estimation of Caloric Expenditure

Metabolic rate may vary markedly even within single disease categories and from hour to hour, so that precise determinations would require almost continuous monitoring.[45] Such an approach is unrealistic, however, and metabolic rate is usually estimated by one of several methods. The Harris-Benedict formula, developed in 1919, has proven to be remarkably accurate for determining basal metabolic expenditures. This value may be multiplied by a "stress factor" and an "activity factor" to correct for disease-related increments (Table 10–3). This approach is accurate only within broad limits and should be used only if objective measurements are not available. Oxygen consumption may be calculated from cardiac output and arterial-venous oxygen differences in patients with pulmonary artery catheters, but the results may be in error by more than 20% (Table 10–4). Oxygen consumption and carbon dioxide production may be directly measured by collecting expired gases and volumes, but frequent measurements may be necessary because of rapidly changing metabolic

TABLE 10–3.
Estimation of Metabolic Rate When Indirect Calorimetry Is Not Available.

HARRIS-BENEDICT FORMULA Estimated resting metabolic expenditure for a normal unstressed individual.

For men, $BMR = 66 + 13.7 \times \text{wt in kg} + 5 \times \text{ht n cm} - 6.8 \times \text{age}$

For women, $BMR = 655 + 9.6 \times \text{wt in kg} + 1.7 \times \text{ht n cm} - 4.7 \times \text{age}$

Kcal/kg METHOD Assuming average height to weight ratio and age 20–60, approximately 25 kcal/kg for men and 20 kcal/kg for women.

STRESS FACTOR

ELECTIVE SURGERY	SKELETAL TRAUMA	BLUNT TRAUMA	TRAUMA WITH STEROIDS	SEPSIS	BURNS	NORMAL
1.24	1.35	1.37	1.61	1.60	2.10	1.0

ACTIVITY FACTOR

CONFINED TO BED	OUT OF BED
1.2	1.3

Caloric requirements = BMR × Stress Factor × Activity Factor

Note that metabolic rate may vary markedly based on stage of illness. Thus, for example, assignment of a stress factor of 1.6 is not correct for all phases of sepsis and potentially could be harmful (see text). Stress and activity data adapted from Long, CL, Schaffel N, Geiger JW, et al: Estimation of energy and protein needs from indirect calorimetry and nitrogen balance *JPEN* 1979; 3:452–456.

TABLE 10–4.
Estimation of Metabolic Rate by Hemodynamic Measurement*

$\dot{V}O_2$ (ml/min) = 13.4 × Hb × CO × ($SaO_2 - S\bar{v}O_2$) + 0.0031 × CO × ($PaO_2 - P\bar{v}O_2$)

$\dot{V}O_2$ (1/day) = (1.44) ($\dot{V}O_2$ ml/min)

RME (keal/day) = 3.94 × $\dot{V}O_2$ (1/day) + 1.11 × $\dot{V}CO_2$ (1/day)

assuming a respiratory quotient of 1.0, $\dot{V}O_2 = \dot{V}CO_2$ therefore

RME = (3.94 + 1.11) (1.44) ($\dot{V}O_2$ ml/min) = 7.27 ($\dot{V}O_2$ ml/min)

*Accuracy depends on accurate measurements of hemoglobin, cardiac output SaO_2 and $S\bar{v}O_2$ expect error of approximately 20%.

rates (Table 10–5). In addition, expired air collections are difficult in patients receiving ventilatory support, and errors are common. An overestimation of caloric expenditure must be avoided in patients who are hypotensive since, overfeeding leads to an increase in oxygen requirements (see below); such individuals may have metabolic rates even lower than predicted by the Harris-Benedict formula. In fact it may be wise to discontinue feeding for such patients until hemodynamic stability has been restored.

Glucose Versus Fat

A fat-glucose regimen has been found to be as effective as an all-glucose regimen for promoting anabolism in unstressed malnourished patients.[46] Amino acids even in the absence of other caloric intake, have been found to promote positive nitrogen balance in some studies of catabolic patients.[47,48] One study of a few highly catabolic patients failed to demonstrate an increase in nitrogen balance as a result of fat infusion.[49] However, a number of other studies of seriously ill individuals have found formulas containing as much as 75% lipid emulsion calories to be as effective as calorically equivalent all-glucose formulas.[50] These studies do not clearly demonstrate whether the addition of fat to glucose regimens improves nitrogen balance. Exogenous insulin has been found to improve nitrogen balance in highly catabolic but not mildly catabolic patients, and the greater stimulation of endogenous insulin by all-glucose solutions may explain some of the variation observed.

The issue of lipid versus glucose calories involves more than a question of nitrogen balance, however. Lipid produces a smaller increment in carbon dioxide production than carbohydrate and is less likely to produce hepatic abnormalities. On the other hand, long-chain triglycerides (contained in most intravenous emulsions) may suppress immunity[51] or impair oxygenation.[52] Since the precise mixture of fat and glucose is a trade-off, the best compromise appears to be to individualize support for specific clinical settings. A patient with respiratory failure who is nonseptic and who is weaning from mechanical ventilation, for example, may benefit from a formula with a low carbohydrate and high lipid content,

TABLE 10–5.
Measurement of Metabolic Rate by Indirect Calorimetry (Measurements Made at Rest).

Caloric requirements = REE × activity factor

REE = 3.94 × $\dot{V}O_2$ + 1.11 × $\dot{V}CO_2$

while a stable postoperative patient will not be adversely affected by an all-glucose formula. Neither glucose nor long-chain triglyceride emulsion appear to be optimal materials, and other caloric substrates are currently under study.

In any event, it is necessary to provide at least 500 cc of 10% lipid emulsion composed of long-chain fatty acids twice weekly for patients receiving hypertonic glucose in order to prevent essential fatty acid deficiency (EFAD). Interestingly, EFAD does not develop in patients who are starved; apparently the elevated insulin levels which are stimulated by all glucose regimens prevent mobilization of essential fatty acids from peripheral stores.

A reasonable approach in patients with critical illness may be to slightly overestimate caloric intake and provide 25–50% of calories by lipid emulsion each day. Infusion of glucose at rates higher than 5–7 mg/kg/min, even in the most hypermetabolic patients, has not been shown to increase glucose oxidation. Even at this rate of infusion, as little as 50% of glucose was oxidized.[53,54] Septic patients, especially those with mixed venous oxygen tensions greater than 40 mm Hg, may be unable to oxidize infused glucose and may exhibit respiratory quotients higher than 1.0 even when glucose is infused at less than the metabolic rate.[55]

Exogenous Insulin

Several studies have convincingly demonstrated improved nitrogen balance for highly catabolic patients (but not mildly catabolic patients) when exogenous insulin is infused to maintain blood sugar in the 75–150 gm/dl range, presumably due to its action on skeletal muscle.[14,16] Few side effects are observed if glucose is not infused at excessive rates and if adequate amounts of amino acids are also infused. Progressively increasing insulin requirements are often an early indication of sepsis or other untoward event. Conversely, the patient recovering from illness may unexpectedly develop hypoglycemia; this should alert the physician that "stress metabolism" is ongoing, possibly due to unrecognized sepsis.

Determination of Protein Requirements

The minimum amount of protein required for maintenance of body protein is not known with certainty. The World Health Organization has suggested that 0.6 grams of protein/kg/day be considered the minimum daily amount necessary, but this level has not been universally accepted. Not surprisingly, the optimal amount of protein required for individuals with critical illness is even less well understood. For optimal protein synthesis, amino acids should be administered in the molar proportions necessary for protein synthesis. Deficiency of any one essential amino acid renders a proportion of the remaining amino acids unusable for incorporation into body stores.

Relationship Between Nitrogen Intake and Nitrogen Balance

Increasing nitrogen intake, at constant caloric intake, produces a linear increase in nitrogen balance similar to the relationship between caloric intake and nitrogen balance.[56] Studies of normal individuals at steady state consistently have shown, even under the most rigorous experimental conditions, that increasing nitrogen intake to rates commonly infused into highly catabolic patients produces markedly positive nitrogen balance on the order of 10 grams of nitrogen per day.[57] After several days of high protein intake, the positive nitrogen balance falls to one to three grams of positive nitrogen balance without any increase in body mass. Thus, increasing nitrogen balance by increased protein feeding itself may not necessarily have an anabolic effect. While study of total body protein synthetic rate has been attempted,[58] methodologic problems prevent complete acceptance of their results.[59] Isotope dilution techniques suffer from the fact that lean body mass is calculated from total body exchangeable potassium; since potassium may become repleted more rapidly than nitrogen during the initiation of nutritional support, the technique may not be applicable to the study of nitrogen balance.

Defective Net Protein Utilization During Highly Catabolic States

It is unclear why net protein utilization, a measure of the proportion of an ingested protein load which is incorporated into protein stores, is defective during highly catabolic states.[60] This defect appears to be corrected by infusing greater than normal quantities of amino acids, suggesting either a relative deficiency of one or more essential amino acids or impaired ability to utilize amino acids for protein synthesis. Diminished uptake of amino acids by muscle of septic individuals has been demonstrated.[61]

It is difficult to determine the appropriate infusion rate of amino acids in highly catabolic patients. In the absence of convincing information, however, it appears wise to maximize the chances of efficacy by infusing higher than normal quantities of amino acids. The presence of a negative nitrogen balance is good evidence that endogenous protein stores are diminishing. Generally, 1.5–2.0 grams of amino acids per kilogram per day are recommended for septic,[62] multiple trauma,[56] and burn[57] patients based on nitrogen balance studies.

BCAA-enriched Formulas

The idea of enriching conventional amino acid formulas with branched-chain amino acids arose in part from the observation that catabolic muscle appears to consume its own BCAA. In addition leucine, a BCAA, appears to enhance muscle protein synthesis both directly and by stimulating insulin secretion. The advantage of BCAA has not been accepted by all investigators, since conventional formulations administered in the proper proportions can generally reduce apparent nitrogen loss to acceptable levels, even in highly catabolic individuals. A recent study in septic patients demonstrated that administered leucine was cleared from the circulation while clearance was impaired for other amino acids. This difference was observed in patients who ultimately died but not in those who survived.[63]

The studies which have prospectively compared nitrogen balance during infusion of conventional versus BCAA-enriched formulas have had mixed results; some have shown improved nitrogen retention with BCAA while others have not. The differences between the two techniques have been small, however, and may not be clinically significant. Since the cost of BCAA-enriched mixtures is substantial, and the results not clearly better than those with conventional mixtures, their use should probably be limited to experimental situations.[59]

Hepatic Formulations

Hepatic encephalopathy has generally been associated with large protein loads, although the pathogenesis of the disorder is not well understood. Treatment usually requires malnutrition-inducing therapy. One theory of pathogenesis is related to the inability of the diseased liver to clear those amino acids not metabolized by skeletal muscle, kidneys, and GI tract. Aromatic amino acid concentrations rise while BCAA are relatively low. Aromatic amino acids may serve as substrates for the synthesis of false neurotransmitters, and their high concentration in the circulation may be one reason for the development of encephalopathy. Since aromatic and BCAA compete with each other for passage across the blood-brain barrier, a high aromatic to BCAA serum level may predispose to encephalopathy.[64,65] Amino acid formulations supplemented with BCAA and deficient in aromatic amino acids have been developed to test the hypothesis that shifting the unfavorable amino acid ratio might improve encephalopathy. Studies evaluating the efficacy of BCAA-enriched and deficient aromatic amino acids supplements have not revealed impressive results.

Renal Formulations

Nutritional support programs for patients with acute renal failure are complicated because blood urea levels are related to amino acid catabolic rates as well as excretory function. Blood urea will rise in the absence of nutritional support because of the catabolism of endogenous amino acids. If conventional amino acid support is used, however, urea levels rise even faster because of defective net protein utilization in catabolic patients. Formulas containing only essential amino acids and adequate calories reduce and may stop the progressive rise in urea concentration that would otherwise occur. Most likely, the majority of these amino acids are utilized for protein synthesis while those amino acids released from endogenous protein breakdown may be scavenged and used for synthesis of the remaining nonessential amino acids. These formulas contain twice the amount of essential amino acids found in conventional amino acid mixtures and are, therefore, twice as effective.[66] Provision of excessive quantities may cause the blood urea to rise since there is a limit to the quantity which can be incorporated into native protein; however, inadequate quantities are ineffective, and the BUN also rises. The optimal amount of essential amino acid supplementation has not been determined with great accuracy, but it is probably appropriate to administer approximately half the quantity of conventional amino acids that would normally be given to a patient with the same disease-state without renal failure. The administered amount can be decreased if the BUN rises rapidly. More than 0.75 grams per kilogram per day should not be administered however, because hyperammonemic encephalopathy has been reported.

The problem is even more complicated when oliguria or anuria occurs. The amino acid support necessary to keep the BUN at manageable levels almost always leads to fluid overload. Dialysis or ultrafiltration is the price that must be paid for adequate nutritional intervention. If frequent dialysis becomes necessary for volume overload, it may be less expensive and equally effective to use conventional amino acid formulations.

Ions

Fuel and protein are valueless unless essential nutrients required for their utilization are also available. Those ions which are sequestered primarily in the intracellular space—phosphorous, potassium and magnesium—are particularly important. Profoundly diminished serum levels may follow within hours of initiating nutritional support, particularly for emaciated patients as the intracellular ion concentrations become rapidly repleted. Failure to anticipate this phenomenon may lead to unexpected complications. As much as 100 millimoles of phosphorus or magnesium and even greater quantities of potassium may be required in the initial 24 hours; thus, it is important to check serum levels of these substances within six hours of initiation of nutritional support in those patients who are most malnourished. Only usual amounts of these ions should be placed in the initial formula; supplemental quantities may be infused separately. Concentrations of ions should then be checked daily until stable. Generally, approximately 10–15 millimoles each of calcium, magnesium, and phosphorous are required per day when steady state has been reached.

A variety of humoral and hemodynamic responses lead to the retention of electrolytes and fluid in critically ill patients. Administration of standard volumes of nutritional formula frequently necessitates administration of a diuretic. Since hyponatremia commonly occurs with diuretic therapy, sodium must be added to the nutritional support formula. Metabolic acidosis with or without an anion gap is frequently observed in critically ill patients.[67] Sodium administered as the acetate rather than the chloride salt is useful since it is converted to bicarbonate within the liver.

Vitamins

Premixed solutions containing all the vitamins necessary for normal patients are commercially available. Whether these may adequately serve the needs of various critically ill populations is not clear. Increased quantities of vitamin C may enhance wound healing. Vitamin A may counter the deleterious effect on wound healing for those patients who require steroids.

Trace Elements

Mixtures of trace elements are also available commercially. Caution should be exercised when providing these to patients with acute renal failure who cannot excrete zinc or chromium, and for patients with biliary obstruction who may not excrete copper and manganese. Acutely catabolic patients and those with increased intestinal losses may have increased requirement for zinc. The Expert Panel for Nutrition Advisory Group of the American Medical Association recommends that an additional 2 mg of zinc be infused per 24 hours for adults in acute catabolic states but recommends frequent serum monitoring.[68]

MODES OF DELIVERY

Full nutritional supplementation may be provided orally, enterally, or through a peripheral or central venous catheter. Most critically ill patients are not capable of maintaining adequate oral intake.

Enteral Alimentation

Enteral feeding compared to intravenous feeding is considerably less expensive and generally safer when proper precautions are taken. Comparative studies have found that enteral intake (when absorbed) is at least as effective as intravenous supplementation. Thus, this option should always be considered first.

Sites of Delivery

Pulmonary aspiration is the greatest danger of this form of therapy, particularly for ventilator-dependent patients during weaning trials and other patients experiencing respiratory distress. Deviation of blood flow from the GI tract to the respiratory musculature (a well-recognized phenomenon during exercise) may produce a degree of gastric atony while the pumping action of the diaphragm on the stomach may then lead to regurgitation. Frequent assessment of gastric residual volume may prevent this potentially disastrous complication. Failure to check even a single residual volume at high infusion rates may result in the accumulation of a large gastric volume.

Duodenal or jejunal placement of the feeding tube fluorosopically may circumvent this problem. The stomach and large bowel are generally the first to succumb to and the last to recover from ileus. Thus, even when the stomach is atonic, nutrients may be absorbed from the small bowel. Even this approach is not entirely satisfactory, since critically ill patients may develop paralytic ileus without warning. Duodenal feeding may also occasionally result in aspiration. One approach that circumvents this problem is the use of two lumens, one ending in the duodenum for infusion of nutrients and one in the stomach to check residual volumes and administer antacids. This approach may occupy both of the patient's nostrils and should be reserved for patients at greatest risk.

Factors Predisposing to Diarrhea

Severe diarrhea frequently limits the effectiveness of enteral formulations despite intact propulsive function of the GI tract. The catabolism of critical disease-states frequently leads to villous atrophy and diminished ability of the intestine to synthesize lactase and other digestive enzymes. Antibiotic administration may lead to bacterial overgrowth or pseudomembranous colitis. Formulations containing a good deal of fat or of high osmolarity often cause diarrhea, even at lower infusion rates. One approach to the treatment of diarrhea in this setting is the reduction of osmolarity by dilution or the use of powdered rice formula (long-chain polymers of low osmotic strength) for part of the administered calories. Provision of bacterial spores (Lactinex) is occasionally beneficial for patients who have received courses of broad spectrum antibiotics. Only lactose-free formulas should be provided. Medium-chain triglyceride oil is less likely to produce diarrhea than LCT (safflower) oil. Kaopectate is occasionally useful. Narcotic agents occasionally become necessary; however, they frequently lead to prolonged ileus.

Premixed Versus Modular Formulations

Availability of premixed formulations should not be an excuse to avoid calculating or delivering required nutrients. A number of protein, fat, and carbohydrate supplements are available that can be added to premixed formulas in order to achieve desired goals. In addition, a complete modular enteral feeding system recently has become available.

Peripheral Venous Administration Delivery

Long-term ICU patients most in need of nutritional support are frequently the same ones who lack peripheral venous access.

Protein Sparing Therapy

One approach to reducing the administered volume of fluid has been the administration of glucose and amino acids. While this protects part of endogenous protein, it is not applicable to most critically ill patients. Two hundred grams of glucose per day markedly curtails nitrogen loss for normal individuals by suppressing gluconeogenesis from endogenous amino acids, but has little impact on the quantity of nitrogen lost by highly catabolic patients. Isolated amino acid infusion at 1.7 gm/kg/24 hours has been shown to produce near nitrogen equilibrium in several studies of postoperative patients; however, few have attempted to correct for the marked rise in BUN that generally occurs.[47,48] A failure to excrete synthesized urea may be one reason for a near zero nitrogen balance. On the other hand, a number of investigators have documented an increase in protein synthetic rate when amino acids are infused in the absence of additional caloric intake. The applicability of this form of therapy for highly catabolic critically ill patients is unclear.

Full Support

It is possible to infuse 2,250 calories and 82 grams of protein in a three liter volume; 1,500 of these calories are derived from the lipid emulsion. The addition of one unit of heparin per cc of solution and the infusion of 10% lipid emulsion at the same rate as the amino acid-dextrose solution produces a final osmolality of 900 mOsm/liter. This mixture is generally tolerated by most veins and can be made by mixing equal volumes of D_{20} and 10% amino acids.

Central Venous Alimentation

In many respects, central venous infusion is the most direct approach to hyperalimentation, since volumes may be minimized, calculations are easier, and there is usually no question regarding absorption. It is safe and effective in the hands of the experienced clinician; however, occasional complications are unavoidable, and the choice between enteral and central venous support should be made with care.

Sites of Delivery

Cannulation of the subclavian vein is preferable because it is easier to apply a truly occlusive dressing at this site, since it allows free rotation of the neck and because, in males at least, growth of hair is slower here. However, the internal jugular vein is also frequently used. The tip of the catheter should be positioned in the superior vena cava. The choice of larger vessels with relatively high flow rates reduces the likelihood of irritation and thrombosis associated with solutions of high osmolarity. Perforation of the ventricle has been reported when stiff catheters are inserted to excessive lengths, and fluoroscopy should be utilized when available. Solutions for total parental nutrition (TPN) can be infused through the proximal port of Swan-Ganz catheters, but infusion of hypertonic glucose-insulin-potassium through the distal port has resulted in pulmonary infiltrates. It is not clear whether cellophane sheaths maintain true sterility of the transdermal portion of the Swan-Ganz catheter, so it may be prudent not to infuse TPN solutions through introducer sheaths even though there is no information indicating that solutions containing crystalline amino acids are any more likely to become infected than are other glucose containing solutions (see below).

TPN Associated Sepsis

The TPN associated sepsis rate is approximately 2% or less in most institutions where hyperalimentation teams stress strict aseptic technique. Careful line insertion and a precise protocol for the meticulous changing of dressings by a well trained and experienced team is necessary to achieve this low rate. Most evidence indicates that the most important cause of these infections is infection of the dermal tunnel through which the catheter passes. Blood and other material favorable to bacterial growth should be removed prior to application of the dressing. The skin and exposed catheter should be treated with antiseptic to prevent infection of the dermal tunnel, and a new dressing applied every two days (see chapter 11).

Total parenteral nutrition may lead to infection in other ways. Amino acid-glucose solutions suppress growth of most organisms, although *Candida* grows well. Lipid emulsions support the growth of many organisms that may enter through the air portal, which is protected by a millipore filter. The internal lumen of the catheter may become colonized, particularly when the line is violated repeatedly; for this reason lumens committed to TPN should be used for no other purpose. Finally, after several days, a fibrin sheath forms on the intravascular portion of most catheters; during an episode of bacteremia this may become colonized and subsequently protect bacteria from antibiotic action. Thus, catheters should be removed after periods of known or suspected bacteremia.

It seems likely that as long as the nutrient solution is mixed aseptically, TPN lines are no more likely to lead to catheter associated sepsis than other central venous lines except that they usually are left in place for longer periods of time. Knowledge of pathophysiology and careful attention to detail should reduce sepsis rates to acceptable levels (less than 2%).

COMPLICATIONS CAUSED BY NUTRITIONAL SUPPORT

A number of iatrogenic complications occur with TPN. Decreased serum levels of the various ions, volume overload, essential fatty acid deficiency, pulmonary aspiration, hyperglycemia, and catheter sepsis have been discussed above. Several additional problems have also been observed.

Increased Oxygen Consumption

The term specific dynamic action is used to describe the normal increase in oxygen consumption following ingestion of a meal that is required to convert excess fuel intermediates into glycogen or fat. This increase in unstressed patients is generally small. Oxygen consumption may increase by as much as 20–30% in injured or septic patients infused with glucose at rates 1.75 to 2.25 times the fasting metabolic rate.[43] Such increases in O_2 consumption may overly burden a circulatory system impaired by sepsis, shock, or acidosis. Caloric replacement in such patients should be limited to the amount calculated from the Harris-Benedict equation and should not include extra calories added for presumed stress. Since lipids do not appear to raise oxygen consumption to the degree observed with carbohydrates, mixtures prepared for individuals with hemodynamic compromise should not contain more than half of their calories as glucose.

Increased CO_2 Production

Nutritional supplementation may also produce large increases in carbon dioxide excretion. This may be partly due to increased oxygen consumption, but two other factors are also important in patients receiving large quantities of carbohydrate. The respiratory quotient for carbohydrate oxidation is 1.0 compared to 0.7 for fat. Since the respiratory quotient for a starving patient is generally near 0.8, raising the respiratory quotient to 1.0 with exogenous carbohydrate will, even without raising O_2 consumption, increase carbon dioxide excretion by 25%. In addition, only about 50% of infused glucose is oxidized; a portion of the remainder may be converted to lipid. During lipogenesis from glucose, only four of every six carbons are used for lipid synthesis; the rest enters the circulation and is part of the up to 50% increase in CO_2 production observed in injured or septic patients.[43] Infusion of glucose at high rates in hypermetabolic septic patients with mixed venous oxygen saturations greater than normal increased the respiratory quotient to 1.2.[55]

The degree to which increased CO_2 production requires increased minute ventilation depends upon the dead space to tidal volume ratio (VD/VT). A patient with a

VD/VT of 0.66 must increase minute ventilation twice as much as a patient with a VD/VT of 0.33 in order to achieve the same P_{CO_2}. Infusion of carbohydrate at twice the metabolic rate has resulted in a doubling of minute ventilation for ICU patients.[43] Nutritional regimens rich in lipid produce lesser degrees of CO_2 excretion and lower respiratory quotients.

Azotemia

Elevated urea levels may be due to either decreased excretion or to increased synthesis. Increased synthesis may be due to either an increased endogenous catabolic rate or to administration of exogenous protein at a rate in excess of the patient's ability to incorporate it into endogenous stores. Administration of nutritional support will generally increase urea synthesis because of defective protein utilization and mobilization of amino acids from the periphery. Nitrogen balance, however, may increase and should be measured at regular intervals and at varying amino acid intakes. Nitrogen balance is not an accurate reflection of urea synthesis in patients with rising BUN (see above), but can be corrected by estimating changes in the total body urea pool. This can be done by weighing patients at 24-hour intervals, estimating total body water, and multiplying by serum urea concentration. Essential amino acids should be considered if uremia becomes excessive.

Abnormal Hepatobiliary Function

Liver function abnormalities have been observed in patients receiving parenteral but not enteral hyperalimentation. The wide range of proposed etiologic agents—dextrose, lipid emulsion, amino acid solutions, endotoxin, choline deficiency— suggest a multifactorial process. Biopsy specimens have revealed fatty infiltration and glycogen accumulation; histologic inflammation is unusual. Calculus or acalculus cholecystitis is a recognized complication of long-term TPN and is occasionally observed in ICU patients who may be asymptomatic.[69] Rising bilirubin, alkaline phosphatase, or transaminase should prompt a reevaluation of caloric and amino acid requirements. Substitution of some of the calories with lipid emulsion in patients receiving high glucose concentrations may reverse enzyme changes.

REFERENCES

1. Cuthbertson DP: Observations on the disturbance of metabolism produced by injury to the limbs. *Q J Med* 1932; 1:233–246.

2. Reifenstein EC, Fuller A, Wells SL: The accumulation, interpretation, and presentation of data pertaining to metabolic balances, notably those of calcium, phosphorus, and nitrogen. *J Clin Endocrinology* 1945; 5:367–393.

3. Cahill GF: Starvation in man. *N Engl J Med* 1970; 282:668–675.

4. Wolfe BM, Culegras JM, Sim AJW, et al: Substrate interaction in intravenous feeding. Comparative effects of carbohydrate and fat on amino acid utilization in fasting man. *Ann Surg* 1977; 186:518–540.

5. Long CL, Kinney JM, Geiger JW: Nonsuppressability of gluconeogenesis by glucose in septic patients. *Metabolism* 1976; 25:193–201.

6. Rennie MJ, Millward DJ: 3-methylhistidine excretion and the urinary 3-methylhistidine/creatinine ratio are poor indicators of skeletal muscle protein breakdown. *Clin Sci* 1983; 65:217–225.

7. O'Donnell TF, Clowes GHA, Blackburn GL, et al: Proteolysis associated with a deficit of peripheral energy fuel substrates in septic man. *Surgery* 1976; 80:192–200.

8. Clowes GHA, Randall HT, J Cha C: Amino acid and energy metabolism in septic and traumatized patients. *JPEN* 1980; 4:195–205.

9. Daly JM, Mihranian MH, Kehoe JE, Bren-

nan MF: Effects of postoperative infusion of branched chain amino acids on nitrogen balance and forearm muscle substrate flux. *Surgery* 1983; 94:151–158.

10. VanderWoude P, Morgan R, Kosta JM, et al: Addition of branched-chain amino acids to parenteral nutrition of stressed critically ill patients. *Crit Care Med* 1986; 14:685–688.

11. Clowes GHA, Hirsch E, George BC: The significance of altered protein metabolism regulated by proteolysis inducing factor, the circulating cleavage product of interleukin-1. *Ann Surg* 1985; 202:446–458.

12. Levenson SM, Watkin DM: Protein requirements in injury and certain acute and chronic diseases. *Fed Proc* 1959; 18:1155–1190.

13. Bessey PQ, Watters JM, Aoki TT, Wilmore DW: Combined hormonal infusion stimulates the metabolic response to injury. *Ann Surg* 1984; 200:264–281.

14. Woolfson AMJ, Heatley RV, Allison SP: Insulin to inhibit protein catabolism after injury. *N Engl J Med* 1979; 300:14–17.

15. Hinton P, Allison SP, Littlejohn S, Lloyd J: Insulin and glucose to reduce catabolic response to injury in burned patients. *Lancet* 1971; 767–769.

16. Brooks DC, Bessey PQ, Black PR, et al: Insulin stimulates branched chain amino acid uptake and diminishes nitrogen flux from skeletal muscle of injured patients. *J Surg Res* 1986; 40:395–405.

17. Arora NS, Rochester DF: Effect of body weight and muscularity on hyman diaphragm muscle mass, thickness and area. *J Appl Physiol* 1982; 52:64–70.

18. Arora NS, Rochester DF: Respiratory muscle strength and maximal voluntary ventilation in undernourished patients. *Am Rev Respir Dis* 1982; 126:5–8.

19. Marcotte JE, Canny GJ, Grisdale R, et al: Effects of nutritional status on exercise performance in advanced cystic fibrosis. *Chest* 1985; 90:373–379.

20. Faulk WP, Demaeyer EM, Davies AJS: Some effects of malnutrition on the immune response in man. *Am J Clin Nutr* 1974; 74:638–646.

21. Keenan RA, Moldawer LL, Yang RD, et al: An altered response by peripheral leukocytes to synthesize or release endogenous mediator in critically ill, protein-malnourished patients. *J Lab Clin Med* 1982; 100:844–856.

22. Leiter LA, Marliss EB: Survival during fasting may depend on fat as well as protein stores. *JAMA* 1982; 18:2306–2307.

23. Abel RM, Beck CH, Abbott WM, et al: Improved survival from acute renal failure after treatment with intravenous essential l-amino acids and glucose. Results of a prospective, double-blind study. *N Engl J Med* 1973; 288:695–699.

24. Baek SM, Makabali GG, Bryan-Brown CW, et al: The influence of parenteral nutrition on the course of acute renal failure. *Surg Gynecol Obstet* 1975; 141:405–408.

25. Giacchino JL, Geis P, Wittenstein BH, et al: Surgery, nutritional support and survival in patients with end-stage renal disease. *Arch Surg* 1981; 116:634–640.

26. Rapp RP, Young B, Twyman D, et al: The favorable effect of early parenteral feeding on survival in head-injured patients. *J Neurosurg* 1983; 58:906–912.

27. Esgaib AS: Parenteral nutrition (PN) as a useful method on weaning patients off mechanical ventilation (MV). *JPEN* 1978; 2.

28. Bassili HR, Dietal M: Effect of nutritional support on weaning patients off mechanical ventilators. *JPEN* 1981; 5:161–163.

29. Sganga G, Siegel JH, Brown G, et al: Reprioritization of hepatic plasma protein release in trauma and sepsis. *Arch Surg* 1985; 120:187–199.

30. Dahn MS, Jacobs LA, Smith S, et al: The significance of hypoalbuminemia following injury and infection. *Am Surgeon* 1985; 51:340–343.

31. Rothschild MA, Oratz M, Schreiber SS: Albumin synthesis. *N Engl J Med* 1972; 286:748–757 and 286:816–821.

32. Courtney ME, Greene HL, Folk CC, et al: Rapidly declining serum albumin values in newly hospitalized patients; prevalence, severity, and contributory factors. *JPEN* 1982; 6:143–145.

33. Starker PM, Gump FE, Askanazi J, et al: Serum albumin levels as an index of nutritional support. *Surgery* 1982; 91:194–199.

34. Fischer JE, Ghory MJ: Protein deficiency and immunity in the hospitalized patient, in Wright RA and Heymsfield S (eds): *Nutritional Assessment.* Blackwell Scientific Publications Inc, 1984.

35. Seltzer MH, Flecher S, Slocum BA, Engler PE: Instant nutritional assessment in the intensive care unit. *JPEN* 1981; 5:70–72.

36. Kelly SM, Rosa A, Field S, et al: Inspiratory muscle strength and body composition in patients receiving total parenteral nutrition therapy. *Am Rev Resp Dis* 1984; 130:33–37.

37. Heymsfield SB, McManus II, CB, Setiz SB, et al: Anthropometric assessment of adult protein-energy malnutrition, in Wright RA, Heymsfield SB (eds): *Nutritional Assessment.* Blackwell Scientific Publications Inc, 1984.

38. Heymsfield SB, Arteaga C, McManus C, et al: Measurement of muscle mass in humans: Validity of the 24-hour urinary creatinine method. *Am J Clin Nutr* 1983; 37:478–494.

39. Long CL, Schaffel N, Geiger JW, et al: Metabolic response to injury and illness: Estimation of energy and protein needs from indirect calorimetry and nitrogen balance. *JPEN* 1979; 3:452–456.

40. Weissman C, Kemper M, Askanazi, et al: Resting metabolic rate of the critically ill patient: measured versus predicted. *Anesthesiology* 1986; 64:673–679.

41. Field S, Kelly SM, Macklem PT: The oxygen cost of breathing in patients with cardiorespiratory disease. *Am Rev Resp Dis* 1982; 126:9–13.

42. Savino JA, Dawson JA, Agarwal N, et al: The metabolic cost of breathing in critical surgical patients. *J Trauma* 1985; 25:1126–1133.

43. Askanazi J, Rosenbaum SH, Hyman AI, et al: Respiratory changes induced by the large glucose loads of total parenteral nutrition. *JAMA* 1980; 243:1444–1447.

44. Brennan MF, Fitzpatrick GF, Cohen KH, Moore FD: Glycerol: Major contributor to the short term protein sparing effect of fat emulsion in normal man. *Ann Surg* 1975; 182:386–394.

45. Van Lanschot JJB, Feenstra BWA, Vermeij CG, Brunining HA: Calculation versus measurement of total energy expenditure. *Crit Care Med* 1986; 14:981–985.

46. Jeejeebhoy KN, Anderson GH, Nakhooda AF, et al: Metabolic studies in total parenteral nutrition with lipid in man. *J Clin Invest* 1976; 57:125–136.

47. Freeman JB, Stegink LD, Wittine MF, Thompson RG: The current status of protein sparing. *Surg Gynecol Obstet* 1977; 144:843–849.

48. Blackburn GL, Flatt JP, Clowes GHA, O'Donnell TE: Peripheral intravenous feeding with isotonic amino acid solutions. *Am J Surg* 1973; 125:447–454.

49. Kirkpatrick JR, Dahn M, Lewis L: Selective versus standard hyperalimentation. *Am J Surg* 1981; 141:116–121.

50. Baker JP, Detsky AS, Steward S, et al: Randomized trial of total parenteral nutrition in critically ill patients: metabolic effects of varying glucose-lipid ratios as the energy source. *Gastroenterology* 1984; 87:53–59.

51. Hamawy KJ, Moldawer LL, Georgieff M, et al: The effect of lipid emulsions on reticuloendothelial system function in the injured animal. *JPEN* 1985; 9:559–565.

52. Hageman JR, Hunt CE: Fat emulsions and lung function. *Clin Chest Med* 1986; 7:69–77.

53. Burke JF, Wolfe RR, Mullany CJ, et al: Glucose requirements following burn injury; parameters of optimal glucose infusion and possible hepatic and respiratory abnormalities following excessive glucose intake. *Ann Surg* 1979; 190:274–285.

54. Elwyn DH, Kinney JM, Malayappa J, et al: Influence of increasing carbohydrate intake on glucose kinetics in injured patients. *Ann Surg* 1979; 190:117–127.

55. Giovannini I, Boldrini G, Castagneto M, et al: Respiratory quotient and patterns of substrate utilization in human sepsis and trauma. *JPEN* 1983; 7:226–230.

56. Iapichino G, Radrizzani D, Solca M, et al: The main determinants of nitrogen balance during total parenteral nutrition in critically ill injured patients. *Intensive Care Med* 1984; 10:251–254.

57. Soroff HS, Pearson E, Artz CP: An examination of the nitrogen requirements for equilibrium in burned patients. *Surg Gynec Obstet* 1961; 159–172.

58. Wolfe RR, Goodenough RD, Burke JF, Wolfe MH: Response of protein and urea kinetics in burn patients to different levels of protein intake. *Ann Surg* 1983; 197:163–171.

59. Brennan MF, Cerra F, Daly JM, et al: Report of a research workshop: Branched-chain amino acids in stress and injury. *JPEN* 1986; 10:446–452.

60. Iapichino G, Sloca M, Radrizzani D, et al: Net protein utilization during total parenteral nutrition of injured critically ill patients; an original approach. *JPEN* 1981; 5:317–321.

61. Hasselgren PO, Janes JH, Fischer JE: Inhibited muscle amino acid uptake in sepsis. *Ann Surg* 1986; 302:360–365.

62. Long CL, Crosby F, Geiger JW, Kinney JM: Parenteral nutrition in the septic patient: nitrogen balance, limiting plasma amino acids, and calorie to nitrogen ratios. *Am J Clin Nutr* 1976; 29:380–391.

63. Pittiruti M, Siegel JH, Sganga G, et al: Increased dependence of leucine in posttraumatic sepsis: Leucine/tyrosine clearance ratio as an indicator of hepatic impairment in septic multiple organ failure syndrome. *Surgery* 1985; 98:378–386.

64. Jones EA: The enigma of hepatic encephalopathy. *Postgrad Med J* 1983; 59:42–54.

65. Schenker S, Hoyumpa AM: Pathophysiology of hepatic encephalopathy. *Hosp Pract* 1984; 99–121.

66. Tempel G, Jelen S, Jekat F: Investigation of protein metabolism with respect to amino acid administration. *JPEN* 1985; 9:725–731.

67. Kushner RF: Total parenteral nutrition—associated metabolic acidosis. *JPEN* 1986; 10:306–310.

68. Guidelines for essential trace element preparations for parenteral use—A statement by the Nutrition Advisory Group of the American Medical Association. *JPEN* 1979; 3:263–267.

69. Roslyn JJ, Pitt HA, Mann L, et al: Parenteral nutrition-induced gallbladder disease: A reason for early cholecystectomy. *Am J Surg* 1984; 148:58–63.

11 SPECIFIC ETIOLOGIC FACTORS IN CRITICAL ILLNESS

SEPSIS

Almost any acute disease process or physical agent can lead to critical illness. The consequences of these morbific agents have been described in the preceeding pages. Certain of these primary etiologic factors are common enough for special consideration.

Sepsis is often linked to the development of multiple organ system failure because of derangements of organ perfusion, oxygen extraction, and cellular metabolism (chapter 2). Many patients are free of sepsis upon entry into the intensive care unit (ICU) but develop an infection during their stay, which either prolongs their illness or leads directly to their death. An infection rate in ICUs of 18% was documented in the University of Virginia Hospital between 1979 and 1981.[1] Rates of nosocomial infection in units vary markedly, of course, depending on the types of patients, time of sampling, and the degree to which prophylactic measures are enforced. However it is clear that nosocomial infections are extremely common among critically ill patients and contribute significantly to morbidity and mortality.

Immune Depression of ICU Patients

The immune function of most critically ill patients is impaired. Trauma,[2,3] sepsis,[3] burns,[4] malignancy,[5] and malnutrition[6–10] are conditions strongly associated with cutaneous anergy; cutaneous anergy in turn is a powerful predictor of sepsis, morbidity, and mortality in a wide variety of patient groups regardless of its cause.[2,5,6,11,12] Other measures of immune function are frequently also abnormal. Burns greater than 20% of body surface area may produce decreased serum complement, immunoglobulin levels, and other measures of immune function independent of nutritional status.[4] Trauma and burns are associated with defective lymphocyte blast transformation,[13–15] neutrophil chemotaxis,[16–18] and increased numbers of suppressor T cells.[19–21] In addition, fibronectin, a protein which enhances opsonization of gram-positive organisms, frequently is deficient in ICU patients.[21,22] The compromised immune system coupled with the large number of invasive devices implanted or invasive procedures performed on these patients accounts for the high infection rates in the ICU compared to other parts of the hospital (with the possible exception of the hematology/oncology service).

The Gastrointestinal Tract

A sometimes poorly recognized but important source of infection in ICU patients is the gastrointestinal tract. The gut harbors large numbers of bacteria; preventing free access of these organisms to adjacent organ systems are several mechanisms. The *epiglottis* normally prevents aspiration of oral contents. Insertion of an endotracheal tube prevents massive aspiration but permits leakage of small quantities of posterior pharyngeal contents into the trachea.[23] Similarly, impairment of the gag reflex of spontaneously breathing patients for any reason may lead to introduction of pathogenic organisms into the trachea. The acid pH of the *stomach* normally sterilizes gastric contents between feedings; however, the accepted practice of gastric acid neutralization for stress ulcer prophylaxis may permit pathogenic bacteria to proliferate; the stomach has been found to be a significant source of tracheal colonization and subsequent infection in mechanically ventilated patients.[23] Infusion of enteral feedings which have become contaminated may increase this risk.[24] For this reason it is recommended that enteral feeding solutions and equipment be changed at frequent intervals.[25] The *gall bladder* is normally sterile, due in part to the frequent contraction of this organ. Patients receiving long-term TPN have an increased incidence of gallstones and/or biliary sludge and, consequently, calculous and acalculous cholecystitis.[25A] This may be due in part to the lack of enteral stimulation to contract. The *intestinal epithelium* normally prevents entry of intestinal bacteria into the portal circulation; a possible role of an impaired intestinal epithelial barrier in critically ill humans is suggested by animal studies.[26,27] Intestinal mucosal integrity may become impaired during ischemia[28] or because of catabolism of the gastrointestinal mucosa.[29] The *liver and hepatic reticuloendothelial system* may play an important role in protecting the systemic circulation from gastrointestinal tract-derived endotoxin; portal venous endotoxemia is common even in otherwise normal individuals postoperative from elective surgery.[30] Matuschak et al. found 100% mortality among patients with end-stage liver failure who developed hypoxemic respiratory failure, and postulated the existence of a liver-lung axis.[31] Matuschak, Rinaldo, and Van Thiel have subsequently injected endotoxin into the peritoneal space of rats; rats pretreated with N-acetylgalactosamine to produce liver injury manifested a markedly greater mortality rate and acute neutrophilic lung inflammation than mice without liver impairment.[32] Finally, use of broad- spectrum antibiotics predisposes to infection with Clostridium difficele; pseudomembranous colitis is unusual in the ICU population but occasionally does occur. Patients with unexplained diarrhea should be investigated for this pathogen.

The Respiratory Tract

Colonization of the respiratory tract occurs when bacteria are permitted to adhere to host respiratory epithelium; adherence of bacteria to tracheal cells of patients with tracheostomies correlated both with bacterial colonization of the upper respiratory tract and with nutritional status.[33] Colonization of the respiratory tract predisposes to nosocomial pneumonia.[34] Bacteria may be introduced into the respiratory tract from the oropharynx or stomach (see above). The majority of critically ill patients are intubated and exhibit a depressed level of consciousness so that aspiration of greater than normal quantities of bacteria is common. Huxley et al. found that 70% of patients with depressed consciousness aspirated radiolabeled indium injected into the posterior pharynx.[35] In addition to aspiration, bacteria may be introduced into the respiratory tract from contaminated respiratory equipment. For this reason, it is important to maintain asepsis during endotracheal suctioning and to change ventilator tubing and humidifying devices frequently. Many ICU patients develop regional atelectasis due to decreased inspiratory effort or extrinsic compression. Collapsed segments often subsequently become infected. Incentive spirometry, when feasible, is the most effective means of preventing this atelectasis postoperatively. Most endotracheal tubes are constructed of polyvinyl chloride, a substance to which bacteria adhere particularly well.[36] For all these reasons, sputum of intubated ICU patients is rarely sterile. However, since all intubated patients with positive sputum cultures do not develop respiratory infection, the clinician must be guided by the appearance of infiltration on chest radiographs, by the degree of sputum production, and by the appearance of granulocytes on sputum gram stain. Although simple bronchitis rarely produces fever, granulocytosis, or the sepsis syndrome, intubated ICU patients with copious amounts of purulent sputum should be treated with appropriate antibiotics since upper respiratory infections frequently exacerbate bronchospasm and/or delay weaning in the patient who is too weak to clear his airways. Sputum may be collected by several methods. Baigelman recently compared the results of three methods of harvesting sputum from intubated patients with new pulmonary infiltrates; in 12 of 12 patients, the same organisms grew from the sputum obtained by suction through a fiberoptic bronchoscope directed to the area of infiltration, by double-lumen protected sheath brush passed through the bronchoscope or by ordinary endotracheal suction catheters.[37]

Patients intubated nasally with either tracheal or gastric tubes are at increased risk of sinusitis since these cavities may not drain freely. Sinusitis not infrequently is discovered on CAT scans which were ordered to rule out CNS lesions. The fever work-up of any patient who is nasally intubated should include portable sinus films.

The Urinary Tract

Urinary tract infections of varying degrees of severity are common in ICU patients due to the high frequency and duration of bladder catheterization. Organisms may migrate through the urethral meatus around the outside of the catheter or may enter the bladder through the lumen of the tubing. After 10 days of catheterization, the incidence of bacteruria may reach 50%. Bacteruria predisposes to infection but, of itself, is not indicative of infection. Systemic fever, leukocytosis, or other clinical signs of sepsis should not be attributed to a urinary tract infection unless pyuria also is demonstrable (unless the patient is granulocytopenic). Antibiotics usually are not indicated in the bacteruric patient without evidence of pyuria, since resistant strains of organisms are likely to arise. An exception is colonization with Candida; the low toxicity of amphotericin bladder wash compared with the considerable toxicity of systemic amphotericin may justify early treatment of patients with candiduria.[38] Urinary tract infections in patients with nonoliguric renal failure may be somewhat more difficult to treat due to diminished antibiotic penetration of the bladder; for such patients intermittent catheterization may be preferable to continuous indwelling urinary catheterization.

The Central Nervous System

Meningitis does not commonly arise *de novo* in ICU patients unless the subarachnoid space has been disrupted by fracture or by an invasive device. Presence or absence of a stiff neck is of little value in diagnosis. Patients with basilar skull fracture, CSF leak, and brain swelling are particularly difficult to manage; these patients are almost invariably febrile whether or not an infection is demonstrable, they are clearly predisposed to meningitis, and lumbar puncture risks brain herniation. Some clinicians elect to treat such patients based on changes in the clinical examination. Other CNS infections such as brain abscess occasionally arise in bacteremic ICU patients.

Catheter Sepsis

Catheter sepsis arises by one of four basic mechanisms. Most common is migration of organisms down the dermal tunnel formed by the catheter.[39,40] Colonization of the skin surrounding the site of insertion precedes such infections.[41] For this reason, it is essential that dressings be changed frequently and aseptically; this is equally as important as maintaining sterile technique during catheter insertion. Nelson et al. found retrospectively that patients experienced a 28% rate of catheter sepsis when a surgical house officer performed central venous catheter dressing changes compared to a 3.3% rate when a trained nurse performed this task.[42] The second mechanism by which sepsis may arise from a catheter is by bacterial colonization of the tip; a fibrin sheath forms around the intravascular portion of most catheters within three days; following an episode of bacteremia, roughly 20% of catheters will become colonized with bacteria, which then may be shielded by systemic antibiotics.[43–46] The third mechanism of catheter sepsis is colonization of the "hub" or intraluminal segment of the catheter.[46,47] For this reason, it is wise to reduce line invasion to a minimum. Finally, the infusate may become infected. Although TPN solutions are commonly suspect, these actually are less likely than many other fluids to become infected, particularly when they contain crystalline amino acids.[48]

Unfortunately, erythema and induration are both nonspecific and insensitive indicators of catheter sepsis.[49–51] In general, all catheters (including peripheral catheters) which have been in place for three or more days should be replaced in patients who become clinically septic. When the index of suspicion is very low, a catheter may be changed over a guidewire; the intradermal segment of the catheter can be cultured by the semiquantitative method of Maki, Weise, and Sarafin.[39] Should the removed catheter prove to be infected, the site may be changed. At the time of catheter removal, an attempt should be made to express pus from the insertion site; such a finding should raise the clinician's index of suspicion of septic thrombophlebitis, a condition which may be fatal if the vein is not surgically excised.[48,52] Central vein suppurative phlebitis may be managed as endocarditis; surgical intervention should be reserved for recurrent septic pulmonary emboli or refractory sepsis in spite of medical therapy.[48]

Catheter materials, construction, and introduction devices tend to change so rapidly that clinical studies largely have failed to keep pace. Therefore findings of investigators who studied older versions of arterial, central venous, and pulmonary arterial catheters may not apply to newer devices. Nevertheless, most clinicians agree on the following guidelines. Peripheral IV catheters should be changed every 72 hours; centers where they are routinely left in place longer than 72 hours experience infection rates between 2% and 5%.[49] Intra-arterial catheters for blood pressure monitoring should be changed every four days.[43,48] Little data concerning the optimal timing for changing pulmonary arterial catheters is available; Appelfeld et al. studied nonseptic postoperative patients who were monitored with PA catheters; no patient whose catheter was discontinued in less than three days and whose catheter was repositioned less than three times developed positive blood culture.[53] Unfortunately the etiology of sepsis in those patients who manifested positive blood cultures was not clearly catheter-related.[48] The stagnant column of fluid within the low-compliance tubing of pressure monitoring devices and the transducer dome were frequent causes of epidemic sepsis in earlier days; transducers, domes, heparin flush, and tubing administration sets should be changed every 48 hours.[48] Catheters used for total parenteral nutrition become infected more frequently than other catheters, primarily because they are routinely left in place longer. Since these catheters do not become infected with predictable regularity, most experts do not recommend replacement of TPN catheters on a routine basis unless there is suggestive evidence of sepsis.[48] "Triple lumen" catheters recently have been introduced and are suited particularly to the needs of ICU patients who often have limited venous access and who require a multitude of intravenous infusions. Some groups have noted higher infection rates for these catheters than for single-lumen catheters.[54,55] Others, however, have documented infection rates which are similar to those for single lumen catheters.[56,57] A possible reason for the difference in documented infection rates may be the frequency of dressing changes; Pemberton et al.[54] changed dressings one to three times per week while Kelly et al. changed dressings daily or every other day.[56]

Catheters frequently are changed over guidewires in order to spare the patient the risk and discomfort of a new puncture. This is a safe technique if the removed catheter is cultured and the new catheter removed promptly should the removed catheter prove to have been infected.[48] Bozzetti et al. recently changed central venous catheters over guidewires even when the catheters were found to be septic; although they reportedly documented resolution of catheter infection by this method, they cultured catheter tips in broth,[58] a nonspecific method.[39] This practice makes little sense in view of the current understanding of the pathogenesis of catheter sepsis.[48]

The clinician who suspects catheter sepsis, in addition to culturing the blood percutaneously, should send the catheter tip and intradermal segment for culture.[48] A presumptive diagnosis of catheter sepsis is made when 15 or more colonies of bacteria grow by the semiquantitative method and when the identical organisms are grown from blood obtained from a distant site.[39] Maki recommends antibiotic therapy for 7–10 days for critically ill patients with documented catheter sepsis.[48]

Surgical Wounds

Surgical wound infections usually occur relatively late. Streptococcal or Clostridial infections can occur on the first or second postoperative day. However, Staphylococcal infections tend to occur on the third to fourth postoperative day, mixed bacterial infections on the fourth to sixth postoperative day and isolated gram-negative bacterial infection after a week.[59] Intra-abdominal infections that occur as a consequence of bowel leakage are characteristic of the source of leakage. The stomach is generally sterile but may contain aerobic and anaerobic species similar to the mouth. Bile may contain aerobic gram-negative bacilli, enterococci, Clostridium species, or Bacteroides fragilis. The small bowel contains aerobic gram-negative bacilli. The colon contains anaerobes, enterococci, and gram-negative bacilli.[60] The abdominal exam is frequently not helpful for diagnosis, particularly in elderly patients or ICU patients with a diminished level of consciousness. CT scan of the abdomen is often helpful for localizing collections of fluid. Undrained pus almost never is treated adequately with antibiotics alone. Solomkin, Flohr, Quie, and Simmons[61,62] and Marsh et al.[63] have presented evidence that mixed flora infections which contain Candida should be treated with at least low-dose amphotericin.

Management of Septic Shock

The sudden onset of fever, leukocytosis, and hypotension suggests septic shock. It is common in ICU patients. When urine output is maintained within acceptable limits and oxygenation has not deteriorated significantly, right heart catheterization usually is not necessary. Cardiac output is almost always greater than normal. Mixed venous oxygen saturation Sv_{O_2} is generally normal or increased and usually does not vary with oxygen delivery in septic patients. Therefore Sv_{O_2} should not be utilized as a guide to the adequacy of oxygen transport in the septic patient (p. 30). Oxygen consumption tends to increase linearly with oxygen delivery, suggesting that oxygen delivery should be maximized.

The single most important approach to septic shock is volume resuscitation, since the basic circulatory defect is increased capacitance of the vascular bed. Dopamine or dobutamine are useful adjuncts to treatment, usually in doses of 5–15 ug/kg/min, but should not be used unless adequate intravascular volume replacement has been accomplished and further increments in pulmonary capillary wedge pressure do not lead to improved cardiac output. The clinician should not assume, even though calculated systemic vascular resistance is low, that the circulation is uniformly vasodilated. Resistance may be low in some vascular beds which receive increased perfusion, and high in others which are poorly perfused. Administration of a vasoconstrictor agent could further reduce perfusion of a critically underperfused vascular bed. Nevertheless, vasoconstrictor agents such as dopamine or norepinephrine are occasionally necessary in order to maintain adequate pressure to perfuse vital organs. High doses of vasoconstrictors should only be used when arterial pressure falls to extremely low levels, since these drugs may cause regional ischemia. Occasional patients respond with increased blood pressure and urine output despite large doses of norepinephrine; to the extent that renal perfusion mirrors other organ perfusion, urine output may be used as a physiologic guide to vasoconstrictor therapy. Naloxone therapy recently has been found to be useful, at least temporarily, for patients who cannot be weaned from vasopressors. A recommended starting dose is 0.03 mg/kg bolus followed by 0.03 mg/kg/hr continuous infusion.[64] It is usually ineffective in patients with profound shock.

Certain patients, following a prolonged period of septic shock, develop a hemodynamic profile characterized by low cardiac output, increased systemic vascular resistance, and low mixed venous oxygen saturation. Whether such individuals could benefit from higher oxygen transport is usually a moot point, since maximal quantities of fluids and vasopressor agents do not improve performance.

The *sine qua non* of treatment is the selection of proper antibiotic agents and the surgical drainage of abscesses. Failure to choose the correct regimen renders other resuscitative efforts futile. The patient with candida sepsis, for example, who does not receive amphotericin will die despite all other resuscitative efforts. Similarly, undrained pus will provide a continued source of endotoxin and endogenous mediators, which will perpetuate hemodynamic and metabolic abnormalities and cellular dysfunction.[65] The clinician must culture all likely sources rapidly and efficiently and must *immediately* administer antibiotics that will treat effectively all likely etiologic organisms. Antibiotic therapy can be adjusted when culture results become available.

Choice of the best antibiotic agent varies from one hospital to another because of development of characteristic resistance patterns; therefore no recommendations can apply to all situations. Knowledge that the patient in an adjacent bed is colonized with a resistant Pseudomonas, for example, may influence the choice of antibiotics for a patient who develops pneumonia. In general, however, abdominal infections should be treated initially with aminoglycoside, a semisynthetic penicillin, and clindamycin. Pulmonary and urinary tract infections should be treated with a semisynthetic penicillin and an aminoglycoside. Enterococcus must be treated with a semisynthetic penicillin. Catheter sepsis usually is due to staphylococci unless the patient has received multiple antibiotics, where gram-negative bacteria or candida are likely pathogens.

CARE OF THE BURNED PATIENT

A large body surface area burn is one of the most severe stresses which can be borne by the human organism. Loss of the dermal barrier exposes the body almost continuously to life-threatening insults to the immune, thermoregulatory, oxygen transport, protein synthetic, and emotional/psychological apparatus; each of these defense mechanisms may be stressed to the highest tolerable degree, often simultaneously. It is not surprising, therefore, that survival is best among the young and previously healthy; the old and the very young rarely survive a large injury.

The importance of transporting severely burned patients to the nearest burn center cannot be overemphasized. General hospitals which do not contain committed burn units cannot provide optimal care due to lack of proper facilities, specialized medical supplies, and properly trained physicians, nurses, and technicians, each of whom plays a vital role. The intensivist who has not received training in a burn center may not understand the importance of seemingly trivial signs, symptoms, and principles of management.

Initial Evaluation

Dermal damage commonly results from steam, flame, hot liquids, hot objects, chemicals, or electricity. The percentage of body surface area (BSA) which has been injured and the degree of injury of all areas should be estimated and recorded during the initial physical examination. This information is necessary for estimating prognosis, outlining the treatment plan, and anticipating the severity of illness likely to follow. Minor burns (dermal burns of less than 10–15% of body surface area) may be managed on an outpatient basis if provisions can be made for changing dressings regularly by sterile technique and if expert physician follow-up is available. The physician to be responsible for outpatient coverage should be contacted before the patient is sent home. Patients with burns of the face, hands, feet, or perineum may, however, require hospitalization; should a burn in one of these locations become infected, disfiguring or incapacitating scars may result. In addition, patients with circumferential burns around an extremity should be hospitalized; as fluid "leaks" through the disturbed capillary-endothelial barrier, the resulting eschar may swell, leading to compression and devascularization of the distal extremity. In general, patients with burns larger than 10–15% BSA should be hospitalized since "burn shock" (see below) or subsequent septic shock is much more likely to occur with large burns.

In addition to estimating the size of the burn, each burned area should be classified according to the estimated density of viable epithelial regenerative cells. This, of course, is related to the time-honored "degree" of burn and affords an estimate of the likelihood and time needed to attain complete skin regeneration. Epidermal (first degree) burns spare the basal layer of epidermis more or less entirely, permitting complete and rapid regeneration; unlike more serious burns, hyperesthesia is common. Dermal (second degree) burns are characterized by fluid-containing vesicles. Sensation of pinprick may be intact and the underlying wound may blanch with light pressure, indicating preservation of innervation and vascularity. Nests of epidermal cells in hair follicles in deeper layers of the skin permit reconstruction of the dermal barrier within one to three weeks (provided that local infection does not intervene). Deeper dermal burns retain the capability of ultimate dermal regeneration; however, residual epidermal cells are fewer, sensation is not present and the likelihood of scarring is greater. Subdermal (third degree) burns are the most serious, due to total destruction of epidermal regenerative cells. Vesicles may be present, and the skin may appear normal. Sensation is absent.

In addition to the skin, the examiner must pay careful attention to elements of the history and physical examination that suggest injury to other organ systems. *Carbon monoxide poisoning* is common and impairs oxygen transport by diminishing oxygen carrying capacity of the blood. Carboxyhemoglobin levels by Cooximeter should be determined for those patients with suspected inhalation injury. PaO_2 and oxyhemoglobin saturation will be normal.[66] Damage to the *upper airways* should be suspected in any patient with facial burns, singed nasal hairs, hoarseness, carbonaceous sputum, or erythema or edema of the oropharynx. Patients with suspected upper airway injury should be hospitalized and should undergo fiberoptic bronchoscopy by a bronchoscopist familiar with this type of injury.[67] Damage is caused not by direct thermal injury, but rather by irritating gases, chemicals, or particulate matter. Clinical signs of upper airway obstruction may appear abruptly as late as two to three days from the time of injury and may progress to total airway obstruction within a period as brief as 30 minutes; such a course usually is observed in patients with large burns who require large volumes of intravenous fluid for resuscitation. The *pulmonary parenchyma* may be injured independently of the upper airways. The adult respiratory distress syndrome may appear 48–72 hours after the initial injury and may be due to chemical injury of the alveoli or to sepsis occurring at later periods. Although the burn itself often receives the most attention, careful consideration must be given to the possibility of additional *traumatic injuries*, as suggested by a careful history and physical examination. Patients with circumferential burns around an extremity must be examined at frequent intervals to ensure that the distal circulation is intact.

Acute Management

Prior to transport to a burn center, several temporary measures should be considered to ensure continuity of care. Carboxyhemoglobin levels greater than 20% should be treated with inhalation of 100% oxygen; this measure decreases the half-life of carbon monoxide from four hours (breathing room air) to 30 minutes. Patients with stridor or severe respiratory distress should be intubated immediately. Patients with circumferential burns of the thorax are at particularly high risk for respiratory failure as the eschar progressively limits respiratory excursions. Wounds should be covered with dry sterile dressings. Hypovolemic shock may develop rapidly as fluid and proteins leak through the damaged capillary-endothelial barrier; a Foley catheter should be inserted for monitoring urine flow rate, which may serve as a guide to fluid resuscitation. Isotonic saline or lactated Ringer's should be infused at a rate to maintain urine output at 0.5 cc/kg/hour for adults and 1.0 cc/kg/hour for children during transport. Patients with large body surface area burns may require upwards of 20 liters of fluid during the initial 24 hours. A nasogastric tube should be placed in patients with large body surface area burns since adynamic ileus almost invariably is present and predisposes to pulmonary aspiration.

Initial Management in the Intensive Care Unit

Severely burned patients often appear stable in the early hours following admission to the burn unit. The clinician must not be lulled into an unwarranted sense of security, however, since a number of catastrophic events may follow simultaneously or in rapid succession with little warning; hypovolemic or septic shock, airway obstruction, respiratory failure, or loss of distal circulation to a limb. The importance of frequent auscultation of the chest cannot be overemphasized.

Resuscitation

As stated, "burn shock" is the result, partially at least, of extensive loss of plasma from the intravascular space during the first one to three days. This is due to "capillary leak" in both burned and unburned tissues. Maldistribution of blood flow did not appear responsible for shock in a canine model of burn shock; renal and splanchnic flow fell markedly following a 40% dermal burn and were restored nearly to normal following resuscitation.[68] Serum proteins leak from the intravascular space during the initial 24 hours; plasma volume increased spontaneously during the second 24 hours of one clinical study, suggesting a partial improvement of capillary permeability during this period.[69]

In addition to proteins, sodium is also lost from the extracellular space following severe burn injury. This apparently is due to impaired ability of cells within and distant to burned tissues to maintain the normal gradient between intracellular and extracellular sodium and potassium.[70,71] This loss of the transmembrane sodium gradient is observed in other forms of injury as well as burns and contributes to the hypovolemia observed clinically.[70,71]

Colloid appears to play little role in the initial resuscitation of the burned patient. Pruitt, Mason, and Moncrief found no evidence that colloid-containing solutions augmented blood volume more effectively than crystalloid solutions during the early postburn period,[72] suggesting that capillary permeability is increased. Monafo and Ayvazian[73] have reviewed the use of hypertonic saline in patients with increased vascular permeability. Numerous studies have since demonstrated the effectiveness of hypertonic saline solutions in the burn population with regard to decreasing the volume of fluid required for resuscitation.[74–77] Hypertonic saline solutions do not attempt to raise plasma oncotic pressure and increase plasma volume but attempt to shift fluid from the intracellular space to the extracellular space. This treatment is beneficial in situations where increased water administration may be harmful (accumulation of fluid within eschars). During hypertonic saline resuscitation, serum sodium concentration usually is allowed to rise as high as 160; at that point isotonic fluid is substituted for the duration of the resuscitation. This method of resuscitation has been used at a number of institutions and complications other than thirst are rarely observed.

The end-point of resuscitation may be determined by several methods. Many clinicians use urine output as a physiologic guide to the adequacy of volume expansion. Adequate urine flow, it is reasoned, should correlate with adequate renal blood flow. Since renal blood flow is sensitive to a relative or absolute decrease in cardiac output, urine flow should correlate with the adequacy of intravascular volume. Urine output of 0.5 cc/kg/hour for an adult is the minimum volume required to excrete the average quantity of waste generated by a normal individual, assuming normal concentrating ability. The same approach may be used to determine the adequacy of urine flow in burned patients. Increased secretion of ACTH and aldosterone following a severe burn may reduce urine output independently of renal blood flow so that this method might overestimate the quantity of fluid required for resuscitation. Burned patients resuscitated in this manner, however, rarely develop renal insufficiency or other organ dysfunction during the initial period, although randomized prospective studies have not been performed. Another method is the use of formulas to determine the optimal volume of fluid for resuscitation per surface area of burned tissue. Formulas, however, do not allow for individual variability of fluid requirements. Pulmonary artery balloon flotation catheters may be indicated for patients with unexplained low urine flow rates, refractory hypotension, or unexplained pulmonary edema. Long intravascular catheters, however, are associated with an increased incidence of catheter sepsis, possibly due to the increased frequency of bacteremia in these patients. Inotropic or pressor agents occasionally are required for patients with preexisting cardiac disease or for patients who develop septic shock.

Oxygen Transport

Pulmonary artery balloon flotation catheters are generally not necessary since the decreased blood pressure and urine output, due to burn or septic shock, may be improved by volume administration and small infusions of dopamine or dobutamine. Patients who fail to respond rapidly to this therapy may require invasive hemodynamic monitoring. Oxygen transport data, when available, provide a fascinating perspective from which to view the physiology of a critically ill hypermetabolic patient. Burned patients, to a greater degree than most other critically ill patients, consume supranormal quantities of oxygen in the resting state; oxygen consumption as high as three times normal has been documented,[78] although lower values more commonly are observed under resting conditions.[79] A number of reasons for the increased oxygen consumption are apparent. First, loss of the dermal barrier permits loss of considerable quantities of heat. In a classic study, Wilmore demonstrated that oxygen consumption varied in the opposite direction of the ambient temperature; the highest levels of ambient room temperature were associated with the lowest rates of oxygen consumption. Higher rates of oxygen consumption in turn were associated with increased urinary catecholamine excretion. However, when the patients were given alpha and beta blocking agents simultaneously, metabolic rate diminished. Of interest was the finding that all patients who were unable to maintain body temperature subsequently died.[78] Increased oxygen consumption is also thought to be related to increased protein synthetic rate,[80] to increased hepatic metabolic rate,[81] to elevated catecholamine levels,[78] to increased sodium-potassium ATPase activity, and to increased work in breathing.

It is important to recognize the implications of increased oxygen requirements of burned patients when evaluating hemodynamic profiles; a cardiac index of 2.5 liters per minute is rarely adequate to satisfy the oxygen requirements of such patients and generally is associated with hypotension, diminished urine output, and low mixed venous oxygen saturation. The situation is analogous to exercise; burned patients often demonstrate diminished urine output when cardiac output is "normal." Raising cardiac output therapeutically to high levels is often necessary to raise renal and other organ perfusion to acceptable levels.

Infection Control

Following initial resuscitation and stabilization, patients with burns of large body surface areas remain continuously at risk of death from sepsis until an effective dermal barrier is synthesized. Organisms invade the skin and produce systemic signs of sepsis when their concentration approaches 100,000 per gram of tissue.[82] Septic shock often develops with surprising rapidity.

Burned patients are prone to infection markedly, not only because of loss of the dermal barrier, but also because of severe impairment of the immune system. Nearly every imaginable immune defect has been documented, including decreased antibody and complement levels, impaired chemotaxis and phagocytic activity of neutrophils, diminished function of T cells, increased circulating immunosuppressors, decreased macrophage activity, and decreased fibronectin. Burns increase suppressor T cell activity and decrease helper activity, resulting in a shift of the ratio of OKT-4 to OKT-8 cells.[83]

It is obvious, therefore, that considerable effort must be directed at promoting rapid wound healing and preventing infection.[84] Wounds which are clearly devoid of epidermal regenerative cells are usually grafted with split thickness autologous skin as soon as possible. Heimbach demonstrated that early excision and autologous grafting reduced the length of hospitalization and mortality in patients where wound healing was predicted to take more than three weeks.[85] Devitalized tissue is removed (using general anesthesia) as completely as possible. Skin 7–10/1,000 of an inch thick is harvested from normal skin with a dermatome. Coverage is improved by making multiple parallel linear incisions with a meshing device to produce a "fish net" appearance. The wound is covered with a thin gauze dressing which has been soaked with silver nitrate solution. The dressing is soaked with silver nitrate solution every two hours until the first dressing change to keep the skin moist. Wounds which are not grafted with autologous skin may be covered temporarily with synthetic or cadaveric grafts after wound excision.[86,87]

Cultures of uncovered burned tissue should be performed three times weekly; a 2 × 2 inch gauze pad is placed directly on the wound, wetted with sterile lactated Ringer's and cultured[88] A colony count greater than 100,000 is associated with wound invasion and sepsis. Surveillance cultures of all burned areas provide the clinician with early warning of infection, identification of responsible organisms, and drug sensitivities. Ungrafted wounds must be covered with topic antimicrobial agents, usually silver sulfadiazene, at 12 hour intervals. This topical ointment may occasionally produce leukopenia, which does not seem to be associated with an increased infection rate. At the next dressing change, all foreign material must be removed and dead tissue debrided. The wound again is covered with antibiotic ointment, wrapped with sterile gauze dressings of five to six layers, and protected with "Ace" bandages. Dressing changes are extremely painful, and ketamine anesthesia is occasionally necessary. Sterile gloves, cap, mask, and gown are indicated for all dressing changes. Antimicrobial ointments do not sterilize a burn wound, but reduce bacterial growth considerably.

Nutritional Support

Although prospective, randomized clinical trials have not been performed, it generally is agreed that protein-rich nutritional supplementation is essential to survival of this illness. In fact, current knowledge about nutritional support in critically ill patients is based on studies of burned patients. Although attention often is focused on the quantity of calories administered, recent studies have demonstrated that the number of calories burned by most patients is probably not as great as previously suspected.[71] The markedly increased quantity of protein that the patient must synthesize is obvious. Large quantities of protein-rich fluid are lost in burn dressings. A new layer of skin must be synthesized, as must increased quantities of leukocytes, complement, antibodies, platelets, and other proteins. Precursors for this new protein must arise from endogenous stores unless provided exogenously. Urinary protein losses reported for burned patients are greater than any other illness; urinary nitrogen losses as high as 60 grams (equivalent to 375 grams of protein) have been documented.

Spontaneous oral feedings are preferable, and a high protein, high caloric diet should be provided for those individuals able to eat it. Milk shakes including raw eggs should be provided ad lib. Nasogastric feedings, preferably through a duodenal feeding tube should be initiated early in patients unable or unwilling to eat spontaneously. Care must be taken to check gastric residuals frequently since ileus secondary to sepsis is common and may result in pulmonary aspiration. Increasing protein intake to as high as 3 grams per kilogram per day may be beneficial as long as serum urea levels do not rise. For those individuals unable to tolerate either oral or nasoduodenal feeding, intravenous nutritional support must be provided.

Sufficient supplemental insulin to maintain serum glucose between 100 and 150 g/dl has been found to improve nitrogen balance markedly in a prospective randomized study of burned patients.[89] On the other hand, both Burke et al.[90] and Elwyn et al.[91] have found that increasing glucose infusion rates are associated with progressively decreasing glucose oxidation, and that supplemental insulin may lead to accumulation of fat in the liver. All of these findings are consistent with the recent finding that increasing insulin effectively decreases muscle catabolism without necessarily increasing glucose oxidation in highly catabolic patients.[92] Increasing glucose infusion rate may influence nitrogen balance primarily by its effect on skeletal muscle; the glucose-stimulated release of endogenous insulin or infusion of exogenous insulin may be beneficial for skeletal muscle although it promotes accumulation of fat within the liver.

Hyperglycemia almost always is found with severe burn injuries. Normally, glucose infusion stimulates increased insulin secretion. Increased insulin levels in turn alter the glucagon to insulin ratio and block hepatic gluconeogenesis. In addition, increased insulin concentrations lead to increased uptake of glucose by skeletal muscle, an organ system which uses little if any glucose under fasting conditions. The concentration of insulin required to suppress hepatic gluconeogenesis is roughly half the concentration required to increase muscular uptake. Thus, gluconeogenesis is suppressed before peripheral utilization is increased.[93] During burn injury, glucose production is markedly elevated. Superimposition of sepsis causes further increments in the rate of gluconeogenesis. Increased gluconeogenesis is due to hepatic clearance of amino acids, which are released at an accelerated rate from skeletal muscle,[94] to increased Cori cycle activity,[95] and to increased serum concentrations of catecholamines and glucagon. Burned patients clear exogenous glucose less readily than normal patients due to resistance of peripheral tissues to insulin and, in addition, manifest less suppression of hepatic gluconeogenesis.[93]

TRAUMA

Sudden unintended injury is responsible for more loss of potential years of life before age 65 than any other cause. This index differs markedly from the cause-specific mortality per 100,000 population and is sensitive to problems with high prevalence in younger groups. This analysis is important because it specifies a national agenda for health care. The years of potential life lost from unintentional injury are 2,308,000 while the mortality rate is 40.1/100,000. For comparison, malignant neoplasms and diseases of the heart are the second and third causes of lost years; cancer leads to 1,803,000 lost years (191.6/100,000), while cardiovascular diseases lead to 1,563,000 lost years (324.4/100,000). Suicides and homicides are fourth with 1,247,000 years lost (20.6 deaths/100,000). Homicide and suicide rates are highest in young males; more individuals die each year in the United States from automobile accidents than died in the entire Korean war. Peacetime trauma death rates are so high that death rates for young males actually *decline* during wartime.

Wartime experiences have demonstrated the importance of early treatment of severe injuries (see chapter 2), but the advantages of on-site triage and early transportation to appropriate levels of acute care are not generally available during peacetime. Death in injured patients is usually due to the same types of organ failure observed in other critically ill patients. Shoemaker, Appel, and Kram,[96] express the view of a final common pathway leading to death in the following way:

> The major premise is that death in critical illness follows well-defined cardiorespiratory patterns that are independent of the specific clinical diagnosis, accidental or operative traumatic lesions, etc. That is, irrespective of illness or injury, there are a finite number of physiologic events that mark the downhill lethal course and distinguish it from that of survivors. For example, the lethal renal, cardiac, or respiratory failures after pelvic fracture from blunt trauma are not measurably different from these failures after extensive ablative surgery for carcinoma.

While many attempts have been made to rapidly transport injured people to appropriate institutions, the present-day care of injured patients represents a major unfulfilled national health priority. It is one area where medical science is clearly in front of the organizing ability of industrial societies.

Wounds may be penetrating or blunt. The damage produced by stab wounds is usually limited to the tract of entry. Gunshot wounds, in contrast, may produce damage of multiple organs. The damage created by a bullet is related to its weight and the square of its velocity, so that a rifle bullet may produce much more damage than a slowly moving pistol bullet. Blunt trauma leads to the crushing of tissue, to fractures and to deceleration injuries as movable structures move on impact and tear at their attachment to fixed tissues. Hematomas cause problems because of loss of blood from the vascular bed, local compression of vital structures, and the release of vasoactive substances.

The details of surgical care for the traumatized patient are beyond the scope of this text, although the importance of the restoration of oxygen delivery is the key to patient survival. Indeed, the suddenly injured but otherwise healthy individual provides an important model of critical illness. Much early understanding of severe illness was based on the wartime work of Wiggers and his associates in experimental hemorrhagic shock and is detailed in Chapter 2. The Committee on Trauma of the American College of Surgeons has developed an organized approach to the treatment of trauma known as the advanced trauma life support system or ATLS. Initial care is divided into four stages: (1) initial management of immediate life-threatening problems, (2) rapid examination of the entire patient, (3) continued monitoring, and (4) definitive care. A detailed review of this approach has recently been provided by Wilson.[97]

Oxygen delivery must be restored by maintaining ventilation and blood flow. Airway management has been detailed in Chapter 7. Early attempts at airway control, particularly in the field or in the emergency room, must consider the possibility of cervical spine fractures. Extension of the neck must be avoided until radiographic examination has been completed. Foreign bodies including dentures must be removed from the mouth and the tongue must be moved foreward by moving the mandible foreward (the tongue muscles are attached to the anterior mandible). The mandible may be moved foreward by (1) grasping the chin between the index finger and thumb (chin lift), (2) grasping the anterior mandible by placing the thumb inside the mouth behind the incisors (jaw lift) or (3) placing the thumbs behind the mandibular angle (jaw thrust). Other useful devices for maintaining an open airway include the oral airway, the nasopharyngeal airway, and the esophageal obturator airway.

The adequacy of ventilation must be immediately evaluated. Respiratory difficulty may be caused by central nervous system involvement, airway obstruction, contusions of chest wall and lung, pneumothorax, distended abdomen, and injury to the diaphragm. Respiratory failure developing hours after injury is usually due to the adult respiratory distress syndrome (see chapter 7). ARDS following trauma was called "traumatic pulmonary collapse" during World War I and "the wet lung" during World War II. McAslan and Cowley[98] demonstrated the importance of early intubation and mechanical ventilation to prevent respiratory failure and death in their studies at the Maryland Institute for Emergency Medical Services Systems (MIEMSS). They intubated patients based on their integrated clinical evaluation rather than on arterial respiratory gas analysis alone. Patients were intubated and placed on mechanical ventilation if they met the following criteria: (1) history of high speed automobile accident, (2) suspicion of major blunt trauma, (3) a mean arterial pressure less than 60 mm Hg at any one time, no matter how brief, and (4) replacement of more than 20% of blood volume. In addition, patients with impaired consciousness or evidence of pulmonary contusion were also intubated. This "preventive" approach eliminated respiratory failure as a cause of death in trauma and significantly reduced mortality.

The syndrome of fat embolism may resemble ARDS and indeed may itself be considered a cause of ARDS. Wilson et al.[99] studied a group of patients with fractures and found thrombocytopenia, increased circulating fat levels, and decreased arterial oxygen tensions in almost all. The classic fat embolus syndrome occurs 24–48 hours after injury and is characterized by respiratory and central nervous system dysfunction. Conjunctival and cutaneous petechiae, particularly across the upper chest and axilla, are due to thrombocytopenia and deposition of dermal fat. It seems likely that circulating fat particles lead to platelet activation. While increased blood and urinary fat, petechiae and reduced factors V and VII may suggest fat embolism but could also occur in ARDS associated with fractures. Classic ARDS and fat embolism are probably closely related; pharmacologic doses of corticosteroids are probably indicated if the clinical setting fits the criteria for the latter diagnosis.

Certain consequences of chest trauma require special consideration. Several fractures in a single rib produce a flail chest; the affected area bulges paradoxically inward with inspiration. Initial management consists of applying a sandbag over the unstable chest wall region. Mechanical ventilation maintains alveolar ventilation in patients with flail chests, but is not necessary unless there is evidence of abnormal respiratory gas exchange or the patient has evidence of severe trauma.[100] Hemothorax, pneumothorax, or hemopneumothorax usually indicates severe parenchymal injury with potential connections between the airway and pleural space. Subcutaneous emphysema results from the dissection of air either through tears in the parietal pleura or around peribronchial spaces into the hilum and pleural space. Chest tubes should be used to drain blood and control pneumothoraces. Chest tube position should be checked by lateral and posteroanterior chest radiographs in the upright position. Negative pressure is maintained by a water seal bottle which should be 1–2 feet below the patient's chest. The tube should not be clamped since a continuing airway leak could produce a tension pneumothorax. Atelectasis and pulmonary embolism also complicate trauma and are considered in pages 254 and 259.

Alterations in blood flow following trauma produce hypotension or shock. It is almost always due to hypovolemia and must be treated with vigorous fluid resuscitation. The application of military antishock trousers (MAST) in the field delivers 300–1,000 ml of blood from the lower body and may preserve vital organ function during transportation. At least two intravenous lines should be inserted as soon as possible; one should be used to measure central venous pressure. Wilson[97] points out that a subclavian line should be inserted on the injured side of the chest if chest injury is present so that potential complications will not involve the uninjured lung. Arterial blood pressure serves as a guide to fluid replacement. Usually three liters of crystalloid such as Ringer's lactate are infused within 20–30 minutes in hypovolemic and hypotensive patients. Failure to raise blood pressure to 80–90 mm Hg suggests uncontrolled bleeding and is an indication for immediate surgery. Blood should be started after initial resuscitation with crystalloid in an amount equal to the estimated blood loss.

A rapidly falling blood pressure may also be due to pericardial tamponade, tension pneumothorax, or myocardial contusion. Blind insertion of a chest tube (4th or 5th intercostal space, in the axilla) should be performed if there is evidence of respiratory distress. Persistent hypotension with elevated venous pressure suggests pericardial tamponade, which should be immediately treated by pericardiocentesis. Myocardial contusion is diagnosed by evidence of ventricular dysfunction and is best treated with an inotrope such as dobutamine.

Continuing blood loss from lacerated blood vessels is one of the most common causes of traumatic death. Rupture of the thoracic aorta usually produces death within minutes, but some patients with incomplete rupture and an expanding hematoma may survive for one or more hours. Chest trauma is sometimes minimal, and an aortogram is indicated if rupture is suspected. Abdominal bleeding may be difficult to diagnose in patients with blunt trauma but can be identified by peritoneal lavage. Laparotomy is generally performed because of intra-abdominal bleeding and visceral damage. Wilson[97] has listed a series of indications for the procedure: (1) any gunshot wound which may have damaged the peritoneal cavity, (2) penetration of the peritoneum identified by direct vision or by radiographic study, (3) severe and continuing blood loss not explained by other injuries, (4) severe or increasing abdominal tenderness or rigidity, (5) general deterioration, (6) evidence of peritonitis, (7) peritoneal free air, (8) blood in the peritoneal lavage, or (9) an enlarging peritoneal mass.

Wound infection, particularly following abdominal trauma, is a major problem which can be minimized by initial careful surgical care. Unrecognized abscesses may produce nonbacteremic sepsis (chapter 2), and anaerobic infections provide therapeutic challenges. Tetanus can be avoided by prior immunization and the use of immune serum, but other clostridia present perplexing diagnostic and therapeutic problems. Wound botulism, for example, produces cranial nerve dysfunction, may escape detection, and requires treatment with specific antisera. The principles presented earlier in this chapter apply equally to the traumatized patient.

THE ACQUIRED IMMUNODEFICIENCY SYNDROME (AIDS) AND PNEUMOCYSTIC PNEUMONIA

Acute respiratory failure associated with the parasite *Pneumocystis carinii* has become a relatively common reason for hospital admission in recent years. Prior to 1983, most of these patients were recipients of kidney transplants and had been immunosuppressed with cyclosporin. Since then, there has been a striking increase in pneumocystis pneuemonia because of a national epidemic of immunodeficiency produced by infection with the HTLV-III virus now called the human immunodeficiency virus (HIV). Many of these patients are critically ill, but admission patterns to intensive care units vary widely. Fifteen percent of 111 patients admitted to the San Francisco General Hospital for AIDS[101] were admitted to the intensive care unit during the second quarter of 1984. By the last quarter in 1985, 160 patients had been admitted, but only 3% of these were treated in the intensive care unit. Sixty-nine of 415 patients with pneumonia due to *P. carinii* were admitted to the ICU in the years 1983–1985, usually for mechanical ventilation. The hospital death rate for these patients was 87% and averaged 20% per month for all hospitalized patients with the disease. It has never been clear whether patients with respiratory failure associated with severe pneumonitis should be considered to have the adult respiratory distress syndrome although they exhibit the same clinical presentation as other patients with ARDS (dyspnea, cough, diffuse pulmonary infiltrates and severe hypoxemia). Suffredini et al.[102] studied 12 patients with *P. carinii* following renal transplant. Six of these required mechanical ventilation because of progressive respiratory failure and had the clinical criteria for ARDS; five of these survived. Maxfield,

Sorkin, and Fazzini[103] obtained lung biopsies from patients with acute respiratory failure due to *P. carinii.* The alveolar spaces were filled with relatively acellular proteinaceous material and microorganisms with little interstitial infiltration. Patients with ARDS, in contrast, had interstitial and alveolar edema and cellular infiltration.

The Centers for Disease Control first become aware of the AIDS epidemic in the spring of 1981 when 26 cases of Kaposi's sarcoma and 15 cases of *P. carinii* were found in previously health homosexual men from San Francisco and New York City. By December 1982, 878 cases of AIDS had been reported; the cumulative case number increased to 28,098 by December 1986. The CDC[104] estimates that there will be 270,000 reported cases by 1991. Although public concern over casual transmission and infection has reached near hysteria levels, the risk factors for AIDS have been relatively stable. In December 1986, 97% of AIDS patients were either homosexual or bisexual men, IV drug users, persons with hemophilia or other coagulopathies, or heterosexual partners of persons with AIDS or at risk from AIDS. Transmission of HIV among heterosexual partners has been clearly demonstrated. Fischl, Dickinson, and Scott[105] studied the spouses and children of 45 adults with AIDS. 50% of female spouses and 71% of male spouses were antibody positive. Fifteen of 109 children had AIDS, ARC, or persistent generalized lymphadenopathy, and all of these were born to HIV-positive mothers. One percent of all cases in males and 10% of cases in women were associated with transfused blood or blood components. A small and constant percentage of individuals with AIDS does not fall into the recognized risk groups, but continued study of these individuals frequently reveals evidence of other sexually transmitted diseases. A cluster of patients with AIDS in economically deprived areas of Western Palm Beach, Florida suggested arthropod bore infection, but no evidence of this was found. Indeed, the case rate in that area (295/100,000 population) is comparable to that in San Francisco (316/100,000) or New York City (270/100,000). Health workers are not at risk even when they are in close contact with patients with AIDS. Positive antibodies for HIV were not found in over 1,000 health workers who experienced needle sticks while caring for AIDS patients, although three patients with positive antibodies following needle sticks were subsequently reported. This extremely low incidence is in contrast to the infectivity of hepatitis B following inadvertent needle stick.

HIV has an affinity for mononuclear cells and destroys both macrophages and T lymphocytes. Macrophage infection with virus particles could explain the involvement of the brain and other organs. The primary target, however, is the T lymphocyte. Fluorescent-tagged monoclonal antibodies (OKT or leu antibodies) have shown a depletion of T-helper cells ($OKT4^+$) producing an inverted T-helper/T-suppressor cytotoxic ($OKT4^+/OKT8^+$) ratio. A decrease in absolute number of T-helper lymphocytes appears most diagnostic of AIDS, but other conditions can also reduce either the T-helper cell population or invert the ratio.[106,107] Skin test anergy and reduced proliferative responses to in vitro mitogens are also found in AIDS, but may occur later in the disease than abnormalities in T cell subsets. Changes in T-lymphocyte function may also affect B-lymphocyte function, and the common finding of increased immunoglobulins suggests marked changes in B cell function.

The presence of Kaposi's sarcoma, primary lymphoma of the brain, and a group of opportunistic infections (*Pneumocystic carinii,* toxoplasmosis, cryptococcosis, atypical mycobacteriosis, cytomegalic virus, and others) are considered "moderately predictive" of cellular immune deficiency by the CDC. Antibodies to HIV, lymphopenia, skin test anergy to common antigens, and inversion of T-helper/T-suppressor ratios by increasing the suppressor lymphocyte population confirm the diagnosis. Other patients from risk groups with chronic generalized lymphadenopathy, unexplained weight loss, fever, profound malaise and lethargy, thrombocytopenia, and lymphopenia are considered to have the AIDS-related complex (ARC). Thus, patients with antibodies to HIV may be asymptomatic carriers. Three cohort studies in infected homosexuals followed for up to 72 months suggest that 23–26% contracted ARC, and 7–15% contracted AIDS.[108] Polk et al. followed 1,835 men over a median follow-up of 15 months.[109] Fifty-nine developed AIDS. A decreased number of helper T-lymphocytes, an increased number of suppressor lymphocytes, a low level of antibody to HIV, a high titer of cytomegalovirus antibody, and a history of sex with someone who developed AIDS independently predict the subsequent development of AIDS.

Pneumocystis carinii pneumonia has been found in 64% of the 25,834 men reported by the CDC through December 8, 1986. Thus, by the end of 1986, there were somewhat more than 16,000 patients with *P. carinii* pneumonia. *By 1991, the cumulative case total could be more than 150,000 or 100,000 per year with that disease, making it the most common cause of acute respiratory failure.*

Murray et al.[110] estimated in 1982 that 25% of patients with *P. carinii* pneumonia required intubation and mechanical ventilation because of hypoxemic respiratory failure. Physiologic studies in seven such patients were recently described by Maxfield, Sorkin, and Fazzini.[103] Arterial Po_2 averaged 62 mm Hg with an average inspired oxygen concentration close to 50%. The physiologic shunt averaged 43% of cardiac output; the anatomic shunt 34%. These measurements were made with an average of 2 cm H_2 of PEEP. Increase in PEEP to an average of 11 cm H_2 increased arterial Po_2 to 72 mm Hg and decreased the physiologic and anatomic shunts to 37% and 30% of cardiac output, respectively. The arterial-venous oxygen difference was lower than normal (3.1 ml/dl) and did not change with PEEP. Compliance did not change with added PEEP, suggesting either that increased oxygenation was not due to recruitment of additional alveolar units, or that recruitment was not reflected by compliance changes at the level of PEEP studied.

The diagnosis of *P. carinii* should be confirmed by recovery of the agent before treatment is instituted. Bigby et al.[111] showed that the inhalation of a mist of 3% saline generated by an ultrasonic nebulizer produced 2–5 ml of sputum. If microscopic examination of the stained specimens were negative, bronchoscopy and bronchoalveolar lavage were performed. Ninety-three of 113 patients studied were ultimately found to have *P. carinii*; the parasite was found in the sputum in 78% of these individuals. Either trimethoprim-sulfamethoxazole or pentamidine has been used in treatment. Wharton et al.[112] compared the two agents in 41 patients. Death rates during the 21 day treatment period were 25% for trimethoprim-sulfamethoxazole and 5% for pentamidine. Seventy percent of the former group and 55% of the later group developed major complications that included neutropenia and thrombocytopenia, azotemia, increased liver enzymes, severe rash, or toxic delirium. None of the treatment differences reached statistical significance, and the authors concluded that the two agents are "probably of equal effectiveness in treating pneumonia caused by *P. carinii* in patients with

AIDS. Although the rates of adverse reactions are nearly identical, the kinds of reactions are somewhat different."

Since there are no known survivors from AIDS, the ethical implications of admission to ICUs become critically important. Forty of the 45 patients with *P. carinii* who were intubated and mechanically ventilated at the San Francisco General Hospital died. The median survival for the five patients who left the unit was seven months and the medial survival for all hospitalized patients with *P. carinii* was eight months. This is strikingly different from outcomes in patients with *P. carinii* following renal transplantation. Reduction in pharmacologic immunosuppression permits the emergence of cell-mediated immunity, and five of the six patients with respiratory failure reported by Suffredini et al. survived.[102]

The San Francisco General Hospital group supported the right of competent patients to decide whether they wished to undergo potentially painful and probably futile treatment. A study of 188 patients with AIDS by Steinbrook et al.[113] revealed that 45% would not want intubation and mechanical ventilation, even though their answers to a questionnaire indicated they were unrealistically optimistic over the outcome of such care, believing that 53% survived hospital care compared to the actual 13%. Physicians expressed similar views.[101] Most of the resident (82%) and attending (62%) medical staff stated that they would not wish to be intubated if they had pneumocystis pneumonia and AIDS themselves. They also admitted that their views had changed remarkably over the preceding two years since 80% of the physicians questioned would have recommended intubation earlier. These attitudes on the part of both physicians and patients explains why the ratio of unit to hospital admission for pneumocystic pneumonia declined from 21% to 4% between 1984 and 1985. This experience provides an important lesson for others charged with the care of hopelessly ill but mentally competent young adults. The predicted doubling of incidence over the next five years suggests close to 100,000 patients each year with Pneumocystis pneumonia by 1991. The 11.2 day length of stay reported by the San Francisco group could cripple critical care facilities by requiring more than one million patient days nationally at a cost of more than one billion dollars annually. Increased investigative efforts to eliminate the causal agent and the more general use of out-of-hospital (hospice) care seem to be the logical approaches to this frightening health care cataclysm.

Drug Overdosage

Drug overdosage must be considered in any individual exhibiting drowsiness, coma, hyperactivity, or other behavioral disturbance. A careful history from patient, family, and friends must evaluate possible ingestion of prescription or nonprescription drugs, controlled substances, cleaning fluids, solvents, and other chemicals.

Lavage and induced vomiting are time-tested techniques for preventing absorption of toxic materials. The stomach normally empties in 2–4 hours so that lavage after that time is useless. Instillation of large volumes of fluid hasten gastric emptying so that dilution of ingested material is not indicated. Lavage of irritant materials such as alkali may injure the esophagus, and aspiration of gastric acid may cause a severe chemical pneumonitis. Intubation or careful positioning and suctioning is necessary to prevent lung damage. Ipecac may be used if the patient is alert. Activated charcoals decrease absorption of most drugs except solvents and inorganic salts.[114] These agents continue to adsorb toxic materials as they pass through the small intestine. A dose of 1 gm/kg up to a maximum of 60 gm every six hours[115] should be administered as soon as the stomach is emptied.

Dopamine-induced or osmotic diuresis will hasten the excretion of many drugs. Ascorbic acid is used to acidify the urine and hasten excretion of basic materials such as phencyclidine and amphetamine. Alkalinization with bicarbonate or acetazolamide increases the excretion of phenobarbital and salicylates. Hemodialysis may be necessary in certain critically ill individuals; direct mixing of blood with a variety of absorbent material (hemoperfusion) removes material much more rapidly than hemodialysis.[116]

Chemical pneumonitis following aspiration leads to a severe form of the acute respiratory distress syndrome. An example of almost unbelievably abnormal arterial blood gases is shown in Figure 11–1. This patient died soon after admission despite intubation and controlled ventilation. There is little evidence that corticosteroids are effective in preventing chemical pneumonitis, and there is some suggestion that they increase the likelihood of secondary infections. Bronchoscopy is indicated if there is evidence of collapse of a major segment or lobe. Bacterial infection of injured bronchoalveolar surfaces is common and should be identified by frequent microscopic evaluation of tracheal aspirate; antibiotics should be added whenever appropriate, but are probably not indicated on a prophylactic basis.

Another complication of drug ingestion is pulmonary edema due to hypoxic or chemical damage in pulmonary capillaries. While a number of agents may alter capillary permeability, opiates have been shown to produce a particularly resistant variety of pulmonary edema, perhaps due to pulmonary venous constriction. Table 11–1 shows acute respiratory failure in a young man who ingested a large quantity of methadone. An elevated pulmonary capillary wedge pressure in the presence of a normal cardiac silhouette and absence of auscultatory evidence of left ventricular failure suggests the possibility of pulmonary venous constriction.

The characteristics of a few relatively common toxic substances are discussed below.

Ethyl Alcohol

Intoxication with ethyl alcohol frequently complicates critical illness, especially head trauma. Experimental studies and clinical observations suggest that head injury in intoxicated individuals has a greater mortality than head injury alone. Alcohol depresses ventilation and myocar-

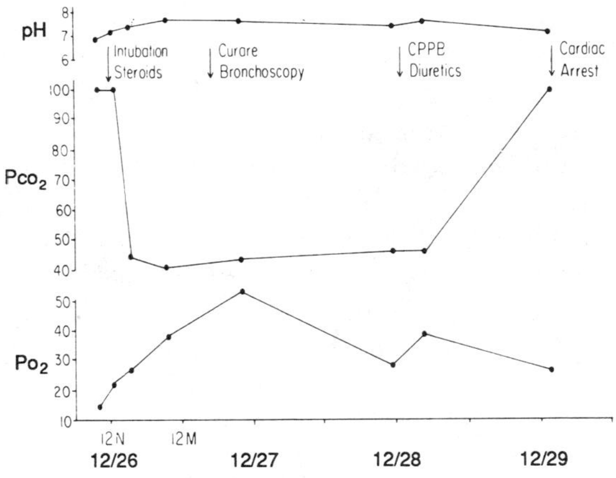

FIG 11–1.
Acute respiratory failure in patients with drug overdosage and massive aspiration pneumonitis. Arterial oxygen tension was 12 mm Hg on admission. This high carbon dioxide tension on admission reflects drug-induced depression of the respiratory center. Artificial ventilation with a volume cycle ventilator readily returns carbon dioxide tension to normal. Uncontrolled hypoxemia due to venoarterial shunting persisted throughout the entire admission. All oxygen tension values obtained while breathing 100% oxygen. In spite of vigorous treatment, the patient could not be adequately oxygenated and cardiac arrhythmias, ventricular fibrillation, and death ensued.

TABLE 11–1.
Pulmonary Edema and Acute Respiratory Failure Probably Due to Pulmonary Venoconstriction in a 26-year-old Methadone Addict

PARAMETER	PATIENTS	NORMAL
PO_2 breathing 100% O_2^a (mm Hg)	30	650
PCO_2 (mm Hg)	37	40
pH (units)	7.45	7.40
Right atrium (mm Hg)	10	< 5
Pulmonary artery (mm Hg)	35/25	25/5
Pulmonary wedge[b] (mm Hg)	27	< 10

[a]Patient intubated and ventilated by an Emerson respirator with 100% oxygen.
[b]Pulmonary wedge pressure is markedly elevated and together with normal heart size suggests pulmonary venoconstriction.

dial contractility. Mental deterioration increases as blood alcohol levels increase from 0.5 mg/m to 1.5 mg/ml. Coma is seen at concentrations of 5 mg/ml.

Withdrawal of alcohol in the hospitalized alcoholic may lead to a withdrawal syndrome characterized by tremulousness and hallucinations within 36 hours.[117] Delirium tremens is characterized by severe agitation, tachycardia, sweating, hyperthermia, and abusive behavior. The syndrome can be prevented when subtle evidence of irritability is treated with a sedative like diazepam (Valium). Oral doses of 5–10 mg are useful in patients with early evidence of alcohol withdrawal; infusions of 1 mg/min are necessary when severe agitation is present, but careful monitoring is necessary to prevent hypoventilation or cardiac depression. A major problem with the use of diazepam is its long half-life which, together with its metabolites, may exceed 1–2 days. The use of lorazepam (Ativan), a benzodiazepine with a mean half-life of about 16 hours and inactive metabolites, reduces the likelihood of central nervous system depression associated with the accumulation of drugs. Many of the manifestations of alcohol withdrawal are due to increased sympathetic nervous system activity, and Kraus et al[118] have recently shown that the beta blocking agent, atenolol, reduced mean length of hospital stay and the use of benzodiazepines in patients with the syndrome.

Tricyclic Antidepressants and Other Anticholinergics

Acute overdoses of tricyclic antidepressants are extremely common, accounting for 37% of toxic substances admissions to intensive care units.[119] Tricyclic antidepressants (amitriptyline, desipramine, doxepin, and imipramine) and phenothiazines (chlorpromazine, prochlorperazine, and promethazine) block cholinergic receptors and produce syndromes suggesting sympathetic excess. They both produce respiratory center depression and coma. In addition, phenothiazines are associated with muscle rigidity and torticollis, while the tricyclics produce widening of the QRS complex and life-threatening cardiac arrhythmias. These agents produce extensive receptor blockade. Cholinergic blockade produces tachycardia, fever, dilated pupils, flushed skin, dry mucous membranes, urinary retention, hallucinations, and coma. Tricyclics also block the reuptake of norepinephrine, producing adrenergic dysfunction. Phenothiazines block dopaminergic receptors so that dopamine used either as a diuretic or a vasopressor may be ineffective.

Seizures, ventricular arrhythmias, and death are common with tricyclic overdosage.[119] Boehnert and Lovejoy[120] prospectively studied 49 patients divided into two groups on the basis of limb lead QRS intervals. Seizures were observed in 34% and ventricular arrhythmias in 14% of patients with a QRS duration of 0.10 sec or longer while drug levels failed to predict their occurrence. Seizures occurred at any degree of QRS prolongation, but ventricular arrhythmias were only seen when the QRS complex exceeded 0.16 sec. Ventricular arrhythmias should be treated with propranolol to blunt adrenergic hyperactivity. Administration of sodium bicarbonate and potassium and hyperventilation increase intracellular potassium and stabilize membrane potentials.[121] Drugs such as quinidine, procaine amide, or lidocaine should not be used since they increase the conduction defect. Hypotension following ingestion of either phenothiazines or tricyclic antidepressants is treated with volume expansion.

The cholinergic agonist, physostigmine, reverses central nervous system abnormalities, but the reversal is of short duration. Two-thirds of patients awaken following administration of the agent,[122] but it is not clear whether cardiac arrhythmias are reversed.[123] Seizures complicate the use of physostigmine, and patients must be carefully monitored in critical care units. Neither forced diuresis, hemodialysis, nor charcoal hemoperfusion is useful in treating the receptor blockade associated with tricyclics.

Cocaine

Cocaine and its purified derivative, crack, have become the most common recreational drugs in the United States. Cocaine is a potent sympathomimetic agent that stimulates the central nervous system and increases both heart rate and blood pressure. Amphetamines produce similar sympathomimetic effects. Cocaine is absorbed intranasally within 20 minutes and produces an excitable state with dilated pupils, tachycardia, tachypnea, hypertension, vomiting, and hallucinations. Increasing doses may produce hyperthermia, respiratory arrest, seizures, and ventricular arrhythmias. Isner et al.[124] reported clinical and pathologic findings in seven patients. The recreational use of nonintravenous cocaine was associated with acute myocardial infarction, ventricular tachycardia and fibrillation, myocarditis, sudden death, or a combination of these abnormalities. The authors suggested that cocaine-mediated small vessel constriction and increased myocardial oxygen requirements associated with sympathetic hyperactivity were pathogenetic factors.

Patients with cocaine overdosages are seriously ill. Continuous physiologic monitoring is necessary, since excitability may be rapidly replaced by respiratory depression. Hyperactivity should be treated with sedatives such as intravenous diazepam, 5 mg, or barbiturates. Neuroleptics such as halperidol or chlorpromazine should not be administered in the acute stages since they lower the seizure threshold.[125] The early treatment of seizures and acidosis may be life saving.[126] Propranolol is useful for the treatment of tachycardia and arrhythmias; lidocaine should probably be avoided since it may cause seizures. Naloxone may be necessary if there is evidence of concurrent opiate intoxication, but the agent potentiates the action of cocaine when given within 30 minutes of its use.

Phencyclidine (PCP)

PCP and its congeners are readily manufactured and are effective when taken by ingestion, injection, or inhalation.[127] Its psychedelic properties produce a variety of manifestations requiring a high index of diagnostic suspicion.[128] Wide mood swings may suggest psychiatric illness. Violent behavior leading to assault and homicide, withdrawal states, flushing, excessive salivation, seizures, neurologic abnormalities, hypertensive crises, and other phenomena may be observed. Treatment includes administration of activated charcoal, ascorbic acid to acidify the urine, furosemide, diazepam, and propranolol.

REFERENCES

1. Donowitz LG, Wenzel RP, Hoyt JW: High risk of hospital-acquired infection in the ICU patient. *Crit Care Med* 1982; 10:355.

2. McLoughlin GA, Wu AV, Saporoschetz I, et al: Correlation between anergy and a circulating immunosuppressive factor following major surgical trauma. *Ann Surg* 1979; 190:297–304.

3. MacLean LD, Meakins JL, Taguchi K, et al: Host resistance in sepsis and trauma. *Ann Surg* 1975; 182:207–216.

4. Munster AM, Winchurch RA: Infection and immunology. *Crit Care Clin* 1985; 1:119–127.

5. Griffith CDM, Ross AHM: Delayed hypersensitivity skin testing in elective colorectal surgery and relationship to postoperative sepsis. *JPEN* 1984; 8:279–280.

6. Hiebert JM, McGough MM, Rodeheaver G, et al: The influence of catabolism on immunocompetence in burned patients. *Surgery* 1979; 86:242–274.

7. Faulk WP, Demaeyer EM, Davies AJS: Some effects of malnutrition on the immune response in man. *Am J Clin Nutr* 1974; 74:638–646.

8. Law DK, Dudrick SJ, Abdou NI: The effects of protein calorie malnutrition on immune competence of the surgical patient. *Surg Gynecol Obstet* 1974; 139:257–266.

9. Bistrian BR, Blackburn GL, Scrimshaw NS, Flatt JP: Cellular immunity in semi-starved states in hospitalized adults. *Am J Clin Nutr* 1975; 28:1148–1155.

10. Edelman R: Cell-mediated immune response in protein-calorie malnutrition—A review, in Suskind P (ed): *Malnutrition and the Immune Response*. New York, Raven Press, 1977.

11. Meakins JL, Pietsch JB, Subenick O: Delayed hypersensitivity: indicator of acquired failure of host defenses in sepsis and trauma. *Ann Surg* 1977; 186:241–250.

12. Johnson WC, Ulrich F, Meguid MM: Role of delayed hypersensitivity in predicting postoperative morbidity and mortality. *Am J Surg* 1979; 137:536–542.

13. Keane SM, Birmingham W, Shatney CM, et al: Prediction of sepsis in the multitrauma patient by assays of lymphocyte responsiveness. *Surg Gynecol Obstet* 1983; 136:163.

14. Munster AM, Wirzhurch RA, Birmingham WJ, et al: Longitudinal assay of lymphocyte responsiveness in patients with major burns. *Ann Surg* 1980; 192:772.

15. Dawson CW, Ledgerwood AM, Rosenberg JC, et al: The effects of total parenteral nutrition on immunodepression due to malnutrition. *Ann Surg* 1977; 185:467.

16. van Dijk WC, Varbrugh HA, van Rijswijk REN, et al: Neutrophil function, serum opsonic activity and delayed hypersensitivity in surgical patients. *Surgery* 1982; 92:21.

17. Deitch EA, Gelder F, McDonald JC: Prognostic significance of abnormal neutrophil chemotaxis after thermal injury. *J Trauma* 1982; 22:199.

18. Warden GD, Mason AD, Pruitt BA: Suppression of leukocyte chemotaxis in vitro in thermally injured patients. *J Clin Invest* 1974; 54:1001.

19. Munster AM: Post traumatic immunosuppression is due to activation of suppressor T-cells. *Lancet* 1976; 1:1329.

20. McIrving AJ, O'Mahony JB, Saporoschetz BS, et al: Depressed immune response in burn patients. *Ann Surg* 1982; 196:297.

21. Saba TM, Jaffee E: Plasma fibronectin (opsonic glycoprotein): Its synthesis by vas-

cular endothelial cells and role in cardiopulmonary integrity after trauma as related to reticuloendothelial function. *Am J Med* 1980; 68:577–594.

22. O'Connell MT, Becker KM, Steele BW, et al: Plasma fibronectin in medical ICU patients. *Crit Care Med* 1984; 12:479–492.

23. Pingleton SK, Hinthorn DR, Liu C: Enteral nutrition in patients receiving mechanical ventilation. *Am J Med* 1986; 80:827–832.

24. Van Enk RA, Furtado D: Bacterial contamination of enteral nutrient solutions: Intestinal colonization and sepsis in mice after ingestion. *JPEN* 1986; 10:503–507.

25. Anderson KR, Norris DJ, Godfrey LB, et al: Bacterial contamination of tube-feeding formulas. *JPEN* 1984; 8:673–678.

26. Roslyn JJ, Pitt HA, Mann L, et al: Parenteral nutrition-induced gallbladder disease: a reason for early enolecystectomy. *Am J Surg* 1984; 146:58–63.

27. Howerton EE, Kolmen SN: The intestinal tract as a portal of entry of pseudomonas in burned rats. *J Trauma* 1972; 12:335–340.

28. Deitch EA, Maejima K, Berg R: Effect of oral antibiotics and bacterial overgrowth on the translocation of the GI tract microflora in burned rats. *J Burn Care Rehab* (in press).

29. Iriyama K, Hichiwaka H, Asami H, et al: Effects of total parenteral nutrition on the development of intestinal endotoxemia in rats: a comparison between glucose and lipid. *JPEN* 1986; 10:413–415.

30. Mochiauke H, Trocki O, Dominioni L, et al: Mechanism of prevention of postburn hypermetabolism and catabolism by early enteral feeding. *Ann Surg* 1984; 200:297–308.

31. Prytz H, Holst-Christensen J, Korner B, Liehr H: Portal venous and systemic endotoxaemia in patients without liver disease and systemic endotoxaemia in patients with cirrhosis. *Scand J Gastroenterol* 1976; 11:857–863.

32. Matuschak GM, Rinaldo JE, Van Thiel DH, Pinsky MR: Acute respiratory failure with pre-existing end stage hepatic insufficiency is irreversible. *Am Rev Resp Dis* 1985; 131 (part 2):A:135.

33. Matuschak GM, Rinaldo JE, Van Thiel DH: Influence of D-galactosamine-induced liver dysfunction on mortality and the liver-lung interaction in ARDS, in preparation.

34. Niederman MS, Merrill WW, Ferranti RD, et al: Nutritional status and bacterial binding in the lower respiratory tract in patient with chronic tracheostomy. *Ann Intern Med* 1984; 100:795–800.

35. Johanson WG, Pierce AK, Sanford JP, Thomas SD: Nosocomial respiratory infections with gram-negative bacilli. *Ann Intern Med* 1972; 77:701–706.

36. Huxley EJ, Vorosla J, Gray WR, et al: Pharyngeal aspiration in normal adults and patients with depressed consciousness. *Am J Med* 1978; 64:564.

37. Sottile FD, Harrie TJ, Prough DS, et al: Nosocomial pulmonary infection: Possible etiologic significance of bacterial adhesion to endotracheal tubes. *Crit Care Med* 1986; 14:265–270.

38. Baigelman W, Bellin S, Cupples A, Berenberg MJ: Bacteriologic assessment of the lower respiratory tract in intubated patients. *Crit Care Med* 1986; 14:864–868.

39. Wise GJ, Goldberg P, Kozinn PJ: Genitourinary candidiasis: diagnosis and treatment. *J Urol* 1976; 116: 778–780.

40. Maki D, Weise CE, Sarafin HW: A semiquantitative culture method for identifying intravenous-catheter-related infection. *N Engl J Med* 1977; 296:1305–1309.

41. Snydman DR, Murray BA, Mornfeld S, et al: Total parenteral nutrition-related infections: Prospective epidemiologic study using semiquantitative methods. *Am J Med* 1982; 73:695–699.

42. Snydman DR, Pober BR, Murray BA, et al: Predictive value of surveillance skin cultures in total parenteral nutrition related-infection. *Lancet* 1982; 1385–1388.

43. Nelson DB, Kien CL, Mohr B, et al: Dressing changes by specialized personnel reduce infection rates in patients receiving

central venous parenteral nutrition. *JPEN* 1986; 10:220–222.

44. Band JD, Maki D: Infections caused by arterial catheters used for hemodynamic monitoring. *Am J Med* 1979; 67:735–740.

45. Harris JA, Cobbs, CG: Persistent gram-negative bacteremia: Observations in twenty patients. *Am J Surg* 1973; 125:705–717.

46. Henzel JG, DeWeese MS: Morbid and mortal complications associated with prolonged central venous cannulation. *Am J Surg* 1971; 121:600–605.

47. Sitges-Serra A, Puig P, Linares J, et al: Hub colonization as the initial step in an outbreak of catheter-related sepsis due to coagulase negative staphylococci during parenteral nutrition. *JPEN* 1984; 8:668–672.

48. Sitges-Serra A, Linares J, Perez JL, et al: A randomized trial on the effect of tubing changes on hub contamination and catheter sepsis during parenteral nutrition. *JPEN* 1985; 9:322–325.

49. Maki DG: Infections associated with intravascular lines, in Remington JS, Swartz MN (eds): *Current Clinical Topics in Infectious Disease.* New York, McGraw Hill Book Co, 1982; 309–363.

50. Maki DG, Goldman DA, Rhame FS: Infection control in intravenous therapy. *Ann Intern Med* 1973; 79:867–887.

51. Altemeier WA, McDonough JJ, Fullen WD: Third day surgical fever. *Arch Surg* 1971; 103:158–166.

52. Freeman R, King B: Recognition of infection associated with intravenous catheters. *Br J Surg* 1975; 62:404– 406.

53. Jarrett F, Maki DG, Cahn CK: Management of septic thrombosis of the inferior vena cava caused by candida. *Arch Surg* 1978; 113: 637–639.

54. Appelfeld JJ, Caruthers TE, Reno DJ, Civetta M: Assessment of the sterility of long-term cardiac catheterization using the thermodilution Swan-Ganz catheter. *Chest* 1978; 4:377–380.

55. Pemberton LB, Lyman B, Lander V, Covinsky J: Sepsis from triple vs single lumen catheters during total parenteral nutrition in surgical or critically ill patients. *Arch Surg* 1986; 121:591–594.

56. McCarthy MC, Shives J, Robison RJ, Broadie TA: Prospective evaluation of triple and single lumen catheters in total parenteral nutrition. *JPEN* 1986; 10:83.

57. Kelly CS, Ligas JR, Smith CA, et al: Sepsis due to triple lumen central venous catheters. *Surg Gynecol Obstet* 1986; 163:14–16.

58. Misny P, Erp F, Marein D, Steiger E: Complications of single versus multilumen temporary central venous catheters for total parenteral nutrition. *JPEN* 1986; 10:17a.

59. Bozzetti F, Terno G, Bonfanti G, et al: Prevention and treatment of central venous catheter sepsis by exchange via a guidewire: A prospective controlled trial. *Ann Surg* 1983; 192:48–52.

60. Stone HH: Infection in postoperative patients. *AM J Med* 1986; 81(suppl 1A):39–44.

61. Stone HH, Kolb LD, Geheber CE: Incidence and significance of intraperitoneal anaerobic bacteria. *Ann Surg* 1975; 181:705–710.

62. Solomkin JS, Flohr AB, Quie PG, Simmons RL: The role of candida in intraperitoneal infections. *Surgery* 1980; 88:524–530.

63. Solomkin JS, Flohr AB, Simmons RL: Candida infections in surgical patients: Dose requirements and toxicity of amphotericin B. *Ann Surg* 1982; 195:177–185.

64. Marsh PK, Tally FP, Kellum J, et al: Candida infections in surgical patients. *Ann Surg* 1983; 198:42–47.

65. Sprung CL, Schein BMH, Long WM: Controversies in the management of sepsis and septic shock: Corticosteroids, naloxone, and nonsteroidal anti-inflammatory agents, in Sibbald WJ, Sprung CL (eds): *New Horizons: Perspectives on Sepsis and Septic Shock.* Fullerton, CA, Society of Critical Care Medicine, 1986.

66. Heideman M: Bacteremia and multiple organ failure: The role of injured tissue and abscesses, in Ninnemann JL (ed): *Traumatic Injury: Infection and Other Immunologic Sequelae.* Baltimore University Park Press, 1983.

67. Cahalane MC, Demling RH: Early respiratory abnormalities from smoke inhalation. *JAMA* 1984; 251:771–774.

68. Jurkovich GJ, Moylan JA: Inhalation injury: A major burn complication. *Hospital Physician* 1983; 92–98.

69. Asch MJ, Meserol PM, Mason AD, Pruitt BA: Regional blood flow in the burned unanesthetized dog. *Surg Forum* 1971; 22:55.

70. Pruitt BA, Mason AD, Moncrief JA: Hemodynamic changes in the early postburn patient: The influence of fluid administration and of a vasodilator. *J Trauma* 1971; 11:36.

71. Curreri PW, Wilmore DW, Mason AD, Newsome TW: Intracellular cation alterations following major trauma: Effect of supranormal caloric intake. *J Trauma* 1971; 11:390–396.

72. Flear CTG, Battacharya SS, Singh CM: Solute and water exchanges between cells and extracellular fluids in health and disturbances after trauma. *JPEN* 1980; 4:98–120.

73. Pruitt BA, Mason AD, Moncrief JA: Hemodynamic changes in the early postburn patient: The influence of fluid administration and of a vasodilator. *J Trauma* 1971; 11:36.

74. Monafo WW, Ayvazian VH: Significance of sodium loading in blood replacement, in Malinin TI, Zeppa R, Crucker WR, Callahan AB (eds): *Acute Fluid Replacement in the Therapy of Shock*. New York, Stratten Intercontinental Medical Book Corp, 1974, pp 185–189.

75. Monafo WW: The treatment of burn shock by intravenous and oral administration of hypertonic lactated saline solution. *J Trauma* 1970; 10:575–586.

76. Simazake S, Yoshioka T, Tanaka N, et al: Body fluid changes during hypertonic lactated saline solution therapy for burn shock. *J Trauma* 1977; 17:38–43.

77. Caldwell FT, Bowser B: Critical evaluation of hypertonic and hypotonic solutions to resuscitate severely burned children. *Ann Surg* 1980; 198:546–552.

78. Monafo WW, Halverson JD, Schechtman K: The role of concentrated sodium solutions in the resuscitation of patients with severe burns. *Surgery* 1984; 95:129–134.

79. Wilmore DW, Long JM, Mason AD, Skreen RW, Pruitt BA: Catecholamines: Mediator of the hypermetabolic response to thermal injury. *Ann Surg* 1974; 180:653.

80. Saffle JR, Medine A, Raymond J, et al: Use of indirect calorimetry in the nutritional management of burned patients. *J Trauma* 1985; 25:32–39.

81. Kein CL, Young VR, Rohrbaugh DK, Burke JF: Increased rates of whole body protein s ynthesis and breakdown in children recovering from burns. *Ann Surg* 1978; 187:383–391.

82. Wilmore DW, Goodwin CW, Aulick LH, et al: Effect of injury and infection on visceral metabolism and circulation. *Ann Surg* 1980; 192:491–499.

83. Lindberg RB, Moncreif JA, Mason AD: Control of experimental and clinical burn wound sepsis by topical application of sulfamylon compounds. *Ann NY Acad Sci* 1968; 150:950–960.

84. Munster AM, Winchurch RA: Infection and immunology. *Crit Care Clin* 1985; 1:119–127.

85. Luterman A, Dasco CC, Curreri PW: Infections in burn patients: *Am J Med* 1986; 81(1A):45–52.

86. Heimbach D: The results of early primary excision. *J Trauma* 1981; 21:732.

87. Frank DH, Wachtel T, Frank HA, Sanders R: Comparison of biobrane, porcine, and human allograft as biologic dressings for burn wounds. *J Burn Care* 1983; 4:186–190.

88. Achauer BM, Martinez SE: Burn wound pathophysiology and care. *Crit Care Clin* 1985; 1:47–58.

89. Brentano L, Moyer CA, Gravens DL, Monafo WW: Bacteriology of large human burns treated with silver nitrate. *Arch Surg* 1966; 93:456–460.

90. Hinton P, Allison SP, Littlejohn S, Lloyd J: Insulin and glucose to reduce catabolic response to injury in burned patients. *Lancet* 1971; 767–769.

91. Burke JF, Wolfe RR, Mullany CJ, et al: Glucose requirements following burn injury. Parameters of optimal glucose infusion and possible hepatic and respiratory abnormalities

following excessive glucose intake. *Ann Surg* 1979; 190:275–285.

92. Elwyn DH, Kinney JM, Malayappa J, et al: Influence of increasing carbohydrate intake on glucose kinetics in injured patients. *Ann Surg* 1979; 190:117–127.

93. Brooks DC, Bessey PQ, Black PR, et al: Insulin stimulates branched chain amino acid uptake and diminishes nitrogen flux from skeletal muscle of injured patients. *J Surg Res* 1986; 40:395–405.

94. Wolfe RR: Glucose metabolism in burn injury: A review. *J Burn Care* 1985; 6:408–418.

95. Wilmore DW, Goodwin CW, Aulick LH, et al: Effect of injury and infection on visceral metabolism and circulation. *Ann Surg* 1980; 192:491–499.

96. Wilmore DW, Aulick LH, Mason AD, Pruitt BA: Influence of the burn wound on local and systemic responses to injury. *Ann Surg* 1977; 186:444–455.

97. Shoemaker WL, Appel PL, Kram HB: Role of oxygen transport patterns in the pathophysiology, prediction of outcome, and therapy of shock, in Bryan-Brown CW, Ayres SM (eds): *Oxygen Transport and Utilization*. Fullerton, CA, Society of Critical Care Medicine, 1987.

98. Wilson RF: Trauma, in Shoemaker WC, Thompson WL, Holbrook PR (eds): *Textbook of Critical Care*. Philadelphia, WB Saunders, 1984.

99. McAslan TC, Cowley RA: The preventive use of peep in major trauma, in *The American Surgeon*, Philadelphia, JB Lippincott, 1979.

100. Wilson RF, McCarthy B, LeBlanc LP, et al: Respiratory and coagulation changes after uncomplicated fractures. *Arch Surg* 1973; 106:395.

101. Trinkle JK, Richardson JD, Franz JL, et al: Management of flail chest without mechanical ventilation. *Ann Thorac Surg* 1975; 19:355.

102. Wachter RM, Luce JM, Turner J, et al: Intensive care of patients with the acquired immunodeficiency syndrome: outcome and changing patterns of utilization. *Am Rev Resp Dis* 1986; 134:891.

103. Suffredini AF, Tobin MJ, Wajszczuk CP, et al: Acute respiratory failure due to Pneumocystis carinii pneumonia: Clinical, radiographic, and pathologic course. *Crit Care Med* 1985; 13:237.

104. Maxfield RA, Sorkin IB, Fazzini EP: Respiratory failure in patients with acquired immunodeficiency syndrome and Pneumocystis carinii pneumonia. *Crit Care Med* 1986; 14:443.

105. Centers for Disease Control: Update: Acquired Immunodeficiency Syndrome–United States. *MMWR* 1986; 35:757.

106. Fischl MA, Dickinson GM, Scott GB: Evaluation of heterosexual partners, children, and household contacts of adults with AIDS. *JAMA* 1987; 257:640.

107. Schleifer SJ, Keller SE, Camerino M, et al: Suppression of lymphocyte stimulation following bereavement. *JAMA* 1983; 250:374.

108. Bach MA, Bach JF: Imbalance in T-cell subsets in human diseases. *Int J Immunopharmacol* 1981; 3:269.

109. Francis DP, Jaffe HW, Fultz PN, et al: The natural history of infection with the lymphadenopathy-associated virus/human T-lymphotropic virus type III. *Ann Intern Med* 1985; 103:719.

110. Polk BF, Fox R, Brookmeyer R, et al: Predictors of the acquired immunodeficiency syndrome developing in a cohort of seropositive men. *N Engl J Med* 1987; 316:61.

111. Murray JF, Felton CP, Garay S, et al: Pulmonary complications of the acquired immunodeficiency syndrome: Report of a National Heart, Lung and Blood Institute workshop. *N Engl J Med* 1984; 310:1682–1688.

112. Bigby TD, Margolskee D, Curtis JL, et al: The usefulness of induced sputum in the diagnosis of Pneumocystis carinii pneumonia in patients with the acquired immunodeficiency syndrome. *Am Rev Resp Dis* 1986; 133:515–518.

113. Wharton JM, Coleman DL, Wofsey CB, et al: Trimethoprim-sulfa-methoxazole or pentamidine for Pneumocystis carinii pneumonia in the acquired immunodeficiency syndrome: A prospective randomized trial. *Ann Intern Med* 1986; 105:37.

114. Steinbrook R, Lo B, Moulton J, et al:

Preferences of homosexual men with AIDS for life-sustaining treatment. *N Engl J Med* 1986; 314:457–460.

115. Greensher J, Mofenson HC, Piccioni AL, et al: Activated charcoal updated. *JACEP* 1979; 8:261.

116. Crome P, Dawling S, Braithwaite RA, et al: Effect of activated charcoal on absorption of nortriptyline. *Lancet* 1977; 1:1203–1206.

117. Ehlers SM, Zaske DE, Sawchuk RJ: Massive theophylline overdose: Rapid elimination by charcoal hemoperfusion. *JAMA* 1978; 240:474.

118. Thompson WL: Management of alcohol withdrawal syndromes. *Arch Intern Med* 1978; 138:278.

119. Kraus ML, Gottlieb MD, Horwitz RI, et al: Randomized trial of atenolol in patients with alcohol withdrawal. *N Engl J Med* 1985; 313:905.

120. Rosen MJ: Tricyclic antidepressant overdosage: Clinical features and management. *Heart Lung* 1983; 12:222–225.

121. Boehnert MT, Lovejoy FH: Value of the QRS duration versus the serum drug level in predicting seizures and ventricular arrhythmias after an acute overdosage of tricyclic antidepressants. *N Engl J Med* 1985; 313:474.

122. Giller EL Jr, Bialos DS, Bocherty JP, et al: Chronic amitriptyline toxicity. *Am J Psychiatry* 1979; 136:458.

123. Newton RW: Physostigmine salicylate in the treatment of tricyclic antidepressant overdose. *JAMA* 1975; 231:941.

124. Bigger JT Jr, Kantor SJ, Glassman AH, et al: Is physostigmine effective for cardiac toxicity of tricyclic antidepressant drugs? *JAMA* 1977; 237:1311.

125. Isner JM, Estes NAM II, Thompson PD, et al: Acute cardiac events temporally related to cocaine abuse. *N Engl J Med* 1986; 315:1438.

126. Gay GR: You've come a long way, baby! Coke time for the new American lady of the eighties. *J Psychoactive Drugs* 1981; 13:297.

127. Jonsson S, O'Meara M, Young JB: Acute cocaine poisoning: Importance of treating seizures and acidosis. *Am J Med* 1983; 75:1061–1064.

128. Thompson WL: Recognition, treatment, and prevention of poisoning, in Shoemaker WC, Thompson WL, Holbrook PR (eds): *Textbook of Critical Care*. Philadelphia, WB Saunders, 1984.

129. Stillman R, Petersen RC: The paradox of phencyclidine (PCP) abuse. *Ann Intern Med* 1979; 90:428.

12 DYSFUNCTION OF OTHER ORGANS

THE LIVER

Alterations of the liver in the critically ill are common but poorly understood. All 18 patients with multiple organ failure following ruptured abdominal aneurysm had chemical or clinical jaundice.[1] Typically, SGOT rose to 400–600 units within the first few days and then returned to normal. Total and direct bilirubin began to rise as the SGOT began to fall, and it continued to rise in an almost linear manner until death occurred. Levels as high as 35 mg/dl were reported in one patient. Centrilobular necrosis, bile stasis, congestion, and fatty infiltration were found at post mortem. Forty percent of the patients with multiple organ failure studied by Coalson[2] had moderate to severe hepatic necrosis, while 22% had fatty infiltration. The sinusoids were distended and lined by prominent Kupfer cells. Sepsis appears to produce early changes in liver function, and Meakins et al.[3] have suggested that unexplained hyperbilirubinemia in critically ill patients may suggest unrecognized infection.

The liver carries out many hundreds of identifiable and important chemical functions. These include: (1) regulation of energy metabolism by storing and releasing glycogen and fats, (2) synthesis of a large number of proteins, (3) detoxification of drugs, (4) regulation of salt and water metabolism, and (5) storage of vitamins and heavy metals. These functions are performed in parenchymal cells bound to each other by fusion of the plasma membranes of adjacent cells. Bile canaliculi are located within these fused membranes. Single layers of cells surround blood-filled sinusoids which are lined by endothelial cells. Large openings in sinusoidal walls permit ready passage of large molecules from the sinusoids to the interstitial spaces of Disse. Specialized liver macrophages called Kupfer cells are located within the sinusoids and detect the presence of a variety of substances returning to the liver via the portal circulation. The liver cords are arranged around a central vein and form a lobule. The radiating cords extend to form a hexagonal structure with six corners. A portal triad with portal vein, hepatic artery, and biliary duct is found at each corner. Oxygen tension decreases as portal and hepatic arterial blood courses through sinusoids to the hepatic vein. These gradients have been divided into three arbitrary zones with the highest oxygen tensions in the periportal areas (zone C) and the lowest near the central vein (zone A). Functional stratification within the lobule is related to oxygen tensions; enzymes required for the synthesis of glucose are much more plentiful in the periportal zone C, while glycolytic enzymes occur in the oxygen deficient zone A.

Hepatic blood flow is about 25% of the cardiac output and is affected by posture, exercise, alimentation, and autonomic neural activity. Seventy percent of the blood flow is provided by the portal vein and the remainder by the hepatic artery. Portal pressure averages 10 mm Hg, and its oxygen tension is much lower than that of arterial blood. Hepatic arterial and portal streams meet in the low pressure hepatic sinusoids and jointly perfuse the hepatocytes.

If the kidney is considered the major regulator of body fluids and electrolytes, then the liver is the major regulator of body fuel sources. Either glucose or fatty acid can be utilized by the body, and the liver matches fuel availability to metabolic need as well as determining whether the primary fuel at any moment should be sugar or fat. The liver metabolizes about 50% of the ingested glucose and synthesizes glucose between meals to maintain blood glucose levels within close limits. The *glycolytic* enzymes of the liver, in the presence of adequate insulin, catalyze the oxidation of glucose to pyruvate in the glycolytic (Embden-Myerhof) cycle. Pyruvate is oxidized to acetyl coenzyme A and enters the Krebs citric acid cycle. Oxidized nicotinamide-adenine dinucleotide (NAD) carries electrons from both glycolytic and Krebs cycle to the respiratory enzymes in the mitochondria. Lactate produced by the skeletal muscles is converted to pyruvate by the liver and oxidized in the citric acid cycle. Lactate produced by skeletal muscle is either oxidized in the liver to pyruvate or used to produce glucose (Cori cycle). Glucose delivered to the liver in excess of metabolic need is stored as glycogen or converted into fat.

The liver maintains glucose availability during periods of increased need or glucose deficit by *gluconeogenetic* pathways. Glucagon, glucocorticoids, and growth hormone reverse glycolytic pathways and produce glucose from glycogen, amino acids, lactate, and glycerol.

An important third fate for ingested glucose is the synthesis of five-carbon sugars through the *pentose pathway*. This pathway uses NAD phosphate (NADP) as an electron carrier to produce the five-carbon sugars needed for the synthesis of nucleic acids, glycoproteins, and glycolipids. Reduced NADP (NADPH) provides electrons for the one-electron reduction of oxygen to O_2-, the superoxide anion (see chapters 1 and 2).

Fat provides most of the metabolic fuel in adequately fed individuals. The liver oxidizes fatty acids to produce ketone bodies, stores fat, and converts excess glucose and amino acids to fatty acids. An important continuous circulation between the periphery and the liver delivers fatty acids to the liver. Triglycerides formed from these fatty acids become the building blocks of lipoproteins.

The liver synthesizes dozens of proteins for its internal use as enzymes and for external transport as plama proteins. These exported proteins include albumin, lipoproteins, transferrin, ceruloplasmin, haptoglobin, clotting factors, antiproteases, certain complement factors, and C-reactive protein. The reductions in circulating albumin and prothrombin concentrations in advanced parenchymal failure are evidence of the importance of these synthetic functions.

Decreased synthesis of clotting factors is one of the most serious consequences of liver damage. The liver synthesizes fibrinogen, prothrombin, factor V (proaccelerin), factor VII (proconvertin), factor IX (Christmas, factor X [Stuart]), factor XI (plasma thromboplastin antecedent), and factor XIII (fibrin stabilizing factor). Prothrombin and factors VII, IX, and X require vitamin K for their synthesis. Half-lives of these clotting factors determine the likelihood of a deficiency in acute hepatic failure. Factor VII has the shortest half-life (4–6 hours), and its deficiency accounts for a prolonged prothrombin time with normal albumin in acute hepatic necrosis. Prothrombin and factors VII, IX, and X require vitamin K for final assembly of a carboxyl residue to the glutamic acid. Vitamin K does not correct the prothrombin time if the problem is due to defective protein synthesis.

Hypotension or shock leads to a drop in pressure and flow to both hepatic artery and portal vein. Decreased portal vein oxygen tensions and increased portal vein concentrations of carbon dioxide, hydrogen ion, lactic acid, and ammonia are found in shock. Portal vein pressure rises, suggesting intrahepatic venous obstruction. Kupfer cell and hepatocyte dysfunction can be identified as early as 60–90 minutes after experimental shock.[4] Vasoconstriction further reduces hepatic blood flow, and the resultant hypoxia leads to the release of proteolytic enzymes and a decrease in Kupfer cell phagocytosis.[5] Cowley et al.[6] studied a large number of patients in shock admitted to the Maryland Institute for Emergency Medical Services and found that evidence of hepatic dysfunction suggested a poor prognosis. Reductions in clotting factors, elevations of ammonia, and hepatic enzymes were much greater in nonsurvivors compared to survivors. The concentrations of liver enzymes began to fall as liver failure progressed. Pathologic studies in these patients revealed the appearance of intracellular lipid within the first 24 hours. Sinusoidal dilitation and congestion were common and were most marked in the central zones, spreading to the midzones in more profound shock. The periportal areas were relatively normal. Characteristic centrilobular necrosis was observed in patients dying after several days in profound shock.

The amount of centrilobular necrosis varies with the intensity and severity of the perfusion deficit. Seeley et al.[7] described patients with infarction of an entire hepatic lobe, but these situations appear uncommon. In one study, hepatic necrosis was found in 9% of patients in shock for less than 10 hours, 22% in shock for 10–24 hours and 93% in those in shock for more than 24 hours.[8]

Careful monitoring of bilirubin concentrations and liver enzymes may alert the physician to major changes in patient status. Hepatic venous congestion due to right ventricular failure is associated with a large palpable liver and modest elevations of unconjugated bilirubin. Hepatic enzymes such as the SGOT are usually normal or mildly elevated in chronic right ventricular failure. Interpretation of elevated enzymes in patients with multiple system dysfunction is often difficult. Killip and Payne,[9] for example, observed markedly elevated SGOT concentrations in patients with acute myocardial infarction in shock. The marked elevations were not due to the infarcted myocardial tissue, but to centrilobular hepatic necrosis.

Experimental hemorrhagic shock produces a profound decrease in hepatic high energy phosphate synthesis, which is associated with mortality.[10] Similar declines in hepatic ATP levels and increases in lactate/pyruvate ratios in late sepsis suggest decreased hepatic blood flow and organ hypoxia.[11] In contrast, hepatic mitochondrial ATP synthetic activity increases in early sepsis[12] in response to increased metabolic requirements. When hypotension progresses, ATP concentrations decline.

THE SPLANCHNIC CIRCULATION

The blood supply to the stomach and intestines contains a rich alpha-adrenergic innervation. Hypoperfusion and shock lead to selective vasoconstriction in the mucosal layer, while other layers of the gut are relatively spared.

Endotoxin produces vasoconstriction in the dog, but produces vasodilatation in the human splanchnic circulation, so that many of the early studies on shock cannot be directly applied to man.[13]

Gastointestinal ischemia leads to a loss in effectiveness of its barrier function, allowing septic material from the lumen to reach the circulation. In addition, there may be loss of water, electrolytes, and protein into the lumen; severe protein loss produces a serious oncotic and nutritional deficiency termed "exudative enteropathy." Ischemic ulcers commonly produce bleeding from almost any region of the gut, although the stomach, jejunum, and ileum are the most commonly involved. Prompt restoration of oxygen delivery with avoidance of vasoconstrictor agents (where possible) reduces the prevalence of gastointestinal lesions in the critically ill, although these lesions are common in patients who develop multiple organ failure. Few clinical observations on the effects of dopamine on the splanchnic circulation have been made, but it is likely that the prominent renal dilatation produced by the catecholamine is shared by blood vessels supplying the liver, gastointestinal tract, and pancreas.

THE PANCREAS

Pancreatic involvement is common in shock and multiple organ failure (chapter 2). Acute or intermittent chronic hypoperfusion leads to acinar cell necrosis with zymogen granule activation, loss of the limiting membrane, and release of pancreatic enzymes into the circulation. Release of such enzymes may be a significant factor in the development of the shock syndrome.[14] Acute pancreatitis is a risk factor for the development of the adult respiratory distress syndrome, perhaps because of the release of pancreatic enzymes.[15] Hypoxia and hypercapnia have profound effects on pancreatic blood flow,[16] emphasizing the importance of maintaining overall oxygen delivery.

HEMOSTASIS AND DISSEMINATED INTRAVASCULAR COAGULATION

The evolution of knowledge concerning hemostasis parallels the development of modern techniques of cell biology. Early investigators using the formation of a clot discovered and named a group of clotting factors which appeared to play a predominant role in coagulation. More recent research demonstrates that at least four separate systems have evolved to prevent loss of blood from the vascular system: (1) the vascular wall and endothelium, (2) the coagulation cascade, (3) platelets, and (4) the fibrinolytic mechanism. Until recently, research into hemostasis centered on blood reactions that were observed in test tubes. Since a container that completely inhibits blood coagulation has not been found, the vascular lining must contain substances promoting fluidity of the blood. Important studies over the past decade have established that endothelial cells synthesize and release powerful anticoagulant factors; when endothelial damage occurs, these factors are inactivated and thrombosis occurs.

The Coagulation Cascade

The coagulation cascade is a series of inactive proteins that are successively activated to become proteolytic enzymes, which in turn activate the next protein in the cascade. Amplification occurs as each successive enzyme activates more protein than the previous one. The coagulation cascade, like the complement cascade, represents a controlled reaction that can be regulated at multiple sites. Vascular injury, factor XII (Hageman factor), epinephrine, and other agents produce platelet adherence and aggregation. A small amount of adenosine diphosphate is then released and promotes additional aggregation with release of additional ADP, serotonin, platelet phospholipid for platelet factor 3 and thromboxane A_2. The platelets interact with the coagulation cascade by providing binding sites for factors V, VIII, and activated X. They also activate factor XI and secrete calcium.

Endothelial damage appears to promote procoagulant and reduce anticoagulant activity of the vascular wall. Factor XII, prekallikrein and high molecular weight kinogen are assembled on a negatively charged surface like the damaged vascular wall, and they then activate factor XI (plasma thromboplastin antecedent). High molecular weight kinogen is a large nonenzymatic template that binds the other three molecules, which are all single chain polypeptides of about 80,000 molecular weight. Prekallikrein is activated to kallikrein, which appears to have at least two functions: it releases bradykinin from high molecular weight kinogen and activates factor XII, which then activates the entire coagulation cascade.

Activated factor XII activates factor XI which, in turn, activates factor IX. Activated factor IX in the presence of factor VIII, calcium, and lipid activates factor X. This sequence of factor activation is termed the intrinsic pathway; factor X may also be activated by thromboplastin and factor VII. Activated factor X then converts prothrombin to thrombin in a reaction catalyzed by factor V, calcium, and lipid. Thrombin then splits fibrinopeptides A and B from the fibrinogen molecule to form fibrin and also leads to platelet aggregation. Thrombin activity is balanced by a group of naturally occurring antithrombins. The overall activity of the intrinsic system is tested by measuring the whole clotting time or the partial thromboplastin time. The prothrombin time measures the activity of the extrinsic pathway (Fig 12–1). All of the clotting factors except VIII and V are synthesized in the liver; factor VIII is produced by endothelial cells.

Endothelial anticoagulant substances were identified much later than plasma clotting factors.[17] An endothelial receptor protein called thombomodulin binds thrombin formed by the coagulation cascade and inactivates it. Thrombomodulin also activates a recently discovered vitamin K-dependent plasma protein termed protein C. Protein C exerts an anticoagulant effect by inactivating factors V and VIII in the presence of phospholipid and calcium ions.

The fibrin clot is enzymatically degraded by the proteolytic enzyme plasmin. Plasminogen, the precursor of plasmin, is closely bound to fibrinogen so that the thrombolysis is preordained and begins

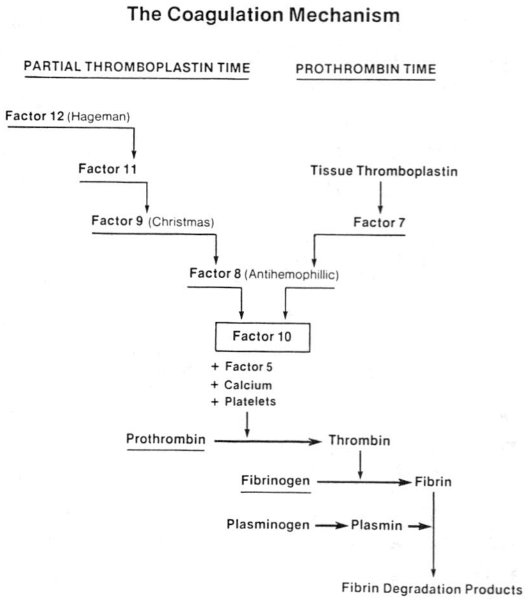

FIG 12–1.
The coagulation mechanism. Underlined factors are consumed by clotting reaction and are decreased in disseminated intravascular coagulation.

as soon as fibrin is formed. The formation of plasmin is stimulated by a group of plasma and endothelial substances; tissue plasminogen activator has become an important pharmacologic agent for the early treatment of thrombosis; urokinase is a naturally occurring plasminogen activator. Fibrinolysis is recognized by the measurement of fibrin degradation products, which may be fragments of either fibrin or fibrinogen. The fragments may be measured by radioimmunoassay and exert a direct inhibitory effect on the coagulation process.

Disseminated Intravascular Coagulation

Fibrinolysis following physiologic hemostasis is termed "primary fibrinolysis." Platelet and fibrinogen turnover are increased by surgical trauma, venous thrombosis, neoplasia, bacteremia, and obstetrical bleeding.[18] Platelet counts and fibrinogen concentrations are frequently within normal limits, demonstrating that enhanced production may compensate for increased consumption. Since all of the known coagulation factors except for factor VIII are synthesized by the liver, and factor VIII may also be of liver origin, decreased liver perfusion may lead to decreased production of clotting factors. Increased thrombosis may also be caused by antithrombin-3, one of the most important antithrombins. This physiologic inhibitor falls dramatically following severe trauma.[19] The anticoagulant activity of thrombomodulin may also be altered in critical illness; Moore et al.[20] have found that sepsis stimulates a tissue factor which promotes coagulation by decreasing thrombomodulin activity.

Disseminated intravascular coagulation (DIC) or consumption coagulopathy is an important consequence of those morbific factors leading to multiple organ failure. Activation of the coagulation cascade goes hand in hand with activation of the complement cascades, monocytes, and granulocytes (see chapter 2) and is enhanced by abnormalities in the physiologic inhibitors discussed above. Differentiation of this serious coagulopathy from purposeful coagulation is sometimes difficult. DIC is characterized by widespread activation of the fibrinolytic system with rapid lysis of newly formed clots. Diffuse bleeding from wounds, venopuncture sites and the urinary tract is associated with fibrinogen and platelet consumption. Mild DIC may be asymptomatic and may be recognized by prolongation of the prothrombin (PT) and partial thromboplastin (PTT) times. Classically, severe DIC is diagnosed when bleeding is associated with thrombocytopenia, elevated PT and PTT, decreased fibrinogen, and increased concentration of fibrin split products. Thrombocytopenia in sepsis may be from an immune mechanism, so that DIC should not be diagnosed unless hypofibrinogenemia and increased split products are present. Bleeding is associated with widespread thrombosis which may produce vital organ malfunction.

Severe bleeding is uncommon, however, in the critically ill patient, even though coagulation abnormalities may be identified by laboratory test. Mant and King[21] studied 47 patients with severe DIC who had fibrinogen levels below 150 mg/100 ml and platelet counts below 100,000. PT and PTT were usually abnormal. The three leading causes were sepsis, shock, or trauma. These authors felt that DIC was rarely the major cause of death; skin and mucous membrane bleeding was common but not serious. Bleeding from wounds, the gastrointestinal tract, and the lung were usually due to local abnormalities but were thought to contribute to death in 26% of patients.

Treatment requires correction of underlying abnormalities (see Table 12–1). The presence of asymptomatic coagulation disturbances in critically ill patients

TABLE 12–1.
Life Threatening Insults

Blood and fluid loss
Hypoxia
Tissue injury
Chemical imbalance

demands reevaluation of therapeutic strategy, particularly if abnormalities increase in magnitude. The use of heparin is controversial. It inhibits the actions of thrombin on fibrinogen and will decrease coagulation, but will, of course, lead to bleeding if the vascular bed is disrupted. Heparin should only be used with an intact vascular bed and is contraindicated in patients with injury, cerebral bleeding, or vasculitis. Initial loading should be with a relatively low dose of 2,000 units in a 70 kg person. Factor replacement is also controversial since many believe it may enhance the coagulation process. One approach has been the use of heparin to inhibit thrombin activity followed by factor replacement.

Therapy with Clotting Factors

The most common indication for transfusional therapy is the replacement of shed blood by stored red blood cells so that oxygen delivery can be augmented. Indications for blood transfusion must be precisely stated since the undesirable effects of transfusion are not uncommon. The acquired immunodeficiency syndrome, hepatitis, syphilis, and malaria can be transmitted by human blood. In one study conducted by the Veterans Administration in 1975, posttransfusion hepatitis was found in 11.3%; 80% of these were anicteric.[22] Antibody to HIV was found in 92% of individuals with hemophilia A and 52% of those with hemophilia B, suggesting widespread exposure;[23] by September 1986, 238 cases of hemophilia-acquired AIDS had been reported. Hemolytic transfusions in properly matched blood are, in contrast, quite rare but sometimes difficult to diagnose in the unconscious patient.

Red blood cell packs have an average hematocrit of 70%, and the administration of each pack increases the hematocrit by 3–5%. The shelf-life of red cells is 21 days, but freezing to −81° allows them to be stored almost indefinitely. Stored blood becomes progressively acidotic; the pH falls to 6.89 at 14 days. Potassium rises to 20 meq/L and 2,3 DPG falls from 12.5 to 7 ug/gm hemoglobin. Perfluorochemical emulsion Fluosol-DA has been proposed as a substitute for red blood cells that would be stable for long periods of time and not transmit infectious agents. Unfortunately, it is not an effective oxygen carrier. Gould, Rosen, and Sehgal[24] administered up to 40 ml/kg of a 20% preparation to patients with hemoglobin concentrations averaging 7.2 gm/dl. Arterial oxygen content increased only 0.7 ml/dl and the half-life for the material was 24.3 hours.

Fresh frozen plasma contains almost all necessary coagulation factors. Clotting factors are standardized to a normal 70 kg adult so that each ml of plasma contains one unit of each factor. Each unit of frozen plasma also raises the fibrinogen level by 26 mg/dl. Freezing and thawing of plasma to 4°C contains all coagulation factors but increased amounts of factors VIII, fibrinogen, and fibronectin. Cryoprecipitate is made from pooled plasma, so that the risk of infectious agents is many times greater than with a single unit of fresh frozen plasma. Platelet infusions are indicated if bleeding from thrombocytopenia is present, or if therapeutic procedures are anticipated in individuals with marked reduction in platelet counts. A single unit of platelets will raise the circulating platelet count by about 10,000/mm^3, and packs prepared from 8 units by 50,000 to 100,000/mm^3. The shelf-life of platelets is low, and only 20% are viable after 24 hours of storage.

ENDOCRINE DYSFUNCTION

The release of counterregulatory hormones including cortisol, epinephrine, and glucagon has been detailed in Chapters 1 and 2. The release of aldosterone, antidiuretic hormone, and atrial polypeptide (atrin) produces salt and water retention and has been described in Chapter 8. Abnormal secretion of other humoral agents may also modify the evolution of critical illness.

Thyroid Dysfunction and the Sick-Euthyroid Syndrome

Thyroid hormone (T_4) is normally bound to serum protein and converted in the peripheral tissues by the enzyme 5′ deiodinase to triiodothyronine (T_3). Decreased protein binding and activity of 5′ deiodinase in serious illness leads to a decrease in T_4 and T_3 with an increase in L-reverse triiodothyronine (rT_3). Decreased protein binding leads to increases in the free fractions of T_4 and T_3. Most patients with serious illness have normal thyroid stimulating hormone concentrations and are presumably euthyroid. Decreases in thyroid hormone concentrations may be an adaptive process that limits the increased oxygen consumption and protein catabolism that characterizes serious illness. The TSH level does not always rise in seriously ill patients even if they are hypothyroid, so that administration of thyrotropin releasing hormone (TRH) may be necessary for diagnosis. The normal two or threefold elevation of TSH following administration of TRH is exaggerated in hypothyroidism. Dopamine and glucocorticoids inhibit TSH secretion and may further confuse the interpretation of thyroid evaluation.

Adrenocortical Dysfunction

Adrenal hypofunction may be observed in multiple organ failure and in patiens with adrenal hemorrhage due to sepsis or to acquired coagulopathy. Much more common is hypoadrenalism secondary to the use of exogenous steroids. Patients who have received corticosteroid preparations for more than two weeks may have adrenal atrophy. Administration of ACTH in normal individuals leads to increases of more than 7 ug/dl from baseline. In severe stress, the rise above baseline may be more than 18 ug/dl. Severe adrenal insufficiency (adrenal crisis) should be treated with dexamethasone (10 mg) or methylprednisolone (50 mg). Both hyponatremia and hypoglycemia are hallmarks of adrenal failure and should be treated by the administration of 5% dextrose in normal saline.

REFERENCES

1. Tilney NL, Bailey GL, Morgan AP: Sequential system failure after rupture of abdominal aortic aneurysms: An unsolved problem in postoperative care. *Ann Surg* 1973; 178:117–112.

2. Coalson JJ: Pathology of sepsis, septic shock and multiple organ failure, in Sibbald SJ, Spruce CL (eds): *New Horizons. Perspectives in Sepsis and Septic Shock.* Fullerton, CA, Society of Critical Care Medicine, 1985.

3. Meakins JL, Wicklund B, Forse RA, et al: The surgical intensive care unit: Current concepts in infection. *Surg Clin North Am* 1980; 50:117–132.

4. Carlson RP, Lefer AM: Hepatic cell integrity in hypodynamic states. *Am J Physiol* 1976; 231:1408.

5. White RR, Mela L, Bacalzo V, et al: Hepatic ultrastructure in endotoxemia, hemorrhage, and hypoxia: Emphasis on mitochondrial changes. *Surgery* 1973; 73:525.

6. Cowley RA, Hankins JR, Jones RT, et al: Pathology and pathophysiology of the liver, in Cowley RA, Trump BF (eds): *Pathophysiology of Shock, Anoxia, and Ischemia.* Baltimore, Williams and Wilkins, 1982.

7. Seeley TT, Blumenfeld DM, Ikeda R, et al: Hepatic infarction. *Hum Pathol* 1972; 3:265.

8. Ellenberg M, Osserman KE: The role of shock in the production of central liver cell necrosis. *Am J Med* 1951; 11:170.

9. Killip T III, Payne MA: High serum transaminase activity in heart disease. Circulatory failure and hepatic necrosis. *Circulation* 1960; 21:646.

10. Ozawa K, Ida T, Kamano T, et al: Different response of hepatic energy charge and adenine nucleotide concentrations to hemorrhagic shock. *Res Exp Med* 1976; 169:145.

11. Chaudry IH, Wichterman KA, Baue AE: Effect of sepsis on tissue adenine nucleotide levels. *Surgery* 1979; 85:205–211.

12. Ohkawa M, Chaudry IH, Clemens MG, et al: Hepatic mitochondrial responses to sepsis and septic shock. *Circ Shock* 1983; 10:273–274.

13. Brobmann G, Ulano HB, Hinshaw LB, Jacobson ED: Mesenteric vascular responses to endotoxin in the monkey and dog. *Am J Physiol* 1970; 219:1464.

14. Manabe T, Suzuki T, Honjo I: Role of the pancreas in organ blood flow during shock. *Surg Gynecol Obstet* 1978; 146:577–582.

15. Interiano B, Stuard ID, Hyde RW: Acute respiratory distress syndrome in pancreatitis. *Ann Intern Med* 1972; 77:923–926.

16. Broadie TA, Devedas M, Rysavy J, et al: The effect of hypoxia and hypercapnia on canine pancreatic blood flow. *J Surg Res* 1977; 27:114–118.

17. Clouse LH, Comp PC: The regulation of hemostasis: The protein C system. *N Engl J Med* 1986; 314:1298.

18. Harker LA, Slichter SJ: Platelet and fibrinogen consumption in man. *N Engl J Med* 1972; 287:20.

19. Seyfer AE, Seaber AV, Dombrose FA, et al: Coagulation changes in elective surgery and trauma. *Ann Surg* 1981; 193:210.

20. Moore KL, Andreoli SP, Esmon NL, et al: Endotoxin enhances tissue factor and suppresses thrombomodulin expression of human vascular endothelium in vitro. *J Clin Invest* 1987; 79:124–130.

21. Mant MJ, King EG: Severe, acute disseminated intravascular coagulation. *Am J Med* 1979; 67:557–563.

22. Seeff LB, Zimmerman HJ, Wright EC, McCollum RW: VA cooperative study of post-transfusion hepatitis, 1969–1974: Incidence and characteristics of hepatitis and responsible risk factors. *Am J Med Sci* 1975; 270:355.

23. Centers for Disease Control: Surveillance of hemophilia-associated acquired immunodeficiency syndrome. *MMWR* 1986; 34:669.

24. Gould SA, Rosen AL, Sehgal LR: Fluosol-DA as a red cell substitute in acute anemia. *N Engl J Med* 1986; 314:1653.

13 THE CARE OF THE CRITICALLY ILL

The preceding pages of this text have emphasized the importance of a pathophysiologic framework for the treatment of critically ill patients. Most patients in critical care units exhibit markedly abnormal organ function, and the support of those dysfunctional systems while curative measures are applied forms the basis of present day practice. The text has also emphasized the likely cellular abnormalities that lead to organ dysfunction in the belief that more fundamental interventions, such as the use of monoclonal antibodies to bind bacterial toxin or inhibit destructive enzyme activity, may restrain the forces leading to organ failure. At the moment, however, care of the critically ill is extraordinarily complex and requires the creative efforts of a talented team of health professionals if the patient's chance of meaningful survival is to be pushed to the limit.

Most of the public, and many health professionals, focus on the technological nature of critical care. In truth, the training, commitment, experience, interpersonal skills, and organization of people at the bedside make the difference between effective and ineffective critical care. The first edition of this text, published in 1967, emphasized that "a constant, dedicated, and intelligent nurse is the most important ingredient of the modern intensive care unit," and nothing in the years that followed has challenged this view. Unfortunately for the patient, however, the potentially life-giving resources available to seriously ill or injured people are dispensed in a manner not substantially different from that practiced by physicians who travelled to their patients by means of horse and buggy. Any discussion of the present day opportunities for improved patient care must be embedded in a discussion of hospital practice in the last quarter of the twentieth century.

The application of evaluative techniques that measure the outcome of hospital care has revealed striking disparities in the quality of that care, and has provided a preliminary glimpse at the reasons underlying that disparity. Knaus and his associates[1] at the George Washington University Medical Center have used their physiologic evaluation system (APACHE) to predict the likelihood of death in individual patients after admission to critical care units. They studied the actual mortality in 5,030 patients admitted to 13 different hospitals and found that it ranged from 59% to 158% of that predicted. Their description of the hospital with the very best and worst mortality experience provides an unusually clear picture of the importance of the organization of critical care. They found that the hospital with the best mortality experience:

relied on carefully designed clinical protocols implemented by senior level in-unit physicians. This hospital also had the most comprehensive nursing educational support system. Clinical specialists with masters degrees and extensive experience in intensive care units had, as their primary responsibility, the orientation and development of the nursing staff. Educational programs were targeted not only to the staff nurse as a care giver but also to the charge nurse as manager. As a result of this educational program, the nursing staff at Hospital 1 had independent responsibilities within the clinical protocols. Excellent communication between physicians and nursing staff was ongoing to ensure that all patient care needs were met. For example, Hospital 1 was the only institution that had a routine policy to cancel major elective surgery if adequate nursing staff was not available—a decision that could be made by the unit nurse in charge. A similar degree of respect extended to other physician and nursing interactions.

In contrast, the hospital with the poorest performance:

> had no dedicated unit physician staff to direct admission, discharge, or treatment policy . . . (it) also lacked a comprehensive nursing organization and functioned without a consistent centralized nursing authority, formal educational program, or provision for continuity of patient care through primary nursing or other form of staff assignment. Also during this study, admitting physicians and unit nursing staff communicated poorly. No policy was established for routine discussion of patient treatment, and there was no direct coordination of staff capabilities with clinical demands. Frequent disagreements about the ability of the nursing staff to treat additional patients occurred, and there was an atmosphere of distrust..

Studies like these suggest that advances in scientific understanding of human illness have not been matched by parallel developments in the sociopolitical aspects of medical practice. It is not unreasonable to explain this paradox by suggesting that scientific and nonscientific ideas do not mature at the same rate. The rates of growth of the two branches of human thought are quite different and rarely in phase. Until very recently, the world of letters and political thought was clearly ahead of that of science. At some point, science moved ahead of nonscientific thought and created an imbalance with serious implications for mankind.

Morgagni[2] published the anatomic features of human disease in his work "De Sedibus et Causis Morborum" (The Seats and Causes of Disease) at a time (1769) when the periods of renaissance and enlightenment were in full flower. In the publication year of Morgagni's masterpiece, Samuel Adams organized the first Committee of Correspondence to deal with English tyranny, and Handel's Messiah was performed in New York City for the first time.

By 1799, well after the writing of the Declaration of Independence and the United States Constitution, George Washington was bled to death by physicians who removed several quarts of blood and additionally dehydrated him with violent purges and cathartics. His presumed obstructive pharyngitis led to airway obstruction so that volume contraction and arterial hypoxemia must have markedly diminished his oxygen delivery. The suggestions of a young physician that tracheostomy might be useful were brushed aside by older colleagues. That same year, Thomas Jefferson wrote "The state of medicine is worse than that of total ignorance. Could we divest ourselves of everything we suppose we know in it, we should start from a higher ground and with fairer prospects. From Hippocrates to Brown we have had nothing but a succession of hypothetical systems each having its day of vogue, like the fashions and fancies of caps and gowns, and yielding in turn to the next caprice."[3]

But light was beginning to shine on the practice of medicine. Two years before the death of Washington, Edward Jenner innoculated a boy with material from a cow pox blister and showed that the subsequent exposure to small pox did not lead to disease. A half-century later, Verdi and Wagner had created some of the most beautiful operatic music ever to grace the human mind while Oliver Wendell Holmes was jeered by his professional colleagues for suggesting that child-bed fever was caused by the transmission of infectious material from other patients. The French Impressionist painters held their first exhibit in Paris at about the same time Koch identified the anthrax bacillus and Pasteur showed that a chemically modified bacillus could be used to produce immunity against specific diseases. Shortly after the beginning of the Twentieth Century, Picasso had entered his Pink Period, Albert Einstein had formulated the Special Theory of Relativity, and the first successful antimicrobial agent was developed by Paul Ehrlich.

The Twentieth century discoveries of nuclear explosives and molecular biology provided poisons and fruits that outstripped the creative efforts of sociologists and political scientists. The imbalance between the promise of medical science and the organization of health care emphasizes the urgent need to articulate a modus operandi that can focus the resources of the intensive care unit on individual patient needs.

Evaluation of Critical Care Practice

The overriding goal of contemporary practice is the support of failing organ systems. The APACHE method developed by Knaus et al[4] generates an acute physiology score based on a set of 12 objective physiologic measurements that assess the function of individual organs. In addition, the patient's long-term health status and age are considered. Both specific etiology and physiologic dysfunction determines the probability of death but a close relationship exists between mortality and physiologic score within each diagnostic category except for diabetic ketoacidosis. One interpretation of that finding may be that most physicians adequately evaluate and quickly treat patients with diabetic ketoacidosis, or that those physicians who do not are quick to refer to appropriate specialists. The mortality rate, for example, in septic shock is about 25% when the APACHE score is under 6, but rises to 75% when it is greater than 21.

A number of investigators have attempted to determine the cost and effectiveness of critical care. More than ten years ago, Cullen et al[5] studied 226 unstable postoperative patients requiring intensive physician and nursing care in an acute care unit at the Massachusetts General Hospital. They measured the intensity of therapy by their therapeutic-intervention scoring system (TISS) and stratified their recovery room population into four groups: (1) routine wakeup (5 TISS points and no mortality) (2) close observation (11 points and 15% mortality) (3) intensive nursing care (23 points and 21% mortality) and (4) the study group which required intensive physician and nursing care and consumed 43 TISS points. More than half of the class 4 patients were dead in one month, and 73% were dead at the end of one year. At one month, most survivors were still hospitalized and, at one year, 11 of the 62 survivors were still hospitalized. Striking differences in hospital charges were observed. Patients dying within one month stayed in the hospital for an average of 16.1 days, and the total hospitalization charge per patient was $10,109. The cost was $14,377 for those who fully or partially recovered by twelve months, and $24,327 for those who were alive after one month but either died or were seriously disabled by one year. Costs associated with blood replacement accounted for about 25% of costs during the first month; the costs were published in 1976 and would be several fold higher in 1987.

Scheffler et al[6] used the APACHE classification system to demonstrate a U-shaped relationship between therapeutic intervention and the likelihood of survival. The first portion of the curve included 45% of admissions and 19%of TISS points. Mortality rates declined sharply as the intensity of therapeutic intervention increased. Clearly critical care was effective for these patients. Death rates remained constant in spite of increasing intensity of intervention in the second segment of the curve, which included 46% of the patients. Nine percent of admissions were included in the third segment, where death rates rose rapidly in spite of increasing therapeutic intensity. This third segment accounted for 24% of the total TISS points delivered in the intensive care unit.

Data such as those presented above suggest that certain patients admitted to critical care units are not salvageable. Care in high-level critical care units is useless, adds to the distress of both patient and family, and, according to the analysis of Scheffler et al,[6] accounts for more than 25% of the cost incurred by critical care units. While some individuals are too sick for care in critical care units, others are not sick enough! Thibault et al[7] found that 77% of 2693 consecutive admissions to a medical intensive care unit required continuous electrocardiographic monitoring or frequent measurement of vital signs, but not active interventions such as mechanical ventilation, invasive hemodynamic monitoring, or use of parenteral agents requiring constant monitoring. Only 10% of patients admitted for monitoring rather than intervention subsequently required major diagnostic or therapeutic procedures. Knaus et al[8] found that 49% of admissions and 65% of nursing shifts were for close nursing care, and that 86% of patients admitted for monitoring never required active treatment prior to discharge. Obviously a two-level system of care is inadequate for most hospitals. Intermediate units where patients can be admitted for close observation and electrocardiographic monitoring with rapid transfer to critical care units when necessary are obviously important for both patient comfort and economy of care.

Many medical interventions lead to unexpected and adverse side effects and could actually increase hospital mortality in seriously ill patients. Trunet et al[9] studied 325 patients admitted to an intensive care unit in Paris and found that 12.6% had been admitted for iatrogenic disease. Illness in 19 of the 41 patients was potentially avoidable and included untoward responses to drugs, medical misjudgements, and complications of procedures. Steel et al[10] found that 36% of 815 consecutive patients admitted to a general medical service of a university hospital had one or more iatrogenic illnesses. There were a total of 497 unexpected reactions, and 43% of patients had between 2 and 7 complications. The incident was considered major in 9% of all patients studied and contributed to death in 2%. The drugs most commonly implicated in major incidents were anticoagulants, propranolol, digoxin, and antihypertensives. Diagnostic and therapeutic procedures accounted for 175 of the total 497 complications. The National Institutes of Health Consensus Conference on Critical Care,[11] held in March 1983, concluded that "The risk of iatrogenic morbidity and mortality for all patients must be included in consideration of ICU effectiveness. Complications associated with major interventions are not infrequent despite the concentration of skilled personnel in the ICU . . . Technical difficulties, errors in interpretation, and increased interventions induced by continuous monitoring, facilitated by immediate availability of personnel and equipment, are potential hazards for the monitored patient. Iatrogenic illness rates in the ICU are not known with any precision. This gap in our knowledge contributes substantially to our uncertainty about the effectiveness of ICU care."

Critical Care Practitioners: The Nurses

The most important practitioner in the critical care unit is the critical care nurse. These nurses, mostly women, evolved during the nineteen sixties and seventies during a period that saw the traditional captaincy of the physician questioned, the role of the traditional bedside nurse expand and dramatically change, and women demand equality in both workplace and family. Women had traditionally played subordinate roles in most societies, and the relationship between nurse and physician was not dissimilar to that between pilot and flight attendant or priest and nun! The emergence of the highly skilled critical care nurse is certainly the single most important event in the evolution of the critical care concept.

Millar[12] has pointed out that ordinarily new graduates should not move directly to critical care units because they do not possess the clinical experience and maturity necessary for the extremely stressful unit environment. She studied a group of new nursing graduates entering the Massachusetts General Hospital and was surprised to learn that "a disturbing number of these new graduates were unfamiliar with routine clinical skills: 53% stated they were unable to monitor neurologic vital signs, 63% could not administer oxygen via a face mask, 77% could not monitor central venous pressure, 78% could not perform cardiopulmonary resuscitation, 78% were unable to monitor peripheral pulses, 85% could not recognize basic arrhythmias and 95% were unable to insert an airway. An extensive postgraduate educational experience is clearly necessary, and the American Association of Critical Care Nurses has taken leadership in developing programs that lead to certification. The coveted award of critical care certification (CCRN) identifies an experienced nurse; units staffed with large numbers of certified nurses function at a much higher level of expertise than others. CCRN certification should become a national standard and should be part of the description of an accredited unit.

It has been difficult to recruit adequate numbers of trained critical care nurses because of increasing demand and the lure of other more autonomous professions. A recent survey of 556 nurses listed ten qualities that would attract nurses to remain in critical care.[13] In rank order they were:

1. Patient/nurse ratio of 3:1 or less
2. Intellectual challenge
3. Opportunities for learning
4. Other reasons
5. Variety and excitement
6. Proficient use of skills
7. Being a member of an effective team
8. Recognition and respect
9. Learning to handle emergencies
10. Pay differential.

It is interesting that pay differential was well down the list. It is important, however, to financially reward nurses for varying levels of educational achievement and experience.

The nursing profession, just like the medical profession, is rooted in both science and art. The two professions overlap in many areas but are autonomous. The courts have held that the physician is not the "captain of the ship" and that nurses, too, have independent and autonomous roles. The nurse is not the hand-maiden of the physician. Respect and cooperation among nurses and physicians is the first requirement of any successful unit. The combined talents of physicians and nurses have led to the evolution of many important critical care principles. Certain of these were developed primarily by nursing professionals after careful physiologic study. At times, physicians were reluctant to encourage the application of these principles in patients under their care. Educational programs for both physicians and nurses have frequently been necessary to convince health professionals of their importance.

The education of critical care nurses is vital for improved patient care, improved function of the critical care team, and for the personal satisfaction of individual nurses. Millar[12] has described the six-week program developed by nurse educators at the Massachusetts General Hospital. Performance expectations, knowledge base, and clinical skills were detailed and presented over a six-week period divided into three increasingly complex segments. Much of the nurse's practice involves observation and monitoring of patients; indeed, the ability of a skilled nurse to recognize early evidence of organ failure might be considered the hallmark of the critical care nurse. Other activities include the implementation of physician-initiated interventions, although many interventions result from team consensus. Other activities demonstrate the unique contributions of nursing research to patient care. Several important examples of these contributions follow.

Prevention of Atelectasis

The introduction of the oxygen electrode into clinical medicine revealed the surprising frequency of arterial hypoxemia in seriously ill patients. It was first treated by the administration of oxygen, and clinical studies soon identified its relationship to microatelectasis and venoarterial shunting. Measurement of arterial oxygen tension, not the use of chest radiography, become the accepted method for identifying the presence of diffuse alveolar collapse. Nursing, much more than medicine, understood how to prevent atelectasis in the hospitalized patient. While physicians tended to turn to intermittent positive pressure breathing devices, nurses learned that instruction in deep breathing and coughing prevented pulmonary complications in most hospitalized patients. Bedside experience emphasized the importance of a deep breath before the cough, flexion of the knees if in bed, and other individualized cough techniques.[14] Other important preventive measures included the careful use of oxygen with adequate humidification, avoidance of excessive sedation, and early mobilization. While physicians tended to insist that patients remain in bed, nurses argued that bed rest was inherently dangerous and should be prescribed with great care.[15]

The management of excessive secretions in seriously ill patients requires a group of techniques. Purposeful coughing with good expiratory airflow is the most effective method for clearing secretions. Nasotracheal suctioning is occasionally useful, but the catheter cannot reach secretions beyond the carina. Fiberoptic bronchoscopy may be used to visualize the larynx for precise placement of a nasopharyngeal catheter and the visualization of segmental airway to determine areas of local obstruction. Proper positioning in bed is essential for the adequate clearance of secretions. The old-fashioned jack-knife position for "postural drainage" required strong leg muscles and placed the patient's head close to floor dust. Proper positioning in bed will selectively drain bronchial segments and is more effective and comfortable than the traditional head-down position.

Four positions are generally selected

for clearing secretions. Not all patients require these positions, and many cannot tolerate them for long periods of time. The principles of each position, however, may be used in the routine positioning of all patients. In some patients, firm but gentle clapping with cupped hands over the affected area facilitates the loosening of mucus plugs. Generally, the combination of adequate humidification, deep breathing, and purposeful coughing while in the appropriate positions is sufficient. The upper lobes are drained in the sitting position. Leaning foreward about 15 degrees drains the posterior segments while leaning backward clears anterior segments. Figure 13–1**A** shows the patient positioned to drain the right middle lobe. The patient is in the Trendelenburg position lying on his left side. He leans back about 15 degrees and is supported by a pillow extending from axilla to thigh. Figure 13–1**B** shows drainage of the lateral basal segments of either lower lobe. The patient is lying on the unaffected side with the head lowered 45 degrees. A pillow is placed under the lateral lumbar region. Figures 13–1**C** and 13–1**D** show drainage of anterior and posterior segments of the lower lobes by either supine or prone positioning.

Positioning and Physical Therapy

The critical care nurse, frequently working together with a physical therapist, arranges frequent position changes (at least every hour) to prevent the accumulation of secretions in the dependent positions of the lung.[16] Stasis of secretions in the bases and periphery of the lungs is enhanced by the all too frequently observed supine semi-Fowler's position. In this upright position, it is difficult if not impossible for secretions to ascend from the bases to the mainstem bronchi where they can be reached by the aspirating catheter.

Right and left lateral positioning, with the head of the bed gradually lowered, is tolerated by most patients connected to a ventilator. It must be emphasized that the patient's position in bed dictates which portions of the lungs are ventilated and perfused. Although there is increased perfusion in the lower portions, the terminal bronchioles may be filled with secretions owing to gravity drainage; this situation interferes with normal blood gas exchange. Many pillows must be used to ensure that the patient is indeed positioned in a normal, comfortable, therapeutic position.

Active or passive exercises to the arms and legs are essential to maintain muscle tonus, joint range of motion, and prevent thromboembolism. A program of breathing retraining and strengthening exercises should begin as soon as possible in patients with chronic airway obstruction who require ventilatory assistance. Deconditioning may be prevented and exercise tolerance increased by various arm and leg exercises, which should be synchronized with the breathing pattern while the patient is being assisted by the ventilator.

As soon as the patient is medically stable, he should sit in a chair even if only for brief periods of time. The chair treatment for acute myocardial infarction was introduced over forty years ago and should be applied to most critically ill patients, where possible, since it produces both psychologic and physiologic improvement. This can be accomplished even while the patient is receiving mechanical ventilation, but care must be taken to prevent pulling or twisting of airway tubing. Before returning to bed, the patient should stand for a few moments and, if possible, bend slightly at the knees several times to regain leg muscle function. A walker equipped with a small pressure-cycled ventilator allows early ambulation while continuing mechanical ventilation (Fig 13–2), and a variety of in-bed exer-

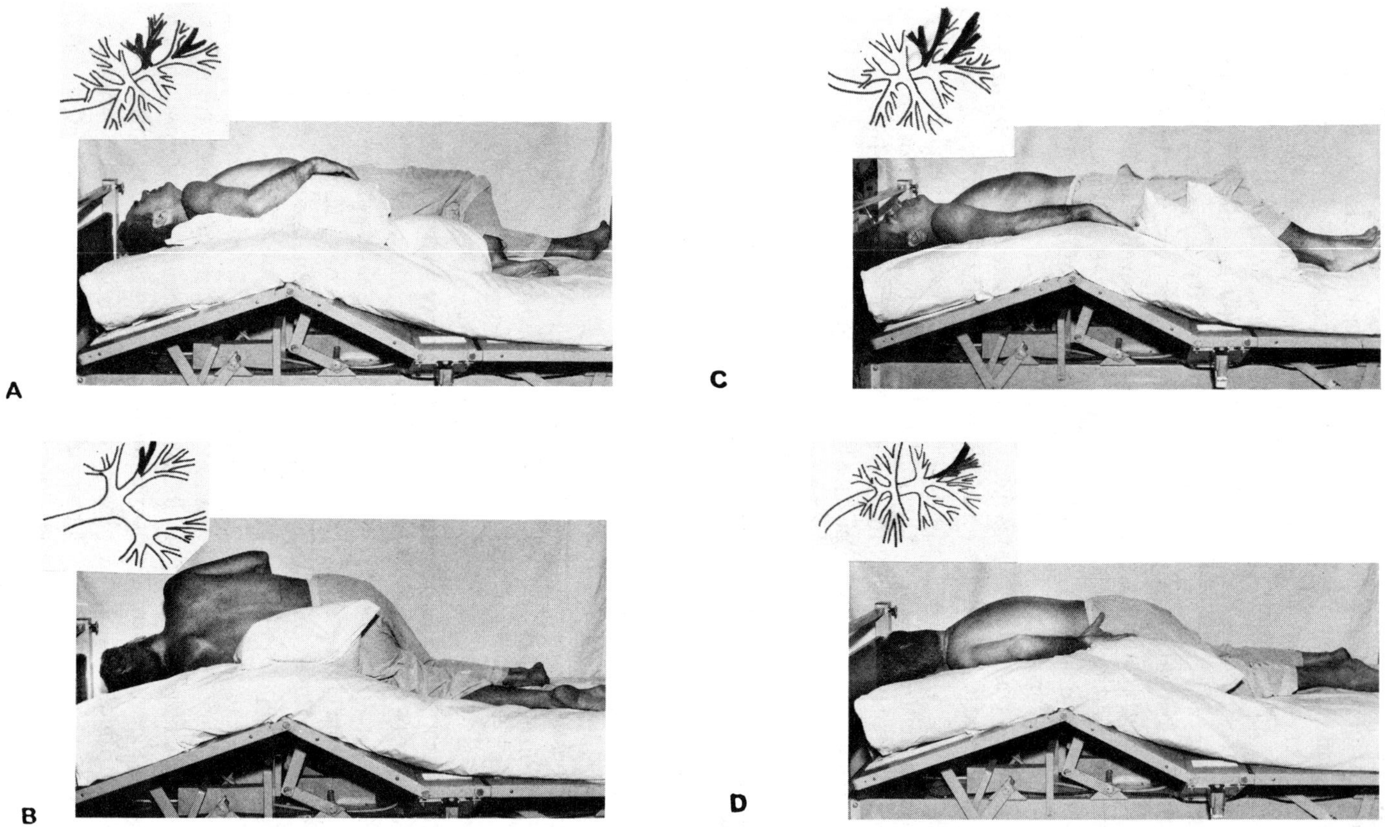

FIG 13–1.

Recommended positions for draining discrete bronchial segments. Those segments expected to drain by gravity are hatched in the inset. See text for complete description. (**A**) Optimal position for draining right middle lobe. The same position with the patient on his right side allows drainage of the lingular segment of the left upper lobe. (**B**) Drainage of lateral basal segment of either right or left lower lobe. The patient is placed on the unaffected side. Recommended positions for draining discrete bronchial segments. Those segments expected to drain by gravity are hatched in the inset. See text for complete description. Recommended positions for draining discrete bronchial segments. Those segments expected to drain by gravity are hatched in the inset. See text for complete description. (**C**) Drainage of the anterior basal segment of right lung and anterior and medial basal segments of left lung. (**D**) Drainage of posterior segments of right or left lower lobe bronchi. Apical segments may be drained in the same position if the bed is not placed in gatch.

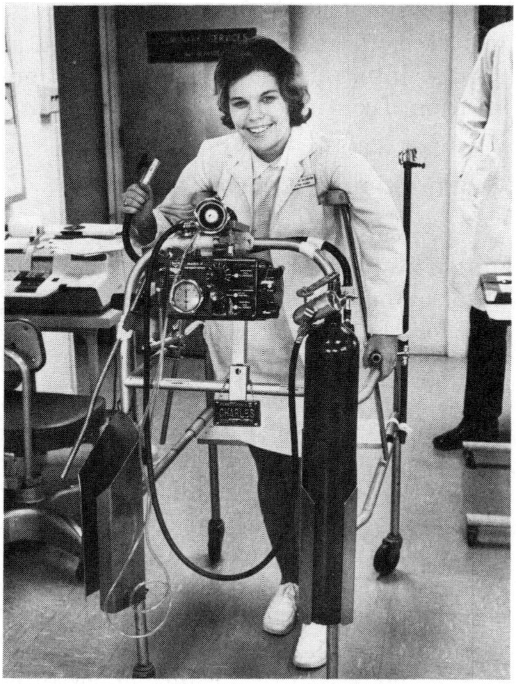

FIG 13–2.
Early ambulation prevents loss of skeletal muscle tone and may be achieved even during mechanical ventilation with a walker equipped with a small pressure cycled ventilator. (Courtesy of William Rexrode, M.D., and Leon Shirk, A.R.I.T., York Hospital, York, Pa.)

cise devices are available. Elastic stockings should be worn to prevent thromboembolic complications.

Critical Care Practitioners: The Physicians

Issues surrounding the training, certification, and privilege delineation of physicians caring for critically ill patients have become even more contentious than those concerning nursing roles. The development of specialty board certification is a relatively new idea for the medical profession; even now it is not universally recognized that graduation from medical school does not necessarily imply expertise in all aspects of medicine. Medical practitioners have divided themselves into type of practice (medicine or surgery), age of patient, gender of patient, or organ system involved. The evolution of critical care medicine has demonstrated that certain physicians must devote most of their practice to the care of seriously ill hospitalized patients. Most physicians engage in comprehensive practice; ambulatory care occupies a considerable proportion of their activities. Experience gained through years of trial and error has clearly shown that the amount of day-to-day participation in critical care practice is as important as the initial professional preparation. Just as busy surgeons perform better than those who operate infrequently, so does the busy intensivist practice more effectively than individuals who only rarely follow patients in intensive care units.

The Society of Critical Care Medicine has been deeply involved in the education of critical care practitioners and has attempted to be *inclusive* rather than *exclusive* in its membership. Indeed, the present leadership in critical care medicine was drawn from the ranks of anesthesiology, surgery, pediatrics, pulmonary medicine, cardiovascular medicine, general internal medicine, and others. The Society of Critical Care Medicine urged a group of specialty boards to consider the training and certification of specialists in that field and, in 1980, the American Boards of Anesthesiology, Internal Medicine, Pediatrics, and Surgery petitioned the American Board of Medical Specialties (ABMS) to recognize critical care medicine as a unique corpus of medical knowledge. The ABMS provided an important definition of critical care medicine that illuminates much of the confusion surrounding the nature of its practice.

> Critical care medicine (CCM) is a multidisciplinary endeavor that crosses traditional department and specialty lines, inasmuch as the problems encountered in the criti-

cally ill patient encompass various aspects of many different specialties. The CCM physician is a specialist whose knowledge is of necessity broad, involving all aspects of management of the critically ill patient, and whose base of operation is the ICU. The CCM physician must have completed training in a primary specialty and, in addition, must have had training in the CCM aspects of many disciplines to enable him: to work in concert with various specialists on the patient care team in the ICU; to utilize recognized techniques for life support; to teach other physicians, nurses, and health professionals the practice of intensive care; and to foster research. Thus, CCM is a multidisciplinary subspecialty, based in the ICU, with its primary concern being the care of the patient with critical illness.

The ABMS authorized formation of a joint committee on critical care medicine which was formed in 1980. The JCCCM had two members each from the four primary boards and two members from the Society of Critical Care Medicine. While substantial progress toward the development of joint certification was made, it soon became apparent that critical care medicine was too central to the mission of each individual board to allow a common examination and certification. In early 1985, the JCCCM found itself unable to agree on common training requirements and shortly thereafter became inactive. Each of the primary boards decided to offer its own examination in a move that marks the evolution of critical care into a full-fledged medical subspecialty.

The diversity of primary board preparation for critical care medicine guarantees a dynamic and creative future for the new specialty. General surgeons, anesthesiologists, chest physicians, other medical specialists, and broadly trained intensivists graduating from programs in critical care will all seek certification and add a new dimension of expertise to the care of seriously ill patients. Certified critical care physicians would be expected to spend much of their time in intensive care units, and recertification would be required at regular intervals and be based on demonstration of continued active involvement.

Organization of Critical Care Units

The first step in organizing a critical care unit or system is the development of a hospital committee to establish detailed policies for the delivery of care within the unit. Admission and discharge policies, the role of medical and nursing directors, the required credentials of physicians, and the behavior of consultants must be clearly outlined so that all participating in the unit can understand their roles. An ongoing quality assurance program, educational programs for nurses and physicians, and regular case management conferences help evaluate patient care.

The medical director has major clinical, educational, and administrative responsibilities. This individual may be full-time in larger institutions but is usually part-time in smaller hospitals. The medical director should also be responsible for the education and evaluation of resident physicians during their assignment to the unit. Greenbaum[17] surveyed 7,500 units in American hospitals and found that cardiologists were medical directors in about 50% of units. Chest physicians directed 20% of units, and only 1% of directors in small hospitals and 4% of directors in large hospitals had formal critical care training. Medical directors must have significant management and communication skills in addition to their professional expertise.

The unit nursing director should have advanced training in critical care. The nursing director is responsible for reviewing and supervising standards of nursing practice. She, or he, negotiates much of the unit budget with hospital administration, determines staffing patterns, coordinates nursing activities with those of physicians and supporting services, and is responsible for an ongoing educational program for nurses. Frequently a nurse-educator will actually manage the educational programs but will report to the nurse director of the unit.

Unit leadership must focus all available resources on individual patient problems. The coordination of individual admitting physicians, a group of consultants, and the activities of physical therapists, respiratory therapists, dietitians, and others require flexible but carefully delineated lines of responsibility. The unit directors frequently must serve as gatekeepers, controlling admissions and discharging patients who no longer need or can benefit from critical care.

The Council of the Society of Critical Care Medicine and the Board of Directors of the American Association of Critical Care Nurses developed a task force on collaboration that recommended a series of important principles:

1. Responsibility and accountability for effective functioning must be vested in physician and nurse directors who are on an equal decision-making level.
2. These directors must be appropriately prepared and educated. In addition to competence in patient management, they need knowledge and experience in the following areas: management principles, resource management, and skills in interpersonal relations including conflict resolution.
3. The organizational structure of a critical care unit must ensure that physicians are autonomous when dealing with issues that solely affect medical practice.
4. The organizational structure of a critical care unit must ensure that nurses are autonomous when dealing with issues that solely affect nursing practice.
5. Most aspects of patient care require interdependence between physicians and nurses. These aspects must be identified and addressed jointly.
6. Every critically ill person requires medical and nursing care. The services of additional disciplines may also be required in specific situations. In order to provide a holistic approach, the care delivered by other health team members must be coordinated by the physician and nurse directors.
7. Unit support services must be organized to enable the directors to carry out their primary responsibility in the practice of their relative disciplines in an optimal manner.
8. The directors are accountable for the evaluation of care on a timely basis.
9. The directors are responsible for creating and maintaining an environment in which individuals have opportunities to realize their potentials.
10. Close collaboration between the directors is essential for successful management. This collaboration can be enhanced by daily rounds, weekly meetings, and other means that will ensure continuous, open communication.

These organizational arrangements apply to most intensive care units even though they are in small hospitals. Greenbaum's survey[17] indicated that 37% of the units were in hospitals with less than 100 beds, while 17% were in hospitals with more than 400 beds. Most hospitals have a single multidisciplinary unit caring for all types of patients. While the approach to organization described above is useful for most hospitals, the types of patients found in community hospitals are quite different from those in university hospitals. Draper, Wagner, and Knaus[18] recently compared 223 consecutive medical-surgical admissions to a 300 bed community hospital and 613 admissions to the multidisciplinary ICU at the George Washington Medical Center. The mean physiology and treatment intensity scores for the community hospital were 7 and 27, respectively, compared to 17 and 27 for the university hospital. These observations led Zimmerman[19] to reflect that there may be too much emphasis on critical care in the community hospital. "It is unlikely," he wrote, "that the hospital that sees only a few critically ill patients each year can maintain the equipment and skills needed for optimal care. Therefore, while there is a need for every hospital to have a place for concentrated care, monitoring, and immediate resuscitation, the small proportion of unstable, critically ill patients must best be cared for by safe transfer to a larger center. At present, only 3–4% of admissions to tertiary care ICU's are transferred from other hospitals."

There is general agreement that intensive care units should have no more than 8–12 beds. Twelve bed units can be clustered together so that they can share a variety of support services, but individual units should probably not have more than 12 beds. The NIH Consensus Conference[11] proposed a classification of units and recommended staffing patterns for each:

Level I. This is a comprehensive and multisystem critical care unit. A physician-director or qualified designee is immediately available to the unit at all times. The nurse-patient ratio is 1:1 or greater depending on the severity of the patient's condition. All necessary invasive and noninvasive monitoring is available. There is a teaching and research obligation.

Level II. This unit is a multipurpose or a specific purpose unit. Examples include respiratory, coronary care, mixed medical-surgical and others. A physician-director or qualified designee is available in the hospital. This unit can perform therapeutic interventions based on invasive and noninvasive monitoring and has a nurse-patient ratio of 1:1, 1:2, or 1:3, depending upon the severity of the patient's condition.

Level III. This unit provides for limited use of invasive monitoring and therapeutic interventions such as assisted ventilation. A physician-director or qualified designee must be readily available. In-hospital coverage must be available from a physician who is credentialed by the hospital in life support, airway, and ventilator management. Nurse-patient ratio is 1:2, 1:3, or 1:4, depending on the severity of the patient's condition.

Level IV. This is a specialty unit, but does not meet the definition of an ICU. This unit provides noninvasive monitoring for those patients who may have arrhythmias and the potential for complications. A unit director or designee is provided and will respond as needed. Arrhythmia monitoring and basic CPR skills are provided. The nurse-patient ratio is 1:4 or 1:5, depending on the patient's condition. This ratio does not apply if the number of patients is less than four. Larger hospitals might have several units, and level IV units might serve as intermediate care units.

Delegation and Autonomy in the Critical Care Unit

The organizational structure described above requires great maturity among physicians, nurses, and other health professionals. Indeed, inappropriate autonomous behavior on the part of physicians is frequently the cause of most conflict situations within the ICU. The sociologist Wendy Carlton has studied interpersonal relationships in a large university hospital and summarized her observations in a chapter entitled "Delegation and Autonomy: The Tensions of Giving and Taking."[20]

Physicians have difficulty in giving up tasks that could be performed by other health professionals because they fear "role deprivation." Carlton defined role deprivation as the "perception of a loss of self-esteem or status because a meaningful component of professional role definition has been lost through the delegation or usurpation of task function. For example, while students or house staff frequently attend routine deliveries, the obstetrician, in his interaction with the father, may still attempt to convey the impression that he has delivered the baby." She emphasized that most physicians interpret autonomy to mean to "do what they please, as long as it does not blatantly conflict with a professional code of ethics, such as the AMA code, and as long as it does not displease a limited number of other physicians who act in supervisory capacities, such as chiefs of services. In other words, autonomy is a function of professional consensus, which is protected by the self-contained nature of professional circles."

Carlton's observation of physicians in action convinced her that there was frequently little professional consensus even in presumably objective situations such as selection of an antibiotic. She concludes that serious opportunities for conflict exist because of the "extensive professional autonomy granted to physicians by their peers as well as by their patients. While there may be institutionalized means of review . . . most cases do not come under the review of supervisory agencies with any significant role in constraining physicians." And, of course, the situation is perpetuated in medical education as students learn to prize their autonomy as a privilege of their lofty professional achievements.

A successful unit moderates autonomy by carefully specifying levels of delegation in published policies accepted by the medical staff in advance: "the unit director can decide who to admit and who to discharge when beds are filled" or "the nurse director decides if staffing is sufficient for elective surgical procedures." The unit promotes consensus development by the liberal use of protocols for most dysfunctional organs and the graphic display of physiologic data so that critical decisions can be made in a logical manner and on a timely basis. Siegel et al,[21] for example, used a computer-generated data base and a group of protocols to manage seriously ill patients on the surgical service at the Buffalo General Hospital. Mortality rates from trauma decreased from 25% in 1973 to 7.5% in 1978, and much of the improved survival was attributed to the enhanced consensus development.

Stress in the Critical Care Unit

The problems of autonomy and delegation discussed above appear to be a leading cause of stress in the intensive care unit. Bailey and Steffen[22] reported on studies with 1,800 ICU nurses and found that the three most stressful factors were (1) conflicts with other health professionals, (2) inadequate staffing, and (3) lack of support in dealing with death and dying. So-called "burnout" is common, and some nurses are unable to work in units for more than six months. Studies have shown that ICU nurses show more evidence of anxiety, depression, and hostility than non ICU nurses.

Physician stress is equally common but may be expressed as desensitization to patient suffering and death. Physicians who appear hardened and insensitive to the needs of patient and family may actually be protecting themselves against their loss of self esteem in the face of what many construe as failure.

A certain amount of stress is unavoidable in health professionals working closely with life and death issues. The personal rewards are great when patients survive; introspection, guilt, and depression may occur in the face of unexpected death. The unit functions best and protects its staff from unnecessary stress when strong medical and nursing leadership create a highly motivated and communicative team. There is simply no substitute for regular team conferences, explicit discussions of psychosocial and philosophical as well as clinical issues, and occasional interaction with psychologists, ethicists, and other nonhealth professionals.

Patients and Families

Intensive care units are not pleasant places for either patients or their families. Successful treatment frequently requires unfamiliar experiences such as intubation, mechanical ventilation, and the insertion of vascular lines. Patients are exposed to long periods of uncertainty, general emotional distress, sensory deprivation, and monotony. Psychologic needs are as important as physiologic requirements.

A few simple techniques are extremely useful. All procedures must be explained to the patient, and to the family. What is being done? What results are anticipated? How can the patient most effectively participate? A well-informed family member will transmit less anxiety to a patient than one who is apprehensive and unsure of the patient's status. Patients and their families are often frustrated by communication problems associated with endotracheal intubation. The use of a magic slate or pencil and paper is useful if the intravenous apparatus has been placed in the patient's nonwriting arm. Medical discussions must take place outside of the patient's room since misinterpretation of health professionals' discussions are commonplace.

Adequate provision for sleep and rest is essential to prevent fatigue, exhaustion, confusion, and disorientation. If the patient is constantly bombarded by strange and obtrusive auditory and visual stimuli produced by oxygen apparatus, ventilators, and various types of monitors all with their buzzers and flashing lights, behavior disturbances can be anticipated. The artificial elimination of the day and the night sequence, sleep deprivation, almost continuous sensory stimulation, and monotony are not well tolerated by patients with prolonged illnesses. They generally have a diminished capacity to cope with any additional stress. Every effort should be made to organize care in such a way as to permit the patient to have disturbance-free rest periods during the day and quiet nights interrupted only when necessary for clinical evaluation or treatment.

A small vase of flowers can do much to brighten the patient's immediate environment. The sight of a familiar object may relieve some of the anxiety produced by unfamiliar and frightening surroundings. Normal orientation may be enhanced by a visible clock and a large wall calendar marking off each day as it passes. Background music interrupts the rhythmic monotony of ventilators cycling and monitors beeping and helps to relieve tension in both patients and staff.

Physicians fare no better than nonphysicians when they are patients in the critical care setting. Dr. Edward Viner was a 34-year old hematologist when he spent 120 days in the hospital; 6 weeks were spent in the ICU, and he was intubated and mechanically ventilated for 31 days. His eloquent comments were recently recorded,[23] and should be studied by all who would work in the intensive care unit:

> . . .neither we doctors, nor any health professionals, have any idea what we ask of our patients, physically, and emotionally, at a time when they are least able . . . I started

strong and thought I was tough. It was important to me to be a good patient; that meant you did what you were told, you tried to cooperate. But by the end of this there was nothing left—I couldn't cooperate even though I wanted to.

The doctor may think he's the most important person in the cast of characters, but very often he's not. Understand, I was cared for in an intensive care unit by a surgical staff who was in the OR much of the day. We didn't have the new critical care intensivist type that would have been there all of the time. So the person I lived with through each 24 hour period was the nurse.

I had a lot of time for reflections while I lay there on a respirator . . . I decided I could quickly tell whether the nurse, the doctor, the house officer, whoever it was, really cared or not and that was in a very obvious nonverbal communication. I think you can tell in 30–60 seconds—it just emanates out of those who have it—and it doesn't out of those who don't . . . I decided there were two kinds of nurses—angels and bitches—and the same applied to the housestaff. Some just didn't care.

I also had a lot of frustration with the rotation of the nurses. Every nurse, every shift, three shifts a day, 7 days a week, that's 21 first dates in a week theoretically, and you have to get to know each other, and I got paranoid. I'd have a nurse I liked one or two shifts and she'd be gone. Was I a bad patient? Did I smell bad? Didn't I cooperate? What was the problem?

I resented inappropriate behavior on the floor—raucous laughter. You see a lot of funny things going on in the middle of the night at the nursing station. I saw boobs caressed and bottoms pinched, and all kinds of things, and I resented it because I was dying and the rationale, the raison d'etre of the whole unit, as far as I was concerned, was to keep me from dying.

. . . my life would have been different if people had listened to me. The night I vomited and aspirated in the ICU, I tried to explain that I was aspirating. I was supposed to be on an endotracheal tube with a balloon that doesn't let that happen. I tried to explain, 'even so it's going down my lungs'. I was drowning. 'My, my, don't we know a lot about ourselves,' I was told.

Dr. Viner concluded his comments with a challenge to his colleagues that are fitting final words for this text:

> We must not be a battery of specialists rendering superior treatment while care is absent. We must not make patients the victims rather than the benficiaries of what we have to offer. We must always keep our perspective, not get lost in the maelstrom of our technology, and always keep track of where we are with our machines—not only medically and scientifically, but economically, legally, morally, and humanly.

Dr. Francis Peabody was dying from carcinoma of the stomach when his transcendental essay, "The Care of the Patient" was written.[24] He closed his essay with the memorable phrase: "One of the essential qualities of the clinician is interest in humanity, for the secret of the care of the patient is caring for the patient." Dr. Peabody's timeless statement might be paraphrased by a modern emphasis that the *care of the critically ill is caring for the critically ill.*

REFERENCES

1. Knaus WA, Draper EA, Wagner DP, et al: An evaluation of outcome from intensive care in major medical centers. *Ann Intern Med* 1986; 104:410.

2. Morgagni, *De Sedibus et causis morborum* (The seats and causes of disease), translated by Benjamin Alexander, Millar and Cadell, London, 1769.

3. Jefferson, T: Letter to William Green Munford, June 18, 1799, in *Thomas Jefferson: Writings*. New York, Literary Classics of US, 1984.

4. Knaus WA, Zimmerman JE, Wagner DP, et al: APACHE—Acute physiology and chronic

health evaluation: A physiologically based classification system. *Crit Care Med* 1981; 9:591.

5. Cullen DJ, Ferrara LC, Brigs BA, et al: Survival, hospitalization, charges and follow-up results in critically ill patients. *N Engl J Med* 1976; 294:282.

6. Scheffler RM, Knaus WA, Wagner DP, et al: Severity of illness and the relationship between intensive care and survival. *Am J Public Health* 1982; 72:449.

7. Thibault GE, Mulley AG, Barnett GO, et al: Medical intensive care: Indications, interventions, and outcome. *N Engl J Med* 1980; 302:938.

8. Knaus WA, Wagner DP, Draper EA, et al: The range of intensive care services today. *JAMA* 1981; 246:2711.

9. Trunet P, Le Gall J-R, Lhoste F, et al: The role of iatrogenic disease in admissions to intensive care. *JAMA* 1980; 244:2617.

10. Steel K, Gertman PM, Crescenzi C, et al: Iatrogenic illness on a general medical service at a university hospital. *N Engl J Med* 1981; 304:638.

11. Parrillo JE, Ayres SM (eds): *Major Issues in Critical Care Medicine.* Baltimore, Williams & Wilkins, 1984.

12. Millar S: Staffing of a critical care unit, in Parrillo JE, Ayres SM (eds): *Major Issues in Critical Care Medicine.* Baltimore, Williams & Wilkins, 1984.

13. Stephen S, Bailey J: Sources of stress and satisfaction in ICU nursing. *Focus on AACN* 1969; 6:26.

14. Lagerson JB: The cough—Its effectiveness depends on you. *Resp Care* 1973; 18:434.

15. Lagerson JB: The bed and the breath. *Resp Care* 1973; 18:190.

16. Cardus D: Oxygen alveolar-arterial tension differences after 10 days recumbency in man. *J Appl Physiol* 1967; 23:934.

17. Greenbaum D: Standards for critical care medicine, in Shoemaker W, Thompson WL, Holbrook P (eds): *Textbook of Critical Care.* Philadelphia, WB Saunders, 1983.

18. Draper EA, Wagner DP, Knaus WA: The use of intensive care: A comparison of a university and community hospital. *Health Care Financ Rev* 1981; 3:49.

19. Zimmerman J: Administration structure of a critical care unit, in Parrillo JE, Ayres SM (eds): *Major Issues in Critical Care Medicine.* Baltimore, Williams & Wilkins, 1984.

20. Carlton W: *"In Our Professional Opinion . . .": The Primacy of Clinical Judgment over Moral Choice.* Notre Dame: Univ Notre Dame Press, 1978.

21. Siegel JH, Cerra FB, Moody EA, et al: The effect on survival of critically ill and injured patients of an ICU teaching service organized about a computer-based physiologic CARE system. *J Trauma* 1980; 20:558.

22. Bailey JT, Steffen M: Perceptions of stress: 1800 nurses tell their stories, in Claus KE, Bailey JT (eds): *Living with Stress and Promoting Well Being: a Handbook for Nurses.* St. Louis, C.V. Mosby, 1980.

23. Viner E: Living with critical care. *Concern Soc of Crit Care Med* Winter, 1987.

24. Peabody F: The care of the patient. *JAMA* 1927; 88:877.

APPENDIX

EXPLANATION OF SYMBOLS

A series of standardized symbols has been used throughout this book to describe certain physiologic variables. Although the symbols appear imposing to the uninitiated, they were introduced by a group of physiologists in 1950 to simplify the description of complex cardio-respiratory processes. The complete report on standardization of definitions and symbols in respiratory physiology may be found in Federation Proceedings, 9:602, 1950.

Each symbol is composed of a group of symbols standing for specific variables, locations, or molecular species.

General variables are described by capital letters.

V = gas volume in general
$\dot{V}$ = gas volume per unit time
P = gas pressure in general
$\dot{Q}$ = volume flow of blood
C = concentration in blood phase

(The dot above a general variable indicates a time derivative.)

Localization of the general variable is indicated by a small capital letter for the gas phase or a lower case letter for the blood phase. This letter is not subscripted.

$P\textsc{a}$ = Alveolar gas pressure
$P\textsc{i}$ = Inspired air gas pressure
Pa = Arterial pressure
$P\textsc{v}$ = Venous pressure

Molecular species is denoted by the full chemical symbol printed in small capital letters immediately following the general variable. This is **not** subscripted when it is the only symbol following the general variable.

$P\textsc{co}_2$ = partial pressure of carbon dioxide
$P\textsc{o}_2$ = partial pressure of oxygen

When both location and molecular species are specified, the localizing letter is used first, followed by the symbol for molecular species. In this situation, the chemical symbol appears as a **subscript**.

Pa_{CO_2} = partial pressure of carbon dioxide in arterial blood

In contrast, the negative logarithm of the hydrogen ion concentration is represented by a lower case p and an upper case H.

pH

INDEX

Abdominal bleeding, 367
Acalculous cholecystitis, 353
Accelerated idioventricular rhythm, 167
Acceleration, 68
Acetazolamide, 92, 202, 243, 292
Acetoacetate (AcAc), 60
Acetylcholine, 99, 188, 313
Acetylcholinesterase, 99
Acetyl CoA, 34
Acetylcysteine, 247
Acidemia, 301
Acidification (of urine), 298
Acidifying agents, 292
Acidosis
  and carbon dioxide tension, 215
  cellular, 21
  combined, 304
  compensated respiratory, 302
  and diaphragmatic function, 203
  double, 304
  hypercholemic, 289, 292
  hyperkalemic, 287, 299
  hypokalemic, 300
  intracellular, 15
  lactic, 61, 124, 303
  affect of lidocaine on, 159
  metabolic, 30, 50, 54, 60, 124-125, 155, 203, 280, 287, 303 344
  and myocardial contractility, 71, 134, 158, 199
  and oxygen consumption, 347
  and oxyhemoglobin dissociation curve, 8-9
  during renal failure, 282
  respiratory, 155, 206, 223, 241, 298, 301-302, 304
  vasoconstrictive effects of, 97
  and ventricular dysfunction, 116, 119, 127
Acid pH, 353
Acids, 293
Acinus, 180
Acquired Immunodeficiency Syndrome. *See* AIDS
Actin, 70
Action potential, 150-151
Activated charcoal, 370, 374
Activity factor, 339
Acute aortic dissection, 148
Acute interstitial nephritis, 281
Acute myocardial infarction, 126, 128-133, 135-148, 159, 160, 164, 199, 241-255, 323, 373, 382
Acute obstructive lung disease, 216
Acute-phase proteins, 31, 35, 335
Acute pulmonary embolism (APE), 259-261
Acute renal failure, 276-283, 283, 286, 287, 336, 344
Acute respiratory collapse, 235
Acute respiratory distress syndrome, 28, 147, 207, 216-217, 219, 229, 239, 371
Acute respiratory failure, 206-207, 216-217, 222, 227, 232, 237, 239-244, 255, 367, 369
Acute tubular necrosis (ATN), 277, 278-281
Acute ventilatory failure, 216
Adenosine diphosphate (ADP), 33, 71, 82, 89, 384
Adenosine triphosphate (ATP), 70, 90, 101, 120, 130, 153, 316
  concentrations of, 33
  depletion of, 20
  generation of, 3-4, 33, 46, 316, 382
  inhibition of, 158
  loss of, 15
  synthesis, 1, 22, 27, 36
Adenylate cyclase, 16, 19, 103
ADP. *See* Adenosine diphosphate
Adrenal crisis, 387
Adrenal hypofunction, 387
Adrenalin. *See* Epinephrine
Adrenal insufficiency, 284
Adrenergic agonists, 105, 258

Adrenergic blockade, 105
Adrenergic innervation, 382
Adrenocortical dysfunction, 387
Adrenocorticotrophin (ACTH), 19, 100, 276, 313, 361, 387
Adult respiratory distress syndrome (ARDS)
in burn patients, 359
identification of, 44
mechanical ventilation, 225-231, 237-238
and oxygen extraction, 49
and pancreatitis, 383
prevention of, 207
in trauma, 365, 367
treatment for, 209, 223-225, 239-240
venoarterial shunt in, 208
Advanced trauma life support system (ATLS), 365
Aerobic metabolism, 298
Aerosol generator, 245
Afterload, 72, 73, 79, 82, 109, 115-119, 128, 138, 146, 220, 227
Afterload mismatch, 116
Agitation, 372
Agranulocytosis, 291
AIDS, 367-370, 386
AIDS-related complex (ARC), 367-368
Airflow obstruction, 240
Airway, 234-236
Airway collapse, 240
Airway constriction, 173
Airway damage, 236
Airway management, 365
Airway obstruction, 365
Airway obstructive diseases, 216
Airway pressure, 232
Airway resistance, 183
Airway responsiveness, 257
Akinesis, 127
Akinetic mutism, 320
Alanine, 33
Albumin, 289, 336, 381
Albuterol, 246-247
Aldosterone, 17, 268, 274-275, 278, 285, 288, 291, 300, 361, 387
Alkalemia, 301
Alkalinization, 371
Alkalin phosphatase, 348
Alkalosis, 8, 40, 97, 155, 234, 252, 292, 298, 299, 301, 306
All-glucose formulas, 340
Alpha-adrenergic blockers, 188
Alpha-adrenergic receptors, 139, 158
Alpha-adrenergic stimulation, 90, 97, 105
Alpha blocking agents, 97, 120, 361
Alpha receptors, 103, 103-105, 107, 109
Alpha receptor stimulation, 103
Alveolar air, 180
Alveolar-arterial gradient for carbon dioxide, 192
Alveolar-arterial oxygen difference (Aa_{DO_2}), 191, 196, 228, 255
Alveolar-capillary
block syndrome, 209
gas exchange, 222, 257
gradient, 251
membrane, 186, 187, 297
Alveolar closure, 208
Alveolar collapse, 198
Alveolar dead space, 209
Alveolar duct constriction, 183
Alveolar edema, 220, 232, 368
Alveolar equation, 181
Alveolar hypoventilation, 250
Alveolar integrity, 196-198
Alveolar macrophage, 221
Alveolar oxygen tension, 181, 187, 251
Alveolar pressure, 188-189
Alveolar septa, 180, 188
Alveolar ventilation, 186, 188, 209-210, 239, 241, 243-244, 248, 257, 296, 301, 366
Alzheimer's disease, 314
Ambient temperature, 361
American Association of Critical Care Nurses, 393, 399
American Board of Medical Specialties (ABMS), 397
Amino acids, 33, 36, 313, 334, 342
aromatic, 342
essential, 343
solutions, 335
Aminoglycosides, 39, 276, 280, 307
Aminophylline, 204, 258
Amiodarone, 162
Ammonia, 33, 301
AMP, 33
Amphetamines, 371, 373
Ampillin, 248
Amrinone, 110, 166
Amyloid, 35
Anabolic hormone, 339
Anaerobic glucose consumption, 333
Anaerobic metabolism, 4-5, 30, 46, 54, 124-125, 130, 155-156, 201, 298, 303
Anaphylaxis, 19
Anemia, 94, 122, 286
Anergy, 28, 29, 352, 368
Anesthesia, 92, 97, 198, 235, 321, 363
Angina pectoris, 125, 129, 141, 142, 249
Angiocardiography, 260
Angioplasty, 141-142, 144, 147
Angiotensin, 16, 48, 116, 119, 120
I, 98, 268
II, 17, 98, 100, 188, 268-269
Anoxia, 317
Anoxic anoxia, 317
Antibiotics, 243, 247-248, 358
Anticoagulant factors, 383
Anticoagulant therapy, 135, 392

Antidiuretic hormone (ADH), 274, 275, 284-285, 387
Antihypertensives, 291, 392
Antithrombins, 384, 385
Aortic baroreceptors, 119
Aortic body, 201, 242
APACHE classification system, 389, 391, 392
Apallic syndrome, 320
Aphasia, 319
Apnea, 203, 307, 324
Apnea test, 324-325
Arachidonic acid, 18
Arachnoid, 312
Archadonic acid, 224
Archadonic metabolism, 224
Argon, 176, 228
Arousal, 319, 323
Arterial blood gases, 54, 190, 199, 233, 324, 371
Arterial blood pressure, 51, 59, 91, 97, 116, 117, 121, 176, 211, 268, 282, 321
Arterial carbon dioxide tension, 211, 233
Arterial constriction, 118
Arterial desaturation, 187
Arterial hypoxemia, 134, 136
Arterial lactate, 142
Arterial oxygen content, 11, 46, 47, 91
Arterial oxygen saturation, 53-54, 59, 64, 94, 97
Arterial oxygen tension, 198, 207-208, 212, 228-230, 241, 242, 248-252, 253, 260, 276, 366
Arterial-venous gradient, 167
Arterial-venous oxygen content, 249
Arterial-venous oxygen content difference, 369
Arteriolar resistance, 93
Arterioles, 88
Arteriovenous anastmosis, 89, 203
Arteriovenous oxygen difference, 8, 29, 83, 88
Arteriovenous shunting, 49, 85. *See also* Venoarterial shunt
Ascorbic acid, 371, 374
Assist-control (A/C) ventilation, 233-234, 237
Asthma, 246, 256-259
Astrocytes, 311
Asynchrony, 127
Asyneresis, 127
Atelectasis, 64, 196-198, 208, 219, 227, 232, 250, 253-254, 366, 394-395
Atenolol, 372
Atheromatous embolic diseases, 281
Atmospheric pressure, 176, 179, 226
ATP. *See* Adenosine triphosphate
ATPase, 70, 338, 362
Atrial arrhymthias, 162
Atrial fibrillation, 162, 167
Atrial natiuretic factor, 269, 275
Atrial systole, 77, 156
Atrin, 269, 276
Atrioventricular junction (AV), 152-153
Atropine, 99, 259
Autocannabalism, 34, 36
Autologous grafting, 362
Autolysis, 322
Autolytic enzymes, 21
Automaticity, 150, 154, 156-157
Automobile accidents, 364
Autonomic nervous system, 99-100
Autoregulation, 90, 93, 98, 148, 180, 311, 315, 317, 321
Axon, 311
Azotemia, 291, 369

Bacteremic shock, 221
Bacterial contamination, 246
Bacterial spores, 345
Bacteruria, 354
Barbituates, 322
Barometer, 176
Baroreceptors, 101, 160
Barotrauma, 232
Barrier function, 382
Bartter's syndrome, 285
Base deficit, 124
Basilar skull fracture, 354
Beclamethasone, 259
Bernard, Claude, 17
Beta-adrenergic
 activation, 268
 agonists, 188, 246, 258, 307
 receptors, 139, 157
 stimulation, 97
Beta blockade, 135, 136, 160
Beta blockers, 154, 157, 160, 361, 372
Beta endorphin, 19, 313
Betahydroxybutyric (BOHB), 60
Beta receptors, 90, 103, 105, 107-108
 Beta-1, 103, 105, 108, 110
 Beta-2, 103, 108, 110
Bicarbonate, 10, 92, 166, 202, 210, 214-215, 241, 286-287, 290, 297, 300, 305, 373
Bicarbonate-carbon dioxide curve, 305
Bicarbonate ion concentration, 296, 298, 304, 321
Bicarbonate-P_{CO_2} diagram, 306
Bicarbonate replacement, 124
Bile, 356
Bile canaliculi, 380
Bile stasis, 380
Bilirubin, 348
Biventricular failure, 147
Bladder catheterization, 354
Blood-brain barrier, 202, 203, 316-317, 321
Blood cultures, 27
Blood flow
 alveolar pressure, 188-189
 cerebral, 62, 87, 90-91, 119, 214, 314-315, 318, 321
 changes in, 61, 90, 235
 coronary, 87, 90, 92-94, 107, 119, 129-130, 138, 142, 144-145, 153-156, 165, 167
 cortical, 315

in critical illness, 338
cutaneous, 90, 107
determinants of, 11, 85-86
during exercise, 82
and emphysema, 190
hepatic, 109, 381-382
improving, 249
inadequate, 223
increases in, 92, 211, 214
maintenance of, 51, 190
maldistribution of, 360
measuring, 45
myocardial, 90
and oxygen delivery, 44
pulmonary, 94-96, 209, 241, 314
rate of, 191
rationing of, 48
reducing, 214, 229
regional, 140, 190, 211, 315
regulating, 84, 87, 180
renal, 44, 52, 62, 87, 98, 107-110, 124, 144, 214, 268-269, 273, 276-278, 279, 282, 291, 361
resistance to, 86
restoration of, 47
during shock, 91
skeletal, 87, 90, 107
splanchnic, 87, 90, 97-99, 107-109, 119, 382-383
during stress, 97
systemic, 44, 226
and trauma, 365-366
velocity of, 226
Blood gas tensions, 186
Blood transfusions, 366, 386
Blood volume, 97, 240, 275, 278, 291, 365
"Blue bloater," 190, 241
Blunt trauma, 364, 367
Body fluids, 269-273, 286
Body water, 275, 286, 290, 336
Bohr relationship, 183
Bowditch, H. P., 84
Boyle's law, 179
Bradycardia, 158, 323
Bradykinin, 120, 188
Brain damage, 286, 321-325
Brain death, 322-325
criteria for, 325
Brain dysfunction, 319
Brain failure, 319
Brain lactate content, 316
Brain metabolic requirements, 321
Brain oxygen consumption, 311
Brain reserve, 319
Brain resuscitation, 322
Brain stem
functions, 323
reflexes, 324
Branched-chain amino acids (BCAA), 33, 333, 342-343
Bretylium tosylate, 161
Bronchioles, 180, 187, 240, 255
Bronchiolitis, 240
Bronchitis, 241
Bronchoalveolar lavage, 221, 232
Bronchopleural fistulae, 233
Bronchopneumonia, 241
Bronchospasm, 256-259, 354
Bubble-jet humidifier, 245
Buffer base, 305
Buffer capacity, 215
Buffering, 215, 293-294, 297, 302-303
BUN (nitrogen of urea), 277, 280, 281, 282, 286, 343, 345, 348
Bunsen coefficient, 177
Burn centers, 358
Burn injury, 360
Burns, 352, 358-364
Burn shock, 358-359, 360, 361
Burn therapy, 335

Cachectin, 23
Caffeine, 204
Calcitonin, 308
Calcium, 16, 17, 21, 67, 70, 103, 142, 149, 278, 306, 344
Calcium-activated calmodulin mechanism, 317
Calcium cascade, 316, 322
Calcium channel, 153
blockers, 142, 157, 160, 322
Calculous cholecystitis, 353
Calmodulin, 102-103
Calmodulin-dependent protein kinases, 16, 102-103
Caloric expenditure, 338
Caloric intake, 277, 338-339, 341, 346
Caloric requirements, 338
Campbell, E. J. Moran, 243
Candida, 354
Candida sepsis, 357
Cannon, Walter, 15, 17
Capacitance vessel, 90
Capillaries, 88, 98, 175, 188, 203, 251, 296
Capillary blood flow, 89, 208
Capillary-endothelial barrier, 288
Capillary leakage, 218, 220, 360
Capillary permeability, 360
Captopril, 120
Carbachol, 257
Carbamino compounds, 10
Carbohydrates, 337
Carbon dioxide, 176, 177, 288, 296-297, 315
concentrations of, 43, 201, 214, 382
in dead space, 183
exchange, 181
excretion of, 347
inhalation, 202
production, 209-210, 339
retention, 202, 302
transfer, 175
transport, 6-10, 296-297
Carbon dioxide combining power, 304
Carbon dioxide dissociation curve, 210
Carbon dioxide tension
and alveolar ventilation, 186, 189-192, 198-204, 239, 241, 249, 301
arterial, 44, 91-92, 209, 232
in asthma, 257
decreases in, 8-10, 303, 315

Carbon dioxide tension
  and alveolar ventilation—cont'd.
  increases in, 155, 304
  measurement of, 45
  as a symptom of disease, 123-124, 207, 210-215, 242-243, 255, 259
Carbon dioxide titration curve, 304-306
Carbonic acid, 10, 293, 295
Carbonic anhydrase inhibitors, 291, 296
Carbon monoxide poisoning, 359
Carboxyhemoglobin, 359
Cardiac arrest, 317, 321, 324
Cardiac arrhythmias, 149-167, 241, 245, 258, 306, 372
  causes of, 146
  consequences of, 245, 258
  in the critically ill, 149-155, 167-168, 210,
  development of, 154-155
  digitalis-induced, 161
  electrical pacing for, 164-165
  electrical termination of, 163-164
  and metabolic acidosis, 124
  resuscitation, 165-167
  treatment of, 156-162
Cardiac contractility, 118
Cardiac conversion, 164
Cardiac depression, 372
Cardiac dysfunction, 144-145
Cardiac index, 132, 142, 144, 223, 239, 362
Cardiac muscle, 335
  work, 338
Cardiac output
  adjusting, 240
  in arrhythmias, 155-156
  in burn patients, 289
  calculation of, 7, 43, 44
  changes in, 227
  in chronic obstructive lung disease, 249
  in critical illness, 37
  decreases in, 32, 48, 50, 96, 132, 134, 213, 220, 226, 229, 282, 321
  effect of drugs on, 110, 138-139, 141
  evaluation of, 120
  and exercise, 83-84
  increases in, 45, 49, 60, 99, 107, 110, 147, 211, 212
  and intrathoracic pressure, 229, 230
  low, 51, 59, 61
  manipulation of, 226
  measuring, 55, 78
  and oxygen consumption, 46, 81, 88
  and oxygen extraction ratio, 47
  in patients with hypertension, 148
  and perfusion, 268, 272
  and pulmonary blood flow, 95
  rate of, 115
  and renal failure, 62, 277-278
  and shock, 194, 357
  sudden cessation of, 165
  urine output, 362
  and venoarterial shunts, 122, 208
Cardiac rupture, 143
Cardiac transplantation, 147
Cardiac work, 69, 211
Cardiogenic pulmonary edema, 219, 220, 256
Cardiogenic shock, 108, 115, 117, 120, 135, 137, 142-143, 144, 146
Cardiomyopathies, 144, 145-146
Cardiopulmonary resuscitation, 165-167, 324, 329
Carnitine deficiency, 334
Carotid body, 200, 203, 242
Carotid sinus, 101
Casts, 280
Catabolic states, 342
Catabolism, 332-333, 336
Catalase, 22-23
Catecholamine inotropes, 139, 155
Catecholamines, 17, 31, 63, 71, 93, 100, 102, 105-106, 110, 124, 127, 139, 158, 167, 259, 364, 383
Catheter removal, 355
Catheters, 355, 356
Catheter sepsis, 52, 355-356, 358
Cause-specific mortality, 364
Cell body, 311
Cell death, 15, 20-23, 30, 116, 120, 318
Cell injury, 20-23
Cell membrane, 16, 150, 270, 288
Cell regulation, 16-17
Cell replication, 29
Cell to cell adhesion, 21
Cellular buffers, 297
Centers for Disease Control, 368, 369
Central cyanosis, 122
Central nervous system failure, 26, 37, 332-333, 354
Central veins, 275
Central venous infusion, 346
Central venous pressure, 285
Centrilobular emphysema, 190, 240
Centrilobular necrosis, 380, 382
Cerebral bleeding, 386
Cerebral blood flow, 62, 87, 90-91, 119, 214, 314-315, 318, 321
Cerebral circulation, 61-62, 91-92
Cerebral death, 326
Cerebral edema, 214, 316-317, 321
Cerebral function, 123-124
Cerebral ischemia, 11, 318
Cerebral ischemic syndromes, 318
Cerebral oxygen delivery, 213
Cerebral vascular accident, 148
Cerebrospinal fluid, 312
  bicarbonate concentration, 92
Ceruloplasmin, 381
Charles' law, 179
Chemical messengers, 16
Chemical pneumonitis, 371
Chemoreceptors, 119, 201-202, 242, 303

Chemotaxis, 21, 29, 352
Chest radiographs, 354
Chest trauma, 366-367
Chest tubes, 366
Chest wall compliance, 184
Cheyne-Stokes aspiration, 203, 324
Chloride, 270, 274, 291
Chloride shift, 297
Cholecystokinin (CCK), 19, 314
Cholinergic blockers, 322, 372
Cholinergic neural activity, 319
Cholinergic neurons, 314
Chromium, 344
Chronic airflow obstruction, 240
Chronic airways obstruction, 216, 241-261
 acute respiratory failure associated with, 240-241, 242-244
Chronic anemia, 94
Chronic lung disease, 194
Chronic obstructive lung disease, 206, 216, 240
Chronic renal failure, 278
Chronic respiratory failure, 240
Chvostek signs, 307
Cimetidine, 237
Circulatory congestion, 115
Circulatory insufficiency, 115
Circulatory monitoring, 43-64
 arterial blood pressure, 51
 arterial oxygenation and, 54-55
 cardiac hemodynamics, 55-59
 circulatory compensation, 58
 invasive, 52
 oxygen extraction, 47
 oxygen transport, 53
 physical examination for, 50-51
 sphygmomanometry, 51-52
Circumferential burn, 358
Cis-platinum, 307
Citric acid cycle, 4
Clinical sepsis, 38
Clonidine, 105, 149
Closed chest massage, 165, 166-167
Closing capacity, 240
Clotting factor, 381, 383, 386
Coagulation cascades, 17, 222, 383-385
Coagulation, intravascular, 384-386
Cocaine, 373
Colitis, 282
Collagenase, 223
Collateral circulation, 129
Colligative property, 272
Colloid resuscitation, 289
Colloid solutions, 38
Colonization, 353, 355
Coma, 286, 319, 323, 325, 372
Coma vigil, 320
Combined acidosis, 304
Common ion effect, 294
Compensated respiratory acidosis, 302
Compensation, 215
Complement cascades, 17, 21, 222
Complement levels, 221
Complete heart block, 164
Compliance, 217, 227, 233, 236, 369
 chest wall, 184
 diastolic, 80-81
 dynamic, 231
 lung, 184, 229
 myocardial, 57
 pulmonary, 96, 198, 218, 225, 255
 ventricular, 75, 80, 81, 118, 129, 138, 145
Compression, 63
Conduction, 151, 157, 162
Conductive zone, 180
Confusion, 286
Congestion, 380
Congestive atelectasis, 208
Congestive heart failure, 241, 278, 291
Conjugate base, 293
Conjunctival oxygen monitoring, 62
Constrictive pericarditis, 144, 145
Consumption coagulopathy, 385
Content, 319
Continuous distending pressure, 229
Continuous negative pressure, 229
Continuous positive airway pressure (CPAP), 239
Continuous positive-pressure breathing, 96
Contractile element, 72
Contractile failure, 115,116, 118
Contractility, 73, 79, 84, 96, 100, 110, 118, 127, 132, 134, 155, 158, 160, 249, 372
Controlled breathing, 231
Controlled mechanical ventilation (CMV), 233, 259, 371
Convulsions, 286, 318
Cori cycle, 381
Corneal reflex, 325
Coronary artery disease, 125
Coronary artery thrombi, 142
Coronary blood flow (CBF), 87, 90, 92-94, 97, 107, 109, 119, 129-130, 138, 142, 144-145, 153-156, 165, 167
Coronary bypass surgery, 143, 147
Coronary shock, 93, 128, 133, 255
Coronary sinus, 133, 140, 146, 156
Coronary thrombosis, 125, 127, 135, 165
Coronary vascular resistance (CVR), 130
Coronary vasospasm, 135
Cor pulmonale, 241
Corticosteroids, 32, 39, 224, 242, 252, 259, 322, 366, 371
Corticotropin releasing factor (CRF), 100
Cortisol, 32, 100, 334, 387

Coughing, 394
Countercurrent multiplier system, 275
Counterregulatory hormones, 387
Crack, 373
Cranium, 314
C-reactive protein, 35, 381
Creatine kinase, 140
Creatine phosphate, 2, 4, 46, 120
Creatinine, 43, 109, 224, 273, 276, 277, 280, 282
  clearance, 277
  /height index, 337
Critical care
  certification (CCRN), 393
  cost of, 391
  medicine (CCM), 397
  nurses, 393-394, 401
  physicians, 397-398, 401
Critical care units, 389, 392
  autonomy in, 400-401
  organization of, 398-400
  stress in, 401
Critical closing pressure, 130, 134
Critically ill, treatment of, 389-403
Cromolyn, 259
Cryoprecipitate, 21, 386
Crystalloid solutions, 37, 288
CSF leak, 354
CT scan, 356
Cuff pressure, 235
Cultures, 27, 362
Cutaneous anergy, 352
Cutaneous blood flow, 90, 107
Cyanosis, 50, 122-123, 186, 203, 237
Cyclic adenosine monophosphate (cAMP), 16-17, 19, 71, 100, 102-103, 110, 153, 204
Cyclic guanine monophosphate (cGMP), 100
Cyclooxygenase, 18, 39, 222, 224, 268
  inhibitors, 220, 225, 269
Cyclosporin, 367
Cytotoxic, 316
Dalton's law, 176
Damping, 52
Dark adaptation, 315
Dead space, 181, 183, 185, 192, 209, 219, 254
Decarboxylation, 4
Decerebrate behavior, 324
Decremental conduction, 152
Deefferented syndrome, 326
Deep breathing, 255, 394
Dehydration, 245, 273, 274, 278, 280, 286, 292, 297, 301, 308
Delirium, 320
Delirium tremens, 372
Dementia, 320
Dendrites, 311
Deoxyribonuclease, 247
Dependent segments, 190
Depolarization, 153, 158, 163, 316
Dermal barrier, 358, 372
Dermal burns, 359
Dexamethasone, 387
Dextro-dobutatmine, 108
Dextrose solutions, 288
Diabetes insipidus, 287
Diabetic ketoacidosis, 124
Diaphragm, 203-204, 227, 335, 365
Diaphragmatic muscle, 335
  fatigue, 336
Diarrhea, 345
Diastolic arterial pressure, 142
Diastolic compliance, 80
Diastolic depolarization, 153, 158, 163
Diastolic overload, 116
Diazepam, 372, 373, 374
Diazoxide, 149, 188
Diethylenetriamine pentasacetic acid, 220
Diffuse bleeding, 385
Diffusion, 175, 178, 179, 186-187, 192, 202, 239, 296
Diffusion block, 187, 209, 251
Diffusion gradient, 187
Digestive enzymes, 345
Digitalis, 139, 153, 159, 162-163
Digoxin, 141, 163, 164, 307, 392
Diphenylhydantoin, 161-162
Direct current cardioversion, 163
Direct current defibrillation, 165
Direct stimulation, 202
Disequilibrium, 286
Disse, 380
Disseminated intravascular coagulation (DIC), 385
Distal tubular activity, 274, 276, 291
Distribution, 179, 188, 190
Diuretics, 138, 243, 256, 269, 278, 284-285, 288, 291-292, 306, 321, 344
Dobutamine, 38, 64, 106, 107-110, 118, 128, 138, 140-141, 143, 163, 357, 367
"Doll's head" phenomenon, 325
Dopamine, 38, 64, 97, 101, 106, 107-110, 140-141, 357, 373, 383, 387
Dopamine (DA-1) receptor, 105, 313
Doppler echocardiography, 55
Double acidosis, 304
Down-regulation, 32, 105
Doxapram, 238
DPN. *See* NAD
DPNH. *See* NADH
Drug overdosage, 370-371
DuBois, Eugene, 29
Duodenal feeding, 345
Durable powers of attorney, 328
Dura mater, 312
Dynamic compliance, 231
Dysfunction, 207, 227, 257, 288, 319, 335, 361, 366, 372
Dyskinesis, 127, 128, 313
Dyspnea, 185

Echocardiography, 59, 128, 137, 143

Edema, 285
alveolar, 220, 232, 368
cardiogenic pulmonary, 219, 220, 256
cerebral, 214, 316-317, 321
pulmonary, 98, 110, 115, 122, 136, 148, 194, 206, 208, 216, 220, 248, 255-256, 283, 284, 292, 371
Educational programs, 390, 394
EEG monitoring, 62
Effective refractory period, 151
Ejection fraction, 80, 116, 118, 138, 145, 317
EKG monitoring, 63
Elastase, 223
Elastic resistant, 183
Electrical countershock, 167
Electrical impedance cardiography, 55
Electrical pacing, 164-165
Electrolytes
changes, 215
composition, 269
concentrations, 269-270, 272, 282, 283
deficits, 290
disorders, 283
disturbances, 280, 288
imbalance, 158, 167
monitoring, 288
Embden-Myerhof cycle, 381
Embolization, 52
Emergency tracheostomy, 237
Emphysema, 184, 187, 190, 202, 240, 366
End-capillary oxygen tension, 187
End-diastolic fiber length, 76, 79, 84
End-diastolic pressures, 56, 59, 74, 76-77, 129, 138
End-diastolic volume (EDV), 77-78, 145
End-expiratory distending pressure, 229
Endocrine dysfunction, 386-387
Endogenous pyrogen, 28
Endomyocardial biopsy, 145
Endoplasmic reticulum, 16
Endothelial anticoagulant substances, 384
Endothelial cells, 221
Endothelial damage, 384
Endothelial injury, 220
Endotoxic shock, 19, 203
Endotoxin lung damage, 225
Endotracheal intubation, 234, 237, 256
Endotracheal tubes, 236, 237, 353, 354
End-systolic pressure-volume relationship, 119
End-systolic volume (ESV), 77, 83-84
Energy, 69
Energy deficits, 333
Enteral alimentation, 344-345
Enteral feedings, 353
Enterococcus, 358
Entropy, 69
Epidermal burns, 359
Epinephrine, 31, 93, 98, 100-102, 105-106, 107-108, 120, 188, 257, 258, 313, 334, 383, 387
Epithelial cells, 180
Equilibrium, 176, 178, 271, 294
Erectile property, 198
Erythropoietin, 212
Eschars, 360
Essential fatty acid deficiency (EFAD), 341
Ethacrynic, 291
Ethacrynic acid, 291-292
Ethical problems, 328-329, 370
Ethyl alcohol, 307, 371-372
Excitability, 151
Exercise, 82-85, 88, 98, 116, 155, 198, 209, 362, 395
Exogenous insulin, 341
Exogenous steroids, 387
Expiration, 183, 184, 197, 225, 233, 239, 241, 254
Expiratory collapse, 227-229
External cardiac work, 68
Extracorporeal membrane oxygenation (ECMO), 147-148, 233
Extracorporeal support for respiratory insufficiency (ECMO), 27
Extubation, 238
Exudative enteropathy, 383

Facial burns, 359
Factor replacement, 386
False neurotransmitters, 342
Fasciotomy, 63
Fat embolism, 365-366
Fatigue, 306, 336
Fatty infiltration, 380
Fiber contraction, 72
Fiberoptic bronchoscopy, 394
Fiberoptic reflectometry, 61
Fiber shortening, 72, 79, 93-94, 108, 138
Fibrin degradation products, 385
Fibrinogen, 35, 142, 385
Fibrinoid changes, 148
Fibrinolysis, 385
Fibrinolytic mechanism, 383
Fibrinolytic system, 385
Fibrinopeptides A and B, 384
Fibrin split products, 385
Fibronectin, 21,335, 352, 362
Fick principle, 7, 43, 61, 77, 87-88
"Fight or flight" response, 15, 17, 99
Finch, Clement, 44
"First messenger," 102
Flaccidity, 324
FLAVH, 4
"Floppy" cuff construction, 235
Fluid overload, 282
Fluid retention, 238, 276
Fluorocarbons, 63
Fluosol-DA, 386
Force, 68
Forced expiratory vital capacity (FEV), 257
Force-velocity relationship, 72-73, 84, 118
Fractional shortening, 118

Frank-Starling law, 57, 71, 75, 83
Free fatty acids, 33
Free oxygen radicals, 14
Free radicals, 223, 316
Free-radical scavengers, 142, 322
Free water excretion, 283, 288
Freezing point, 272
Fresh frozen plasma (FFP), 289, 386
Frictional resistance, 184
Frozen plasma, 63
Functional residual capacity, 229, 239
Functional residual volume, 229
Furosemide, 256, 286, 290, 292, 321, 374

Gag reflex, 353
Gall bladder, 353
Gamma-aminobutyric acid (GABA), 314
Gases, 175-180, 238, 339
Gas exchange, 175, 185, 192, 209, 218-220, 228, 242, 257, 278, 366
Gastric acid neutralization, 353
Gastrin, 19
Gastrointestinal bleeding, 14, 27, 120
Gastrointestinal ischemia, 383
Gas volume, 254
Gated system model, 153
"Gates," 153
Gentamicin, 280
Geometric factor, 138
Gibbs-Donnan principle, 272
Global hypoxia, 317
Global ischemia, 317-318
Glomerular capillary pressure, 268
Glomerular filtration, 269, 273, 277
Glomerular filtration rate (GFR), 277, 279, 285
Glomerular vascular pressure, 98
Glucagon, 19, 31, 32, 333, 334, 364
Glucocorticoids, 247, 387
Glucocorticosteroids, 224
Gluconeogenesis, 31, 33, 36, 333, 345, 363, 364
Gluconeogenetic pathways, 381
Glucose
  deficits, 333
  flux, 33
  oxidation, 333
  synthesis, 333
Glutamine, 33, 301
Glycogenolysis, 36, 67
Glycolysis, 4
Glycolyte enzymes, 381
Glycolytic cycle, 4-5
Goblet cells, 180
  metaplasia, 241
"Golden hour," 28, 135
"Grace period," 166
Grace, William, 165, 166
Gram-negative bacterial infection, 356
Gram-negative endotoxin, 220
Granulocytes, 221, 222, 223
Growth hormone, 32
Guanine-nucleotide binding proteins, 16
Gunshot wounds, 364

Hageman factor, 383
Haldane effect, 11
Half-normal saline solution, 289
Hallucinations, 373
Halolperidol, 313
Haptoglobin, 381
Harris-Benedict formula, 339, 347
Harvey, William, 67, 327
Headache, 214
Heart disease, 241
Heart failure, 26, 37, 115, 125, 129, 147, 240, 241, 283-284, 291
Heated aerosol generator, 253
Hematocrit, 43,63, 212, 286
Hematomas, 367
Hemodialysis, 21, 26, 221, 282, 371
Hemodynamic instability, 277-278, 281, 282
Hemodynamic monitoring, 37, 137, 361
Hemoglobin, 7, 13, 43, 46, 53-54, 63, 94, 97, 122, 186, 212, 248, 281, 296-297, 302
  concentration, 44, 47, 53, 59, 212
Hemoglobin dissociation curve, 212
Hemopneumothorax, 366
Hemorrhagic diathesis, 282
Hemorrhagic shock, 288, 365, 382
Hemostasis, 383
Hemotalogic failure, 37
Hemothorax, 366
Henderson-Hasselbach equation, 294, 298, 306
Henry's law, 177
Heparin, 135, 260, 283, 346, 386
Hepatic arterial flow, 98
Hepatic artery, 381, 382
Hepatic blood flow, 109, 381-382
Hepatic cirrhosis, 278
Hepatic-derived protein, 336
Hepatic dysfunction, 382
Hepatic encephalopathy, 342
Hepatic failure, 26, 99
Hepatic high energy phosphate synthesis, 382
Hepatic necrosis, 27, 382
Hepatic venous congestion, 382
Hepatic venous flow, 98
Hepatitis, 386
Hepatocyte dysfunction, 382
Hepatorenol syndrome, 278
Hering-Breuer reflexes, 200
Hetastarch, 289
High energy phosphates, 316
High frequency ventilation (HFV), 232
High molecular weight kinogen, 384
Hill equation, 54, 69, 72
H influenzae, 248
Hippocampus, 311
His electrocardiogram, 152

His-Purkinje system, 152, 161
Histamine, 188
Histotoxic anoxia, 317
Homicides, 364
Homosexuals, 368-369
Hospital death rate, 367
Host defenses, 332, 334-335
Human immunodeficiency virus (HIV), 367, 386
Humidification, 244-247
  devices for, 354
Humoral regulation, 188
Huntington's Chorea, 314
Hyaline membrane disease, 232
Hydralazine, 128, 149, 188
Hydration, 272, 301
Hydrogen ion concentration, 202, 214, 288, 292-295, 297-298, 301, 303, 305, 315, 382
Hydrogen ion response, 215, 242
Hydrostatic pressure, 219
Hydroxyl radical, 23, 225
Hyperactivity, 373
Hyperalimentation, 332, 346, 348
Hyperbilirubinemia, 27, 380
Hypercalcemia, 282, 287, 307-308
Hypercapnia, 98, 123, 155, 167, 199, 202, 204, 206, 207, 210, 214-215, 241-242, 255, 259, 275, 302, 306
Hypercarbia, 54, 238
Hyperchloremic acidosis, 289, 292
Hyperemia, 90
Hyperfusion, 280
Hyperglycemia, 284, 287, 291, 363
Hyperkalemia, 155, 215, 280, 282-283, 287
Hyperkalemic acidosis, 299
Hyperlipidemia, 284
Hypermagnesemia, 282, 308
Hypermetabolism, 210
Hypernatremia, 278, 286-287, 289
Hyperosmolarity, 286
Hyperosmolar nonketotic coma, 287
Hyperparathryoidism, 307
Hyperphosphatemia, 280, 282, 307
Hyperplasia, 277
Hyperproteinemia, 285
Hypertension, 51, 101, 148-149, 188, 211, 226, 247, 259, 277, 315, 317, 321, 323
  cardiac output during, 148
  malignant, 148
  pulmonary, 116
Hypertensive emergencies, 148-149
Hypertensive enchephalopathy, 148
Hyperthermia, 372
Hypertonic saline, 360
Hypertrophic cardiomyopathy, 145
Hyperuricemia, 291
Hyperventilation, 50, 91, 124, 199, 202-203, 210-211, 215, 234, 241, 245, 253, 258, 301, 302, 306, 315, 321
Hypervolemia, 285
Hypoadrenalism, 387
Hypoalbuminemia, 278
Hypocalcemia, 116, 280, 282, 306-307
Hypocapnia, 91, 199, 202, 206, 210-211, 214, 306, 315
Hypochloremia, 215, 289, 292
Hypochloremic alkalosis, 291, 292, 299
Hypoglycemia, 341, 387
Hypokalemia, 155, 158, 215, 281, 285, 287-288, 291, 307
Hypokalemic acidosis, 299
Hypomagnesemia, 158, 283, 307
Hyponatremia, 278, 283-286, 290, 292, 344, 387
Hypoosmolarity, 284, 285
Hypoperfusion, 28, 32, 39, 277, 289, 382
Hypophosphatemia, 116
Hypophysis, 274
Hypotension, 98-99, 100, 119, 127, 277, 279, 316, 362, 366, 382
  and arterial blood pressure, 51
  and brain damage, 321, 323
  caloric requirements for, 340
  cardiac output during, 55
  causes of, 137, 203, 236
  from drugs, 159
  effects of, 201
  and ischemia, 317
  "pre-shock" syndrome, 141
  in renal failure, 282-283
  in shock, 91
  in silent sepsis, 27
  as a symptom, 111, 143
  treatment of, 134, 290
Hypotensive therapy, 148
Hypothalamus, 312
Hypothemia, 321
Hypothermia, 325
Hypoventilation, 123, 167, 202, 207, 215-216, 242, 250, 253, 303, 324, 372
Hypovolemia, 28, 30, 40, 51, 53, 55, 64, 115, 137, 144, 223, 278, 282, 366
Hypovolemic shock, 117, 120, 137, 360
Hypoxemia, 48, 167, 199, 201, 233, 303, 324, 367
  arterial, 134, 136
  in asthma, 259
  body response to, 17
  cardiovascular responses to, 211-213
  causes of, 64, 188, 212, 217, 220
  and cerebral flow, 91
  in heart disease, 127
  and oxygen tension, 13, 193, 253, 255
  and renal blood flow, 98
  and respiratory dysfunction, 206-209, 241
  in silent sepsis, 27
  symptoms of, 54
treatment for, 223, 249, 251
Hypoxemic drive, 201

Hypoxia
blood flow and, 180
brain response to, 316, 324
in cardiovascular dysfunction, 153, 155, 158, 167
causes of, 248
cellular, 82
diseases associated with, 214, 256
global, 317
myocardial, 94, 130
and renal failure, 275
symptoms of, 202
tissue, 13-14, 89, 123, 248
vasoconstrictor response to, 49, 50, 97, 109, 202
Hypoxia-medicated peripheral dilation, 211
Hypoxic drive, 242
Hypoxic vasodilation, 315

Ibuprofen, 220, 225
I/E ratio, 232
Immobilization, 307
Immune adherence, 21
Immune function, 335, 352
Immune status, 28, 29
Immune system, 20, 222, 259, 313, 358, 362
Impedance plethysmography, 259
Impermeability, 270
Impulse conduction, 151-152
Incentive spirometry, 354
Incompetence, 328
Indicator-dilution methods, 56, 77
Indomethacin, 269
Induced vomiting, 370
Infarction, 259, 319. *See also* Acute myocardial infarction
Infarct size, 134, 135, 139
Infection, 247, 281, 356
Inotropes, 139, 144,204, 367
Inotropic support, 139-141
Inspiration, 96, 180, 197, 200, 225, 229, 230-232, 233-234, 248-249, 254
Inspiratory flow period, 232
Insulin, 16, 17, 31, 32, 34, 333, 341, 363
Insulin resistance, 334
Insulin secretion, 342
Interleukin-1, 20, 28, 34, 36, 222, 334, 335
Interleukin-2, 20, 223, 224
Intermittent mandatory ventilation (IMV), 217, 230-231, 232, 234, 237, 238, 240
Intermittent positive-pressure breathing, 96, 190, 206, 234, 244, 258
Interstitial space, 269
Intestinal epithelium, 353
Intra-aortic balloon counterpulsation (IACP), 127, 130, 132-133, 142, 144, 146, 167
Intracellular space, 269
Intracerebral pressure tracings, 320
Intracranial pressure (ICP), 214, 314, 317, 320, 321, 323
monitoring of, 62
Intragastric pH, 237
Intrapleural pressure, 229, 239
Intrathoracic pressure, 96, 165, 226, 229, 230
Intravascular space, 269, 289
Intraventricular catheter, 320
Intraventricular pressure, 74
Intrinsic sympathetic agonist, 160
Intubation, 223, 234-235, 236, 239, 243, 254-255, 259, 354, 359, 365, 369-370, 371
Inverse ratio ventilation, 232
Ion pumps, 270
Ion transport, 270
Ischemia, 11, 19, 51, 63, 90, 100, 141, 160, 317-318, 353
Ischemic anoxia, 317
Ischemic heart disease, 127-128, 132, 135, 141
Ischemic myocardium, 322
Ischemic penumbra, 320-321
Ischemic ulcers, 383
Isoetharine, 246
Isometric contraction, 72, 73
Isoproternol, 94, 97, 103, 107, 129, 132, 139, 147, 158, 183, 188, 204
Isotonic contraction, 73
Isotonicity, 276
Isotonic solutions, 360
Isovolumic contraction, 74
IV drug use, 368

Jaundice, 380
JCCCM, 398
Jeopardized (heart regions), 320
Juxtaglomerular cells, 98, 268, 276
Juxtamedullary nephrons, 268
Juxtamedullary tubes, 98

Kantrowitz, Adrian, 142
Kaposi's sarcoma, 368
Keith-Wagener retinopathy, 148
Ketamine anesthesia, 363
Ketone bodies, 332
Keyexalate, 282
Kidney transplants, 367
Kinetic energy, 176
Kocher-Cushing reflex, 101
Krebs cycle, 33, 130, 277, 381
Krogh, August, 192
Kupfer cells, 380
Kussmaul breathing, 203

Labetalol, 149
Lacerated blood vessels, 367
Lactate concentrations, 316
Lactate extraction, 131, 132
Lactate metabolism, 141
Lactase, 345
Lactic acid, 4, 6, 9, 43-44, 59, 60, 97, 124, 304, 382
Lactic acidosis, 124,303
Lamellar bodies, 180
Laparotomy, 367
LaPlace principle, 74,116, 131, 138, 139, 197
Large airway disease, 240
Laryngeal dysfunction, 257
Laryngeal spasm, 307
Lavage, 221, 232, 367, 370

Lee-White clotting time, 260
Left heart bypass, 147
Left ventricular failure, 148, 165, 257
Left ventricular outflow resistance, 142
Left ventricular volume, 77
Left ventricular wall tension, 79
Lenfant, Claude, 44, 213
Lethargy, 286
Leucine, 342
Leukocyte endogenous mediator, 28
Leukocyte pyrogen (LP), 34
Leukocytosis, 280
Leukopenia, 222
Leukotrienes, 17, 19, 22, 39, 222-223, 224
Levo-dobutamine, 108
Levophid. *See* L-norepenephrine
Lidocaine, 136, 156, 159-160, 161, 168, 235, 373
Limb of Henle, 291
Lipid emulsion, 341, 346, 348
Lipids, 347
Lipogenesis, 347
Lipoprotein lipase deficiency, 334
Lipoproteins, 381
Lipoxygenase, 19, 222, 224
Lithium, 313
Livedo reticularis, 281
Liver, 380-387
Living wills, 328
L-norepinephrine, 107, 130, 132, 144
Locked-in syndrome, 326
Long-chain fatty acids, 341
Loop diuretics, 269, 284, 291, 321
Loop of Henle, 98, 268, 273, 275, 291
Lorazepam, 372
Low-flow oxygen therapy, 201, 243
Lown, Bernard, 163
Lung biopsies, 368
Lung compliance, 184, 229
Lung damage, 222, 225
Lung injury, 221
Lung lymph, 219
Lymphocyte counts, 336
Lysozyme, 223

Macrophages, 17, 18, 20, 22, 32, 180, 218, 221, 222, 240, 252, 362, 368
Macula densa, 268
Magdeburg hemispheres, 175
Magnesium, 70, 307, 343
Magnetic resonance spectroscopy, 3, 45
Malaria, 386
Malignant disease, 307
Malignant hypertension, 148
Malnutrition, 203, 332, 335, 352
Mannitol, 287, 321-322
Maryland Institute for Emergency Medical Service Systems (MIEMSS), 232-233, 365
Mass action, law of, 293
Maximum voluntary ventilation, 238
Mean systemic pressure, 226
Mechanical hyperventilation, 321
Mechanical support, 146-147
Mechanical ventilation, 206, 210, 217, 225-239, 324, 338, 353, 365, 369, 370
Medial hypertrophy, 241
Median survival, 370
Medulla, 268, 279, 312
Medullary respiratory centers, 200-202, 243
Membrane attack complex, 21
Memory loss, 319
Meningitis, 354
Mental activity, 315
Mentation, 27
Metabolic acidosis, 124, 155, 203, 280, 287, 303, 344
Metabolic alkalosis, 298, 300, 303
Metabolic rate, 338
Metaproterenol, 246
Metarterioles, 89
Metchnikoff, E., 20
Methacholine, 257
Methoxamine, 134
Methylprednisolone, 224
Microcirculation, 88
Microglia, 311
Midbrain, 312
Military antishock trousers (MAST), 366
Minimal leak technique, 236
Minute ventilation, 83
Mithramycin, 308
Mitochondria, 1,3, 14, 69, 90, 381
Mitochondrial dysfunction, 21
Mitochondrial PO_2, 4
Mixed venous blood, 43, 48, 186, 191
Mixed venous oxygen saturation, 60, 357, 362
Mixed venous oxygen tension, 11, 44, 192, 248, 341
Mobile coronary care units, 136,166
Mobitz abnormalities, 153
Mobitz type II, 164
Molecular weight, 269
Monoamine oxidase, 102
Monoamines, 313
Monocytes, 18
Monokines, 20, 221
Mood swings, 374
Morphine, 136, 238, 256
Morphine sulfate, 202
Mouth breathing, 245
Mucosal carpet, 245
Mucous, 247
Mucous glands, 180, 240
Mucous plugs, 257
Multiple organ failure, 20, 36,40, 147, 218, 276, 319, 383
Multiple organ systems failure (MSOF), 26, 28, 352
Muscarinic, 99
Muscle catabolism, 335
Muscle rigidity, 372
Muscular irritability, 307
Myocardial blood flow, 90
Myocardial circulation, 63
Myocardial compliance, 57
Myocardial contractility, 73,

Myocardial contractility
—cont'd.
79, 84, 96,100, 110, 118, 132, 134, 155, 160, 249, 372
Myocardial contusion, 366
Myocardial depressant factors, 145
Myocardial hypoxia, 94, 130
Myocardial irritability, 155
Myocardial lactate metabolism, 249
Myocardial metabolism, 132, 144, 145, 167
Myocardial necrosis, 42
Myocardial oxygenation, 132, 142, 249
Myocardial oxygen consumption, 93, 107, 127, 129, 135, 139, 140, 155
Myocardial oxygen delivery, 249
Myocardial oxygen extraction, 93, 94, 132, 142, 144
Myocardial oxygen requirements, 127, 131
Myocardial shortening, 140
Myocardial wall tension, 74, 93
Myocardial work, 107
Myocarditis, 373
Myocardium, 74, 167
Myofibroblasts, 188
Myoglobin, 281
Myosin, 70

N-acetylcystein, 23, 225
NAD, 2, 30, 292, 381
NADH, 2, 4-5, 381
NADPH, 22
Naloxone, 19, 357,373
Nasal cannula, 253
Nasotracheal intubation, 235
Nasotracheal suctioning, 394
National Institutes of Health Consensus Conference on Critical Care, 392, 400
Nebulized bronchodilators, 243
Needle sticks, 368
Negative pressure, 238
Neocortex, 311
Nephrons, 268
Nephrotic syndrome, 278
Nephrotoxicity, 281
Neurohumoral responses, 119-120
Neurons, 311, 312
Neurotransmitter molecules, 313
Neurotransmitter release, 317, 322
Neutron activation analysis, 336
Neutrophil chemotaxis, 352
Neutrophil depletion, 225
Neutrophils, 220, 221, 362
Nicotinamide adenine dinucleotide. *See* NAD
Nicotinic effect, 99
Nifedipine, 149
Nitrogen, 76, 177
Nitrogen balance, 338-339, 340, 341, 348, 363
Nitrogen execution rate, 337
Nitrogen intake, 341-342
Nitrogen leak, 332-333
Nitrogen loss, 332, 333, 363
in burn patients, 363
effects of, 335
pathogenesis of, 334
Nitroglycerine, 138-139,144, 165
Nitroprusside, 117, 138, 149
Nonbacteremic clinical sepsis, 27
Nonoliguric renal failure, 279, 280
Norepinephrine, 31-32, 38, 39, 73, 75, 83, 93, 98-101, 105-106, 118, 120, 129, 132, 138, 161, 188, 313-314, 357, 372
Normal saline, 289
Nosocomial infection, 352
Nosocomial pneumonia, 353
Nucleus solitarius, 100
Nutritional assessment, 336, 337
Nutritional formulas, 337-344
Nutritional status, 238
Nutritional support, 332-348
beginning, 337-338
in burn patients, 363-364

Obtundation, 241, 319
Ocular motion, 324
Oculocephalic reflex, 325
Oculovestibular reflex, 325
Ohm's law, 86
Olfactor nerves, 312
Olfactory cortex, 311
Oligodendrocytes, 311
Opioids, 19
Optic nerves, 312
Oral feedings, 363
Organ failure, 207
Orthostatic hypotension, 278
Osler, Sir William, 28
Osmolality, 272, 284, 285
Osmolarity, 272, 273, 274-275, 280, 284, 287, 290
Osmoreceptors, 274
Osmotic diffusion effect, 271
Osmotic diuresis, 371
Osmotic diuretics, 321
Osmotic equilibirum, 271
Osmotic pressure, 89, 219, 271-273
Ouabain, 139
Oxidative breakdown, 2
Oxidative failure, 1
Oxidative metabolism, 3, 203, 292
Oxidative phosphorylation, 1, 2,3, 22,28, 46, 69, 90, 338
Oxygen, 176, 177, 242
toxic effects of, 251-253
Oxygen administration, 250, 253
Oxygenation, 50, 60, 93, 107, 122, 190, 207, 217, 225, 227-228, 230, 232, 234, 240, 248, 256, 340, 369
Oxygen breathing, 19, 250
Oxygen capacity, 7, 212
Oxygen-carbon dioxide diagram, 242
Oxygen concentration, 194-195, 240, 243, 250-251, 253-254

Oxygen consumption
brain, 311
calculating, 43-45, 47, 50, 61, 129, 338-339
cardiac output, 7, 46, 81, 88
in critical illness, 37, 59, 60
decreases in, 30
determinants of, 1
increased, 335, 347, 357, 361
limits on, 14
maintenance of, 213
mechanics of, 72, 199, 242, 256
mental activity and, 315
myocardial, 88, 93, 107-108, 127, 129, 135, 139, 140, 155
in respiratory distress, 289
stimulators of, 22
Oxygen content, 12, 44, 46, 93, 248
Oxygen damage, 252
Oxygen debt, 6
Oxygen deficits, 26, 37, 39, 316
Oxygen delivery, 10-13, 46, 133, 229, 239, 279, 365, 383, 386
and coronary blood flow, 94
deficits in, 26, 256
definition of, 11
determinants of, 53, 317
effects on, 51, 212
evaluation of, 45
during exercise, 99
failure of, 90
in hypoxemia, 213
increases in, 37, 46, 85, 143
maintenance of, 51, 211-212
measuring, 45, 50, 248-249
monitoring, 60, 256
myocardial, 249
rate of, 47
reduced, 14, 50, 63
regional, 213
renal, 214
and shock, 44
Oxygen deprivation, 14, 221, 311
Oxygen enrichment, 248-249
Oxygen exchange, 8
Oxygen extraction, 130
defective, 49, 59
and Fick principle, 61, 87-88
increased, 50, 130, 201
measurement of, 47-48
Oxygen extraction ratio, 11, 14, 47
Oxygen-induced hypoventilation, 251
Oxygen metabolites, 223
Oxygen radicals, 221,225
Oxygen reduction, 223
Oxygen requirements, 339, 362
Oyxgen saturation, 8, 122, 208, 317, 357
Oxygen tension, 8, 11, 14, 44, 53, 92, 122, 130, 132, 136, 181, 186, 191, 192, 195, 202, 212, 232, 238, 242, 314, 315, 318, 382
alveolar, 181, 186, 251
arterial, 11, 194-201, 202, 207, 208, 212, 228, 230, 232, 241, 242, 248-252, 253, 260, 276, 366
in asthma, 258
in cerebral circulation, 92-93, 314-315
decreases in, 8, 122, 130, 136, 382
end-capillary, 187
and hypoxia, 13
maintenance of, 244
measurements, 46, 53
mixed venous, 12, 44, 191-192, 248, 341
myocardial, 156
venous, 213
Oxygen therapy, 206, 244
Oxygen toxicity, 251-253
Oxygen transfer, 175, 179
Oxygen transport, 6-11, 44, 229, 234, 284, 288, 358, 359, 361-362
Oxyhemoglobin concentration, 208
Oxyhemoglobin dissociation curve, 8, 11, 44, 46-47, 48, 53, 122, 186, 213
Oxyhemoglobin saturation, 12, 30, 44, 46-47, 60, 122, 186, 191, 194-195, 201, 210, 239, 250, 359

P-50, 54, 213
Pacing techniques, 164-165
Pancreas, 383
Pancreatic enzymes, 383
Pancreatic failure, 380
Pancreatitis, 383
Panlobular emphysema, 190
Papillary muscles, 143
Papilledema, 123, 147, 214
Paradoxical bulging, 140
Parasympathetic (cholinergic) nervous sytem, 99-100
Parkinson's Disease, 313
Partial thromboplatin time (PTT), 260, 385
Passive elastic component, 72
Pathologic calcium cascade, 316
Peabody, Dr. Francis, 403
Peak airway pressures, 232
Pediatric respiratory distress syndrome, 225, 233
Pentamidine, 369
Pentose pathway, 381
Peptides, 313
Percutaneous transluminal coronaryangioplasty (PCTA), 141
Perfusion, 179, 188, 203, 210, 213, 241, 268, 277, 284, 289, 311, 315-316 318, 382
distribution of, 188-190
Pericarditis, 282
Pericardiocentesis, 366
Pericardial tamponade, 143, 144, 366
Perikaryon, 311
Peripheral airways, 182
Peripheral cyanosis, 123
Periphral dilation, 211
Peritoneal, 282
Peritoneal lavage, 367

Permeability, 30, 220-221, 223-225, 275, 279, 289, 317, 360, 371
Permeability/surface area coefficient (P/S ratio), 220
Peroxidation, 18
Petechiae, 366
PGE2, 188, 222, 223, 225, 269
PGF2, 188
PGH2, 19
PGI2, 17, 19, 188, 220, 222, 224-225, 269
pH, concept of, 294
Phagocytosis, 21
pH-carbon dioxide tension curves, 215
Phencyclidine (PCP), 371, 373-374
Pheno-barbital salicylates, 371
Phenothiazine, 158, 313, 372
Phenoxybenzamine, 105
Phentolamine, 149
Pheochromocytoma crisis, 148
Phlebitis, 355
Phlebotomy, 213
Phosphate potential, 3
Phosphodiesterase F-III, 110
Phosphodiesterasis, 16,110
Phosphoinositol-calmodulin cascade, 100
Phospholipase A2, 18, 224
Phospholipase C, 17
Phosphorus, 343
Physical therapy, 395-397
Physiologic classification, 136
Physiotherapy, 198
Physostigmine, 373
Pia mater, 312
Pi/CrP, 3
"Pink puffer," 190, 241
Plasma chloride level, 299
Plasma creatine, 223
ratio, 280
Plasmalemma, 16, 20, 102
Plasma oncotic pressure, 219
Plasma thromboplastin antecendent, 384
Plasma volume, 289
Plasmin, 142, 384
Plasminogen, 142, 384
Platelet activation factor, 222
Platelet adherence, 384
Platelet depletion, 225
Platelet phospholipid, 384
Platelets, 221, 223, 282, 363, 383, 384-385
Pneumococcus, 248
Pneumocystis pneumonia, 367, 369, 370
Pneumonitis, 207, 216
Pneumothroax, 366
Polycythemia, 203, 212, 241
Polypeptides, 387
Pontine lesion, 326
Portal triad, 380
Portal vein, 381
Positioning, 394, 395, 397
Positive end-expiratory pressure (PEEP), 57, 81, 217, 219, 227-229, 232, 239, 369
Positive pressure ventilation, 226, 236, 276, 288
Positive pressure ventilators, 233
Postischemic ATN, 279
Postsynaptic receptors, 104
Potassium, 149, 215, 270, 273, 284-285, 287, 291, 299, 302, 311, 316, 342, 343, 386
Potassium channels, 154
Potassium-sodium ion pump, 270-271, 274
Potassium-sparing diuretics, 291
Pouseille equation, 86, 117, 213, 314
Prazosin, 105
Precapillary sphincter, 89
Prekallikrein, 384
Preload, 72, 73, 79, 115, 118, 138-139, 227, 256, 278
Preload reserve, 116, 118
Preshock state, 134, 135, 141
President's Commission for the Study of Ethical Problems in Medicine and Biomedical and Behavioral Research, 325, 327-328
Pressure, 68, 175
Pressure-cycled ventilators, 233
Pressure support ventilation (PSV), 234, 238
Pressure-volume curve, 80, 219, 229
Pressure-volume diagrams, 184
Presynaptic receptors, 103, 120
Primary fibrinolysis, 385
Procaine amide, 153, 159, 373
Procoagulant, 384
Prolactin, 19
Prolonged QT, 307
Propranolol, 134, 160-161, 373, 392
Propylene glucol, 247
Prostacyclin, 18, 269
Prostaglandin E2, 269
Prostaglandins, 17, 18, 22,98, 120, 285
Prostanoids, 222-224
Protamine, 260
Protein binding, 387
Protein catabolism, 31, 33, 36, 332-333
Protein kinase C, 17, 22
Protein kinases, 16, 102, 103
Protein-sparing therapy, 345-346
Protein synthesis, 342, 358
Proteolysis, 333
Proteolysis-inducing factor, 334
Prothrombin (PT), 384, 385
Proton donors, 293
Proximal tubular reabsorption, 273
Pseudohyponatremia, 284
Pseudomembranous colitis, 345
Pseudonomas, 358
Psychedelic properties, 374
Pulmonary arterial pressure, 188-189
Pulmonary artery balloon flotation catheter, 56, 62, 361

Pulmonary artery catheter, 78, 137
Pulmonary artery wedge pressure, 144
Pulmonary aspiration, 344
Pulmonary blood flow, 94-95, 209, 241, 314
Pulmonary blood volume, 97
Pulmonary capillary blood, 210, 227
Pulmonary capillary permeability, 221
Pulmonary capillary pressure, 109
Pulmonary capillary wedge pressure (PCWP), 56-58, 76, 80, 107, 109, 116, 118, 138, 144, 146, 217, 256, 371
Pulmonary compliance, 96, 198, 218, 225, 255
Pulmonary edema, 96, 110, 115, 122, 136, 194, 206, 208, 216, 220, 248 255-256, 283, 284, 291, 371
Pulmonary embolization, 190, 192, 209, 366
Pulmonary failure, 136
Pulmonary fibrosis, 184, 216
Pulmonary hypertension, 116
Pulmonary infiltrates, 354
Pulmonary insufficiency, 248
Pulmonary vascular resistance, 94, 109, 218
Pulmonary vascular tree, 187
Pulmonary vasodilator, 247
Pulmonary venous pressure, 187
Pulmonary ventilation, 203
Pupillary dilatation, 318
Pupillary reactions, 324
Pus, 357
Pyramidal neurons, 312
Pyuria, 354

QRS complex, 372
Quinidine, 153, 158-159, 161, 167
Quinlan, Karen, 326, 327-328

Radial and pedal pulses, 121
Radio-contrast media, 281
Radionuclide ventriculography, 137
Ranitidine, 237
Reabsorption, 273, 288, 290, 307
  bicarbonate, 299-300, 301-302
  sodium, 276, 291
Rebreathing mask, 254
Recanalization, 141-142
Receptor, 16
Recruitment, 231
Red blood cell packs, 386
Reentry phenomenon, 136, 154
Reflex simulation, 200-202
Refractoriness, 157
Refractory period, 151, 162
Refractory tissue, 152
Regional circulation, 85-99
Regional perfusion, 213
Renal arteries, 98
Renal blood flow, 44, 52, 62,87, 98, 107-109, 124, 144, 214, 268-269, 273, 276-278, 282, 291, 361
Renal cell damage, 276
Renal circulation, 62, 97-99
Renal cortex, 268, 291
Renal excretion, 298
Renal failure, 26, 37, 55, 99, 124, 146, 278, 337, 343, 344, 354
  and hemodynamic instability, 277-278
  treatment of 281-282
Renal perfusion pressure, 277
Renal tubular dysfunction, 279, 288
Renin, 98, 120, 268, 276, 285
Reperfusion, 142
Reprioritization, 336
Residual volume of the ventricle, 80
Resistance airways, 182
Respiration, 1, 324
Respiratory acidosis, 155, 298, 301-302, 304
Respiratory alkalosis, 155, 298, 302
Respiratory arrest, 54
Respiratory burst, 20, 22
Respiratory center depression, 122, 201-202, 242-243, 372
Respiratory centers, 323
Respiratory distress, 45, 61
Respiratory enzyme oxidation, 3
Respiratory exchange ratio, 181
Respiratory failure, 1, 26, 37, 59, 99, 123, 179, 206, 215-217, 224, 225, 239-240, 250, 255-256, 259, 360, 365
  associated with chronic airway obstruction, 240-241
Respiratory muscle organ consumption, 338
Respiratory quotient, 347
Respiratory shock, 1
Respiratory stimulants, 202, 238
Respiratory therapy, 206, 213
Respiratory tract, 353-354
Respiratory transpor enzymes, 3
Respiratory work, 185
Resting potential, 150
Restrictive cardiomyopathy, 145
Restrictive lung disease, 216
Resuscitation, 165-167, 289, 324, 329, 361
Reticular activating system, 312, 319
Reticuloendothelial system, 20, 353
Revascularization, 135, 144
Reversed inspiratory/expiratory (I/E) ratio, 232
Reverse triiodothyronine (I-T3), 387
Reversible metabolic process, 323
Rhabdomyolysis, 63, 280, 281

Right ventricular end-diastolic volume, 78
Right ventricular failure, 241
Right ventricular infarction, 143
Right ventricular pressure, 260
Ringer's lactate solution, 287, 289, 360, 362
Risk factors, 218
Rouleaux formation, 87
Rupture
of papillary muscles, 143
of the ventricular system, 143

Saikewicz case, 327
Sarcolemma, 69, 153
Sarcomere, 69, 70
Sarcoplasmic reticulum, 70
Sarnoff ventricular function curve, 84
Scribner shunt, 283
"Second messenger," 102
Secretion, 273, 335, 342
Sedation, 242
Segmental ventricular dysfunction, 119
Selye, Hans, 17
Sepsis, 14, 26-27, 28, 45-46, 117, 127, 210, 216, 218, 221, 223, 224, 240, 289, 333, 335, 341, 359, 362, 380
and cardiac dysfunction, 144-145
catheter, 52, 355-356, 358
causes of, 52
clinical, 38
hemodynamic responses to, 29-30
host factors in, 28-29
oxygen delivery during, 59
respiratory failure, 207
symptoms of, 49, 57, 115
syndrom, 354
TPN associated with, 346-347
Septal shift, 81
Septic shock, 28, 30, 39, 40, 120, 145, 218, 224, 288, 358, 361, 362
Sequential system failure, 26
Serotonin, 188, 313, 384
Serum complement, 352
Serum proteins, 336,360
SGOT, 380, 382
Sheep model, 219
Shock, 19, 28, 99, 100, 107, 136, 192, 194, 202, 210, 216, 240, 347, 366, 382
and acute myocardial infarction, 125-144
bacteremic, 221
blood flow during, 91
in burn patients, 358-359, 360-361
cardiogenic, 108, 115, 117, 120, 135, 137, 142, 143, 144-148
coronary, 93, 128-129, 134, 255
endotoxic, 19, 203
hemorrhagic shock, 288, 365, 382
hypovolemic shock, 117, 120, 137, 360
septic, 28, 30, 39, 40, 120, 145, 218, 224, 288, 357-358, 361, 362
traumatic, 43, 44, 63
Shock syndrome, 11, 90, 116-125
Shoemaker, William, 44
Sighing, 198, 227
Silent sepsis, 40
Silver sulfadiazine, 362
Singlet oxygen,225
Sinusitis, 354
Sinusoids, 380
Skeletal blood flow, 87, 90, 107
Skeletal muscle circulation, 62-63
Skin testing, 336
Slow continuous ultrafiltration (SCUF), 282-283
Slow inward current, 154
Small airway disease, 240
Society of Critical Care Medicine, 397, 399
Sodium, 149, 268, 270, 273, 276, 280, 284, 285, 290, 291, 298, 344
Sodium-calcium pump, 316
Sodium channel, 153
blockers, 157, 159
Sodium concentration, 286
Sodium deficit, 290
Sodium nitroprusside, 149
Sodium-potassium ATP activity, 338
Sodium-potassium ATPase pump, 153, 162, 288, 307
Solubilities, 177
Solubility coefficient, 177
Solubility constant (for CO_2), 296
Somatostatin, 19
Sphygmomanometry, 51-52
Spironolactone, 291
Splanchnic blood flow, 87, 90, 97, 107, 109, 119, 382-383
Spontaneous breathing, 230, 324, 353
Sputum production, 354
Stab wounds, 364
Staircase effect, 84
Standard bicarbonate level, 305
Staphylococcal infections, 356
Starling resistor, 189
Starling's law, 74-75, 76, 78, 89, 96, 219
Starvation, 333, 335
Status asthamaticus. *See* Acute respiratory failure
Stiff lung syndrome, 216
Stored blood, 386
Streptokinase, 142
Stress, 17, 21, 29, 53, 63, 85, 88, 97-98, 99, 120
Stress factor, 339
Stress hormones, 35
Stress metabolism, 341
Stress reactor, 90
Stress response, 100
Stress ulceration, 237, 353
Stroke output, 74, 79-81, 93, 106, 109, 116, 117, 128, 145, 168, 278, 335
Strokes, 318

Stroke volume, 77-78, 83,116, 155
Stroke work, 58, 59-60, 74, 76, 84
Stunned myocardium, 142
Stupor, 319
Subarachnoid bleed, 148
Subarachnoid hemorrhage, 323
Subarachnoid screw, 320
Subarachnoid space, 312
Subcutaneous emphysema, 366
Subdermal burns, 359
Subendocardial infarcts, 129
Substance P, 314
Substrate delivery, 338
Sudden death, 125, 246, 254, 373
Suicide rates, 364
Superoxide anion, 14, 21-23, 47, 142, 223, 225
Superoxide dysmutase, 22, 223
Superoxide ion, 20
Supraventricular tacharrhythmias, 136,167
Supraventricular tachycardia, 134, 158, 164
Supreme Court of New Jersey, 327
Supreme Judicial Court of Massachusetts, 327
Surface tension, 197
Surfactant, 180, 183, 197-198, 219, 225, 232, 240
Surgical wound infections, 356-357
Sympathetic excess, 372
Sympathetic (adrenergic) nervous system, 100-105, 211
Sympathetic stimulation, 214
Sympathomimetic drugs, 15, 105, 373
Synaptic connection, 312
Synchronized IMV (SIMV), 234, 237-238
Syndrome of inappropriate ADH secretion (SIADH), 283-284
Syphilis, 386
Systemic defense response, 17
Systemic vascular resistance, 118, 138, 148
Systolic ejection fraction, 77
Systolic overload, 115

Tachycardia, 155, 211, 323, 373
Tachyphylaxis, 106
T cells, 224, 225, 352, 362, 368
Tension pneumothorax, 237, 366
Terbutaline, 204, 246, 258
Terminal airway closure, 190
Terminal airway disease, 240
Terminal bronchiole, 180
Terminal weaning, 238
Tetanus, 367
Tetracycline, 248
Thalamus, 312
T-helper cells, 368
Theophylline, 110, 258
Therapeutic-intervention scoring system (TISS), 391-392
Thermistor catheter, 78
Thermogenesis, 338
Thiazide derivatives, 291
Thomas, Lewis, 15
Thompson, Leigh, 149
3-methoxy-4-hydroxymandelic acid, 102
3-methylistidine, 333
Thrombin, 17, 222, 384
Thrombocytopenia, 27, 110, 225, 260, 291, 366, 369, 385, 386
Thrombolytic therapy, 142
Thrombomodulin, 384, 385
Thrombosis, 52, 237, 259, 260, 383
Thromboxane A2, 17, 18, 224-225, 269, 384
Thromboxanes, 17, 222, 224-225
Thromboxane synthetase inhibitors, 225
Thyroid dysfunction, 387
Thyroid hormone (T4), 387
Thyroid releasing hormone (TRH), 19, 314
Thyrotropin releasing hormone (TRH), 387
Tissue hypoxia, 89, 248
Tissue-plasminogen activator (TPA), 136, 142, 261, 385
Titratable acidity, 301
T lymphocytes, 20
Torricelli, Evangelista, 175
Torsade de pointes, 158, 162
Torticollis, 372
Total artificial heart, 146
Total Parenteral nutrition (TPN), 336, 346, 353, 356
Total parenteral nutrition solutions, 355
Trace elements, 344
Trachea, 180
Tracheal damage, 236
Tracheal stenosis, 236
Tracheobronchial tree, 179
Tracheostomy, 234,236-237
Tracheostomy tubes, 236
Transcutaneous oxygen sensors, 61-62
Transferrin, 21, 381
Transient ischemic attacks, 318
Transmembrane sodium gradient, 360
Transaminase, 348
Transmitters, 312
Transmural infarcts, 129
Transmural pressure, 86, 95
Transmural pressure differences, 226
Transplantation, 146, 323, 324
Transpulmonic pressure, 227
Transvenous pacemakers, 164
Transverse tubular system (T tubules), 69-70
Trauma, 1, 17, 28, 44, 61, 62, 120, 190, 207, 216, 222, 228, 240, 281, 325, 333, 342, 353, 364-367

Traumatic pulmonary collapse, 365
Traumatic shock, 43, 44,63
Triamterene, 291
Triceps skinfold thickness, 336-337
Tricyclic antidepressants, 372-373
Triglycerides, 340
Trimethaphan, 149
Trimethoprin-sulfa methoxazole, 369
Tropinin, 70
Tropomyosin, 70
Trousseau's signs, 306-307
True venoarterial shunt, 190, 195, 209, 250-251
T-tube, 237
Tubular necrosis. *See* Acute tubular necrosis
2, 3 diphosphoglyceric acid, 8, 47, 49, 213
Type I cells, 180
Type II cells, 180

Ultrafiltration, 273, 282-283
Ultrasonic nebulizers, 244-245
Unconsciousness, 316, 318. *See also* Coma
Underperfusion, 50
Underventilation, 191-192
Unequal ventilation-perfusion effect, 191
Unloading tension (P-50), 8, 213
Unstable angina, 142
Unstressed starvation, 335
Upper airway obstruction, 257, 359
Urea, 273, 277, 282
Uremia, 283
Urinary nitrogen loss, 332
Urinary tract infections, 354
Urine concentration, 274
Urine output, 51, 52-53, 55, 62, 124, 144, 256, 273, 276-277, 279, 287, 289, 357,360, 362
Urine sodium excretion, 285
Urokinase, 142, 260, 385

Vagal hyperactivity, 100
Vagal stimulation, 153, 183
Valsalva intervention, 76
Vanillic acid, 102
Van Slyke manometric method, 12,44, 46
Vapor phase, 178
Vapor pressure, 178
Vascular capacitance, 30
Vascular permeability, 219-220, 223,224
Vascular resistance, 51, 58-59, 79, 95, 109, 117, 124, 128,132, 138, 147, 211, 226, 357
  pulmonary, 218
Vascular scaffold, 198
Vascular spasm, 129
Vascular tone, 188
Vascular volume, 275-276
Vascular wall, 383
Vasoconstriction
  causes of, 121, 140, 214, 260
  cerebral, 92, 321
  epinephrine, 91
  increased, 51
  norepinephrine, 93,141
  pulmonary, 188, 219
  regional, 241
  renal, 282
  splanchnic, 107, 383
  sympathetic nervous system-mediated, 48, 100
  and vascular permeability, 220, 225
  and vascular resistance, 58-59, 94, 97, 109, 117
Vasoconstrictor agents, 55, 357, 383
Vasodilation
  autoregulation, 90
  of carbon dioxide, 123
  causes of, 71, 89, 211
  cerebral, 91, 214, 220
  coronary, 94, 130, 160
  and hypotension, 54
  hypoxic, 315
  isoproterenol, 188
  leukotrienes, 223
  mediation of, 105, 108, 110
  in oxygen extraction, 48-49
  in the septic patient, 30
  splanchnic, 383
  and vascular resistance, 58-59, 117
Vasodilator prostanoids, 220
Vasodilators, 39, 98, 256
Vasogenic, 316
Vasomotor paralysis, 288, 317
Vasopressin, 17, 19, 98, 100, 276, 287
Vasopressor agents, 117
Vasopressors, 357, 373
Vaso-vagal response, 32
Vegetative states, 320, 323, 326
Veins, 88, 381
Velocity, 68, 70, 79
  of circumferential fiber shortening, 79, 118
  of conduction, 151, 162
  of shortening, 72-73
Vena caval umbrella, 261
Venoarterial shunt, 122, 190, 192, 193-194, 195,198, 207-208, 218, 220, 225, 228, 247, 250, 252, 254
Venoconstriction, 84, 89, 226
Venous admixture, 190
Venous capacitance, 117
Venous constriction, 117
Venous oxygen tension, 213, 229
Venous pooling, 83
Venous return, 84, 96, 226
Venous return curves, 84
Ventilation, 179, 180-186, 215, 225, 230-239, 241, 242-244, 250, 251
  alveolar, 209-210, 239, 240, 243-244, 245, 248, 250
  artificial, 254
  assist-control (A/C), 233-234, 237
  controlled mechanical, 233, 259, 371
  control of, 198-199, 227, 230
  distribution of, 188
  high frequency, 232
  intermittent mandatory, 217, 230-231, 232, 234, 237, 238, 240

Ventilation—cont'd.
inverse ratio, 232
maximum voluntary, 238
mechanical, 206, 210, 217, 225-239, 324, 338, 353, 365, 369-370
positive pressure, 226, 236
pressure support, 234, 237
pulmonary, 203-204
spontaneous, 231
synchronized IMV, 234, 237-238
Ventilation/perfusion
distribution, 250
imbalance, 209
ratio, 188, 191, 194-195, 209-210, 241
scanning, 260
Ventilators, 232-234
Ventilator tubing, 354
Ventilatory control, 202-203
Ventilatory drive, 241
Ventilatory failure, 216
Ventilatory reserve, 237, 238
Ventilatory response, 198
Ventilatory therapy, 206
Ventilatory work, 184
Ventricular afterload, 227
Ventricular arrhythmias, 136, 149, 162, 287, 373
Ventricular assist device (VAD), 147-148
Ventricular compliance, 75, 80, 81, 118, 129, 138, 145
Ventricular contraction, 74
Ventricular dilatation, 116
Ventricular dimensions, 128
Ventricular distensibility, 75
Ventricular dysfunction, 116, 117-118, 127, 135-136, 144-146, 227, 307, 367
Ventricular end-diastolic volume, 83
Ventricular failure, 136, 257, 371
Ventricular fibrillation, 136,164, 166-167, 168, 186
Ventricular filling pressure, 56
Ventricular geometry, 127
Ventricular interdependence, 81
Ventricular pacing, 158
Ventricular preload, 227,256
Ventricular septum, 143, 227
Ventricular tachycardia, 373
Venturi mask, 253
Venules, 89
Verapamil, 160, 163
Vertebrate lung, 175
Viner, Dr. Edward, 402-403
Viral respiratory infections, 247
Viscosity, 87, 212
Visual acuity, 315
Vital capacity, 238
Vitamin A, 344
Vitamin C, 344
Vitamin D synthesis, 307
Vitamins, 344
Volume-cycled ventilator, 233
Volume loading, 37, 107
Volume overload, 269, 283
Volume resuscitation, 357

Wacker's triad, 260
Wall tension, 74, 79, 139
Wall thickness, 138
Warfarin, 135, 260
Water, 269, 275, 283, 287, 288
Water deficits, 286
Water reabsorption, 273
Water retention, 284, 291
Water vapor, 245
Waveform, 52
Weakness, 306
Weaning, 234, 235, 237, 238
Wenckebach abnormalities, 153
"Wet lung," 365
Wheezing, 257
Williams, Vaughn, 157
Wolff-Parkinson-White Syndrome, 163
Work, 68,72
Work of breathing, 242
World Health Organization, 341
Wound healing, 362
Wound infection, 367

Zinc, 344
Zymogen granule activation, 383

Knowing the partial prs of a gas is useful b/c it is a msr of the concentrat of the gas & indicates the driving force available to dissolve the gas in a liq.

Gas molecules move down partial prs gradients

3 variables determine _ speed of gas diffusion in the body:

1. the gradient in partial prs
2. the surface area available for diffusion
3. the magnitude of the diffusion distance